ADVANCING ONCOLOGY NURSING SCIENCE

EDITORS

Janice M. Phillips, PhD, MS, RN, FAAN
Cynthia R. King, PhD, NP, MSN, RN, FAAN

Oncology Nursing Society
Pittsburgh, Pennsylvania

ONS Publishing Division
Publisher: Leonard Mafrica, MBA, CAE
Director, Commercial Publishing: Barbara Sigler, RN, MNEd
Technical Content Editor: Angela D. Klimaszewski, RN, MSN
Managing Editor: Lisa M. George, BA
Staff Editor: Amy Nicoletti, BA
Copy Editor: Laura Pinchot, BA
Graphic Designer: Dany Sjoen

Advancing Oncology Nursing Science

Library of Congress Control Number: 2008942985
ISBN: 978-1-890504-76-2

Publisher's Note
This book is published by the Oncology Nursing Society (ONS). ONS neither represents nor guarantees that the practices described herein will, if followed, ensure safe and effective patient care. The recommendations contained in this book reflect ONS's judgment regarding the state of general knowledge and practice in the field as of the date of publication. The recommendations may not be appropriate for use in all circumstances. Those who use this book should make their own determinations regarding specific safe and appropriate patient care practices, taking into account the personnel, equipment, and practices available at the hospital or other facility at which they are located. The editors and publisher cannot be held responsible for any liability incurred as a consequence from the use or application of any of the contents of this book. Figures and tables are used as examples only. They are not meant to be all-inclusive, nor do they represent endorsement of any particular institution by ONS. Mention of specific products and opinions related to those products do not indicate or imply endorsement by ONS. Web sites mentioned are provided for information only; the hosts are responsible for their own content and availability. Unless otherwise noted, dollar amounts reflect U.S. dollars.

ONS publications are originally published in English. Publishers wishing to translate ONS publications must contact the ONS Publishing Division about licensing arrangements. ONS publications cannot be translated without obtaining written permission from ONS. (Individual tables and figures that are reprinted or adapted require additional permission from the original source.) Because translations from English may not always be accurate or precise, ONS disclaims any responsibility for inaccuracies in words or meaning that may occur as a result of the translation. Readers relying on precise information should check the original English version.

Printed in the United States of America

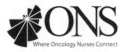

Oncology Nursing Society
Integrity • Innovation • Stewardship • Advocacy • Excellence • Inclusiveness

Contributors

EDITORS

Janice M. Phillips, PhD, MS, RN, FAAN
Manager, Nursing Research
University of Chicago Medical Center
Chicago, Illinois
Preface, Epilogue, Appendix

Cynthia R. King, PhD, NP, MSN, RN,
  FAAN
Professor and Nurse Scientist
Presbyterian School of Nursing
Queens University
Charlotte, North Carolina
*Chapter 4. Advances in Symptoms, Symptom
  Clusters, and Quality of Life by Oncology
  Nurse Scientists*

AUTHORS

Susan L. Beck, PhD, APRN, FAAN,
  AOCN®
Professor and Carter Endowed Chair in
  Nursing
University of Utah, College of Nursing
Salt Lake City, Utah
*Chapter 17. Advancing Oncology Nurs-
  ing Science: Focus on Nursing-Sensitive
  Patient Outcomes*

Ann M. Berger, PhD, RN, AOCN®,
  FAAN
Dorothy Hodges Olson Endowed Chair
  in Nursing
Professor and Advanced Practice Nurse,
  Oncology
University of Nebraska Medical Center,
  College of Nursing
Omaha, Nebraska
*Chapter 15. Accelerating the Research
  Translation Continuum to Improve
  Oncology Patient Outcomes*

Marilyn Bookbinder, RN, PhD
Director of Nursing, Department of
  Pain Medicine and Palliative Care
Beth Israel Medical Center
New York, New York
*Chapter 5. Nursing Science in Palliative
  Care and End-of-Life Care*

Patricia K. Bradley, PhD, RN
Associate Professor
Villanova University, College of Nursing
Villanova, Pennsylvania
*Chapter 10. Nursing Research: Cancer-
  Related Disparities*

Mary K. Canales, PhD, RN
Associate Professor
College of Nursing and Health Sciences
University of Wisconsin-Eau Claire
Eau Claire, Wisconsin
*Chapter 10. Nursing Research: Cancer-
  Related Disparities*

Cynthia Chernecky, PhD, RN, AOCN®, FAAN
Professor
Medical College of Georgia
Augusta, Georgia
Chapter 7. Focus on Lung Cancer

Nessa Coyle, NP, PhD, FAAN
Nurse Practitioner
Supportive Care Program
Pain and Palliative Care Service
Memorial Sloan-Kettering Cancer Center
New York, New York
Chapter 5. Nursing Science in Palliative Care and End-of-Life Care

Linda H. Eaton, MN, RN, AOCN®
Research Associate
Oncology Nursing Society
Pittsburgh, Pennsylvania
Chapter 1. Oncology Nursing Science Priorities

Carol Estwing Ferrans, PhD, RN, FAAN
Professor and Associate Dean for Research
Deputy Director, Center for Population Health and Health Disparities
University of Illinois at Chicago, College of Nursing
Chicago, Illinois
Chapter 13. The Role of National Cancer Institute–Funded Cooperative Groups

Barbara B. Germino, PhD, RN
Professor
University of North Carolina at Chapel Hill, School of Nursing
Chapel Hill, North Carolina
Chapter 12. Conducting Oncology Evidence-Based Intervention Research

Martha L. Hare, PhD, RN
Program Director
National Institutes of Health, National Cancer Institute Center to Reduce Cancer Health Disparities
Bethesda Maryland
Chapter 22. Obtaining Support for a Career in Oncology Nursing Research

Randy A. Jones, PhD, RN
Assistant Professor, Roberts Scholar
University of Virginia, School of Nursing
Charlottesville, Virginia
Chapter 10. Nursing Research: Cancer-Related Disparities

Kathryn Laughon, RN, PhD
Assistant Professor
University of Virginia, School of Nursing
Charlottesville, Virginia
Chapter 18. Qualitative Oncology Nursing Science

Frances Marcus Lewis, RN, MN, PhD, FAAN
Virginia & Prentice Bloedel Professor
University of Washington
Seattle, Washington
Chapter 19. Advancing Family-Focused Oncology Nursing Research

Suzanne M. Mahon, RN, DNSc, AOCN®, APNG
Clinical Professor
Department of Internal Medicine
Division of Hematology/Oncology
School of Nursing
Saint Louis University
St. Louis, Missouri
Chapter 3. Cancer Prevention and Early Detection Nursing Science: 1990–Present

Gail A. Mallory, PhD, RN, NEA-BC
Director of Research
Oncology Nursing Society
Pittsburgh, Pennsylvania
Chapter 14. Role of Professional Organizations and Nonprofit Organizations in Advancing Oncology Nursing Research

Danielle Pierotti May, RN, MSN, AOCN®
Oncology Manager
Northern Westchester Hospital
Mount Kisco, New York
Chapter 17. Advancing Oncology Nursing Science: Focus on Nursing-Sensitive Patient Outcomes

Deborah B. McGuire, PhD, RN, FAAN
Professor and Director, Oncology
    Graduate Program
Director, Developing Center of Excel-
    lence for Palliative Care Research
University of Maryland School of Nursing
Baltimore, Maryland
*Chapter 21. Launching an Oncology
    Nursing Research Career*

Karen Meneses, PhD, RN, FAAN
Professor, Associate Dean for Research
School of Nursing
University of Alabama at Birmingham
Birmingham, Alabama
Chapter 6. Focus on Breast Cancer

Usha Menon, PhD, RN
Associate Professor
Department of Biobehavioral Health
    Science
University of Illinois at Chicago
Chicago, Illinois
*Chapter 16. New Approaches to Conduct-
    ing Oncology Nursing Research Using
    Technology*

Christine A. Miaskowski, RN, PhD, FAAN
Professor and Associate Dean for Aca-
    demic Affairs
Department of Physiological Nursing
University of California
San Francisco, California
*Chapter 11. Development and Maintenance
    of Interdisciplinary Research Teams*

Merle H. Mishel, RN, PhD, FAAN
Kenan Professor of Nursing, Director of
    Doctoral and Postdoctoral Programs
School of Nursing
University of North Carolina at Chapel
    Hill
Chapel Hill, North Carolina
*Chapter 12. Conducting Oncology Evidence-
    Based Intervention Research*

Sandra A. Mitchell, PhD, CRNP, AOCN®
Senior Research Nurse Scientist
National Institutes of Health
Bethesda, Maryland
*Chapter 15. Accelerating the Research
    Translation Continuum to Improve
    Oncology Patient Outcomes*

Maureen E. O'Rourke, RN, PhD
Clinical Professor
University of North Carolina at Greens-
    boro, School of Nursing
Greensboro, North Carolina
Adjunct Assistant Professor of Medi-
    cine-Hematology/Oncology
Wake Forest University School of
    Medicine
Winston-Salem, North Carolina
Chapter 8. Focus on Prostate Cancer

Barbara Parker, RN, PhD, FAAN
Theresa A. Thomas Professor of Nursing
University of Virginia, School of Nursing
Charlottesville, Virginia
*Chapter 18. Qualitative Oncology Nursing
    Science*

Barbara D. Powe, PhD, RN
Director, Underserved Populations
    Research
Behavioral Research Center
American Cancer Society
National Home Office
Atlanta, Georgia
*Chapter 10. Nursing Research: Cancer-
    Related Disparities*

Susan M. Rawl, PhD, RN
Associate Professor
Indiana University School of Nursing
Indianapolis, Indiana
Chapter 9. Focus on Colorectal Cancer

Ellen M. Lavoie Smith, PhD, APRN-BC,
    AOCN®
Assistant Professor
University of Michigan School of Nursing
Ann Arbor, Michigan
*Chapter 13. The Role of National Cancer
    Institute–Funded Cooperative Groups*

Darryl Somayaji, MSN, RN, CCRC
Clinical Nurse Specialist
Department of Nursing
Roswell Park Cancer Institute
Buffalo, New York
Chapter 17. Advancing Oncology Nursing Science: Focus on Nursing-Sensitive Patient Outcomes

Richard H. Steeves, RN, PhD
Madeline Higgenbotham Sly Chair and Professor
University of Virginia, School of Nursing
Charlottesville, Virginia
Chapter 18. Qualitative Oncology Nursing Science

Elizabeth Tornquist, MA, FAAN
Editorial Consultant
Durham, North Carolina
Chapter 20. Introduction to Scholarly Writing

Sandra Underwood, PhD, RN, FAAN
American Cancer Society Oncology Nursing Professor
Northwestern Mutual Life Research Scholar
Professor
University of Wisconsin-Milwaukee
Milwaukee, Wisconsin
Chapter 10. Nursing Research: Cancer-Related Disparities

Claudette G. Varricchio, RN, DSN, FAAN
Consultant
Varricchio Consulting
Wakefield, Rhode Island
Chapter 2. Excellence in Oncology Science: Distinguished Nurse Scientists

Diana J. Wilkie, PhD, RN, FAAN
Professor and Harriet H. Werley Endowed Chair for Nursing Research
Director
Center for End-of-Life Transition Research
Department of Biohavioral Health Science
University of Illinois at Chicago, College of Nursing
Chicago, Illinois
Chapter 16. New Approaches to Conducting Oncology Nursing Research Using Technology

Shanita Williams-Brown, PhD, MPH, APRN
Research Scholar, National Center for Primary Care
Assistant Professor
Department of Community Health and Preventative Medicine
Morehouse School of Medicine
Atlanta, Georgia
Chapter 8. Focus on Prostate Cancer

Contents

Foreword

Advancing Oncology Nursing Science is a timely and important text that provides an assessment of the strengths and gaps in the current field of knowledge of cancer nursing. This text provides a foundation for developing future research directions and synthesizing the science for dissemination and use by oncology nurses and other health professionals. Oncology nursing research has a long history, which has advanced exponentially after the establishment of a stable funding base for nursing research and has strengthened the discipline's opportunities within several institutes at the National Institutes of Health. The professional associations for oncology nursing research have shown a strong focus on the generation and dissemination of nursing research for professional oncology practice. Cancer nursing was one of the first disciplines to develop nursing research priorities and to focus the investigators' endeavors on developing in-depth science in the critical areas needed for practice and health policy. In a short time, those pioneering steps advanced the field of oncology nursing research to the point that a "state-of-the-science" text is required that translates the evolving knowledge base to professional practice and facilitates shaping health policy.

Advancing Oncology Nursing Science not only provides a strong state-of-the-art assessment for cancer nursing research, but it also addresses several other purposes. A vision of oncology nursing and its scientific agenda is developed as part of suggesting future directions for research. The focus on systematically analyzing the current body of knowledge to provide valuable information to nurse leaders for practice, health policy, and educational initiatives, while also generating a thoughtful foundation for setting the future directions for oncology nursing science, is important to this vision. Generating a scientific base for cancer nursing requires understanding the methodologic and research issues, the processes and politics of translating research results into practice and health policy, and the incorporation of multiple disciplines into the study of oncology nursing problems and questions. Practice problems in cancer nursing are very complex and require numerous perspectives and fields of knowledge to gather information that can be valuable in practice settings. Nurse investigators in oncology nursing have been leaders in incorporating multiple health professionals and disciplinary scientists in their research programs. Knowing how to form, lead, and participate in multidisciplinary teams is critical in terms of enriching the scientific base of knowledge for cancer nursing, as well as for other professionals' knowledge bases.

Evidence-based practice (EBP) is a major commitment and initiative for all health professions. *Advancing Oncology Nursing Science* makes a significant contribution to the EBP agenda because it provides synthesized information to all health professionals on bodies of substantiated science that can be translated into clinical practice and health policy. Major areas of knowledge available from cancer nursing research systematically are assessed, including a focus on prevention and detection, symptom management through the continuum, a focus on palliative and end-of-life care, and quality of life through the cancer continuum. Concerns with issues and problems experienced with several site-specific cancers also are addressed, including breast, lung, prostate, and colorectal cancers.

Nursing research and medical research each have different perspectives on the research questions that are consistent with their practice domains and orientation to health care. Nursing research focuses primarily on the person and family experiencing the cancer and asks questions related to how they are preventing, handling, coping with, or responding to the disease, its consequences, and its treatments. Medical research focuses mostly on the disease, its causation, progress, manifestations, and numerous types of treatments. The two types of research are strongly interrelated and strengthen each other. This text illustrates the nursing perspective in terms of oncology nursing research and the science that is generated.

A number of years ago, oncology nursing research focused on prevention and detection of cancer conditions. Multiple studies have provided results on behavioral interventions that can be taken to motivate individuals, families, and communities in adopting healthy lifestyles to prevent cancer. The strong focus on symptom management is evident in the number of nurse investigators studying the side effects and consequences of the disease and its treatments. Numerous reports in nursing research address strategies for handling nausea and vomiting, fatigue, hair loss, mucositis secondary to radiation therapy, and many other symptoms. Quality-of-life and end-of-life issues have been major subjects of study for nurse scientists. A number of quality-of-life measures were developed and tested by nurse scientists, and the end-of-life nursing research programs are influencing end-of-life processes by shaping health policy for terminally ill individuals and their families. These areas all show the professional perspective and commitment of leaders in oncology nursing research.

Addressing the current and emerging issues in oncology science provides an important understanding of the factors influencing the development of the knowledge base and future vision for the field. Multiple factors, such as understanding research results within a cultural context, the use of diverse methodologies for enriching data, the contributions made by nurse investigators, the theoretical and methodologic biobehavioral approaches to oncology nursing research, and the family as part of the oncology experience, as well as other issues, are valuable in understanding the perspectives taken and the richness of oncology nursing science. The preparation of nurse scientists in oncology research and the multiple processes involved in launching and sustaining a research career are basic to the long-term consistent evolution of oncology nursing science and provide important lessons for educational planning and mentoring through predoctoral, postdoctoral, and career-development stages of the research trajectory. Securing funding as part of the preparation is basic to being able to build a long-term research program that will contribute substantiated findings to the body of knowledge. All of these factors are critical to the generation of oncology nursing science.

The initiators of *Advancing Oncology Nursing Science* are to be commended for their foresight and vision in providing the discipline of nursing and the field of oncology nursing with this major contribution to understanding the state of the science and directions for the future. A special word of appreciation to the chapter authors who have contributed their unique expertise and perspective. Many health professionals will benefit. Practitioners will have an evidence base for health care. Nurse investigators', faculty members', and graduate students' careers will be enhanced by the opportunity to build on the knowledge and information provided in this text as oncology nursing science continues its rapid evolution and translation into professional practice and health policy.

Ada Sue Hinshaw, PhD, RN, FAAN
Professor, School of Nursing
University of Michigan

Preface

Advancing Oncology Nursing Science is dedicated to the memory of the many oncology nurse clinicians and scientists who have helped to shape oncology nursing research.

"The greatest accomplishments are those that benefit others."
—Denis Waitley, PhD, Author and Renowned
Productivity Consultant

The need for this book was inspired by a number of factors, including

1. The increasing need for nursing research to inform oncology nursing practice, influence patient outcomes, and advance oncology nursing as an evidence-based specialty
2. The recognition of cancer as an ongoing public health concern
3. The Oncology Nursing Society's (ONS's) commitment to excellence in oncology nursing and quality cancer care
4. The explosion of knowledge generated by oncology nurse scientists over the past two decades.

Cancer will remain a major health concern well beyond the 21st century. Globally, epidemiologists predict that the number of new cancer cases will more than double from 12 million in 2007 to almost 27 million in 2050 (American Cancer Society, 2007). According to the American Cancer Society, approximately 1.4 million new cases of cancer will be diagnosed in 2008. This excludes basal and squamous cell skin cancers and noninvasive cancers of any site except the urinary bladder. Projections indicate that in the United States alone, cancer accounts for one of every four deaths. Increasingly, advancements in cancer care have resulted in improvements in cancer survival. Notably, as of January 2004, the National Cancer Institute estimated that approximately 10.8 million cancer survivors were living in the United States (American Cancer Society, 2008). As we continue to experience advances in cancer detection, diagnosis, and treatment, many more people will be living with cancer as a chronic illness. Research conducted by nurse scientists and other disciplines will continue to play a major role in informing cancer care and the cancer-related experiences of those confronted with the disease.

ONS has a long-standing commitment to transforming cancer care by promoting quality care and excellence in oncology nursing practice; however, transforming care in the 21st century will require new knowledge for a new age. The generation of new knowledge is needed if we are to fully realize ONS's mission of promoting excellence in nursing practice and quality cancer care and its vision of leading the transformation of cancer care. The increased emphasis on evidence-based nursing practice requires up-to-date scientific knowledge that can help to guide oncology nursing practice. The current knowledge base in oncology nursing research provides an excellent foundation on which to build and continue to advance oncology nursing science.

The explosion of oncology nursing research within the past two decades now calls for a well-synthesized discussion on progress and issues related to advancing oncology nursing science. Numerous strides have been made in a number of research areas across the entire cancer continuum, employing diverse populations and disease states. Oncology nurse scientists have made substantive contributions in areas such as cancer symptom management, biobehavioral oncology, cancer communication and decision making, patient-sensitive indicators, and oncology research methodologies, to name a few. We have chosen current experts to create chapters that span the cancer continuum and address a number of trends and issues pertinent to advancing oncology nursing science. *Advancing Oncology Nursing Science* provides an up-to-date discussion on current oncology nursing research and highlights directions for further development of the field. The text is not meant to duplicate the efforts of traditional nursing research texts that focus on the nursing research process and related issues; it is intended as a complement to existing research books. Although aspects of the research process are briefly incorporated throughout the various chapters, the book specifically is designed to

- Highlight the evolution of oncology nursing research
- Identify the current state of the science in oncology nursing science from prevention to palliation
- Examine current and emerging issues of relevance to advancing oncology nursing science
- Discuss future directions for advancing oncology nursing science.

Content

Advancing Oncology Nursing Science is composed of 22 chapters that are divided into four sections, followed by an appendix with resources and an epilogue addressing future directions for the field.

Section I. Foundations and Priorities of Oncology Nusing Science highlights the evolution of oncology nursing science and identifies priorities to further advance the specialty of oncology nursing through research. The book opens with a tribute to distinguished oncology nurse scientists who have ably laid a foundation for oncology nursing science. This section highlights the contributions of a number of oncology nurse scientists whose work continues to shape and inform oncology nursing practice and research.

Section II. Advancing Oncology Nursing Science highlights current advances in oncology nursing research from prevention to palliation. The authors address the state of the science in oncology nursing research, highlighting progress in nursing knowledge regarding prevention, detection, symptom management, end-of-life care, and quality of life. The authors synthesized large bodies of oncology nursing research and highlight directions for future research.

Section III. Leading Causes of Cancer focuses on the progress of research for site-specific cancers. This section highlights research issues regarding breast, lung, prostate, and colorectal cancers. The future of nursing research for each of these cancer types is also discussed.

Section IV. Current and Emerging Issues in Oncology Research provides a timely discussion on a variety of cross-cutting issues relevant to advancing oncology nursing science. Sage oncology nurse scientists address issues such as advancing family-focused oncology nursing research, translating research findings into practice, conducting research using nursing-sensitive patient outcomes, creating and sustaining multidisciplinary research teams, and advancing the field using technology.

Section V. Research Training and Education focuses on advancing oncology nursing science through research, career development, and scholarship. The authors share timely tools of the trade for launching and sustaining a research career in oncology nursing. Opportunities for funding to support oncology nursing research and nursing research training are noted.

Section VI. Selected Resources for Advancing Oncology Nursing Science features useful tips and tools for prospective nurse scientists. This section offers primers on scholarly writing and how to obtain professional and financial support for a career in nursing science, as well as tips as to launch a career in this area. Both veterans and those new to the field can benefit from the resources found in this section.

Epilogue: Looking Into the Future provides some final thoughts on advancing oncology nursing science.

The **Appendix** includes a variety of resources, Web sites, publications, and tools for use when conducting oncology nursing research.

Audience

Advancing Oncology Nursing Science is suitable for a number of audiences, including oncology graduate students and clinicians, faculty members, nurse scientists, and other healthcare professionals with an interest in oncology research. Novice oncology nurse scientists are specifically targeted, as they are encouraged to generate new knowledge that advances oncology nursing science, informs oncology nursing practice, and ultimately aids in transforming cancer care.

References

American Cancer Society. (2007). *Cancer facts and figures, 2007*. Atlanta, GA: Author.
American Cancer Society. (2008). *Cancer facts and figures, 2008*. Atlanta, GA: Author.

Acknowledgments

The editors would like to thank the authors and oncology nurse scientists for sharing their time, talents, and expertise in making this book a reality. A special thanks to Oncology Nursing Society staff Judy Holmes, Barbara Sigler, RN, MNEd, and Laura Pinchot, BA, for their ongoing support and wisdom throughout all phases of this book. We would also like to thank the Oncology Nursing Society for its long-standing and unrelenting commitment to excellence in oncology nursing and quality cancer care. This book provides a beginning synthesis of the contributions made by oncology nurse scientists. It is our wish that *Advancing Oncology Nursing Science* will serve as a significant resource for stimulating ongoing oncology nursing research while helping to solidify oncology nursing as an evidence-based specialty.

SECTION 1

FOUNDATIONS AND PRIORITIES OF ONCOLOGY NURSING SCIENCE

CHAPTER 1

Oncology Nursing Science Priorities

Linda H. Eaton, MN, RN, AOCN®

Introduction

With the rapid advancement in cancer treatment and the continuously changing healthcare environment, nurses constantly are challenged to provide effective patient care. In order to improve cancer care, oncology nursing science must focus on areas of study that address relevant cancer care issues and have a major impact on people with cancer. The establishment of oncology nursing science priorities provides guidance for the generation of new knowledge to direct practice, education, health policy, and ultimately patient care.

Oncology nursing science priorities were established more than 25 years ago. The seminal work of Oberst (1978) was the first to identify priorities, followed by decades of work from national and international authors. This chapter describes the history of establishing oncology nursing science priorities with a specific focus on the Oncology Nursing Society's (ONS's) longstanding history of conducting oncology nursing research priorities surveys. National and international oncology nursing science priorities are reviewed and compared. Lastly, the different ways in which these priorities are used to advance nursing science are described.

Establishing Oncology Nursing Science Priorities

National Priorities

The United States has taken the lead in establishing oncology nursing science priorities. Oberst (1978) used the Delphi technique to delineate priorities among nurses who were working in U.S. cancer centers, general hospitals, and community settings and were interested in the special problems of patients with cancer. The Delphi technique obtains consensus through repeated individual questioning from a group of knowledgeable individuals or an expert in a particular area. Three survey rounds were used to determine priorities for clinical research in cancer nursing. Initially, a panel of 575 nurses was surveyed, and 245 of the nurses completed all three rounds. The 575 nurses who completed at least one survey round identified 1,800 potential research problems that were analyzed and grouped into 101 research topics. The five highest-ranked topics were (Oberst)

1. Relieving nausea and vomiting
2. Nursing interventions for pain
3. Comprehensive discharge planning and follow-up programs
4. Coping with grief and death
5. Prevention and treatment of stomatitis.

These priorities were intended to guide nurse scientists and clinicians in selecting clinical problems to study and in jointly designing innovative ways to improve the nursing care of people with cancer.

In 1992, the Association of Pediatric Oncology Nurses (APON) established research priorities for pediatric oncology nursing using the Delphi technique. Two survey rounds were used, with the second round designed from the results of the first. All APON members were invited to participate (N = 1,528), and 297 members responded with a total of 586 research ideas. The Nursing Research Advisory Committee at St. Jude Children's Research Hospital analyzed these ideas for any overlap or similarity. The resulting 75 research priorities were then rated by importance by 227 APON members. The five most important research priorities were (Hinds et al., 1994)

1. Measuring quality of life (QOL) and late effects in long-term survivors of childhood cancer
2. Evaluating effectiveness of anesthesia, sedatives, or other supportive or educational techniques in reducing patients' anxiety about painful or diagnostic procedures
3. Comparing the safety and effectiveness of different pharmacologic and nonpharmacologic techniques used for pain control
4. Documenting the effects on nurses of exposure to chemotherapeutic agents
5. Identifying factors that influence how children and adolescents comply with treatment regimens and evaluating interventions designed to help family members cope with the treatment process and its outcomes. (These two priorities were both ranked as the fifth priority.)

ONS began establishing oncology nursing science priorities in 1980. Since then, ONS members have been surveyed approximately every four years to identify research priorities. From 1980–1994, the ONS Research Committee surveyed the ONS membership five times to determine the Society's research interests or priorities (Funkhouser & Grant, 1989; Grant & Stromborg, 1981; McGuire, Frank-Stromborg, & Varricchio, 1985; Mooney, Ferrell, Nail, Benedict, & Haberman, 1991; Stetz, Haberman, Holcombe, & Jones, 1995). A goal of the ONS Research Committee is to promote and support collaboration in research among people with shared interests, so initially the survey results were used to create an ONS Directory of Members' Research Activities for members to purchase (Grant & Stromborg). Although the committee organizational structure no longer exists at ONS, project teams convened by the ONS Steering Council and the ONS Board of Directors conducted the ONS Research Priorities Survey in 2000 and 2004 to collect data for the development of the ONS Research Agenda and to establish oncology scientific priorities (Berger et al., 2005; Ropka et al., 2002).

The ONS Research Priorities Survey provides a list of research topics from which respondents can choose. This list was originally developed by members of the ONS Research Committee in 1980 (Grant & Stromborg, 1981), and each subsequent survey has built upon the list of research topics identified in the previous survey. Topics have been added to or deleted from each survey to reflect issues or topics currently relevant to oncology nursing. In 1994, the topics were organized into seven major categories: symptom management, care delivery issues, psychosocial aspects of care, special populations, continuum of care, health promotion behaviors, and treatment decision making (Stetz et al., 1995). These categories also have been modified with each subsequent survey.

When comparing past ONS surveys, methodologic differences in questionnaires, sampling technique and size, and design must be considered. Close comparison of the established research priorities across the surveys is limited because of significant differences in the instructions given to participants (see Table 1-1). For example, in the 1980 and 1984 studies (Grant & Stromborg, 1981; McGuire et al., 1985), participants were asked to identify their top five research interests, whereas subsequent surveys asked participants to identify what they perceive to be the priorities in oncology nursing research. In the 1988 study (Funkhouser & Grant, 1989), participants were asked to identify their top five research priorities, and in the 1991 study (Mooney et al., 1991), they were asked to identify their top 10 research priorities. The past three surveys asked the respondents to use a Likert scale (1 = not at all important and 5 = extremely important) to identify research priorities within a provided list (Berger et al., 2005; Ropka et al., 2002; Stetz et al., 1995).

Sampling approaches also varied. Convenience, random, and a combination of sampling methods were used. *Convenience sampling* uses the most readily available people as study participants, and *random sampling* uses a selection process in which each person has an equal chance of being selected (Polit & Beck, 2004). Initially, the entire ONS membership was surveyed; however, over the years, participants evolved to include two groups: all ONS members who are nurse scientists (doctorally prepared), and a random sample of all other ONS members, primarily consisting of clinicians (Berger et al., 2005; Ropka et al., 2002). This sampling approach promotes clinician and nurse scientist partnerships in advancing oncology nursing science. The priorities of both groups

Table 1-1. Oncology Nursing Society (ONS) Research Priorities Surveys 1981–2004: Methods

Study	Sample	Number Responding	Response Rate	Survey	Instructions Given to Participants
1980 (Grant & Stromborg, 1981)	ONS membership (N = 2,205)	998	45%	One-page mailed questionnaire	Select and rank the five areas in which you hold high research interest.
1984 (McGuire et al., 1985)	ONS members who read the *Oncology Nursing Forum* (sample size not specified)	342	Not reported	Questionnaire printed in the *Oncology Nursing Forum*	Identify from the content the areas in which you are interested in doing research.
1988 (Funkhouser & Grant, 1989)	Convenience sample of ONS members involved in research and leadership (N = 700)	213	30%	Two-page mailed questionnaire	Select and rank the five topics that are priorities in oncology nursing research.
1991 (Mooney et al., 1991)	Convenience sample of ONS members involved in research and leadership (N = 429)	310	70%	Mailed questionnaire	Rank from 1–10 the top 10 priorities for oncology nursing research.
1994 (Stetz et al., 1995)	Random sample of 10% of ONS members who identified patient care as primary functional area, the ONS leadership, and all ONS Advanced Nursing Research Special Interest Group members (N = 2,178)	789	36%	Mailed questionnaire	Rate each of the 93 items using a five-point Likert scale (1 = not at all important to 5 = extremely important) and rank what you perceive to be the top 10 priorities for nursing research.

(Continued on next page)

Table 1-1. Oncology Nursing Society (ONS) Research Priorities Surveys 1981–2004: Methods *(Continued)*

Study	Sample	Number Responding	Response Rate	Survey	Instructions Given to Participants
2000 (Ropka et al., 2002)	Random sample of general ONS membership excluding researchers (n = 1,850) and all ONS researcher members (n = 150)	788	39%	Mailed questionnaire Incentive offered to participants: entry into a drawing for 10 $25 gift certificates for ONS publications of the recipient's choice	Rate each of the 113 topics using a five-point Likert scale (1 = not at all important to 5 = extremely important) in reference to the question "What are the most important issues related to health and health care for individuals affected by cancer that can be addressed by oncology nursing research?"
2004 (Berger et al., 2005)	Random sample of general ONS membership (n = 2,205) and all ONS members in the United States with doctoral degrees (n = 627)	431	15%	Electronic survey Incentive offered to participants: entry into a drawing to win one of three one-year ONS memberships	Rate each of the 117 topics using a five-point Likert scale (1 = not at all important to 5 = extremely important) in reference to the question "How important is it to conduct new research in each of the following topics?"

were considered separately and as a whole, with findings adjusted to remove the effect of the oversampling of the nurse scientist group. The 2000 ONS Research Priorities Survey found that nurse scientist respondents prioritized evidence-based practice, outcomes of cancer care, family issues, and health policy as more important than clinicians did; however, both groups prioritized many areas similarly, such as pain, QOL, early detection, prevention and risk reduction, and fatigue (Ropka et al.). The 2004 ONS Research Priorities Survey found that nurse scientist respondents ranked an additional 10 topics in the top 20 research priorities that the adjusted general membership sample did not rank. These topics were older adults, clustering of symptoms, socioeconomically disadvantaged patients, racial/ethnic/cultural groups, access to cancer care, exercise/physical activity, low health literacy, functional status changes, self-management/self-efficacy, and survivorship (Berger et al.).

In 2004, ONS began using the Internet to survey members about oncology nursing research priorities (Berger et al., 2005). This method is more cost-effective than a mailed survey. Although the response rate for the 2004 electronic survey was lower than previous years when the survey was mailed, it is consistent with response rates from the mailed surveys (Dillman, 2000).

To enhance participation in the survey, participants received a postcard or e-mail reminder in 2000 and 2004. ONS also offered incentives for completing the survey. Participants were entered into a drawing for ONS publication gift certificates and ONS membership (Berger et al., 2005; Ropka et al., 2002). These procedures were based on the Tailored Design Method recommended by Dillman (2000), an authority in survey research.

Although limitations exist in comparing the ONS research priorities identified by past surveys, recognizing priority trends is meaningful for advancing oncology nursing science (see Table 1-2).

Cancer Prevention and Detection: Except for the 1984 survey, cancer prevention and detection always ranked as one of the top 10 research priorities. The continued interest in prevention and early detection is consistent with the healthcare environment's emphasis on health prevention and the National Cancer Institute's (NCI's) cancer control focus. Lifestyle and environmental factors are responsible for a majority of cancer diagnoses, and a dearth of research in these areas exists (NCI, 1997).

Decision Making: Decision making was first recognized in 2000 as the 18th priority. In 2004, decision making about treatment in advanced disease was ranked second, and decision making about treatment was ranked fourth. This reflects the healthcare system's shift to a more consumer-driven system that supports the individual's role in decision making. People with cancer face decisions regarding multiple treatment methods that were not available in the past. Those with advanced cancer often make difficult decisions regarding whether to continue with treatment.

Pain: Despite advancements in the pharmacologic management of pain, this priority has ranked in the top five priorities since the first ONS Research Priorities Survey. Oncology nurses are clearly not satisfied with pain control

Table 1-2. Oncology Nursing Society Research Priorities Surveys 1980–2004: Top 10 Ranked Research Priorities

Rank	1981 (Grant & Stromborg, 1981)	1984 (McGuire et al., 1985)	1988 (Funkhouser & Grant, 1989)	1991 (Mooney et al., 1991)	1994 (Stetz et al., 1995)	2000 (Ropka et al., 2002)	2004 (Berger et al., 2005)
1	Patient or health teaching	Pain control and management	Prevention and early detection	Quality of life[a]	Pain	Pain	Quality of life
2	Coping and stress management	Symptom management	Symptom management	Symptom management[a]	Prevention	Quality of life	Participation in decision making about treatment in advanced disease
3	Pain control and management	Patient or health education	Pain control and management	Outcomes measures for interventions[b]	Quality of life	Early detection	Patient and family education
4	Prevention and early detection	Coping and stress management	Patient or health education[a]	Pain control and management[b]	Risk reduction and screening	Prevention and risk reduction	Participation in decision making about treatment
5	Symptom management	Role of specialist	Coping and stress management[a]	Cancer survivorship	Ethical issues	Neutropenia	Pain
6	Hospice care	Professional issues (certification)[a]	Home care	Prevention and early detection	Neutropenia	Hospice/end of life	Tobacco use and exposure[a]

(Continued on next page)

Table 1-2. Oncology Nursing Society Research Priorities Surveys 1980–2004: Top 10 Ranked Research Priorities (Continued)

Rank	1981 (Grant & Stromborg, 1981)	1984 (McGuire et al., 1985)	1988 (Funkhouser & Grant, 1989)	1991 (Mooney et al., 1991)	1994 (Stetz et al., 1995)	2000 (Ropka et al., 2002)	2004 (Berger et al., 2005)
7	Family support	Patient support systems[a]	Economic influences on oncology	Research utilization	Patient education	Oncologic emergencies	Screening and early detection of cancer[a]
8	Nurse burnout[a]	Characteristics of oncology nurses	Cancer rehabilitation	Cancer rehabilitation	Stress, coping, and adaptation	Suffering	Prevention of cancer and cancer risk reduction
9	Protective mechanisms[a]	Counseling	AIDS	Cost containment[c]	Detection	Fatigue	Palliative care[b]
10	Counseling	Home care	Compliance with treatment	Economic influences[c]	Cost containment	Ethical issues	Evidence-based practice[b]

[a] Tied for rank
[b] Tied for rank
[c] Tied for rank

Note. Based on information from Mooney et al., 1991.

in cancer care. More intervention research is needed in this area, as indicated by almost 60% of the 1994 ONS Research Priorities Survey respondents (N = 789) who indicated the type of research needed for this priority (Stetz et al., 1995). The type of research needed for ranked priorities was not previously reported by ONS Research Priorities Surveys. The distinction between pharmacologic intervention and nonpharmacologic intervention research was not made in identifying the need for more intervention research in pain control. As more nonpharmacologic pain interventions emerge, research in this area is needed.

Patient and Family Education: Teaching patients and families is an essential component of nursing. Patients with cancer and their families require education about many cancer care issues, including diagnosis, treatment, self-care, recurrence, survivorship, and end of life. Patient and family education is consistently ranked as an important research priority among ONS members, and in 1981, it was ranked as the number-one priority.

Quality of Life: This cancer care issue has been ranked in the top three priorities since 1991. It was not listed as a topic area on the 1980 and 1984 surveys but was ranked 31st on the 1988 survey because participants listed this priority in response to the open-ended item of "other priorities" (Funkhouser & Grant, 1989). QOL ranked as the highest priority in the most recent ONS Research Priorities Survey (Berger et al., 2005). The initial high ranking of this cancer care issue in 1991 probably reflected the NCI designation that QOL should be included as an outcome measurement in cancer clinical trials (Mooney et al., 1991).

Tobacco Use and Exposure: Tobacco use and exposure was added to the 2004 Research Priorities Survey and ranked as the sixth research priority (Berger et al., 2005). This new priority is of high importance because of the direct relationship of tobacco use and exposure and the incidence of lung cancer and other cancer-related diagnoses.

Addressing Identified Research Priorities

What progress has been made toward addressing these research priorities topics? Has the knowledge not been generated, or do nurses not know of the research? If the answer is one of poor dissemination to practicing nurses, then dissemination efforts must be examined. Nurses also need to learn to be critical consumers of research in order to integrate evidence-based care into their practice (Waddell, 2002). To gather information on nurses' understanding of the research evidence, the 2004 ONS Research Priorities Survey added a question to address participant familiarity with the current research about each topic category. Data showed that clinicians were most familiar with the cancer symptom management research (Berger et al., 2005).

If progress has not been made in the study of research priorities, the quantity and quality of research needs to be addressed (Waddell, 2002). Graduate schools of nursing should encourage the development of thesis and dissertation research that focuses on identified research priorities. Directors of nursing research in clinical settings should encourage research in the practice environment, as well. Research must contribute to the goal of evidence-based nursing practice.

International Priorities

In Canada, Degner et al. (1987) partially replicated Oberst's study and obtained similar results. Oncology nursing science priorities also are established in Australia, Europe, Ireland, the Netherlands, South Korea, and Norway by the Delphi technique or by a mailed questionnaire (Ambaum, Courtens, & Fliedenes, 1996; Browne, Robinson, & Richardson, 2002; Lee et al., 2003; Murphy & Cowman, 2006; Rustoen & Schjolberg, 2000; Yates et al., 2002).

The five most recent international oncology nursing research priorities studies, including the 2004 ONS Research Priorities Survey, were conducted during the past six years (see Table 1-3). Yates et al. (2002) mailed a survey to all 589 members of the Oncology Nurses Group of Queensland, Australia, with a response rate of 54.2%. Participants responded to an open-ended question to identify five priority areas of research related to oncology/palliative nursing. The top four priority areas as indicated in the table were identified by at least 40% of the participants who responded to this question.

Also in 2002, a Delphi survey identified research priorities of European Oncology Nursing Society members. Participants represented 15 European countries, and 223 nurses responded to the first survey. The second survey asked the participants to rank their top five research priorities, and 117 nurses responded (response rate was not reported for either survey). A recognized limitation to the survey was its translation into multiple languages, including Czech, French, German, Italian, and Spanish (Browne et al., 2002).

In South Korea, the Korean Oncology Nursing Society (KONS) conducted a descriptive study in 2003 to establish oncology nursing research priorities for research agenda development. The survey questionnaire was a revised version of the 2000 ONS Research Priorities Survey, which was translated into Korean. Participants were asked to rank five items in order of research priority. All 219 KONS members received the survey by mail, and the response rate was 33.8% (Lee et al., 2003).

The research priorities of oncology nurses from the Republic of Ireland were determined in 2006. A survey mailed to 119 nurses at a national oncology specialist center achieved a response rate of 66%. Using a Likert scale, the top five research priorities were identified from a list of 57 research areas (Murphy & Cowman, 2006).

Limitations in comparing the research priorities of different countries include cultural differences, translation of surveys, and different healthcare systems. Methodologic differences in questionnaires, sampling, and design also exist. Despite these differences, identifying the trends and patterns of

Table 1-3. International Oncology Nursing Research Priorities: A Comparison of Top Five Priorities 2002–2000

Rank	Australia 2002 (Yates et al., 2002)	Europe 2002 (Browne et al., 2002)	South Korea 2003 (Lee et al., 2003)	United States 2004 (Berger et al., 2005)	Republic of Ireland 2006 (Murphy & Cowman, 2006)
1	Psychosocial support	Communication, information giving, and educational needs	Prevention of cancer and cancer risk reduction	Quality of life	Effectiveness of nurse-led clinics on oncology services
2	Pain management	Symptom management (e.g., pain, nausea and vomiting, fatigue)	Pain	Participation in decision making about treatment in advanced disease	Levels of stress and burnout for cancer nurses
3	Symptom management (e.g., nausea and vomiting, constipation, mucositis, nutrition)	Experiences of disease and its treatment (e.g., psychological experiences)	Quality of life	Patient and family education	Identification of communication issues for patients throughout their cancer journey
4	Health system issues (e.g., funding, access/availability of services)	Cancer nursing research (research facilitation and research utilization)	Hospice/end-of-life care	Participation in decision making about treatment	Continuity of care among hospital, community, and hospice settings
5	Patient and community education	Cancer nursing education issues	Standards of care	Pain	Development of nurse-led interventions for the management of pain

research priorities among different countries is important in increasing awareness regarding nursing research development.

The following research priorities are highlighted because they were (a) ranked highly by more than one country or (b) unique as a result of a change in the country's healthcare delivery focus.

Communication Issues: This cancer care issue ranked as the highest research priority among European oncology nurses and as the third highest priority in the Republic of Ireland (Browne et al., 2002; Murphy & Cowman, 2006). Good communication is recognized as essential in ensuring that patients make informed decisions regarding treatment and how best to manage their disease (Murphy & Cowman). Participation in decision making about treatment and treatment in advanced disease are both high-ranking research priorities in the United States (Berger et al., 2005).

Effectiveness of Nurse-Led Clinics on Oncology Services: The roles of the clinical nurse specialist and the advanced nurse practitioner were recently established in the Republic of Ireland. The ranking of this issue as the most important research priority among oncology nurses in the Republic of Ireland may reflect this change in oncology nurses' roles and responsibilities (Murphy & Cowman, 2006).

Pain: Pain management is ranked in the top five research priorities for Australia, Europe, Korea, the United States, and the Republic of Ireland. Lee et al. (2003) recognized the lack of cancer pain intervention studies in Korea. In the Republic of Ireland, the identified research priority specifically addresses nurse-led intervention for pain management (Murphy & Cowman, 2006). Because pharmacologic management is well established, this is an important focus for pain research.

Prevention of Cancer and Cancer Risk Reduction: Korean oncology nurses ranked cancer prevention and risk reduction as the highest research priority. This may reflect the Korean Ministry of Health and Welfare's 10-Year Plan to Conquer Cancer, which was initiated in 1996 (Lee et al., 2003). As previously recognized, this also is a high-ranking research priority among ONS members.

Psychosocial Support: Psychosocial support was recognized as the number-one priority in Australia and the third research priority in Europe. This is a challenging but essential oncology nursing responsibility because people with cancer face many questions and uncertainties related to their disease and treatment.

Quality of Life: From 1994 to 2000, QOL ranked in the top five research priorities in the Netherlands, Canada, and Norway, as well as the United States (Ambaum et al., 1996; Bakker & Fitch, 1998; Rustoen & Schjolberg, 2000; Stetz et al., 1995). It continues to be the number-one priority in the United States and the third ranking research priority in Korea. With increasingly aggressive treatment regimens, people with cancer experience multiple side effects that affect their QOL.

Use of Oncology Nursing Science Priorities Data

ONS uses the research priorities data for a variety of purposes that further research development both within and outside the Society (see Table 1-4). Identifying research priorities is essential for developing the ONS Research Agenda, providing direction for research grant funding and research initiatives, establishing the focus of nursing education programs and conferences, and providing direction in identifying areas of research study and publication by nurse scientists and clinicians.

Oncology Nursing Society Research Agenda

The first ONS Research Agenda was developed in 2001 to inform the ONS leadership, membership, and external individuals and groups about the scientific priorities of the ONS membership. The goals of the ONS Research Agenda are to
* Increase the knowledge base for oncology nursing practice through identifying cutting-edge and critical priority areas of oncology nursing science and recommend mechanisms of support.

Table 1-4. Oncology Nursing Society: Using Research Priorities	
Type of Use	**Examples**
Determining funding priorities for Oncology Nursing Society (ONS) Foundation small grants and major grants programs	Pain, fatigue, neutropenia, and symptom management
Targeting specific corporate donors for research funds	Fatigue Initiative Through Research and Education (FIRE®)—Ortho Biotech, Inc.
Selecting specific clinical issues for education and research initiatives	FIRE® Project State-of-the-knowledge conferences
Choosing topics for sessions at annual ONS conferences	Symptom management, palliative care, nursing-sensitive patient outcomes, patient and family education
Incorporating research priorities into strategic planning	Research-related strategic goals
Developing the ONS Research Agenda	Guides the development of the agenda
Distributing research priorities to federal, professional, and health-related funding agencies	National Cancer Institute, National Institute of Nursing Research, American Society of Clinical Oncology, American Cancer Society
Giving expert testimony at federal, professional, and health-related advisory boards	National Cancer Advisory Board, American Cancer Society Blue Ribbon Panel

Note. From "Research and Oncology Nursing Practice," by D.B. McGuire and M.E. Ropka, 2000, *Seminars in Oncology Nursing, 16*(1), p. 38. Copyright 2000 by Elsevier. Adapted with permission.

- Prepare future oncology nurse scientists to be well trained and equipped to implement ongoing programs of research and to seek support from major sponsors, such as the National Institutes of Health and the American Cancer Society.
- Prepare clinical nurses as critical consumers of research findings that can be applied to practice.

The agenda is developed through a consensus-building effort of ONS nurse scientists, advanced practice nurses, and a cancer survivor. It is reviewed, evaluated, and revised at two-year intervals that coincide with the biennial ONS National Cancer Nursing Research Conference. Funding of the ONS Research Agenda Conference (2002–2007) is supported through an NCI R13 grant award (1 R13 CA101305-1) funded by NCI and the National Institute of Nursing Research. Donna Berry, PhD, RN, AOCN®, FAAN, is the principal investigator (ONS, n.d.-b) and was a member of the 2004 Research Priorities Survey Project Team. Her goal is to provide continuity between the identification of ONS research priorities and the development of the research agenda (Berger et al., 2005).

The survey results provide the important groundwork for the ONS Research Agenda. The development of the 2005–2009 ONS Research Agenda was guided by the 2004 ONS Research Priorities Survey results, priority research areas of other cancer and nursing research funding organizations, and a review of the state of the science of oncology nursing research. Priority research content areas identified by the agenda are (a) cancer symptoms and side effects, (b) individual- and family-focused psychosocial and behavioral research, (c) health promotion, including primary and secondary prevention, (d) late effects of cancer treatment and long-term survivorship issues for patients and their families, (e) nursing-sensitive patient outcomes, and (f) translational research (ONS, n.d.-b). Priority research topics are identified within each content area. The sixth content area, translational research, is essential to increasing knowledge about the dissemination of research to practice. All populations are relevant for study for all of the content areas, including populations across the life span, families and caregivers, and vulnerable populations related to health disparities in minority groups of all types (ONS, n.d.-b).

The ONS Research Agenda is a critical document for furthering ONS's mission of promoting excellence in oncology nursing and quality cancer care. The ONS leadership and membership and the ONS Foundation use the agenda in identifying research goals, funding, and initiatives.

Oncology Nursing Society Research Funding and Initiatives

ONS and the ONS Foundation are credited with an extensive history of supporting the generation of knowledge. In 1984, the ONS Foundation began its small grants program, a source of seed money for oncology nurse scientists to conduct preliminary work that would lead to larger awards. The majority of the small grant studies funded by the ONS Foundation address topics identified by the investigator; however, some small grant awards are designated for studies that address research priorities such as pain assessment and management and symptom management. Since 1984, the ONS Foundation small grants program provided funding for studies addressing the following ONS research priorities: pain ($241,468), QOL ($124,742), cancer prevention and detection ($110,053), and patient and family education ($97,329). Since the inception of the small grants program, 338 studies have received a total amount of $2,528,014 (ONS Research Team, personal communication, May 9, 2007).

The ONS Foundation major grants program began in 1998. This program provides grant awards of $25,000–$500,000. The focus of many of these grant awards is determined by the ONS Research Agenda and research priorities. Research priorities and agenda content areas addressed by major grant funding include neutropenia, symptom management, nursing-sensitive patient outcomes, and translational research. Since the inception of the major grants program, 37 studies have received a total amount of $3,798,470 (ONS Research Team, personal communication, May 9, 2007).

In 1998, the ONS Foundation Clinical Scholar Program funded a Pain Clinical Research Scholar. The goal of the scholar's program was to improve the care given to patients with cancer and their families by fostering evidence-based practice and the utilization of appropriate research findings by oncology nurses. The scholar was responsible for developing an organizational infrastructure that promotes cancer-related pain research and provides opportunities for other nurses to become involved in research. The scholar also created innovative strategies for transferring pain-related research findings into clinical practice (ONS Research Team, personal communication, May 9, 2007).

A major funding and research initiative that addressed fatigue, a frequently reported symptom of cancer and cancer treatment, was the ONS Fatigue Initiative Through Research and Education (FIRE®) supported by Ortho Biotech, Inc. This 1995–2000 initiative was a three-part project designed to increase nurses' awareness and understanding of cancer-related fatigue and increase the amount of research addressing it. A four-day professional education course was held with more than 200 oncology nursing participants from the United States, Canada, and Europe. A fatigue public awareness campaign and public education project was initiated in conjunction with National Cancer Fatigue Awareness Day in the United States. The ONS Research Committee developed a two-phased research program. Phase I provided funding for three investigator-initiated multi-institutional developmental grants of $50,000 each. Phase II provided funding for one investigator-initiated grant of $500,000, three multi-institutional instrument development grants of $50,000 each, a fatigue clinical research scholar of $70,000, and a state-of-the-knowledge conference. Through these mechanisms, the FIRE® project increased the knowledge base about the effects of fatigue on people with cancer and the effectiveness of fatigue-related nursing interventions (Mock, Nail, & Grant, 1998).

The ONS research priorities are shared with federal agencies and other funding organizations. The 1988 ONS Research Priorities Survey was conducted in response to an invitation from Dr. Ada Sue Hinshaw, then-director of the National Center for Nursing Research (which later became the National Institute of Nursing Research) in the National Institutes of Health, asking nursing organizations to submit their nursing research priorities (Funkhouser & Grant, 1989). The ONS research priorities also are shared through expert testimony at federal, professional, and health-related advisory boards (McGuire & Ropka, 2000). The ONS Research Priorities Survey results and Research Agenda are shared routinely with other organizations and are available on the ONS Web site (www.ons.org/research/information).

Oncology Nursing Society Education Initiatives

The ONS state-of-the-knowledge conferences provide an opportunity for scientists and clinicians to determine the state of the science for priority research areas. Besides providing a synopsis of the research for a particular research priority, these conferences may result in the establishment of research networks and collaborative research in areas that need further study. Since 1994, fatigue, pain, QOL, neutropenia, sleep-wake disturbances, and nursing-sensitive patient outcomes research has been addressed at these conferences. Some of the outcomes of these conferences, including a summary of the knowledge base and direction for research and practice, were published in the *Oncology Nursing Forum* (*ONF*) (King et al., 1997; Nirenberg et al., 2006a, 2006b; Winningham et al., 1994).

The ONS Education Agenda incorporated the ONS research priorities identified in 2000 (Ropka et al., 2002). This document is a source for identifying and developing educational projects and programs within ONS. ONS educational programs have addressed ONS research priorities such as cancer prevention and early detection, pain management, end-of-life care, and neutropenia. ONS annual conferences hold educational and research sessions addressing many of the research priorities. These educational programs and conference sessions are an important method for disseminating research and promoting evidence-based practice.

Direction for Research Studies and Publication

Research priorities provide guidance for nurse scientists and clinicians in identifying areas for research study and topics for publication. ONS publishes two premier journals that provide oncology information to nurses. The *Clinical Journal of Oncology Nursing* (*CJON*) publishes clinically focused articles, and *ONF* provides comprehensive coverage of cutting-edge developments in cancer nursing science and patient care (ONS, n.d.-a). A review of the articles published from 2002 to 2007 was conducted to determine the number of research reports and review articles that addressed the research priorities before and after the 2004 ONS Research Priorities Survey (see Table 1-5). Although this is a rudimentary review because only the title of the article was used to determine if the article addressed a priority, it is useful to see if articles are being disseminated on the priority topics.

- The priority addressed by the highest number of articles was QOL. This was not surprising because QOL has been one of the top three priorities since 1991. Interestingly, two years after the 2004 survey, 15 articles were published in *ONF*, which was the highest number in the five-year period.
- Both journals are disseminating information on education, pain, prevention, and screening. Research reports and clinical articles have been published addressing these priorities.

Table 1-5. A Review of Priority Topics Addressed by Articles Published in the *Oncology Nursing Forum (ONF)* and the *Clinical Journal of Oncology Nursing (CJON)* Journals: 2002–2007

2004 ONS Research Priorities	Number of Articles Published by Year					
	2002	2003	2004	2005	2006	2007
Quality of life	*ONF:* 6 *CJON:* 1	*ONF:* 5 *CJON:* 2	*ONF:* 6 *CJON:* 0	*ONF:* 4 *CJON:* 0	*ONF:* 15 *CJON:* 0	*ONF:* 6 *CJON:* 1
Participation in decision making about treatment in advanced disease	*ONF:* 0 *CJON:* 0	*ONF:* 0 *CJON:* 0	*ONF:* 0 *CJON:* 0	*ONF:* 0 *CJON:* 0	*ONF:* 0 *CJON:* 0	*ONF:* 0 *CJON:* 0
Patient and family education	*ONF:* 2 *CJON:* 2*	*ONF:* 4* *CJON:* 3	*ONF:* 4 *CJON:* 1	*ONF:* 2 *CJON:* 1	*ONF:* 0 *CJON:* 3*	*ONF:* 0 *CJON:* 1
Participation in decision making about treatment	*ONF:* 1 *CJON:* 0	*ONF:* 4 *CJON:* 0	*ONF:* 0 *CJON:* 0	*ONF:* 1 *CJON:* 0	*ONF:* 0 *CJON:* 0	*ONF:* 0 *CJON:* 0
Pain	*ONF:* 4 *CJON:* 1	*ONF:* 9* *CJON:* 1	*ONF:* 3 *CJON:* 1	*ONF:* 4 *CJON:* 1	*ONF:* 4 *CJON:* 1	*ONF:* 6 *CJON:* 2
Tobacco use and exposure	*ONF:* 0 *CJON:* 1	*ONF:* 0 *CJON:* 0	*ONF:* 1 *CJON:* 0	*ONF:* 0 *CJON:* 1	*ONF:* 0 *CJON:* 1	*ONF:* 0 *CJON:* 0

(Continued on next page)

Table 1-5. A Review of Priority Topics Addressed by Articles Published in the *Oncology Nursing Forum (ONF)* and the *Clinical Journal of Oncology Nursing (CJON)* Journals: 2002–2007 *(Continued)*						
	Number of Articles Published by Year					
2004 ONS Research Priorities	**2002**	**2003**	**2004**	**2005**	**2006**	**2007**
Screening and early detection of cancer	*ONF:* 6* *CJON:* 0	*ONF:* 7 *CJON:* 2	*ONF:* 4 *CJON:* 1*	*ONF:* 2 *CJON:* 2	*ONF:* 6* *CJON:* 3*	*ONF:* 7* *CJON:* 0
Prevention of cancer and cancer risk reduction	*ONF:* 0 *CJON:* 0	*ONF:* 2* *CJON:* 1	*ONF:* 0 *CJON:* 2*	*ONF:* 1 *CJON:* 1	*ONF:* 5* *CJON:* 0	*ONF:* 2* *CJON:* 1
Palliative care	*ONF:* 0 *CJON:* 1	*ONF:* 2 *CJON:* 2	*ONF:* 0 *CJON:* 1	*ONF:* 0 *CJON:* 1	*ONF:* 0 *CJON:* 0	*ONF:* 4 *CJON:* 0
Evidence-based prac-tice	*ONF:* 2 *CJON:* 0	*ONF:* 1 *CJON:* 2	*ONF:* 3 *CJON:* 0	*ONF:* 1 *CJON:* 1	*ONF:* 0 *CJON:* 2	*ONF:* 1 *CJON:* 3
*Article addresses more than one research priority topic						

- Very few or no articles were found on decision making and tobacco use; however, these priorities were newly identified by the 2004 ONS Research Priorities Survey. Palliative care, another new priority, was addressed in four *ONF* articles in 2007.
- Evidence-based practice also was a new priority in 2004. Both journals have a strong focus on evidence-based practice, and a column published in *CJON* addresses the clinical practice applicability of research findings from specific studies.

Information on some of the research priority topics clearly is being disseminated through ONS journals. A more thorough review of these articles is necessary to determine if the research studies have generated findings that can be recommended for practice. Perhaps more intervention research is needed in these priority areas. If this is not the case, dissemination of new knowledge to the bedside must be a priority.

Conclusion

Establishing research priorities among practicing nurses and nurse scientists is a very successful method for advancing oncology nursing science.

Focusing oncology nursing research on problems experienced in the real world of nursing practice is important. Research should address established priorities, particularly those common research priorities identified both nationally and internationally, such as pain management, quality of life, and cancer prevention and detection. This will benefit people with cancer throughout the world.

The key to quality cancer care is evidence-based practice. Dissemination of quality research must be common practice among the nurse scientist community. Links must be continually established between nurse scientists and practicing nurses to improve the nursing care of people with cancer. By joining resources to increase the knowledge base of priority cancer care issues, research will advance oncology nursing science.

References

Ambaum, B., Courtens, A., & Fliedener, M. (1996). Research priorities in oncology nursing in the Netherlands [Abstract no. 345]. In International Society of Nurses in Cancer Care (Ed.), *Ninth International Conference on Cancer Nursing, August 12–15, 1996* (p. 118). Brighton, United Kingdom: RCN Publishing.

Bakker, D., & Fitch, M.I. (1998). Oncology nursing research priorities: A Canadian perspective. *Cancer Nursing, 21*(6), 394–401.

Berger, A.M., Berry, D.L., Christopher, K.A., Greene, A.L., Maliski, S., Swenson, K.K., et al. (2005). Oncology Nursing Society year 2004 research priorities survey. *Oncology Nursing Forum, 32*(2), 281–290.

Browne, N., Robinson, L., & Richardson, A. (2002). A Delphi study on the research priorities of European oncology nurses. *European Journal of Oncology Nursing, 6*(3), 133–144.

Degner, L., Areand, R., Chekryn, J., Davies, E., Dyck, S., Kristjanson, L., et al. (1987). Priorities for cancer nursing research: A Canadian replication. *Cancer Nursing, 10*(6), 319–326.

Dillman, D.A. (2000). *Mail and internet surveys: The tailored design method* (2nd ed.). New York: Wiley.

Funkhouser, S.W., & Grant, M.M. (1989). 1988 ONS survey of research priorities. *Oncology Nursing Forum, 16*(3), 413–416.

Grant, M., & Stromborg, M. (1981). Promoting research collaboration: ONS research committee survey. *Oncology Nursing Forum, 8*(2), 48–53.

Hinds, P.S., Quargnenti, A., Olson, M.S., Gross, J., Puckett, P., Randall, E., et al. (1994). The 1992 APON Delphi study to establish research priorities for pediatric oncology nursing. *Journal of Pediatric Oncology Nursing, 11*(1), 20–27.

King, C.R., Haberman, M., Berry, D.L., Bush, N., Butler, L., Dow, K.H., et al. (1997). Quality of life and the cancer experience: The state-of-the-knowledge. *Oncology Nursing Forum, 24*(1), 27–41.

Lee, E.H., Kim, J.S., Chung, B.Y., Bok, M.S., Song, B.E., Kong, S.W., et al. (2003). Research priorities of Korean oncology nurses. *Cancer Nursing, 26*(5), 387–391.

McGuire, D., Frank-Stromborg, M., & Varricchio, C. (1985). 1984 ONS research committee survey of membership's research interests and involvement. *Oncology Nursing Forum, 12*(2), 99–103.

McGuire, D.B., & Ropka, M.E. (2000). Research and oncology nursing practice. *Seminars in Oncology Nursing, 16*(1), 35–46.

Mock, V., Nail, L.M., & Grant, M. (1998). Implementing the FIRE® planning grant. *Oncology Nursing Forum, 25*(8), 1389–1412.

Mooney, K.H., Ferrell, B.R., Nail, L.M., Benedict, S.C., & Haberman, M.R. (1991). 1991 Oncology Nursing Society research priorities survey. *Oncology Nursing Forum, 18*(8), 1381–1388.

Murphy, A., & Cowman, S. (2006). Research priorities of oncology nurses in the Republic of Ireland. *Cancer Nursing, 29*(4), 283–290.

National Cancer Institute. (1997, August 7). *A new agenda for cancer control research: Report of the cancer control review group.* Retrieved August 15, 2007, from http://deainfo.nci.nih .gov/advisory/bsa/bsa_program/bsacacntrlmin.htm

Nirenberg, A., Bush, A.P., Davis, A., Friese, C.R., Gillespie, T.W., & Rice, R.D. (2006a). Neutropenia: State of the knowledge part I. *Oncology Nursing Forum, 33*(6), 1193–1201.

Nirenberg, A., Bush, A., Davis, A., Friese, C.R., Gillespie, T.W., & Rice, R.D. (2006b). Neutropenia: State of the knowledge part II. *Oncology Nursing Forum, 33*(6), 1202–1208.

Oberst, M. (1978). Priorities in cancer nursing research. *Cancer Nursing, 1*(4), 281–290.

Oncology Nursing Society. (n.d.-a). *Publications.* Retrieved August 15, 2007, from http:// www.ons.org/publications

Oncology Nursing Society. (n.d.-b). *Research agenda and priorities—research agenda.* Retrieved April 30, 2007, from http://www.ons.org/research/information/agenda.shtml

Polit, D.F., & Beck, C.T. (2004). *Nursing research: Principles and methods* (7th ed.). Philadelphia: Lippincott Williams & Wilkins.

Ropka, M.E., Guterbock, T., Krebs, L., Murphy-Ende, K., Stetz, K., Summers, B., et al. (2002). Year 2000 Oncology Nursing Society research priorities survey. *Oncology Nursing Forum, 29*(3), 481–491.

Rustoen, T., & Schjolberg, T.K. (2000). Cancer nursing research priorities: A Norwegian perspective. *Cancer Nursing, 23*(5), 375–381.

Stetz, K.M., Haberman, M.R., Holcombe, J., & Jones, L.S. (1995). 1994 Oncology Nursing Society research priorities survey. *Oncology Nursing Forum, 22*(5), 785–789.

Waddell, C. (2002). So much research evidence, so little dissemination and uptake: Mixing the useful with the pleasing. *Evidence-Based Nursing, 5*(2), 38–40.

Winningham, M.L., Nail, L.M., Burke, M.B., Brophy, L., Cimprich, B., Jones, L.S., et al. (1994). Fatigue and the cancer experience: The state of the knowledge. *Oncology Nursing Forum, 21*(1), 23–36.

Yates, P., Baker, D., Barrett, L., Christie, L., Dewar, A.M., Middleton, R., et al. (2002). Cancer nursing research in Queensland, Australia: Barriers, priorities, and strategies for progress. *Cancer Nursing, 25*(3), 167–180.

CHAPTER 2

Excellence in Oncology Science: Distinguished Nurse Scientists

Claudette G. Varricchio, RN, DSN, FAAN

Introduction

The Oncology Nursing Society (ONS) has recognized research as an important component of its mission to ensure excellent care for people with cancer since the Society's inception. In 1992, ONS established and awarded the first Distinguished Researcher Award. The purpose of this award is "to recognize the contributions of a member who has conducted or promoted research that has enhanced the science and practice of oncology nursing" (ONS, n.d.).

The current selection criteria are listed in Figure 2-1. These include a "*sustained* program of *substantive* research" that "advanced the delivery of quality cancer care" and provided "a foundation for research by others" (ONS, n.d.). The criteria have evolved and been refined over time to reflect the state of oncology nursing research but have maintained the same requirement for a rigorous program of research that has contributed to quality cancer care by nurses. Each recipient's publication record confirms her suitability for the honor. At the inception of this award, few senior cancer nurse scientists had an established program of research (Molassiotis et al., 2006). ONS recognized the growth of the field of cancer nursing research, and the competition for the award has increased. Currently, many cancer nurse scientists could present strong applications for this award.

The Recipients

In an attempt to present a profile of this distinguished group of scientists, information about them and their work is summarized in a series of tables to

---

Figure 2-1. Selection Criteria for the Oncology Nursing Society (ONS) Distinguished Researcher Award

The candidate must be a member of ONS with an earned doctorate in nursing or a related field who demonstrates:
1. Evidence of outstanding and major contributions to the scientific foundation for practice.
2. Evidence of a sustained program of substantive research.
3. Evidence of a record of publication in oncology.
4. Evidence that the scientist's research program has advanced the delivery of quality cancer care by nurses.
5. Evidence that the scientist's research program has provided a foundation for research by others.
6. Evidence of documented contributions to ONS.
7. Evidence of documented contributions to the cancer community-at-large.

Note. From *ONS Distinguished Award Winners: Distinguished Researcher Award (RE03),* by Oncology Nursing Society, n.d. Retrieved January 30, 2007, from http://www.ons.org/awards/onsawards/distinguishedResearcher.shtml. Copyright Oncology Nursing Society. Reprinted with permission.

---

facilitate comparisons. Table 2-1 lists the recipients by year, degree, areas of concentration, and institution. Table 2-2 lists the awardees and their affiliation at the time of the award. Table 2-3 lists the areas of focus of the research programs of the Distinguished Researcher Award winners. These data provide an overview of the diversity of the awardees and of their preparation as scientists. The areas of research focus are a direct representation of the areas of science important to oncology nursing science over each year in which Distinguished Researcher Awards were presented. The focus of the research has evolved along with nursing science and clinical practice and has been influenced to some degree by the ONS research priorities and by calls for research applications by funding agencies. An evolution of research methodology also can be observed. Research has evolved from descriptive work, development of methods (e.g., Ferrell et al., 1992; McCorkle et al., 1994, 1997), to the testing of interventions and the exploration of causation (e.g., Miaskowski, 2000; Nail, 2002), to simple clinical trials and, more recently, to multisite clinical trials of the effectiveness of nursing interventions (e.g., Dodd, 1997; Mock, 2003). The research has included behavioral approaches (e.g., Champion, 1994; Champion & Menon, 1997; Degner et al., 1997) and basic physiologic approaches (e.g., Mock et al., 2001; Miaskowski, 1996).

Influence on Nursing Science

The Distinguished Researchers have influenced the development of oncology nursing research and science through their activities as faculty advisers and mentors for graduate students, postdoctoral fellows, and colleagues. This

Table 2-1. Doctoral Preparation of the Oncology Nursing Society Distinguished Researchers

Year	Name	Discipline, Graduation Year	Institution of Degree Completion
1992	Jean E. Johnson	Social Psychology, 1971	University of Wisconsin, Madison
1993	Jeanne Quint Benoliel	Nursing, 1969	University of California, San Francisco
1994	Ruth McCorkle	Mass Communication, 1975	University of Iowa
1995	Barbara A. Given	Higher Education, 1976	Michigan State University
1996	Betty R. Ferrell	Nursing, 1984	Texas Women's University
1997	Marylin J. Dodd	Nursing, 1981	Wayne State University
1998	Frances Marcus Lewis	Sociology of Education, 1977	Stanford University
1999	Marcia M. Grant	Nursing, 1987	University of California, San Francisco
2000	Christine Miaskowski	Physiology, 1987	St. John's University
2001	Victoria Champion	Nursing, 1981	Indiana University
2002	Lillian M. Nail	Nursing, 1983	University of Rochester
2003	Victoria Mock	Nursing Science, 1988	Catholic University
2004	Pamela S. Hinds	Nursing Research, 1985	University of Arizona
2005	Marilyn Frank-Strom-borg	Educational Psychology, 1974 Law, 1994	Northern Illinois University Northern Illinois University
2006	Lesley F. Degner	Nursing, 1985	University of Michigan
2007	Ida M. Moore	Nursing, 1985	University of California, San Francisco
2008	Carol E. Ferrans	Nursing Science, 1985	University of Illinois, Chicago

Table 2-2. Affiliation at the Time of the Oncology Nursing Society Distinguished Researcher Award (1992–2008)

Year	Name	Affiliation
1992	Jean E. Johnson	University of Rochester
1993	Jeanne Quint Benoliel	University of Washington
1994	Ruth McCorkle	University of Pennsylvania
1995	Barbara A. Given	Michigan State University
1996	Betty R. Ferrell	City of Hope Comprehensive Cancer Center
1997	Marylin J. Dodd	University of California, San Francisco
1998	Frances Marcus Lewis	University of Washington
1999	Marcia M. Grant	City of Hope Comprehensive Cancer Center
2000	Christine Miaskowski	University of California, San Francisco
2001	Victoria Champion	Indiana University
2002	Lillian M. Nail	Oregon Health and Sciences University
2003	Victoria Mock	Johns Hopkins University
2004	Pamela S. Hinds	St. Jude Children's Research Hospital
2005	Marilyn Frank-Stromborg	Northern Illinois University
2006	Lesley F. Degner	University of Manitoba
2007	Ida M. Moore	University of Arizona, Tucson
2008	Carol E. Ferrans	University of Illinois, Chicago

can be documented by reviewing the coauthors on these scientists' publications as reported in the PubMed database. This history of influence can be traced by following the trail of authorship. The students and mentees may first appear as coauthors with the researcher as the principal author. Then, related works are published that list the mentee as the principal author with the researcher as coauthor. Eventually, the student/mentee publishes works as the primary author with a new group of coauthors, reflecting the growth of the student/mentee's own program of research (e.g., Miller & Champion, 1993; Champion, 1994; Champion, Rawl, & Menon, 2002; Rawl, Menon, Champion, Foster, & Skinner, 2000).

Perhaps a less direct measure of the influence of the Distinguished Researchers is to examine where they have published their research findings and the number of times these publications have been cited by others in published

Table 2-3. Area of Focus for Distinguished Researcher Award Winners

Year	Award Winner	Area of Research Focus
1992	Jean E. Johnson	Coping with cancer
1993	Jeanne Quint Benoliel	Behavior and symptom management
1994	Ruth McCorkle	Assessment of symptom distress and management of symptoms
1995	Barbara A. Given	Impact of caregiving and supportive care on patients with cancer and their families
1996	Betty R. Ferrell	Quality of life, pain, cancer survivorship
1997	Marylin J. Dodd	Self-care in the management of cancer-related symptoms
1998	Frances Marcus Lewis	The impact of cancer diagnosis and treatment on the family
1999	Marcia M. Grant	Health-related quality of life, symptom management in various populations
2000	Christine Miaskowski	Pain and symptom relief
2001	Victoria Champion	Behavioral oncology across the disease trajectory
2002	Lillian M. Nail	The cancer symptom experience, coping, fatigue, etc.
2003	Victoria Mock	Outcomes in women with breast cancer, exercise, fatigue
2004	Pamela S. Hinds	Adolescent hopefulness
2005	Marilyn Frank-Stromborg	Health-promoting behavior, community care, minority populations
2006	Lesley F. Degner	Patient participation in treatment decision making
2007	Ida M. Moore	Childhood cancers and central nervous system toxicities of cancer treatment
2008	Carol E. Ferrans	Quality of life throughout the spectrum of cancer care, including early detection and treatment, long-term survivorship, end of life, and healthcare disparities

articles. This is a means of judging the extent to which the research has been disseminated to the oncology nursing community and to the healthcare community at large. The number of citations reflects the acknowledgment by authors that their work has been influenced by, or extends the work of, the Distinguished Researchers. In this way, one can see how the work of these scientists was the antecedent of current research by others and how their work led to other lines of inquiry. Furthermore, citations in subsequent published works can document how the findings published by the scientists are influencing clinical practice.

Table 2-4 lists the results of a search of the citation index for each scientist (Institute for Scientific Information [ISI] Web of Knowledge[SM] Cited Reference search provided by Mark Vrabel, MLS, AHIP, ONS Information Resources Supervisor). The search represents data compiled from the Web of Science® portion of the database (http://scientific.thomsonreuters.com/products/wos) and includes publications from 1992 to July 2008.

ISI Web of Knowledge is a valuable multidisciplinary resource for those who are interested in tracking the publication histories of nurse scientists or a specific area of research. This fee-based database provides detailed reports from more than 8,000 journals. More specifically, the Citation Index features trend information that can be displayed graphically and includes details such as the number of results found, total and average times cited, and h-index (the rating for scientific productivity and impact) (Thomson Reuters, n.d.). Because this is a fee-based service, nurse scientists and students should inquire with their local libraries or the libraries within educational or medical institutions about the availability of this resource.

As an alternative search method, Google Scholar (http://scholar.google .com) is a freely available resource that offers cited reference information. Articles authored by each scientist include an accompanying "Cited by" link that shows the total number then allows the display of all the individual citing sources.

When evaluating a scientist's impact on the science, considering the limitations of the citation index reports is important. Only journals and publications included in the Citation Index database are included. Authors with a longer and more prolific publishing history are likely to have more citations than those with a shorter history. However, this does not reflect the importance of the author's body of work. Different results of the number of publications or of actual publications listed in PubMed or similar databases may vary depending on which version of the author's name is used in the search. For example, a search of "Hinds PS" yielded 30 publications, but a search of "Hinds P" yielded 27. The lists may vary as to which publications are included and are not always additive. The most frequently cited article may be an indication of where this author has had the greatest effect on the developing science or on the work of other researchers. Another caveat when looking at citation index numbers is that the reports are limited to journals included in this database. Molassiotis et al. (2006) stated that "as a discipline, nursing is not well represented in the Institute for Scientific Information (ISI) which produces the annual journal citation reports and includes only one cancer nursing-specific journal among the 36 included for the ISI for 2004 (*Cancer Nursing*)" (p. 432). Nurse scientists publish in many journals that target specific specialties

Table 2-4. Web of Science® Citation Report: 1992–2008

Year	Researcher	Most Cited Reference (as of July 2008)	Total Times Cited
1992	Jean E. Johnson	Johnson, 1999	40
1993	Jeanne Quint Benoliel	McCorkle et al., 1998 (contributed as the fifth author)	25
1994	Ruth McCorkle	Zorilla et al., 2001 (contributed as the seventh author)	114
1995	Barbara A. Given	Given et al., 1993 (contributed as the third author)	124
1996	Betty R. Ferrell	Ferrell et al., 1995 (contributed as the second author)	215
1997	Marylin J. Dodd	Dodd et al., 2001 (contributed as the first author)	75
1998	Frances Marcus Lewis	Lewis et al., 1993 (contributed as the first author)	80
1999	Marcia M. Grant	Ferrell et al., 1992 (contributed as the second author)	81
2000	Christine Miaskowski	Max et al., 1995 (contributed as the third author)	267
2001	Victoria Champion	Champion, 1993	85
2002	Lillian M. Nail	Schwartz et al., 2001 (contributed as the fourth author)	69
2003	Victoria Mock	Mock et al., 2001 (contributed as the first author)	111
2004	Pamela S. Hinds	Mock et al., 2000 (contributed as the tenth author)	59
2005	Marilyn Frank-Stromborg	Weinrich et al., 1993 (contributed as the third author)	22
2006	Lesley F. Degner	Degner et al., 1997 (contributed as the first author)	372
2007	Ida M. Moore	Bradlyn et al., 1996 (contributed as the fourth author)	59
2008	Carol E. Ferrans	Ferrans & Powers, 1992	196

and/or scientific interests that may have a narrow focus, which does not lead to a high impact factor.

The Distinguished Researchers have published in four of the 50 journals, in all fields, rated as having an impact factor of 49.794 to 14.325 (higher number = higher impact). They have published in 11 of the 32 "nursing" subject category journals rated by ISI. The impact factors of these journals range from 1.836 to 0.067. *Oncology Nursing Forum* has an impact factor of 1.438 and ranks fifth out of 46 journals in the "Nursing" category (M. Vrabel, personal communication, July 22, 2008).

The Distinguished Researchers have had a less obvious effect on oncology nursing science by their participation in peer review committees of the National Institutes of Heath, Agency for Healthcare Research and Quality, ONS Foundation, American Cancer Society, Susan G. Komen for the Cure, and other granting entities.

These scientists also have served on special advisory committees, work groups, task forces, state-of-the-science conferences, and consensus conferences to recommend or develop research agendas and/or set priorities for research funding by these and other organizations. Some have had leadership roles in National Institute of Nursing Research–funded Centers of Excellence in Research at universities. Others have developed training programs for future scientists or implemented nursing research programs in National Cancer Institute–designated cancer centers, academic medical centers, or community-based programs. The Distinguished Researchers have been consultants to less-experienced scientists in the process of developing projects, writing grants, and implementing studies. They also have collaborated among themselves to implement multisite research projects. These activities have brought new scientists into the field and have fostered the development of new areas of inquiry to strengthen the evidence base for oncology nursing practice. All of these approaches have included the training of successive generations of oncology nurse scientists and the development of collegial working relationships with researchers in other disciplines. These activities have strengthened the status of oncology nursing science in all settings and earned the respect of the broader research and academic communities.

The Distinguished Researchers have had an influence on the development of oncology nursing science through their retrospective and prospective presentations at the time of the awards, which were then published in the *Oncology Nursing Forum*. A report of a systematic review of worldwide cancer nursing research analyzed 619 papers published between 1994 and 2003 (Molassiotis et al., 2006). Forty-one percent were published in journals with a reported impact factor. The authors most often were affiliated with academic institutions. The majority of first authors were from the United States. Most of the studies were quantitative single-site studies and used descriptive methodology. The most frequently reported topics were symptoms, nursing issues/role, psychosocial issues, cancer services, and experiences of patients, caregivers, and nurses. Determining if this report is truly representative of the influence of the Distinguished Researchers is not possible because nursing and nursing research are not well represented in the ISI database, which was the source of information for the report; however, it is consistent with the profile of the Distinguished Research Award winners as a group.

Table 2-5 is a compilation of the recommendations for the future extracted from the publications of the Distinguished Researchers' remarks to the ONS Congress at the time of the award. The evolution of both the topics identified and the structure of these addresses over time is interesting to note. The development of each award recipient's research program over time can be

Table 2-5. Research Areas Recommended at the Time of the Distinguished Researcher Award

Year	Award Winner	Recommendations	Reference
1992	Jean E. Johnson	Testing and verification of patients' representation of a healthcare event focusing on the Self-Regulation Theory and encompassing the trajectory of coping throughout stages of disease. Research also should include the economic impact of nurses who base their efforts on the Self-Regulation Theory, as well as the physiologic impact of interventions that enhance coping and reduce stress.	Johnson, J., personal communication, July 24, 2008
1993	Jeanne Quint Benoliel	Not applicable. Benoliel's remarks at the time of the award focused on the events, people, and ideas that guided her along her career rather than an outlook for the future.	Benoliel, J.Q., personal communication, July 31, 2008
1994	Ruth McCorkle	Focus on improvement of clinical practice through research	McCorkle, R., et al., 1994; McCorkle, 1995
1995	Barbara A. Given	Examination of the mechanisms of family and patient burden and all categories of cost of illness; utilization of services; research-based guidelines	Given, B.A., 1995
1996	Betty R. Ferrell	Quality of life and cancer, methodology development, concept clarity	Ferrell, B.R., 1996
1997	Marylin J. Dodd	Self-care, self-management, intervention development and evaluation	Dodd, 1997
1998	Frances Marcus Lewis	Family-focused program development (intervention testing) of psychoeducational interventions	Lewis, 1998

(Continued on next page)

Table 2-5. Research Areas Recommended at the Time of the Distinguished Researcher Award *(Continued)*

Year	Award Winner	Recommendations	Reference
1999	Marcia M. Grant	Quality of life and symptoms, cross-cultural assessments of quality of life; quality of life during palliative care and end of life	Grant, 1999
2000	Christine Miaskowski	Evaluation of side effects of opioid analgesics; mechanisms of gender differences in responses to analgesics; epidemiologic studies of pain, fatigue, and sleep disturbances	Miaskowski, 2000
2001	Victoria Champion	Development of an infrastructure for behavioral oncology research; incorporation of new technologies into oncology nursing research; focus on special populations, prevention/early detection, and multidisciplinary behavioral research	Champion, 2001
2002	Lillian M. Nail	Collaborative research; new methods to address increasingly complex issues (e.g., symptom clusters, synthesis of current knowledge to apply to clinical practice)	Nail, 2002
2003	Victoria Mock	Development of the science of fatigue; more diverse populations; survivorship and palliative care; more rigorous research designs; theory-based research; identification of mediating variables; development of evidence-based guidelines for practice	Mock, 2003
2004	Pamela S. Hinds	Testing of strategies to influence hopefulness in individuals; translation of research findings into clinical tools and evaluation of usefulness in clinical practice	Hinds, 2004
2005	Marilyn Frank-Stromborg	Multidisciplinary approach; multiethnic perspective; influences on outcomes of care; prevention and early detection; influences of the law on care access and quality	Frank-Stromborg, 2005
2006	Lesley F. Degner	Influences on decision making, including culture	Kent, 2006
2007	Ida M. Moore	Childhood cancers and central nervous system toxicities of cancer treatment	Kent, 2007a
2008	Carol E. Ferrans	Addressing quality of life throughout the cancer spectrum and healthcare disparities	Kent, 2007b

followed by reviewing the topics of the author's current publications in a database such as PubMed. The authorships of the current publications also are an indication of the collaborations established and the scope of the current research projects of the award recipients.

Conclusion

This chapter is an attempt to document, from objective sources, the influence of the recipients of the ONS Distinguished Researcher Award since its inception in 1992. This objective approach tells only a part of the story. The rest of the story lies with the individuals, students, mentees, colleagues, and patients who have been influenced directly or indirectly by these professionals over the years. Interviews with all of these people would be necessary to begin to have an appreciation for how the Distinguished Researchers and their bodies of work have influenced the research programs and clinical practice of current oncology nurse scientists and clinicians.

The lasting influence of this group of nurse scientists will come from future generations of scientists and clinicians, who will carry on programs of research and continue to develop the science of oncology nursing. This includes the systematic testing and evaluation of research findings in clinical practice and the promotion and use of evidence-based models of care.

References

Bradlyn, A.S., Ritchey, A.K., Harris, C.V., Moore, I.M., O'Brien, R.T., Parsons, S.K., et al. (1996). Quality of life research in pediatric oncology: Research methods and barriers. *Cancer, 78*(6), 1333–1339.

Champion, V.L. (1993). Instrument refinement for breast cancer screening behaviors. *Nursing Research, 42*(3), 139–143.

Champion, V.L. (1994). Beliefs about breast cancer and mammography by behavioral stage. *Oncology Nursing Forum, 21*(6), 1009–1014.

Champion, V.L. (2001). Behavioral oncology research: A new millennium. *Oncology Nursing Forum, 28*(6), 975–982.

Champion, V.L., Rawl, S.M., & Menon, U. (2002). Population-based cancer screening. *Oncology Nursing Forum, 29*(5), 853–861.

Degner, L.F., Kristjanson, L.J., Bowman, D., Sloan, J.A., Carriere, K.C., O'Neil, J., et al. (1997). Information needs and decisional preferences in women with breast cancer. *JAMA, 277*(18), 1485–1492.

Dodd, M., Janson, S., Facione, N., Faucett, J., Froelicher, E.S., Humphreys, J., et al. (2001). Advancing the science of symptom management. *Journal of Advanced Nursing, 33*(5), 668–676.

Dodd, M.J. (1997). Self-care: Ready or not! *Oncology Nursing Forum, 24*(6), 983–990.

Ferrans, C.E., & Powers, M.J. (1992). Psychometric assessment of the quality-of-life index. *Research in Nursing and Health, 15*(1), 29–38.

Ferrell, B., Grant, M., Schmidt, G.M., Rhiner, M., Whitehead, C., Fonbuena, P., et al. (1992). The meaning of quality-of-life for bone-marrow transplant survivors: The impact of bone marrow transplant on quality-of-life. *Cancer Nursing, 15*(3), 153–160.

Ferrell, B.A., Ferrell, B.R., & Rivera, L. (1995). Pain in cognitively impaired nursing home patients. *Journal of Pain and Symptom Management, 10*(8), 591–598.

Ferrell, B.R. (1996). The quality of lives: 1,525 voices of cancer. *Oncology Nursing Forum, 23*(6), 909–916.

Frank-Stromborg, M. (2005). A research-driven life: Seeking and developing a nurse scientist role in the rural setting. *Oncology Nursing Forum, 32*(5), 945–958.

Given, B.A. (1995). Believing and dreaming to improve cancer care. *Oncology Nursing Forum, 22*(6), 929–940.

Given, C.W., Stommel, M., Given, B., Osuch, J., Kurtz, M.E., & Kurtz, J.C. (1993). The influence of cancer patients' symptoms and functional states on patient depression and family caregiver reaction and depression. *Health Psychology, 12*(4), 277–285.

Grant, M. (1999). Surviving and thriving: The nurse scientist in the clinical setting. *Oncology Nursing Forum, 26*(6), 1013–1022.

Hinds, P.S. (2004). The hopes and wishes of adolescents with cancer and the nursing care that helps. *Oncology Nursing Forum, 31*(5), 927–934.

Johnson, J.E. (1999). Self-Regulation Theory and coping with physical illness. *Research in Nursing and Health, 22*(6), 435–448.

Kent, J. (2006, February 14). *Lesley F. Degner, RN, PhD, receives 2006 Oncology Nursing Society Distinguished Researcher Award* [News release]. Retrieved April 28, 2008, from http://www.ons.org/media/pdf/awards/2006/021406.pdf

Kent, J. (2007a, March 14). *Ida M. Moore, BSN, MA, DNS, receives 2007 Oncology Nursing Society Distinguished Researcher Award* [News release]. Retrieved July 24, 2008, from http://www.ons.org/media/pdf/awards/2007/Dist%20Researcher%20short%20-%20Moore.pdf

Kent, J. (2007b, December 18). *Carol Estwing Ferrans, PhD, RN, FAAN, receives 2008 Oncology Nursing Society Distinguished Researcher Award* [News release]. Retrieved July 24, 2008, from http://www.ons.org/media/pdf/awards/2007/DistResearcherLH-Ferrans.pdf

Lewis, F.M., Hammond, M.A., & Woods, N.F. (2003). The family's functioning with newly diagnosed breast cancer in the mother: The development of an explanatory model. *Journal of Behavioral Medicine, 16*(4), 351–370.

Lewis, F.M. (1998). Family-level services in oncology nursing: Facts, fallacies, and realities revisited. *Oncology Nursing Forum, 25*(8), 1378–1388.

Max, M.B., Donovan, M., Miaskowski, C.A., Ward, S.E., Gordon, D., Bookbinder, M., et al. (1995). Quality improvement guidelines for the treatment of acute pain and cancer pain. *JAMA, 274*(23), 1874–1880.

McCorkle, R. (1995). Oncology nursing—A challenge not to be taken lightly. *Oncology Nursing Forum, 22*(3), 471–477.

McCorkle, R., Jepson, C., Malone, D., Lusk, E., Braitman, L., Buhler-Wilkerson, K., et al. (1994). The impact of posthospital home care on patients with cancer. *Research in Nursing and Health, 17*(4), 243–251.

McCorkle, R., Robinson, L., Nuamah, I., Lev, E., & Benoliel, J.Q. (1998). The effects of home nursing for patients during terminal illness on the bereaved's psychological distress. *Nursing Research, 47*(1), 2–10.

Miaskowski, C. (1996). Special needs related to the pain and discomfort of patients with gynecologic cancer. *Journal of Obstetric, Gynecologic, and Neonatal Nursing, 25*(2), 181–188.

Miaskowski, C. (2000). Improving pain management: An ongoing journey. *Oncology Nursing Forum, 27*(6), 938–944.

Mock, V. (2003). Clinical excellence through evidence-based practice: Fatigue management as a model. *Oncology Nursing Forum, 30*(5), 787–796.

Miller, A.M., & Champion, V.L. (1993). Mammography in women > or = 50 years of age: Predisposing and enabling characteristics. *Cancer Nursing, 16*(4), 260–269.

Mock, V., Atkinson, A., Barsevick, A., Cella, D., Cimprich, B., Cleeland, C., et al. (2000). NCCN Practice Guidelines for cancer-related fatigue. *Oncology–New York, 14*(11A, Suppl. 10), 151–161.

Mock, V., Pickett, M., Ropka, M.E., Lin, E.M., Stewart, K.J., Rhodes, V.A., et al. (2001). Fatigue and quality of life outcomes of exercise during cancer treatment. *Cancer Practice, 9*(3), 119–127.

Molassiotis, A., Gibson, F., Kelly, D., Richardson, A., Dabbour, R., Ahmad, A.M., et al. (2006). A systematic review of worldwide cancer nursing research: 1994 to 2003. *Cancer Nursing, 29*(6), 431–440.

Nail, L.M. (2002). Illuminating problems, defining processes, and improving outcomes: The essence of oncology nursing research. *Oncology Nursing Forum, 29*(6), 941–947.

Oncology Nursing Society. (n.d.). *ONS distinguished awards: Distinguished Researcher Award (RE03).* Retrieved January 30, 2007, from http://www.ons.org/awards/onsawards/distinguishedResearcher.shtml

Rawl, S.M., Menon, U., Champion, V.L., Foster, J.L., & Skinner, C.S. (2000). Colorectal cancer screening beliefs: Focus groups with first-degree relatives. *Cancer Practice, 8*(1), 32–37.

Schwartz, A.L., Mori, M., Gao, R.L., Nail, L.M., & King, M.E. (2001). Exercise reduces daily fatigue in women with breast cancer receiving chemotherapy. *Medicine and Science in Sports and Exercise, 33*(5), 718–723.

Thomson Reuters. (n.d.). *Web of Science®.* Retrieved July 23, 2008, from http://scientific.thomsonreuters.com/products/wos

Weinrich, S.P., Weinrich, M.C., Stromborg, M.F., Boyd, M.D., & Weiss, H.L. (1993). Using elderly educators to increase colorectal cancer screening. *Gerontologist, 33*(4), 491–496.

Zorilla, E.P., Luborsky, L., McKay, J.R., Rosenthal, R., Houldin, A., Tax, A., et al. (2001). The relationship of depression and stressors to immunological assays: A meta-analytic review. *Brain Behavior and Immunity, 15*(3), 199–226.

SECTION II

ADVANCING ONCOLOGY NURSING SCIENCE

CHAPTER 3

Cancer Prevention and Early Detection Nursing Science: 1990–Present

Suzanne M. Mahon, RN, DNSc, AOCN®, APNG

Introduction

Nursing research is an ever-growing science, which encompasses research conducted by nurses as well as research that promotes and advances nursing science. It is typically, although not exclusively, published in nursing journals. Some nurses also engage in interdisciplinary research, and others engage in what is traditionally considered "bench" research or laboratory research. All of these types of research have important implications for advancing the nursing science of cancer prevention and early detection.

The Oncology Nursing Society (ONS) revises its research agenda on a regular basis. The most recent published agenda is for 2005–2009 (Berry, 2007). Research in health promotion, especially in the areas of primary and secondary prevention, was deemed a priority area. In particular, the ONS Research Agenda recommended much more research regarding tobacco usage and smoking cessation, along with the implementation of cost-effective interventions to increase evidence-based screening for cervical, breast, colorectal, and prostate cancer, based on the findings of the risk assessment. Another item on the agenda involved increasing research to better understand the effects of cancer therapy on long-term survivors. The agenda also stressed the need for more research on the effect of inherited cancer risk on families. The ONS 2005–2009 Research Agenda clearly provides a starting place for considering what research has been completed and what areas need to be fulfilled in the realm of cancer prevention and early detection (Berry).

This chapter focuses on nursing science related to cancer prevention and early detection and also considers the early nursing research in cancer genetics, which is a rapidly emerging subspecialty. The goal of cancer genetics research is to prevent and detect cancer as early as possible in those with a hereditary predisposition. Search strategies for defining this research are described, as well as what currently is known in the realm of cancer prevention and early detection nursing research. Suggestions for future studies in cancer prevention and early detection also are described.

Search Strategy and General Considerations

Search Strategy

The research reviewed in this chapter was conducted by nurses and published in journals with an emphasis on oncology and, in most cases, oncology nursing. This chapter describes the breadth of nursing research related to cancer prevention and early detection, including cancer genetics in literature written in English from 1990 to 2007. Most of this research is from the United States, although literature written in English from other countries is included. Nursing studies in cancer prevention and early detection probably were published in other languages, but they were not reviewed for this chapter.

The review began by using two search engines to access literature most likely written by nurses. First, a search was conducted in CINAHL® (www .cinahl.com), followed by the same search in MEDLINE® (www.nlm.nih.gov/ medlineplus). Search terms included *cancer prevention, cancer detection, cancer screening, cancer genetics,* and *hereditary cancer.* Each was combined with the term *nursing research,* for the years 1990–2007.

More than 2,300 review-type papers written by nurses about cancer prevention and early detection were located. Some of the papers may have suggestions for nursing research but were not reviewed for this chapter. Papers with a specific research focus were much less common. A total of 160 nursing research papers were located with a research focus on the topics of cancer prevention and early detection (see Table 3-1).

Types of Publications

Table 3-2 provides a description of the journals in which nurses published research on cancer prevention and early detection. Clearly, *Cancer Nursing* and *Oncology Nursing Forum* are the journals where nurses were most often published, thus disseminating their research. When nurses select practice-specific nursing journals to submit research, there are both strengths and weaknesses. Nurses may be more likely to read nursing journals. Because

Table 3-1. Number of Publications by Nurse Scientists by Year	
Year	Number of Publications
1990	6
1991	8
1992	8
1993	7
1994	9
1995	8
1996	10
1997	6
1998	8
1999	6
2000	17
2001	13
2002	4
2003	5
2004	17
2005	16
2006	12

N = 160

Note. Information compiled from CINHAL® and MEDLINE® databases.

oncology nurses who are members of ONS automatically receive a subscription to *Oncology Nursing Forum,* they may be more motivated to read it, as it is readily available, and they do not have to actively search for an article. Unfortunately, many non-nurse healthcare providers may not consider a paper published in a nursing journal or take the time to locate such a publication. Of greater concern is that other allied health professionals and physicians may not be aware of significant nursing research simply because it is published in journals accessed primarily by nurses.

Methodologic Considerations for Cancer Prevention and Early Detection Research

Table 3-3 shows a general review of the types of methodology used in the research. Most of the research was survey or descriptive in nature. Reports of the psychometric characteristics of the instruments were variable in the studies. Many of these studies used investigator-developed surveys for which psychometric information was either not available or was described with minimal detail. Most of the randomized controlled trials centered on comparing two or more methods to increase participation in screening, and most of the qualitative studies focused on beliefs regarding cancer screening in various ethnic groups and cultures. The fact that three meta-analyses of literature could be located is encouraging, suggesting that nurses are beginning to develop a body of research on cancer prevention and early detection that is large enough to warrant a meta-analysis.

Sample sizes were variable in the studies. Although a few very large survey studies (greater than 200 participants) were conducted, the sample size generally was less than 100 participants. This might greatly limit the generalizability of the findings from some of the studies. Also, many of the samples were drawn from very discrete populations in a limited geographic area. The majority (74%) were convenience samples.

Table 3-2. Number of Cancer Prevention and Early Detection Articles by Journal 1990–2007

Publication	Number of Publications
Cancer Nursing	43
Oncology Nursing Forum	28
Journal of Advanced Nursing	17
Journal of Cancer Education	13
Cancer Practice	10
Gastrointestinal Nursing	10
Journal of National Black Nurses Association	5
Journal of Nursing Scholarship	4
Preventive Medicine	4
Public Health Nursing	4
Nursing Research	3
Advances in Nursing Science	1
Australian Journal of Advanced Nursing	1
Canadian Journal of Nursing Research	1
Clinical Excellence for Nurse Practitioners	1
Clinical Nurse Specialist	1
Dermatology Nursing	1
Health Education Research	1
ICUs and Nursing Web Journal	1
International Journal of Nursing Studies	1
International Journal of Palliative Nursing	1
Journal of Continuing Education in Nursing	1
Journal of Multicultural Nursing	1
Journal of Nursing Education	1
Journal of Professional Nursing	1
Journal of Transcultural Nursing	1
Nurse Practitioner	1
Qualitative Health Research	1
Research and Theory for Nursing Practice	1
Research in Nursing and Health	1

N = 160

Note. Information compiled from CINHAL® and MEDLINE® databases.

Table 3-3. Types of Nursing Research Studies 1990–2007	
Type of Study	Number of Studies
Survey/completion of an instrument	78
Qualitative approaches	40
Cross-sectional approaches	15
Focus groups	9
Randomized controlled studies	7
Semi-structured interviews	6
Meta-analysis of existing studies	3
Cost-benefit analysis	2
N = 160	
Note. Information compiled from CINHAL® and MEDLINE® databases.	

Research With Special Populations

Many of the papers focused on the screening behaviors, informational needs, and beliefs of various ethnic groups regarding cancer screening (see Table 3-4). The largest subgroups studied were African Americans and Asian groups. The American Cancer Society (ACS, 2008) noted that African Americans are more likely to develop and die from cancer than any other ethnic group. The death rate for African American males is 37% higher than for Caucasian males, at 321.8 deaths per 100,000; the death rate for African American females is 17% higher, at 189.3 per 100,000. This is attributed to disparities in access to prevention and early detection services, inadequate insurance or other financial constraints, and cultural insensitivity. The emphasis today on better understanding the special needs of this population is appropriate.

For Asian Americans, ACS (2008) reported that the overall incidence rates of 359.9 males per 100,000 and 285.8 females per 100,000 are lower than for those of Caucasians (556.7 for males and 423.9 for females), but Asian Americans are more likely to die from cancers related to infections, specifically in cervical cancer and stomach cancer. Thus, targeting this population is appropriate as well.

Areas of Nursing Research Centering on Cancer Prevention and Early Detection

Sixty-two studies dealt with beliefs and knowledge regarding various aspects of cancer prevention. Many of these studies addressed beliefs in defined ethnic

Table 3-4. Research Addressing the Needs of Specific Populations 1990–2007	
Population	Number of Studies
African American	38
Asian	27
Hispanic/Latino	10
Middle Eastern	8
Canadian	4
Australian	1
N = 88	
Note. Information compiled from CINHAL® and MEDLINE® databases.	

or cultural groups. Another group of studies focused on whether individuals intend to be screened or strategies to increase or promote screening or to remove barriers to screening (37 studies). Studies regarding the effectiveness of various approaches to increase awareness of cancer screening benefits constituted another area of research (19 studies).

Promoting screening in those with hereditary risk is an emerging area of nursing research; 11 studies were found addressing this topic. Most addressed issues in hereditary breast and ovarian cancers or hereditary nonpolyposis colorectal cancer. Strategies to increase healthcare professionals' awareness and develop interventions related to cancer prevention and early detection were addressed in 12 studies. Seven studies were found that addressed satisfaction with screening, cost-effectiveness, and tertiary screening. The most common tumor types screened for were breast and/or cervical cancer (see Table 3-5).

Beliefs and Knowledge Regarding Cancer Prevention

Understanding the targeted population's beliefs about cancer and the possibilities for prevention and early detection is a requirement to promoting cancer screening. When such beliefs are understood, theoretically, it is possible to develop appropriate and culturally sensitive tools and strategies to facilitate participation in cancer prevention and early detection activities.

Knowledge deficits about risks and screening recommendations for cancer are a major barrier to screening participation. Powe and Finnie (2004) emphasized this point when studying African Americans at risk for oral cancer. Watts, Merrell, Murphy, and Williams (2004) conducted a meta-analysis of research

Table 3-5. Type of Screening by Site Addressed in Research 1990–2007*

Target Site for Screening	Number of Studies
Breast	61
Cervical	51
Prostate	29
Colorectal	20
Ovarian	6
Skin	4
Lung	3
Oral	2

N = 160
* Some studies addressed more than one site.

Note. Information compiled from CINHAL® and MEDLINE® databases.

literature published between 1996 and 2002. They concluded that healthcare professionals lack an understanding about various minority groups' cultural beliefs, values, and knowledge about cancer screening. This was especially true with regard to myths surrounding screening for breast cancer.

Weinrich et al. (2004) and Weinrich, Weinrich, Boyd, and Atkinson (1998) produced several studies that addressed beliefs and knowledge about prostate cancer. They reported that men, especially African American men, have limited knowledge about prostate cancer symptoms, risk factors, and screening guidelines.

Nursing students may have misconceptions and inadequate information about breast cancer detection (Powe, Underwood, Canales, & Finnie, 2005). Students reported receiving little information about breast cancer screening in their basic curriculum and believed it negatively affected their ability to provide quality care. This is probably true of other cancer types as well.

Few studies have addressed the needs of Native American women in the United States or Canada. Fitch, Greenberg, Cava, Spaner, and Taylor (1998) reported that little is known about the beliefs of Native American women regarding screening behaviors and beliefs, and substantially more research is needed.

Beliefs about mammography, clinical breast examination, and breast self-examination (BSE) are influenced by prior breast biopsies and family history (Lauver, Kane, Bodden, McNeel, & Smith, 1999). Similarly, women may choose not to engage in regular cervical cancer screening because they have had uncomfortable or unpleasant experiences with Pap smear screening in the past (Fitch et al., 1997; Steven et al., 2004).

A large number of studies addressed attitudes and beliefs about breast cancer among African American women (Adams, Becker, & Colbert, 2001; Barroso et al., 2000; Facione, 1999; Facione & Giancarlo, 1998; Foxall, Barron, & Houfek, 2001; Phillips, Cohen, & Moses, 1999; Phillips, Cohen, & Tarzian, 2001; Simonian et al., 2004; Thomas, 2004; Thomas, Saleem, & Abraham, 2005). These studies suggest that African American women are reluctant to participate in breast cancer screening, particularly mammography, because of fears of finding cancer, perceived prejudicial treatment, and financial concerns.

A few studies have addressed beliefs about prostate screening in African American men (Agho & Lewis, 2001; Boyd, Weinrich, Weinrich, & Norton, 2001; Clarke-Tasker & Dutta, 2005; Shelton, Weinrich, & Reynolds, 1999). African American men identified lack of knowledge about screening guidelines, fatalism, and fears of cancer as barriers to participation in cancer screening programs.

Nurse scientists have addressed disparities in cancer prevention and early detection in Hispanics/Latinos. Many Hispanic women are reluctant to undergo breast or cervical cancer screening because they believe screening is unnecessary in the absence of obvious symptoms (Borrayo & Jenkins, 2001; Salazar, 1996; Smiley, McMillan, Johnson, & Ojeda, 2000). Hispanic women may be less likely to follow up on abnormal Pap smear results because they underestimate the seriousness of the condition (Hunt, de Voogd, Akana, & Browner, 1998). Availability of Saturday and evening hours, low-cost screenings, and increased convenience were motivating factors for Hispanic men to participate in prostate cancer screening (Zimmerman, 1997).

Asian Americans' attitudes and participation in cancer screening have been studied extensively, often by doctoral students as part of educational requirements. A strength of many of these studies was the effort to translate interviews and instruments into native dialects and languages. Many Asian American women fail to perceive the seriousness of breast cancer (Hoeman, Ku, & Ohl, 1996; Im, Park, Lee, & Yun, 2004; Kim et al., 1999; Schulmeister & Lifsey, 1999; Twinn & Cheng, 2000). Predictors of breast and cervical cancer screening in Asian American women include being married and having higher levels of education (Han, Williams, & Harrison, 2000; Ho et al., 2005; Sarna, Tae, Kim, Brecht, & Maxwell, 2001; Xu, Ross, Ryan, & Wang, 2005a, 2005b; Yi, 1998; Yu, Kim, Chen, & Brintnall, 2001). A meta-analysis of screening practices in this population reported that the biggest barrier to participating in screening was poor awareness about cancer (Lee-Lin & Menon, 2005). Lack of financial resources and embarrassment were identified as other barriers to participating in screening (Holroyd, Twinn, & Adab, 2004). Problems with language and communication were other identified barriers to Asian and Middle Eastern women's participation in cancer screening (Lee, 2000; Sadler et al., 2001).

Predictors of Participation or Intention to Participate in Cancer Detection Activities

A number of studies have examined whether individuals or populations intend to participate in a recommended prevention or early detection activity. These studies often strive to identify barriers to screening that might be amenable to intervention.

Scientists noted that providing individualized, tailored information about cancer screening increases participation in screening and intention to participate in the short term; however, the long-term benefits are not as clear (de Nooijer, Lechner, Candel, & de Vries, 2004).

Smoking cessation is one of the principal means to reduce mortality, particularly from lung and oral cancers. Although not all authored by nurse scientists, many studies have examined motivation and strategies to quit smoking. Smokers who participate in lung cancer screening may be motivated to participate in a broad range of tobacco cessation programs (Hahn, Rayens, Hopenhayn, & Christian, 2006). As of May 21, 2008, the Cochrane Database of Systematic Reviews and Register of Controlled Trials listed 114 specific reviews under the search term *smoking cessation*. Many of these studies are authored by public health and allied health professionals, including nurses, and provide an excellent starting place when developing smoking cessation programs and examining motivational factors to smoking cessation. The results of a review of studies indicated the potential benefits of smoking cessation advice and/or counseling given by nurses to patients, with reasonable evidence that interventions can be effective (Rice & Stead, 2008). The next phase of research needs to focus on the clinical challenge of incorporating smoking behavior monitoring and smoking cessation interventions as part of standard practice, so that all patients are given an opportunity to provide information about their tobacco use and receive advice and/or counseling to quit along with reinforcement and follow-up (Rice & Stead).

The majority of studies about the intention to participate in cancer screening have centered specifically on breast and/or cervical cancer screening. Nurses should not assume that patients will promptly report symptoms, especially younger women, older women, and women from lower socioeconomic groups (Baldwin, 1996; Bibb, 2001; Facione, Dodd, Holzemer, & Meleis, 1997; Yarbrough & Braden, 2001). Research repeatedly suggests that having a healthcare provider recommend screening might be one of the biggest motivating factors to participating in screening (Champion & Menon, 1997; Lockwood-Rayermann, 2004; Stamler, Thomas, & Lafreniere, 2000). Social isolation also may be associated with a decreased intention to screen (Carruth, Browning, Reed, Skarke, & Sealey, 2006).

Similar findings emerged regarding intention to participate in prostate cancer screening. Recommendations from a healthcare provider may be one of the biggest motivators to participating in prostate cancer screening (Nivens, Herman, Weinrich, & Weinrich, 2001; Oliffe, 2006). The availability of low-cost prostate cancer screening during nontraditional hours, such as evening or Saturday hours, was associated with increased participation and intention to screen (Weinrich, Reynolds, Tingen, & Starr, 2000).

A number of barriers to participating in colorectal cancer screening have been identified, including fear of pain with preparation and examination, embarrassment, fatalism, lack of physician recommendation, and lack of understanding about how to schedule a screening examination (Goel et al., 2004; Green & Kelly, 2004; Sarna & Chang, 2000; Tang, Solomon, & McCracken, 2001). Confusion for both healthcare providers and consumers regarding screening recommendations may be another barrier.

Strategies to Increase Awareness Regarding Cancer Prevention and Early Detection

Nurse scientists attempted to determine and develop strategies to increase both awareness about cancer prevention and early detection and participation in these behaviors. Most of these studies involved specifically defined special populations, which may limit the overall generalizability of the findings, but have contributed to a richer, broader knowledge base and ultimately more culturally sensitive nursing care.

Awareness of risk may or may not increase participation in screening or prevention strategies (Ceber, Soyer, Ciceklioglu, & Cimat, 2006). Efforts to increase awareness have been instituted in church and employment settings with varying degrees of success. Some preliminary suggestions for replication have been offered (Grindel, Brown, Caplan, & Blumenthal, 2004; Hall et al., 2005; Phillips & Belcher, 1999).

Successful strategies to increase awareness include offering not only educational messages but also free screening (Arevian, Noureddine, & Kabakian-Khasholian, 2006; Tingen, Weinrich, Heydt, Boyd, & Weinrich, 1998). Free screening has increased participation in some settings, although it may not provide a reasonable model that is useful for implementation in the general population. Screening for cancer is associated with some financial costs and personnel, so institutions or insurance providers must pay for screening.

Another strategy to increase awareness involves the use of trained volunteers of the same ethnicity as the targeted population to ensure culturally sensitive messages, which is reported to be an effective strategy in some settings (Hansen et al., 2005; Nichols, Misra, & Alexy, 1996; Powe, Ntekop, & Barron, 2004).

Telephone counseling may be an effective means to increase awareness and participation in cancer prevention and early detection behaviors. Champion, Skinner, and Foster (2000) reported that telephone counseling was more than twice as effective at increasing mammography adherence, and in-person counseling was almost three times more effective compared to a control group who received a standard recommendation from the healthcare provider. Individual counseling demonstrated high effectiveness in increasing awareness and participation in screening (Ueland, Hornung, & Greenwald, 2006). This finding reinforces the importance of having a healthcare provider recommend cancer screening or prevention strategies to a patient.

Satisfaction With Cancer Prevention and Early Detection Measures

A number of studies have addressed factors that influence satisfaction or dissatisfaction with screening and its effect on future screening behaviors, particularly in the case of breast and cervical cancer screening. Factors reported to increase satisfaction with screening include respect for privacy, an environment that encourages questions, and caring providers; negative factors include discomfort, fears related to radiation exposure, and financial disparities (Bakker, Lightfoot, Steggles, & Jackson, 1998; Chlan, Evans, Greenleaf, & Walker, 2000; Douglass, Barrison, Powell, & Bramble, 2004; Lalos, Hovanec-Lalos, & Weber, 1997; Sabay, Gray, & Fitch, 2000; Sutherland, Straton, & Hyndman, 1996).

Distress following abnormal screens should not be underestimated. Those with a positive (abnormal) screen may experience significant distress and discomfort; sensitive care during the diagnostic phase may positively influence future decisions regarding screening (Farmer, 2000; Kelly & Winslow, 1996; McGovern et al., 2004; Seckel & Birney, 1996).

Tertiary Screening and Screening for Second Malignancies

Only a few studies have addressed screening for second malignancies. With an ever-growing pool of long-term survivors, efforts need to be expended to provide screening and education to this often-overlooked population. Tertiary screening should include breast and gynecologic screening and, to a lesser extent, colon and skin screening or prevention of complications such as osteoporosis (Mahon & Williams, 2000; Mahon, Williams, & Spies, 2000).

Cancer Prevention and Early Detection in High-Risk Groups

Cancer genetics is a rapidly advancing area of research for nurses. With the commercial availability of testing for some hereditary cancer syndromes, including breast and ovarian cancer, hereditary nonpolyposis colorectal cancer, and hereditary melanoma, nursing interest is increasing about how to best provide care for patients and families who are at risk. Only a limited number of studies addressing genetics and cancer prevention and early detection published by nurse scientists were located. The search strategy may not have located many interdisciplinary studies on hereditary risk that might include nurse scientists. This research is more likely to be reported in a journal that focuses on genetics, including the *Journal of Genetic Counseling* and the *Journal of Human Genetics*, as well as primary care journals.

People with a family history of cancer may greatly over- or underestimate their risk for developing cancer (Hutson, 2003; MacDonald, Sarna, Uman, Grant, & Weitzel, 2005). Consultation with a knowledgeable healthcare provider was considered extremely desirable in several studies exploring issues with cancer genetics counseling (Chalmers, Thomson, & Degner, 1996; Kinney et al., 2001; Loescher, 2003). Those with a family history of cancer may find screening to be a particularly stressful experience and might benefit from supportive interventions (Tiffen, Sharp, & O'Toole, 2005). For some individuals with a hereditary risk for developing cancer, early detection measures may offer hope of control over risk (Chalmers & Luker, 1996; Phelan, Oliveria, & Halpern, 2005); for others, screening may be associated with distress (MacDonald, Sarna, Uman, Grant, & Weitzel, 2006).

Cost-Effectiveness of Cancer Screening

Only a few nurse scientists have addressed issues of the cost-effectiveness of screening. This may be an extremely important area to consider in future studies, especially because of ever-increasing healthcare costs. Studies are needed to better define the actual costs of cancer prevention and early detection strategies (Chang & Eddins, 1996) and how to target screening at groups most likely to benefit (Tsouskas, Noula, & Dimopoulos, 2005).

Professional Issues Associated With Cancer Prevention and Early Detection

Isolated nursing research studies have considered a variety of issues that affect the profession of nursing, the education of nurses, and the delivery of cancer prevention and early detection services and education. Most of these studies are small and need to be replicated, but they provide some introductory insight for developing education programs.

Studies have examined lack of genetic content in Japanese nursing texts (Tsujino, Tsukahara, Frazier, Iino, & Murakami, 2003), training courses in cancer genetics (Masny et al., 2003), education about skin cancer screening (Christos, Oliveria, Masse, McCormick, & Halpern, 2004), lack of screening efforts in rural areas (Lane & Martin, 2005), and effectiveness of partnerships between nursing schools and community agencies (Mundt, Hermann, Conner, & Von Ah, 2006). Other studies have examined patient satisfaction with advanced practice nurses who provide cancer genetics education and role development for nurses in cancer genetics (Bernhardt, Geller, Doksum, & Metz, 2000; Bottorff et al., 2005). The findings from these preliminary studies suggest that nurses can be effective providers of cancer education, as well as cancer prevention, early detection, and cancer genetics services.

Other studies have examined knowledge levels of various groups of nurses regarding cancer prevention and early detection (Beatty, 2000; Howell, Nelson-Marten, Krebs, Kaszyk, & Wold, 1998; Lundgren et al., 2000). Nurses who do not practice exclusively or regularly in the area of cancer prevention and early detection may have significant gaps in their understanding of cancer prevention and early detection strategies and thus may be less likely to discuss these strategies with patients and families at risk. Another study found that nurse practitioners were effective providers of breast care (Coleman, Coon, Fitzgerald, & Cantrell, 2001; Coleman et al., 2004; Mahon, 1997). Nurse endoscopists also can be effective providers of colorectal cancer screening (Wright, 2000).

Recently, attention has been given to developing and validating instruments to assess variables that are important in the study of cancer prevention and early detection. A sampling of these instruments is displayed in Table 3-6. Efforts also have been made to validate these instruments in a variety of ethnic populations (Champion & Scott, 1997; Gozum & Aydin, 2004; Secginli & Nahcivan, 2004). Little research by nurses has addressed ways to recruit individuals to cancer prevention and screening trials. Until this phenomenon is better understood, moving forward with large-scale cancer prevention and early detection trials may be difficult (McKinney, Weiner, & Wang, 2006).

Nurses are beginning to explore the impact of the genetics revolution on cancer prevention and early detection. Advances in molecular and genetic

Table 3-6. Selected Instruments for Research in Cancer Prevention and Early Detection

Instrument	Description	Source
Mammography Pro and Con Scales	Five- to seven-item Likert scales that measure positive and negative attitudes toward mammography	Rakowski et al., 1997
Mammography Stage of Adoption (Stages include precontemplation, contemplation, action, relapse precontemplation, and relapse contemplation.)	Evaluates whether a woman has ever heard of a mammogram, timing of last mammography, number of mammograms in past five years, and intent to undergo mammography in the future	Champion, 1999
Champion Health Belief Model Scale	Scales that examine breast self-examination and mammography beliefs	Champion, 1993
Knowledge of Cancer Warning Signs Inventory	A 25-item self-report questionnaire that yields subscores on the warning signs of cancer, nonwarning signs, and the extent to which one can differentiate between real and false warning signs	Berman & Wandersman, 1991

(Continued on next page)

Table 3-6. Selected Instruments for Research in Cancer Prevention and Early Detection *(Continued)*

Instrument	Description	Source
Perceived Susceptibility Risk: Colorectal Cancer	Scales that measure perceived susceptibility risk, perceived relative risk, and perceived absolute risk for developing colorectal cancer	Manne et al., 2003
Powe Fatalism Inventory	Scales measure four defining attributes of cancer fatalism: fear, predetermination, pessimism, and inevitability of death from cancer. The instrument has been used in relation to screening behaviors.	Powe, 1994, 1995, 1997; Powe & Weinrich, 1999
Colorectal Screening Stage of Adoption	Examines whether individuals have ever had colorectal screening tests, thought about having a test, are planning to have a test, or have an appointment to have a test	Rawl, S.M., et al., 2005

testing are redefining and clarifying individuals who are at very high risk for developing cancer. This will change risk assessment strategies. More research is needed to better understand the most effective ways to convey information about genetic risk, to facilitate adjustment to discussions about genetic testing, and ultimately to form decisions about prevention measures. The impact of genetic testing and hereditary risk is a research priority area for ONS (Berry, 2007). Recommendations for areas of future research include studies that characterize family member involvement in learning about hereditary risk, family communication patterns about hereditary risk, issues related to understanding cancer risk, and psychosocial ramifications of risk assessment and genetic testing. Once these factors are better understood, ONS recommends the development of interventions to facilitate and enhance family communication and evidence-based interventions to address distress and concern about prevention and lifestyle management (Berry).

Conclusion

Nurse scientists are beginning to take an active role in understanding patient motivation, knowledge, and concerns about cancer prevention and early detection. The slow but steady increase in both the number of publications and the research questions addressed is enlightening and encouraging.

The largest area of nursing research centers on differences in screening behaviors and beliefs in different ethnic minority populations. Most of the research has focused on breast and cervical cancer. The degree to which these findings can be extrapolated to other prevention and early detection issues is not clear, although similarities to other cancers are likely.

Nurses may want to consider more interdisciplinary research, especially with psychologists, public health experts, and behavioral scientists. This might lead to dissemination of findings in more diverse journals. The work of Dr. Victoria Champion at Indiana University is a wonderful example of the importance of interdisciplinary research.

Victoria Champion: A Cancer Prevention and Early Detection Nursing Researcher

Victoria L. Champion, DNS, RN, FAAN, received the 2001 ONS Distinguished Researcher Award for her long history of accomplishments in cancer prevention and early detection research. She is an excellent role model and mentor for oncology nurse scientists. Specifically, the evolution of her work in breast cancer early detection demonstrates the significant contributions nurse scientists can make to the science of cancer prevention and early detection. She has published more than 78 research studies that focus on cancer detection, especially breast cancer detection.

In 1984, Champion published an article on instrument development centering on Health Belief Model constructs (Champion, 1984). Much of the success of her research career can be attributed to her early work using a model to guide her research. The Health Belief Model, created by Rosenstock in 1966, provided a framework for Champion to organize research questions about breast cancer detection to understand why women do and do not engage in cancer screening services.

Champion is well known for her instrument development. The development of these instruments began with descriptive, exploratory studies based on the Health Belief Model. As early as 1985, Champion published findings about the use of the Health Belief Model as a predictor of the frequency of BSE practice (Champion, 1985). Subsequent studies about BSE practice built on previous studies (Champion, 1988, 1989, 1993). As the understanding of BSE increased, Champion started to look at the Health Belief Model and mammography utilization (Champion, 1993, 1994, 1995a; Miller & Champion, 1993).

Perhaps one of the most impressive aspects of Champion's work is that she took what she learned from her instrument development and developed intervention studies focusing on BSE proficiency and mammography utilization (Champion, 1995b; Champion, Foster, & Menon, 1997; Champion et al., 2000; Saywell et al., 2003). Champion successfully crossed the bridge from description of a clinical issue to interventional studies—a feat many scientists never achieve.

Champion took what she learned about participation in screening measures and the Health Belief Model and applied this knowledge to colorectal cancer screening (Rawl, S.M., et al., 2005; Rawl, S.R., et al., 2001). Additionally, Champion is studying the ways technology influences modern lives, including health care, and is developing studies that look at integrating technology interventions to increase screening behaviors (Champion, 2001).

More nurse scientists should aspire to the development of a nursing research career focused on a specific area. The National Cancer Institute, ACS, and ONS repeatedly fund Champion's work because she is able to demonstrate how each study builds on what was learned in the previous studies.

Champion provided much insight into behavioral research and how beliefs influence participation in cancer prevention and detection behaviors (Champion, 2001). An understanding of health beliefs guided the interventional studies. Champion is successful because she repeatedly collaborated with a team of other scientists, usually in a multidisciplinary context. This interdisciplinary approach not only contributed to the richness of the data and findings but also encouraged publication of these findings in many different journals. These publications expose more healthcare providers to this substantial body of nursing research and demonstrate how nurse scientists are making a difference in cancer prevention and early detection.

Preliminary research suggests that nurses can be effective providers of cancer prevention and early detection services. Research is needed that clearly supports or refutes that nurses can be competent, effective, and efficient providers of cancer prevention and early detection services and education. This research also needs to evaluate the cost-effectiveness of nurses as providers of these services. More definite proof of the effectiveness would lead to increased demand and roles for advanced practice nurses and would have many implications for professional and graduate education programs.

Long-term survivors of cancer are only recently receiving attention about their risks for late effects of cancer treatment. This is an ONS priority for research (Berry, 2007). In particular, more research is needed to describe the range of potential late effects for cancer survivors and identify modifiable behaviors that can be targeted to minimize late effects of the treatment.

Recommendations for cancer prevention and early detection change over time. In the 1990s, the age at which to begin mammography was controversial. More recently, the recommendations for Pap smear screening for cervical cancer were changed from annually to every three years in some women considered to be at lower risk (ACS, 2008). Different agencies have different guidelines and recommendations for cancer prevention and early detection, which can be accessed at www.guidelines.gov. The extent to which nurses keep current with these guidelines and their implementation of the recommendations when providing patient education is not clear. The degree that periodic changes to these guidelines confuse and possibly affect screening decisions in the general public is unknown as well.

Risk communication strategies ultimately affect decisions about whether to undergo screening. The importance of effective risk communication is increasing because of the ever-growing body of human genetics and genetic testing for predisposition genes. Primary care providers, including nurses, feel many time constraints. Risk assessment is a labor-intensive process. A significant challenge is the development of techniques and strategies that enhance and further a dialogue between patients and healthcare providers without greatly increasing the time spent. ONS recommends descriptive studies to develop and/or test models of risk assessment and to improve risk assessment skills in oncology nurses (Berry, 2007).

Few studies have examined the use of technologic advances in risk communication and education about cancer prevention and early detection (Champion, 2001). Risk communication is more challenging than it appears. Helping people to accurately understand their risk may increase their willingness to participate in cancer screening measures. The growing number of computerized mathematical models to calculate risk of developing a cancer (e.g., the Gail Model) or risk of having a genetic mutation (e.g., BRCAPRO, Berry Model) has changed risk assesment. Computerized risk assessment is available through some Web sites, including the National Cancer Institute's Breast Cancer Risk Assessment Tool (www.cancer.gov/bcrisktool).

The impact of having an abnormal cancer screen merits significantly more research. A small number of studies have described the anxiety and effect of undergoing further diagnostic testing. A better understanding of this experience could lead to the development of strategies to ensure that abnormalities receive diligent and adequate follow-up. Developing strategies that decrease anxiety during diagnostic evaluations may promote participation in screening and compliance with screening recommendations in the future.

The development of standardized instruments to assess issues related to cancer prevention and early detection is necessary to further advance nursing science in this area (Meissner et al., 2004). Most of the instruments currently address breast and colorectal cancer. Instruments need to be developed or refined to measure cancer risk, prevention, and detection issues with other cancers such as skin, prostate, ovarian, uterine, cervical, and oral cancers. Healthcare providers need to develop more standardized outcome measures and routinely implement them, which will increase the generalizability of the findings across cancer subtypes and populations. When using these instruments with randomized controlled intervention studies, the interventions need to be reasonable, streamlined, and cost-effective so that such interventions could be effective and implemented in busy primary care practices.

Another ONS priority area for nursing research addresses issues related to tobacco control (Berry, 2007). Future studies should focus on patterns of tobacco use, continued tobacco use among people diagnosed with cancer and symptom distress, better understanding of the biology of nicotine dependence, variables influencing smoking cessation, effective pharmacologic agents for smoking cessation, and the stigma and blame associated with tobacco-induced malignancy. Once these factors are better understood, evidence-based interventions should be initiated to integrate tobacco prevention into the care and follow-up of survivors of childhood cancer, increase nursing involvement in policy development, enhance the effectiveness of pharmacologic agents in smoking cessation, and promote the role of nurses in community-based tobacco-control programs.

The search strategy used for this chapter may not have been completely inclusive. Undoubtedly, relevant nursing research papers were missed. This review suggests, however, that much has been initiated in cancer prevention and early detection nursing research. Yet, much more needs to be done. Nurses need to continue to look for strategies to increase participation in screening activities. The dissemination of findings in both nursing and multidisciplinary sources should be a priority. Nurse scientists need to find ways to partner with other disciplines, including psychology, genetics, and public health experts, to increase the scope and range of this area of science.

References

Adams, M.L., Becker, H., & Colbert, A. (2001). African-American women's perceptions of mammography screening. *Journal of National Black Nurses Association, 12*(2), 44–48.

Agho, A.O., & Lewis, M.A. (2001). Correlates of actual and perceived knowledge of prostate cancer among African Americans. *Cancer Nursing, 24*(3), 165–171.

American Cancer Society. (2008). *Cancer facts and figures, 2008.* Atlanta, GA: Author.

Arevian, M., Noureddine, S., & Kabakian-Khasholian, T. (2006). Raising awareness and providing free screening improves cervical cancer screening among economically disadvantaged Lebanese/Armenian women. *Journal of Transcultural Nursing, 17*(4), 357–364.

Bakker, D.A., Lightfoot, N.E., Steggles, S., & Jackson, C. (1998). The experience and satisfaction of women attending breast cancer screening. *Oncology Nursing Forum, 25*(1), 115–121.

Baldwin, D. (1996). A model for describing low-income African American women's participation in breast and cervical cancer early detection and screening. *Advances in Nursing Science, 19*(2), 27–42.

Barroso, J., McMillan, S., Casey, L., Gibson, W., Kaminski, G., & Meyer, J. (2000). Comparison between African-American and White women in their beliefs about breast cancer and their health locus of control. *Cancer Nursing, 23*(4), 268–276.

Beatty, R.M. (2000). Health professionals' knowledge of women's health care. *Journal of Continuing Education in Nursing, 31*(6), 275–279.

Berman, S.H., & Wandersman, A. (1991). Measuring knowledge of cancer. *Social Science and Medicine, 32*(11), 1245–1255.

Bernhardt, B.A., Geller, G., Doksum, T., & Metz, S.A. (2000). Evaluation of nurses and genetic counselors as providers of education about breast cancer susceptibility testing. *Oncology Nursing Forum, 27*(1), 33–39.

Berry, D.L. (2007). *Oncology Nursing Society 2005–2009 research agenda*. Retrieved May 1, 2008, from http://www.ons.org/research/information/documents/pdfs/ONSResAgendaFinal10 -24-07.pdf

Bibb, S.C. (2001). The relationship between access and stage at diagnosis of breast cancer in African American and Caucasian women. *Oncology Nursing Forum, 28*(4), 711–719.

Borrayo, E.A., & Jenkins, S.R. (2001). Feeling healthy: So why should Mexican-descent women screen for breast cancer? *Qualitative Health Research, 11*(6), 812–823.

Bottorff, J.L., McCullum, M., Balneaves, L.G., Esplen, M.J., Carroll, J., Kelly, M., et al. (2005). Establishing roles in genetic nursing: Interviews with Canadian nurses. *Canadian Journal of Nursing Research, 37*(4), 96–115.

Boyd, M.D., Weinrich, S.P., Weinrich, M., & Norton, A. (2001). Obstacles to prostate cancer screening in African-American men. *Journal of National Black Nurses Association, 12*(2), 1–5.

Carruth, A.K., Browning, S., Reed, D.B., Skarke, L., & Sealey, L. (2006). The impact of farm lifestyle and health characteristics: Cervical cancer screening among southern farm women. *Nursing Research, 55*(2), 121–127.

Ceber, E., Soyer, M.T., Ciceklioglu, M., & Cimat, S. (2006). Breast cancer risk assessment and risk perception on nurses and midwives in Bornova Health District in Turkey. *Cancer Nursing, 29*(3), 244–249.

Chalmers, K., Thomson, K., & Degner, L.F. (1996). Information, support, and communication needs of women with a family history of breast cancer. *Cancer Nursing, 19*(3), 204–213.

Chalmers, K.I., & Luker, K.A. (1996). Breast self-care practices in women with primary relatives with breast cancer. *Journal of Advanced Nursing, 23*(6), 1212–1220.

Champion, V., & Menon, U. (1997). Predicting mammography and breast self-examination in African American women. *Cancer Nursing, 20*(5), 315–322.

Champion, V.L. (1984). Instrument development for Health Belief Model constructs. *Advances in Nursing Science, 6*(3), 73–85.

Champion, V.L. (1985). Use of the Health Belief Model in determining the frequency of breast self-examination. *Research in Nursing and Health, 8*(4), 373–379.

Champion, V.L. (1988). Attitudinal variables related to intention, frequency and proficiency of breast self-examination in women 35 and over. *Research in Nursing and Health, 11*(5), 283–291.

Champion, V.L. (1989). Effect of knowledge, teaching method, confidence and social influence on breast self-examination behavior. *Image: The Journal of Nursing Scholarship, 21*(2), 76–80.

Champion, V.L. (1993). Instrument refinement for breast cancer screening behaviors. *Nursing Research, 42*(3), 139–143.

Champion, V.L. (1994). Beliefs about breast cancer and mammography by behavioral stage. *Oncology Nursing Forum, 21*(6), 1009–1114.

Champion, V.L. (1995a). Development of a benefits and barriers scale for mammography utilization. *Cancer Nursing, 18*(1), 53–59.

Champion, V.L. (1995b). Results of a nurse-delivered intervention on proficiency and nodule detection with breast self-examination. *Oncology Nursing Forum, 22*(5), 819–824.

Champion, V.L. (1999). Revised susceptibility, benefits, and barriers scale for mammography screening. *Research in Nursing and Health, 22*(4), 341–348.

Champion, V.L. (2001). Behavioral oncology research: A new millennium. *Oncology Nursing Forum, 28*(6), 975–982.

Champion, V.L., Foster, J., & Menon, U. (1997). Tailoring interventions for health behavior change in breast cancer screening. *Cancer Practice: A Multidisciplinary Journal of Cancer Care, 5*(5), 283–288.

Champion, V.L., & Scott, C.R. (1997). Reliability and validity of breast cancer screening belief scales in African American women. *Nursing Research, 46*(6), 331–337.

Champion, V.L., Skinner, C.S., & Foster, J.L. (2000). The effects of standard care counseling or telephone/in-person counseling on beliefs, knowledge, and behavior related to mammography screening. *Oncology Nursing Forum, 27*(10), 1565–1571.

Chang, T., & Eddins, E.R. (1996). Cost-effectiveness of screening against ovarian cancer: The Markov process. *Journal of Multicultural Nursing and Health, 2*(4), 48–54.

Chlan, L., Evans, D., Greenleaf, M., & Walker, J. (2000). Effects of a single music therapy intervention on anxiety, discomfort, satisfaction, and compliance with screening guidelines in outpatients undergoing flexible sigmoidoscopy. *Gastroenterology Nursing, 23*(4), 148–156.

Christos, P.J., Oliveria, S.A., Masse, L.C., McCormick, L.K., & Halpern, A.C. (2004). Skin cancer prevention and detection by nurses: Attitudes, perceptions, and barriers. *Journal of Cancer Education, 19*(1), 50–57.

Clarke-Tasker, V.A., & Dutta, A.P. (2005). African-American men and their reflections and thoughts on prostate cancer. *Journal of National Black Nurses Association, 16*(1), 1–7.

Coleman, E.A., Coon, S.K., Fitzgerald, A.J., & Cantrell, M.J. (2001). Breast cancer screening education: Comparing outcome skills of nurse practitioner students and medical residents. *Clinical Excellence for Nurse Practitioners, 5*(2), 102–107.

Coleman, E.A., Stewart, C.B., Wilson, S., Cantrell, M.J., O'Sullivan, P., Carthron, D.O., et al. (2004). An evaluation of standardized patients in improving clinical breast examinations for military women. *Cancer Nursing, 27*(6), 474–482.

de Nooijer, J., Lechner, L., Candel, M., & de Vries, H. (2004). Short- and long-term effects of tailored information versus general information on determinants and intentions related to early detection of cancer. *Preventive Medicine, 38*(6), 694–703.

Douglass, A., Barrison, I., Powell, A., & Bramble, M. (2004). The nurse endoscopist's contribution to service delivery. *Gastrointestinal Nursing, 2*(8), 21–24.

Facione, N.C. (1999). Breast cancer screening in relation to access to health services. *Oncology Nursing Forum, 26*(4), 689–696.

Facione, N.C., Dodd, M.J., Holzemer, W., & Meleis, A.I. (1997). Help seeking for self-discovered breast symptoms: Implications for early detection. *Cancer Practice: A Multidisciplinary Journal of Cancer Care, 5*(4), 220–227.

Facione, N.C., & Giancarlo, C.A. (1998). Narratives of breast symptom discovery and cancer diagnosis: Psychologic risk for advanced cancer at diagnosis. *Cancer Nursing, 21*(6), 430–440.

Farmer, A.J. (2000). The minimization to clients of screen-detected breast cancer: A qualitative analysis. *Journal of Advanced Nursing, 31*(2), 306–313.

Fitch, M.I., Greenberg, M., Cava, M., Spaner, D., & Taylor, K. (1998). Exploring the barriers to cervical screening in an urban Canadian setting. *Cancer Nursing, 21*(6), 441–449.

Fitch, M.I., Greenberg, M., Levstein, L., Muir, M., Plante, S., & King, E. (1997). Health promotion and early detection of cancer in older adults: Assessing knowledge about cancer. *Oncology Nursing Forum, 24*(10), 1743–1748.

Foxall, M.J., Barron, C.R., & Houfek, J.F. (2001). Ethnic influences on body awareness, trait anxiety, perceived risk, and breast and gynecologic cancer screening practices. *Oncology Nursing Forum, 28*(4), 727–738.

Goel, V., Gray, R., Chart, P., Fitch, M., Saibil, F., & Zdanowicz, Y. (2004). Perspectives on colorectal cancer screening: A focus study group. *Health Expectations, 7*(1), 51–60.

Gozum, S., & Aydin, I. (2004). Validation evidence for Turkish adaptation of Champion's Health Belief Model Scales. *Cancer Nursing, 27*(6), 491–498.

Green, P.M., & Kelly, B.A. (2004). Colorectal cancer knowledge, perceptions, and behaviors in African Americans. *Cancer Nursing, 27*(3), 206–217.

Grindel, C.G., Brown, L., Caplan, L., & Blumenthal, D. (2004). The effect of breast cancer screening messages on knowledge, attitudes, perceived risk, and mammography screening of African American women in the rural South. *Oncology Nursing Forum, 31*(4), 801–808.

Hahn, E.J., Rayens, M.K., Hopenhayn, C., & Christian, W.J. (2006). Perceived risk and interest in screening for lung cancer among current and former smokers. *Research in Nursing and Health, 29*(4), 359–370.

Hall, C.P., Wimberley, P.D., Hall, J.D., Pfriemer, J.T., Hubbard, E.M., Stacy, A.S., et al. (2005). Teaching breast cancer screening to African American women in the Arkansas Mississippi River Delta. *Oncology Nursing Forum, 32*(4), 857–863.

Han, Y., Williams, R.D., & Harrison, R.A. (2000). Breast cancer screening knowledge, attitudes, and practices among Korean American women. *Oncology Nursing Forum, 27*(10), 1585–1591.

Hansen, L.K., Feigl, P., Modiano, M.R., Lopez, J.A., Escobedo Sluder, S., Moinpour, C.M., et al. (2005). An educational program to increase cervical and breast cancer screening in Hispanic women: A Southwest Oncology Group study. *Cancer Nursing, 28*(1), 47–53.

Ho, V., Yamal, J.M., Atkinson, E.N., Basen-Engquist, K., Tortolero-Luna, G., & Follen, M. (2005). Predictors of breast and cervical screening in Vietnamese women in Harris County, Houston, Texas. *Cancer Nursing, 28*(2), 119–131.

Hoeman, S.P., Ku, Y.L., & Ohl, D.R. (1996). Health beliefs and early detection among Chinese women. *Western Journal of Nursing Research, 18*(5), 518–533.

Holroyd, E., Twinn, S., & Adab, P. (2004). Socio-cultural influences on Chinese women's attendance for cervical screening. *Journal of Advanced Nursing, 46*(1), 42–52.

Howell, S.L., Nelson-Marten, P., Krebs, L.U., Kaszyk, L., & Wold, R. (1998). Promoting nurses' positive attitudes toward cancer prevention/screening. *Journal of Cancer Education, 13*(2), 76–84.

Hunt, L.M., de Voogd, K.B., Akana, L.L., & Browner, C.H. (1998). Abnormal Pap screening among Mexican-American women: Impediments to receiving and reporting follow-up care. *Oncology Nursing Forum, 25*(10), 1743–1749.

Hutson, S.P. (2003). Attitudes and psychological impact of genetic testing, genetic counseling, and breast cancer risk assessment among women at increased risk. *Oncology Nursing Forum, 30*(2), 241–246.

Im, E.O., Park, Y.S., Lee, E.O., & Yun, S.N. (2004). Korean women's attitudes toward breast cancer screening tests. *International Journal of Nursing Studies, 41*(6), 583–589.

Kelly, P., & Winslow, E.H. (1996). Needle wire localization for nonpalpable breast lesions: Sensations, anxiety levels, and informational needs. *Oncology Nursing Forum, 23*(4), 639–645.

Kim, K., Yu, E.S., Chen, E.H., Kim, J., Kaufman, M., & Purkiss, J. (1999). Cervical cancer screening knowledge and practices among Korean-American women. *Cancer Nursing, 22*(4), 297–302.

Kinney, A.Y., Croyle, R.T., Dudley, W.N., Bailey, C.A., Pelias, M.K., & Neuhausen, S.L. (2001). Knowledge, attitudes, and interest in breast-ovarian cancer gene testing: A survey of a large African-American kindred with a BRCA1 mutation. *Preventive Medicine, 33*(6), 543–551.

Lalos, A.T., Hovanec-Lalos, C.A., & Weber, B. (1997). Patient satisfaction with conscious sedation for ambulatory colonoscopy in a community hospital. *Gastroenterology Nursing, 20*(4), 114–117.

Lane, A.J., & Martin, M. (2005). Characteristics of rural women who attended a free breast health program. *Online Journal of Rural Nursing and Health Care, 5*(2), 12–27.

Lauver, D.R., Kane, J., Bodden, J., McNeel, J., & Smith, L. (1999). Engagement in breast cancer screening behaviors. *Oncology Nursing Forum, 26*(3), 545–554.

Lee, M.C. (2000). Knowledge, barriers, and motivators related to cervical cancer screening among Korean-American women: A focus group approach. *Cancer Nursing, 23*(3), 168–175.

Lee-Lin, F.M., & Menon, U. (2005). Breast and cervical cancer screening practices and interventions among Chinese, Japanese, and Vietnamese Americans. *Oncology Nursing Forum, 32*(5), 995–1003.

Lockwood-Rayermann, S. (2004). Characteristics of participation in cervical cancer screening. *Cancer Nursing, 27*(5), 353–363.

Loescher, L.J. (2003). Cancer worry in women with hereditary risk factors for breast cancer. *Oncology Nursing Forum, 30*(5), 767–772.

Lundgren, E.L., Tishelman, C., Widmark, C., Forss, A., Sachs, L., & Tornberg, S. (2000). Midwives' descriptions of their familiarity with cancer: A qualitative study of midwives working with population-based cervical cancer screening in urban Sweden. *Cancer Nursing, 23*(5), 392–400.

MacDonald, D.J., Sarna, L., Uman, G.C., Grant, M., & Weitzel, J.N. (2005). Health beliefs of women with and without breast cancer seeking genetic cancer risk assessment. *Cancer Nursing, 28*(5), 372–381.

MacDonald, D.J., Sarna, L., Uman, G.C., Grant, M., & Weitzel, J.N. (2006). Cancer screening and risk-reducing behaviors of women seeking genetic cancer risk assessment for breast and ovarian cancers [Online exclusive]. *Oncology Nursing Forum, 33*(2), E27–E35. Retrieved May 21, 2008, from http://ons.metapress.com/content/h307166720r5525q/fulltext.pdf

Mahon, S.M. (1997). Comparison of methods for the early detection of breast cancer. *Image: The Journal of Nursing Scholarship, 29*(3), 292.

Mahon, S.M., & Williams, M. (2000). Information needs regarding menopause: Results from a survey of women receiving cancer prevention and detection services. *Cancer Nursing, 23*(3), 176–185.

Mahon, S.M., Williams, M.T., & Spies, M.A. (2000). Screening for second cancers and osteoporosis in long-term survivors. *Cancer Practice: A Multidisciplinary Journal of Cancer Care, 8*(6), 282–290.

Manne, S., Markowitz, A., Winawer, S., Guillem, J., Meropol, N.J., Haller, D., et al. (2003). Understanding intention to undergo colonoscopy among intermediate-risk siblings of colorectal cancer patients: A test of a mediational model. *Preventive Medicine, 36*(1), 71–84.

Masny, A., Daly, M., Ross, E., Balshem, A., Gillespie, D., & Weil, S. (2003). A training course for oncology nurses in familial cancer risk assessment: Evaluation of knowledge and practice. *Journal of Cancer Education, 18*(1), 20–25.

McGovern, P.M., Gross, C.R., Krueger, R.A., Engelhard, D.A., Cordes, J.E., & Church, T.R. (2004). False-positive cancer screens and health-related quality of life. *Cancer Nursing, 27*(5), 347–352.

McKinney, M.M., Weiner, B.J., & Wang, V. (2006). Recruiting participants to cancer prevention clinical trials: Lessons from successful community oncology networks. *Oncology Nursing Forum, 33*(5), 951–959.

Meissner, H.I., Vernon, S.W., Rimer, B.K., Wilson, K.M., Rakowski, W., Briss, P.A., et al. (2004). The future of research that promotes cancer screening. *Cancer, 101*(Suppl. 5), 1251–1259.

Miller, A.M., & Champion, V.L. (1993). Mammography in women greater or less than 50 years of age: Predisposing and enabling characteristics. *Cancer Nursing, 16*(4), 260–269.

Mundt, M.H., Hermann, C.P., Conner, A.L., & Von Ah, D.M. (2006). A community partnership model for developing a center for cancer nursing education and research. *Journal of Professional Nursing, 22*(5), 273–279.

Nichols, B.S., Misra, R., & Alexy, B. (1996). Cancer detection: How effective is public education? *Cancer Nursing, 19*(2), 98–103.

Nivens, A.S., Herman, J., Weinrich, S.P., & Weinrich, M.C. (2001). Cues to participation in prostate cancer screening: A theory for practice. *Oncology Nursing Forum, 28*(9), 1449–1456.

Oliffe, J. (2006). Being screened for prostate cancer: A simple blood test or a commitment to treatment? *Cancer Nursing, 29*(1), 1–8.

Phelan, D.L., Oliveria, S.A., & Halpern, A.C. (2005). Patient experiences with photo books in monthly skin self-examinations. *Dermatology Nursing, 17*(2), 109–114.

Phillips, J.M., & Belcher, A.E. (1999). Integrating cancer risk assessment into a community health nursing course. *Journal of Cancer Education, 14*(1), 47–51.

Phillips, J.M., Cohen, M.Z., & Moses, G. (1999). Breast cancer screening and African American women: Fear, fatalism, and silence. *Oncology Nursing Forum, 26*(3), 561–571.

Phillips, J.M., Cohen, M.Z., & Tarzian, A.J. (2001), African American women's experiences with breast cancer screening. *Journal of Nursing Scholarship, 33*(2), 135–140.

Powe, B.D. (1994). Perceptions of cancer fatalism among African Americans: The influence of education, income, and cancer knowledge. *Journal of National Black Nurses Association, 7*(2), 41–48.

Powe, B.D. (1995). Cancer fatalism among elderly Caucasians and African Americans. *Oncology Nursing Forum, 22*(9), 1355–1359.

Powe, B.D. (1997). Cancer fatalism—spiritual perspectives. *Journal of Religion and Health, 36*(2), 135–144.

Powe, B.D., & Finnie, R. (2004). Knowledge of oral cancer risk factors among African Americans: Do nurses have a role? *Oncology Nursing Forum, 31*(4), 785–791.

Powe, B.D., Ntekop, E., & Barron, M. (2004). An intervention study to increase colorectal cancer knowledge and screening among community elders. *Public Health Nursing, 21*(5), 435–442.

Powe, B.D., Underwood, S., Canales, M., & Finnie, R. (2005). Perceptions about breast cancer among college students: Implications for nursing education. *Journal of Nursing Education, 44*(6), 257–265.

Powe, B.D., & Weinrich, S. (1999). An intervention to decrease cancer fatalism among rural elders. *Oncology Nursing Forum, 26*(3), 583–588.

Rakowski, W., Clark, M.A., Pearlman, D.N., Ehrich, B., Rimer, B.K., Goldstein, M.G., et al. (1997). Integrating pros and cons for mammography and Pap testing: Extending the construct of decisional balance to two behaviors. *Preventive Medicine, 26*(5, Pt. 1), 664–673.

Rawl, S.M., Menon, U., Champion, V.L., May, F.E., Loehrer, P., Sr., Hunter, C., et al. (2005). Do benefits and barriers differ by stage of adoption for colorectal cancer screening? *Health Education Research, 20*(2), 137–148.

Rawl, S.R., Champion, V.L., Menon, U., Loehrer, P.J., Vance, G.H., & Skinner, C.S. (2001). Validation of scales to measure benefits of and barriers to colorectal cancer screening. *Journal of Psychosocial Oncology, 19*(3/4), 47–63.

Rice, V.H., & Stead, L.F. (2008). Nursing interventions for smoking cessation. *Cochrane Database of Systematic Reviews 2008,* Issue 1. Art. No.: CD001188. DOI: 10.1002/14651858. CD001188.pub3.

Rosenstock, I.M. (1966). Why people use health services. *Milbank Memorial Fund Quarterly, 44,* 94–124.

Sabay, T.B., Gray, R.E., & Fitch. M. (2000). A qualitative study of patient perspectives on colorectal cancer. *Cancer Practice: A Multidisciplinary Journal of Cancer Care, 8*(1), 38–44.

Sadler, G.R., Dhanjal, S.K., Shah, N.B., Shah, R.B., Ko, C., Anghel, M., et al. (2001). Asian Indian women: Knowledge, attitudes and behaviors toward breast cancer early detection. *Public Health Nursing, 18*(5), 357–363.

Salazar, M.K. (1996). Hispanic women's beliefs about breast cancer and mammography. *Cancer Nursing, 19*(6), 437–446.

Sarna, L., & Chang, B.L. (2000). Colon cancer screening among older women caregivers. *Cancer Nursing, 23*(2), 109–116.

Sarna, L., Tae, Y.S., Kim, Y.H., Brecht, M.L., & Maxwell, A.E. (2001). Cancer screening among Korean Americans. *Cancer Practice: A Multidisciplinary Journal of Cancer Care, 9*(3), 134–140.

Saywell, R.M., Jr., Champion, V.L., Zollinger, T.W., Maraj, M., Skinner, C.S., Zoppi, K.A., et al. (2003). The cost-effectiveness of 5 interventions to increase mammography adherence in a managed care population. *American Journal of Managed Care, 9*(1), 33–44.

Schulmeister, L., & Lifsey, D.S. (1999). Cervical cancer screening knowledge, behaviors, and beliefs of Vietnamese women. *Oncology Nursing Forum, 26*(5), 879–887.

Secginli, S., & Nahcivan, N.O. (2004). Reliability and validity of the breast cancer screening belief scale among Turkish women. *Cancer Nursing, 27*(4), 287–294.

Seckel, M.M., & Birney, M.H. (1996). Social support, stress, and age in women undergoing breast biopsies. *Clinical Nurse Specialist, 10*(3), 137–143.

Shelton, P., Weinrich, S., & Reynolds, W.A., Jr. (1999). Barriers to prostate cancer screening in African American men. *Journal of National Black Nurses Association, 10*(2), 14–28.

Simonian, K., Brown, S.E., Sanders, D.B., Kidd, C.Y., Murillo, V.E., Garcia, R., et al. (2004). Promoting breast cancer screening to women of color. *Nurse Practitioner: American Journal of Primary Health Care, 29*(3), 45–46.

Smiley, M.R., McMillan, S.C., Johnson, S., & Ojeda, M. (2000). Comparison of Florida Hispanic and non-Hispanic Caucasian women in their health beliefs related to breast cancer and health locus of control. *Oncology Nursing Forum, 27*(6), 975–984.

Stamler, L.L., Thomas, B., & Lafreniere, K. (2000). Working women identify influences and obstacles to breast health practices. *Oncology Nursing Forum, 27*(5), 835–842.

Steven, D., Fitch, M., Dhaliwal, H., Kirk-Gardner, R., Sevean, P., Jamieson, J., et al. (2004). Knowledge, attitudes, beliefs, and practices regarding breast and cervical cancer screening in selected ethnocultural groups in Northwestern Ontario. *Oncology Nursing Forum, 31*(2), 305–311.

Sutherland, G., Straton, J., & Hyndman, J. (1996). Cervical cancer: An inpatient screening service. *Australian Journal of Advanced Nursing, 14*(1), 20–27.

Tang, T.S., Solomon, L.J., & McCracken, L.M. (2001). Barriers to fecal occult blood testing and sigmoidoscopy among older Chinese-American women. *Cancer Practice: A Multidisciplinary Journal of Cancer Care, 9*(6), 277–282.

Thomas, E.C. (2004). African American women's breast memories, cancer beliefs, and screening behaviors. *Cancer Nursing, 27*(4), 295–302.

Thomas, V.N., Saleem, T., & Abraham, R. (2005). Barriers to effective uptake of cancer screening among Black and minority ethnic groups. *International Journal of Palliative Nursing, 11*(11), 562, 564–571.

Tiffen, J., Sharp, L., & O'Toole, C. (2005). Depressive symptoms prescreening and post screening among returning participants in an ovarian cancer early detection program. *Cancer Nursing, 28*(4), 325–330.

Tingen, M.S., Weinrich, S.P., Heydt, D.D., Boyd, M.D., & Weinrich, M.C. (1998). Perceived benefits: A predictor of participation in prostate cancer screening. *Cancer Nursing, 21*(5), 349–357.

Tsouskas, L.I., Noula, M., & Dimopoulos, P. (2005, April–June). Practicing an expert system for definition of high-risk group in breast cancer screening. *ICUs and Nursing Web Journal,* (22), 1–5. Retrieved May 21, 2008, from http://www.nursing.gr/protectedarticles/practising.pdf

Tsujino, K., Tsukahara, M., Frazier, L., Iino, H., & Murakami, K. (2003). Genetic content in Japanese language nursing textbooks. *Research and Theory for Nursing Practice, 17*(4), 353–362.

Twinn, S., & Cheng, F. (2000). Increasing uptake rates of cervical cancer screening amongst Hong Kong Chinese women: The role of the practitioner. *Journal of Advanced Nursing, 32*(2), 335–342.

Ueland, A.S., Hornung, P.A., & Greenwald, B. (2006). Colorectal cancer prevention and screening: A Health Belief Model–based research study to increase disease awareness. *Gastroenterology Nursing, 29*(5), 357–363.

Watts, T., Merrell, J., Murphy, F., & Williams, A. (2004). Breast health information needs of women from minority ethnic groups. *Journal of Advanced Nursing, 47*(5), 526–535.

Weinrich, S.P., Reynolds, W.A., Jr., Tingen, M.S., & Starr, C.R. (2000). Barriers to prostate cancer screening. *Cancer Nursing, 23*(2), 117–121.

Weinrich, S.P., Seger, R., Miller, B.L., Davis, C., Kim, S., Wheeler, C., et al. (2004). Knowledge of the limitations associated with prostate cancer screening among low-income men. *Cancer Nursing, 27*(6), 442–453.

Weinrich, S.P., Weinrich, M.C., Boyd, M.D., & Atkinson, C. (1998). The impact of prostate cancer knowledge on cancer screening. *Oncology Nursing Forum, 25*(3), 527–534.

Wright, K.B. (2000). A description of the gastroenterology nurse endoscopist role in the United States. *Gastroenterology Nursing, 23*(2), 78–82.

Xu, Y., Ross, M.C., Ryan, R., & Wang, B. (2005a). Cancer risk factors among Southeast Asian American residents of the U.S. Central Gulf Coast. *Public Health Nursing, 22*(2), 119–129.

Xu, Y., Ross, M.C., Ryan, R., & Wang, B. (2005b). Cancer risk factors of Vietnamese Americans in rural South Alabama. *Journal of Nursing Scholarship, 37*(3), 237–244.

Yarbrough, S.S., & Braden, C.J. (2001). Utility of Health Belief Model as a guide for explaining or predicting breast cancer screening behaviors. *Journal of Advanced Nursing, 33*(5), 677–688.

Yi, J.K. (1998). Acculturation and Pap smear screening practices among college-aged Vietnamese women in the United States. *Cancer Nursing, 21*(5), 335–341.

Yu, E.S., Kim, K.K., Chen, E.H., & Brintnall, R.A. (2001). Breast and cervical cancer screening among Chinese American women. *Cancer Practice: A Multidisciplinary Journal of Cancer Care, 9*(2), 81–91.

Zimmerman, S.M. (1997). Factors influencing Hispanic participation in prostate cancer screening. *Oncology Nursing Forum, 24*(3), 499–504.

CHAPTER 4

Advances in Symptoms, Symptom Clusters, and Quality of Life by Oncology Nurse Scientists

Cynthia R. King, PhD, NP, MSN, RN, FAAN

Introduction

Symptoms and symptom management for individuals with cancer have been important aspects of oncology nursing for decades. More recently, oncology nurse scientists discovered that symptoms often occur in clusters (Dodd, Janson, et al., 2001; Lenz, Pugh, Milligan, Gift, & Suppe, 1997). Oncology nurses play a critical role in the evaluation and improvement of quality of life (QOL) for individuals with cancer. Consequently, they are largely responsible for the increased attention and priority given to symptoms, symptom management, and QOL issues for individuals with cancer. By focusing on symptoms, symptom clusters, and symptom management, nurses have positively affected QOL for this population. This chapter highlights the contributions that oncology nurses have made to advancing nursing science related to symptoms, symptom clusters, and QOL.

Symptoms

For decades, the care of individuals with cancer focused on the medical aspects and advances in tumor pathology, chemotherapy, hormonal therapy, surgical interventions, biotherapy, radiation, hematopoietic stem cell transplant, and technologic advances. Less time and effort were given to patients' experiences of the illness and the physical and psychological symptoms. Because of the attention paid by oncology nurses in assessing and managing symptoms associated with cancer and treatments, significant improvements in the QOL of patients and their families have been made.

As described in Chapter 1, the Oncology Nursing Society (ONS) has been establishing oncology nursing research priorities since 1980 via periodic surveys. Individual symptoms (e.g., pain, fatigue) and symptom management repeatedly have ranked in the top 10 research priorities (see Table 1-2). Based on these priorities, many oncology nurse scientists have conducted studies that have led to significantly improved care and QOL for individuals with cancer.

Among these scientists are ONS Distinguished Researchers who have made outstanding contributions to oncology nursing science and clinical practice. Of particular interest are those scientists who have focused on symptoms and symptom management, including Johnson, McCorkle, Ferrell, Dodd, Grant, Nail, and Mock. (See Chapter 2, Table 2-3, for their specific areas of study.)

For patients with cancer, symptoms and QOL are conceptualized as subjective and multidimensional experiences. In this chapter, a *symptom* is defined differently than a *sign*. Generally, a *sign* is observed by clinicians, whereas a *symptom* is experienced by patients. Nurse scientists have developed several theories to explain the occurrence of symptoms and the relation of symptoms to other factors (Johnson, 1999; Johnson, Fieler, Jones, Wlasowicz, & Mitchell, 1997; Lenz et al., 1997). Johnson, a recipient of the ONS Distinguished Researcher award, developed the Self-Regulation Theory based on work she did with her mentor, Dr. Leventhal, in the 1970s and 1980s. In the Self-Regulation Theory, if individuals with cancer are given concrete, objective information about symptoms, they are able to create a concrete representation (or schema) of what they may experience with cancer treatments. This theory highlights the difference between the occurrence of a symptom (a concrete, objective event) and the emotional response to the symptom. This is an example of early oncology nursing research with symptoms that helped to stimulate advances by many other oncology nurse scientists over the past few decades.

Another one of the first scientists in oncology nursing research to focus on symptoms was Quint (1963). Quint focused on women with breast cancer early in her career. She was one of the first to identify the importance of symptoms and QOL issues. She changed the assumption by healthcare professionals that women with breast cancer were happy to just be alive, even if they suffered from the many serious side effects of radical mastectomy. Quint demonstrated that ongoing symptoms of breast cancer and treatment truly affect QOL. She was recognized as an ONS Distinguished Researcher because she pioneered research in the area of physical symptoms, as well as the psychosocial effects of cancer and its treatment.

Since the work of Quint (1963), Lenz et al. (1997), and Johnson (1999), several dimensions have been discovered to occur across symptoms and populations, including intensity (strength), timing (duration and frequency), level of distress perceived, and quality. Although symptom distress usually is considered separately, the other dimensions (e.g., intensity, timing, quality) are considered to be part of the symptom occurrence (Armstrong, 2003). Most oncology nurse scientists consider *symptom distress* to include the degree or amount of the physical upset, anguish, or suffering experienced because of a specific symptom (Rhodes & Watson, 1987).

Rhodes and Watson (1987) were guest editors of an issue of *Seminars in Oncology Nursing* that focused on symptom distress. The articles in this journal covered a variety of symptoms, including fatigue, insomnia, depression, anxiety, nausea and vomiting, anorexia, elimination problems, and breathing difficulty, and also discussed symptom occurrence and symptom distress and how symptoms should be described in terms of frequency, duration, and severity (Basch, 1987; Gobel & Donovan, 1987; Grant, 1987; Haylock, 1987; McCorkle, 1987; Nail & King, 1987; Rhodes & Watson). The authors wrote that each of these aspects of symptoms might require the use of different measurements or scales in research (Rhodes & Watson).

McCorkle (1987), another ONS Distinguished Researcher, also worked in the 1980s on symptom distress by developing the Symptom Distress Scale. To measure symptoms in patients with cancer, many oncology nurse scientists use instruments that measure symptom occurrence and perceived intensity of the symptoms (Haberman, 1999). Haberman, past director of the ONS Research Team, encouraged oncology nurse scientists to consider the entire symptom experience of individuals with cancer. By *symptom experience*, Haberman means a multidimensional process or a synthesis of symptom occurrence and perceptions of intensity and distress. Distress may be influenced by various factors, including (Armstrong, 2003)

- Age
- Socioeconomic level
- Culture
- Family role
- Education
- Values
- Past experiences.

The symptom experience and the meaning that individuals assign to a symptom or multiple symptoms can profoundly affect their QOL, both positively and negatively. The symptom that is the most distressing to an individual may not be the symptom that is the most meaningful for that individual.

Oncology nurse scientists have demonstrated with their studies over the past few decades that symptoms are relevant clinically across all settings of cancer care (e.g., hospital, outpatient, home care, hospice). For example, Distinguished Researcher Ferrell conducted studies that demonstrated how the homecare setting also requires extensive attention to symptoms. Her results in homecare research showed that the presence of uncontrolled symptoms affects the QOL of both the individual with cancer and the family caregiver (Ferrell & Borneman, 1999, 2000; Ferrell, Grant, Chan, Ahn, & Ferrell, 1995).

Numerous oncology nurse scientists (including several ONS Distinguished Researchers) found that symptoms may affect a variety of health outcomes in patients with cancer. For example, symptoms can affect functional status (Dodd, Miaskowski, & Paul, 2001; Given, Given, Azzouz, & Stommel, 2001; Sarna, 1998), psychological well-being (Cimprich, 1999; McCorkle & Quint-Benoliel, 1983; Molassiotis et al., 1996), healthcare costs (e.g., the undertreatment of pain is very costly because of unreimbursed readmissions to the hospital) (Ferrell & Griffith, 1994; Grant, Ferrell, Rivera, & Lee, 1995), and QOL. The effects of symptoms on QOL will be described later in this chapter.

Symptom Clusters

In the first few decades of published research by oncology nurses, many of the studies were conducted on single symptoms associated with cancer, such as pain, fatigue, and depression. This approach led to significant advances in understanding the assessment and management of many individual symptoms. Focusing on single symptoms is important to continue; however, oncology nurses recognized that patients with cancer rarely present with only one symptom. Thus, they initiated cutting-edge research to evaluate multiple symptoms (e.g., symptom clusters) using cross-sectional and longitudinal designs (Miaskowski, Dodd, & Lee, 2004). This represents a new frontier in symptom management research.

Oncology nurses have recognized for decades that individuals with cancer experience myriad symptoms concurrently caused by the cancer, cancer treatment, or their combination. However, scientists have just begun to realize the importance of assessing the complex relationships between and among symptoms. Symptoms commonly associated with cancer and its treatment are (a) fatigue, (b) nausea and vomiting, (c) pain, (d) depression and/or anxiety, (e) appetite and weight changes, and (f) difficulty sleeping. These symptoms may be caused by cancer, the treatments, or both. In 2001, Dodd, another ONS Distinguished Researcher, called for considering symptoms in clusters versus individually in nursing research (Dodd, Janson, et al., 2001). Considering symptoms in clusters helps to recognize the complexity of the cancer symptom experience. Currently, no single accepted definition of *symptom cluster* exists in oncology nursing research. Dodd and her colleagues have described it as concurrent and related symptoms that may or may not have the same or common etiology (Dodd, Janson, et al.; Dodd, Miaskowski, & Lee, 2004; Dodd, Miaskowski, et al., 2001).

Because the concept of symptom clusters is relatively new to oncology nursing, few, if any, theoretical frameworks are available that directly address this concept. Dodd, Janson, et al. (2001) developed the Symptom Management Model. This conceptual model has a dimension called the *symptom experience,* which comprises the perception, evaluation, and response to symptoms. The plural "symptoms" is used, but symptom clusters are not directly addressed. Other oncology nurses have constructed frameworks or models that focus on a specific symptom and may include other symptoms that contribute to the specific symptom of interest. For example, both Piper and Winningham constructed models focusing on cancer-related fatigue (Piper, 1993; Piper et al., 1998; Winningham et al., 1994). As previously mentioned in the section on symptoms, Lenz et al. (1997) proposed a theory of symptoms that is a middle-range theory of unpleasant symptoms. This theory also describes the presence of multiple symptoms that influence one another. The Theory of Unpleasant Symptoms recognizes physiologic, psychological, and situational antecedents of symptoms and functional outcomes of symptoms. Lenz et al. used the term *multiplicative*, meaning two or more symptoms can have a catalytic effect on one another. For example, fatigue could be perceived to be worse in the presence of one other symptom such as pain, depression, anxiety, or insomnia. However, if fatigue is experienced in the presence of all of the aforementioned symptoms, it would be proportionally more severe. This concept is still theoretical and has not been tested.

Despite the lack of specific theories of symptom clusters, nurse scientists have been able to use other conceptual models and conduct research on specific symptom clusters. Studies have been conducted regarding the correlation between various symptom pairs. For instance, pairs included fatigue and insomnia (Beck & Schwartz, 2000; Miaskowski & Lee, 1999), fatigue and pain (Dodd, Miaskowski, et al., 2001; Gaston-Johansson, Fall-Dickson, Bakos & Kennedy, 1999), pain and depression (Gaston-Johansson et al.), and fatigue and depression (Beck & Schwartz; Dodd, Miaskowski, et al., 2001; Miaskowski & Lee; Redeker, Lev, & Ruggiero, 2000). Gift and colleagues looked at the concurrence and temporal patterning of symptoms as indicators of symptom clustering (Gift, Jablonski, Stommel, & Given, 2004; Gift, Stommel, Jablonski, & Given, 2003). More recently, Beck, Dudley, and Barsevick (2005) demonstrated through a partial mediation model that one symptom can influence another through its effect on a third symptom. The scientists showed that pain affects fatigue directly as well as indirectly through its effect on sleep. Therefore, individuals with cancer who have pain lost sleep and consequently had higher levels of fatigue (Beck et al.).

Researching symptom clusters in oncology nursing continues to be difficult. The individual with cancer may have some symptoms caused by the disease (e.g., nausea from a tumor invading the gastrointestinal tract) and some symptoms caused by the treatment(s) (e.g., decreased appetite and weight loss from chemotherapy). Additionally, individuals may have symptoms secondary to comorbid conditions (e.g., pain and fatigue secondary to rheumatoid arthritis), or the symptoms the individual is experiencing may result in other symptoms (e.g., pain and fatigue can cause anxiety and insomnia). To further complicate the experience, symptoms may interact or be direct or indirect causes of other symptoms. Ultimately, the end result from studying symptom clusters is an increased understanding of the way in which a particular set of symptoms are related, how they affect one another, and how they affect patient outcomes, such as QOL. Potentially, this will lead to new directions for the clinical assessment of symptoms and interventions to improve cancer care and the QOL of individuals with cancer.

Quality of Life

Although the exact number and names of the QOL dimensions continue to be debated, oncology nurses usually recognize physical well-being, psychological well-being, social well-being, and spiritual well-being as the four key dimensions of QOL. These domains interact dynamically (see Figure 4-1). For example, changes in physical well-being such as the development and continuation of symptoms (e.g., pain, fatigue, nausea and vomiting) may have a direct effect on any or all other aspects of QOL (e.g., psychological well-being, social well-being, spiritual well-being).

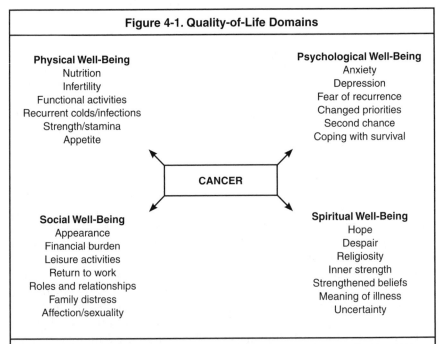

Figure 4-1. Quality-of-Life Domains

Physical Well-Being
Nutrition
Infertility
Functional activities
Recurrent colds/infections
Strength/stamina
Appetite

Psychological Well-Being
Anxiety
Depression
Fear of recurrence
Changed priorities
Second chance
Coping with survival

CANCER

Social Well-Being
Appearance
Financial burden
Leisure activities
Return to work
Roles and relationships
Family distress
Affection/sexuality

Spiritual Well-Being
Hope
Despair
Religiosity
Inner strength
Strengthened beliefs
Meaning of illness
Uncertainty

Note. From "Advances in How Clinical Nurses Can Evaluate and Improve Quality of Life for Individuals With Cancer," by C.R. King, 2006, *Oncology Nursing Forum, 33*(Suppl. 1), p. 6. Copyright 2006 by the Oncology Nursing Society. Reprinted with permission. [Adapted from "Quality of Life in Long-Term Cancer Survivors," by B.R. Ferrell, K.H. Dow, S. Leigh, J. Ly, and P. Gulasekaram, 1995, *Oncology Nursing Forum, 22*(6), p. 916. Copyright 1995 by the Oncology Nursing Society.]

Currently, assessment and measurement of QOL have become important aspects of care provided by nurses to individuals with cancer. For decades, medicine has evaluated the outcomes of cancer treatment by disease-free survival, tumor response, and overall survival. More recently, oncology clinicians and scientists recognized that these outcomes were not adequately assessing the effect of cancer and treatments on individuals with cancer and their daily lives. Furthermore, these outcomes did not help in identifying potential interventions to improve or maintain QOL, including physical well-being, psychological well-being, social well-being, and spiritual well-being.

As reflected in Table 1-2 (see Chapter 1), QOL has repeatedly been ranked in the top 10 research priorities. Thus, numerous oncology nurse scientists developed programs of research focused directly on QOL or on factors that may increase or decrease QOL, such as symptoms and symptom management. ONS has consistently supported efforts for oncology nurses to be involved in activities related to QOL and advancing the science of QOL.

In 1995, ONS, Amgen USA, and Amgen Canada supported the efforts of this author to plan, develop, and lead an ONS State-of-the-Knowledge Conference to address the current knowledge regarding QOL and the cancer experience (King et al., 1997). This international conference was attended by oncology nurses and psychologists from the United States and Canada. ONS and the ONS Foundation have continued to demonstrate support for QOL research. Since 1989, the Foundation has funded many QOL research studies by oncology nurse scientists. ONS has partnered with the Upjohn Corporation since 1988 to support an annual award to recognize nursing excellence in QOL. With help from Dr. Jane Clark and Dr. Cynthia King, ONS established a QOL lectureship at the ONS Annual Fall Institute conference (now called Institutes of Learning). The lectureship was subsequently named the Trish Greene Memorial Quality of Life Lectureship in memory of Trish Greene, who was an oncology nursing leader and nurse scientist. The lectureship was designed to (a) focus ONS membership attention on QOL issues in cancer care, (b) describe the contribution of oncology nursing clinicians, educators, administrators, and scientists to QOL in cancer care, (c) apply QOL-related information to nursing practice, and (d) incorporate QOL philosophy into all aspects of cancer care (Grant & Dean, 2003). Oncology nurse scientists are recipients of this QOL lectureship (King, 2001) and the ONS Publishing Excellence Award for QOL (King, 2006).

In general, oncology nurse scientists have been interested not only in QOL as an outcome but also in how individual symptoms and symptom clusters affect QOL. Ferrell and Grant (2003) discussed some of the research issues in symptom management and QOL. Specifically, they presented symptom items in seven QOL instruments that are used in QOL research. Several of the instruments that help to assess the impact of symptoms on QOL have been developed by oncology nurse scientists (Ferrell, Dow, & Grant, 1995; Grant et al., 1992; McCorkle & Young, 1978). As highlighted in Chapter 2, several of the recipients of the ONS Distinguished Researcher Award conducted research related to symptoms or symptom clusters and how they affect QOL (Ferrell, 1996; Grant, 1999; Hinds, Burghen, Haase, & Phillips, 2006; Mock et al., 2001).

As oncology nurse scientists continue to assess the effect of symptoms and symptom clusters on the QOL of individuals with cancer, ensuring that the symptoms and QOL experience are reported in a reliable and efficient way will be important. One way to do this is via electronic technology to capture patients' self-reporting of symptoms and QOL data (Berry et al., 2004; Mullen, Berry, & Zierler, 2004). Using electronic technology allows for accurate, confidential, and private answering of questions and eliminates many of the steps in retrieving patient interview data.

Conclusion

The oncology nursing research conducted to date clearly demonstrates that symptoms, symptom clusters, symptom management, and how symptoms affect QOL are an integral part of the cancer experience. Through aggressive research and clinical treatment of symptoms, oncology nurses will continue to make significant advances to help to humanize the cancer experience and improve the QOL of individuals with cancer and their families.

References

Armstrong, T.S. (2003). Symptom experience: A concept analysis. *Oncology Nursing Forum, 30*(4), 601–606.

Basch, A. (1987). Symptom distress. Changes in elimination. *Seminars in Oncology Nursing, 3*(4), 287–292.

Beck, S., Dudley, W.N., & Barsevick, A.M. (2005). Pain, sleep disturbance, and fatigue in patients with cancer: Using a mediation model to test a symptom cluster [Online exclusive]. *Oncology Nursing Forum, 32*(3), E48–E55. Retrieved November 15, 2007, from http://ons.metapress.com/content/122n61u334093256/fulltext.pdf

Beck, S.L., & Schwartz, A.L. (2000). Unrelieved pain contributes to fatigue and insomnia [Abstract 195]. *Oncology Nursing Forum, 27*(2), 350–351.

Berry, D.L., Trigg, L.J., Lober, W.B., Karras, B.T., Galligan, M.L., Austin-Seymour, M., et al. (2004). Computerized symptom and quality-of-life assessment for patients with cancer. Part I: Development and pilot testing [Online exclusive]. *Oncology Nursing Forum, 31*(5), E75–E83. Retrieved November 15, 2007, from http://ons.metapress.com/content/c2hn30765683045t/fulltext.pdf

Cimprich, B. (1999). Pretreatment symptom distress in women newly diagnosed with breast cancer. *Cancer Nursing, 22*(3), 185–195.

Dodd, M., Janson, S., Facione, N., Faucett, J., Froelicher, E.S., Humphreys, J., et al. (2001). Advancing the science of symptom management. *Journal of Advanced Nursing, 33*(5), 668–676.

Dodd, M.J., Miaskowski, C., & Lee, K.A. (2004). Occurrence of symptom clusters. *Journal of the National Cancer Institute Monographs, 32*, 76–78.

Dodd, M.J., Miaskowski, C., & Paul, S.M. (2001). Symptom clusters and their effect on the functional status of patients with cancer. *Oncology Nursing Forum, 28*(3), 465–470.

Ferrell, B.R. (1996). The quality of lives: 1,525 voices of cancer. *Oncology Nursing Forum, 23*(6), 909–916.

Ferrell, B.R., & Borneman, T. (1999). Hospice home management of pain and symptoms. *Primary Care and Cancer, 19*(7), 8–10.

Ferrell, B.R., & Borneman, T. (2000). Maintaining quality of life in the home. *Principles and Practice of Supportive Oncology Updates, 3*(5), 1–8.

Ferrell, B.R., Dow, K.H., & Grant, M. (1995). Measurement of the quality of life in cancer survivors. *Quality of Life Research, 4*(6), 523–531.

Ferrell, B.R., & Grant, M.M. (2003). Quality of life and symptoms. In C.R. King & P.S. Hinds (Eds.), *Quality of life: From nursing and patient perspectives: Theory, research, practice* (2nd ed., pp. 199–217). Sudbury, MA: Jones and Bartlett.

Ferrell, B.R., Grant, M., Chan, J., Ahn, C., & Ferrell, B.A. (1995). The impact of cancer pain education on family caregivers of elderly patients. *Oncology Nursing Forum, 22*(8), 1211–1218.

Ferrell, B.R., & Griffith, H. (1994). Cost issues related to pain management: Report from the cancer pain panel of the Agency for Health Care Policy and Research. *Journal of Pain and Symptom Management, 9*(4), 221–234.

Gaston-Johansson, F., Fall-Dickson, J.M., Bakos, A.B., & Kennedy, M.J. (1999). Fatigue, pain and depression in pre-autotransplant breast cancer patients. *Cancer Practice, 7*(5), 240–247.

Gift, A.G., Jablonski, A., Stommel, M., & Given, C.W. (2004). Symptom clusters in elderly patients with lung cancer. *Oncology Nursing Forum, 31*(2), 203–212.

Gift, A.G., Stommel, M., Jablonski, A., & Given, C.W. (2003). A cluster of symptoms over time in patients with lung cancer. *Nursing Research, 52*(6), 393–400.

Given, B., Given, C., Azzouz, F., & Stommel, M. (2001). Physical functioning of elderly cancer patients prior to diagnosis and following initial treatment. *Nursing Research, 50*(4), 222–232.

Gobel, B.H., & Donovan, M.I. (1987). Symptom distress: Depression and anxiety. *Seminars in Oncology Nursing, 3*(4), 267–276.

Grant, M. (1987). Symptom distress. Nausea, vomiting, and anorexia. *Seminars in Oncology Nursing, 3*(4), 277–286.

Grant, M. (1999). Surviving and thriving: The nurse scientist in the clinical setting. *Oncology Nursing Forum, 26*(6), 1011–1022.

Grant, M.M., & Dean, G.E. (2003). Evolution of the quality of life in oncology and oncology nursing. In C.R. King & P.S. Hinds (Eds.), *Quality of life: From nursing and patient perspectives: Theory, research, practice* (2nd ed., pp. 3–28). Sudbury, MA: Jones and Bartlett.

Grant, M., Ferrell, B.R., Rivera, L.M., & Lee, J. (1995). Unscheduled readmissions for uncontrolled symptoms: A health care challenge for nurses. *Nursing Clinics of North America, 30*(4), 673–682.

Grant, M., Ferrell, B., Schmidt, G.M., Fonbuena, P., Niland, J.C., & Foreman, S.J. (1992). Measurement of quality of life in bone marrow transplantation survivors. *Quality of Life Research, 1*(6), 375–384.

Haberman, M. (1999). The measurement of symptom distress. In C.H. Yarbro, M.H. Frogge, & M. Goodman (Eds.), *Cancer symptom management* (2nd ed., pp. 10–19). Sudbury, MA: Jones and Bartlett.

Haylock, P.J. (1987). Breathing difficulty: Changes in respiratory function. *Seminars in Oncology Nursing, 3*(4), 293–298.

Hinds, P.S., Burghen, E.A., Haase, J.E., & Phillips, C.R. (2006). Advances in defining, conceptualizing, and measuring quality of life in pediatric patients with cancer. *Oncology Nursing Forum, 33*(Suppl. 1), 23–29.

Johnson, J.E. (1999). Self-Regulation Theory and coping with physical illness. *Research in Nursing and Health, 22*(6), 435–448.

Johnson, J.E., Fieler, V.K., Jones, L.S., Wlasowicz, G.S., & Mitchell, M.L. (1997). *Self-Regulation Theory: Applying theory to your practice.* Pittsburgh, PA: Oncology Nursing Society.

King, C.R. (2001). Dance of life. *Clinical Journal of Oncology Nursing, 5*(1), 29–33.

King, C.R. (2006). Advances in how clinical nurses can evaluate and improve quality of life for individuals with cancer. *Oncology Nursing Forum, 33*(Suppl. 1), 5–12.

King, C.R., Haberman, M., Berry, D.L., Bush, N., Butler, L., Dow, K.H., et al. (1997). Quality of life and the cancer experience: The state of the knowledge. *Oncology Nursing Forum, 24*(1), 27–41.

Lenz, E.R., Pugh, L.C., Milligan, R.A., Gift, A., & Suppe, F. (1997). The middle-range theory of unpleasant symptoms: An update. *Advances in Nursing Science, 19*(3), 14–27.

McCorkle, R. (1987). The measurement of symptom distress. *Seminars in Oncology Nursing, 3*(4), 248–256.

McCorkle, R., & Quint-Benoliel, J. (1983). Symptom distress, current concerns and mood disturbance after diagnosis of life-threatening disease. *Social Science and Medicine, 17*(7), 431–438.

McCorkle, R., & Young, K. (1978). Development of a symptom distress scale. *Cancer Nursing, 1*(5), 373–378.

Miaskowski, C., Dodd, M., & Lee, K. (2004). Symptom clusters: The new frontier in symptom management research. *Journal of the National Cancer Institute Monographs, 32,* 17–21.

Miaskowski, C., & Lee, K.A. (1999). Pain, fatigue, and sleep disturbances in oncology outpatients receiving radiation therapy for bone metastasis: A pilot study. *Journal of Pain and Symptom Management, 17*(5), 320–332.

Mock, V., Pickett, M., Ropka, M.E., Lin, E.M., Stewart, K.J., Rhodes, V.A., et al. (2001). Fatigue and quality of life outcomes of exercise during cancer treatment. *Cancer Practice, 9*(3), 113.

Molassiotis, A., Van Den Akker, O.B., Milligan, D.W., Goldman, J.M., Boughton, B.J., & Holmes, J.A. (1996). Psychological adaptation and symptom distress in bone transplant recipients. *Psycho-Oncology, 5*(1), 9–22.

Mullen, K.H., Berry, D.L., & Zierler, B.K. (2004). Computerized symptom and quality-of-life assessment for patients with cancer. Part II: Acceptability and usability [Online exclusive]. *Oncology Nursing Forum, 31*(5), E84–E89. Retrieved November 15, 2007, from http://ons.metapress.com/content/l5xq425651537746/fulltext.pdf

Nail, L.N., & King, K.B. (1987). Symptom distress: Fatigue. *Seminars in Oncology Nursing, 3*(4), 257–262.

Piper, B. (1993). *Pathophysiological phenomena in nursing: Human responses to illness* (2nd ed.). Philadelphia: Saunders.

Piper, B.F., Dibble, S.L., Dodd, M.J., Weiss, M.C., Slaughter, R.E., & Paul, S.M. (1998). The revised Piper Fatigue Scale: Psychometric evaluation in women with breast cancer. *Oncology Nursing Forum, 25*(4), 677–684.

Quint, J.C. (1963, November). Impact of mastectomy. *American Journal of Nursing, 63,* 88–92.

Redeker, N.S., Lev, E.L., & Ruggiero, J. (2000). Insomnia, fatigue, anxiety, depression, and quality of life of cancer patients undergoing chemotherapy. *Scholarly Inquiry for Nursing Practice, 14*(4), 275–290.

Rhodes, V.A., & Watson, P.M. (1987). Symptom distress—the concept: Past and present. *Seminars in Oncology Nursing, 3*(4), 242–247.

Sarna, L. (1998). Effectiveness of structured nursing assessment of symptom distress in advanced lung cancer. *Oncology Nursing Forum, 25*(6), 1041–1048.

Winningham, M.L., Nail, L.M., Burke, M.B., Brophy, L., Cimprich, B., Jones, L.S., et al. (1994). Fatigue and the cancer experience: The state of the knowledge. *Oncology Nursing Forum, 21*(1), 23–36.

CHAPTER 5

Nursing Science in Palliative Care and End-of-Life Care

Nessa Coyle, NP, PhD, FAAN, and Marilyn Bookbinder, RN, PhD

Introduction

Many patients living with advanced cancer experience a relatively long period of progressive debilitation and decline, with concomitant and multiple interacting symptoms. These symptoms—physical, psychological, social, spiritual, and existential—may be associated with the cancer, its treatment, or both. Health-related quality of life (HRQOL) for these patients and their families is invariably affected. In addition, technologic advances have made it possible to prolong life even when HRQOL is no longer present. Choices seem endless, responsibility and burden of choice are huge, and communication difficulties regarding transitions in goals of care and site of care are frequent. Further complicating this scenario are an aging society; changing family demographics, with smaller family sizes and limited availability of caregivers; and differing values among a multicultural and diverse ethnic population. All are potential areas for nursing research.

Advances in science have transformed cancer from a usually fatal disease to a curable disease for some and a chronic disease for many others. Acknowledging this fact, in 2002 the World Health Organization (WHO) revised its definition of palliative care:

> Palliative care is *an approach* that improves the quality of life
> of patients and their families facing the problem associated
> with life-threatening illness, through the prevention and relief
> of suffering by means of early identification and impeccable

assessment and treatment of pain and other problems, physical, psychosocial, and spiritual. (WHO, 2002)

The National Cancer Policy Board adopted the new WHO definition, recognizing that palliative care is an integral part of comprehensive cancer care,
beginning at the time of diagnosis and increasing in amount and intensity as
death nears. The National Comprehensive Cancer Network (NCCN, 2008)
expanded upon the WHO definition:

- Palliative care is both a philosophy of care and *an organized, highly structured
  system for delivery of care* to persons with life-threatening or debilitating illness.
- *Palliative care is patient- and family-centered care* that focuses on effective management of pain and other distressing symptoms, while incorporating psychosocial and spiritual care according to patient and family needs, values,
  beliefs, and cultures.
- The goals of palliative care are to prevent and relieve suffering and to support the best quality of life for patients and their families, regardless of the
  stage of their disease or need for other therapies.
- *Palliative care can be delivered concurrently with life-prolonging therapy or as the
  main focus of care* (see Figure 5-1).

NCCN (2008) published guidelines to facilitate the appropriate integration
of palliative care into anticancer therapy. The guidelines addressed symptoms
such as pain, anorexia/cachexia, nausea and vomiting, constipation, malignant
bowel obstruction, and delirium, as well as psychosocial distress, goals and
expectations affecting care, advanced care planning, the imminently dying

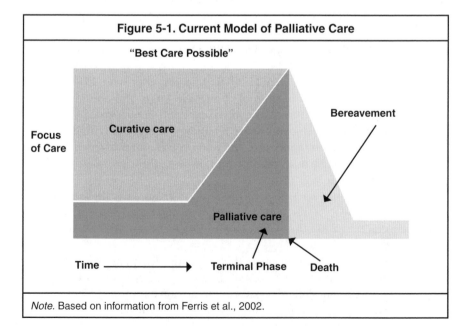

Figure 5-1. Current Model of Palliative Care

"Best Care Possible"

Focus of Care

Curative care

Bereavement

Palliative care

Time ⟶ Terminal Phase Death

Note. Based on information from Ferris et al., 2002.

patient, and care after death. The guidelines are updated annually according to available evidence-based best practices. The work of oncology nurses contributes to this evidence base.

These national and international policy statements and guidelines acknowledge the need to broaden the scope of palliative care beyond end-of-life care and are in concordance that such an approach should be integrated with life-prolonging therapy. The model in which palliative care is intensified at the end of life is the hospice model of care.

State of the Science in Palliative Care and End-of-Life Care

The 1997 Institute of Medicine report *Approaching Death: Improving Care at the End of Life* triggered a series of activities to improve the quality of end-of-life care. By 1999, the National Institute of Nursing Research (NINR), part of the National Institutes of Health (NIH), had begun a series of research solicitations focused on issues related to end-of-life care. Topics included (1) the clinical management of symptoms at the end of life, (2) patterns of communication among patients, families, and providers, (3) ethics and healthcare decision making, (4) caregiver support, (5) the context of care delivery, (6) complementary and alternative medicine at the end of life, (7) dying children of all ages and their families, and (8) informal caregiving.

During this same period, the Study to Understand Prognoses and Preferences for Outcomes and Risks of Treatments (SUPPORT) found that the last six months of life for patients with cancer are characterized by functional decline, poorly controlled severe pain, and confusion (McCarthy, Phillips, Zhong, Drews, & Lynn, 2000). Significant deficits in measuring outcomes of end-of-life care also were identified. These findings, among others, led to the compilation of instruments known as the Toolkit of Instruments to Measure End-of-Life Care (TIME) (Teno, 1997).

To evaluate results of these efforts and the current state of the science in the fields of palliative care and end-of-life care, and to clarify further research priorities, the NINR and the Agency for Healthcare Research and Quality (AHRQ) commissioned an evidence report as the basis for a State-of-the-Science Conference held in Washington, DC, in 2004. Oncology nurse scientists participated in this conference. The following five broad questions were asked (NIH Consensus Development Program, 2004).

1. What defines the transition to end-of-life care?
2. What outcome variables are valid indicators of the quality of the end-of-life experience of the dying person and for the surviving loved one?
3. What patient, family, and healthcare system factors are associated with better or worse outcomes at the end of life?
4. What processes and interventions are associated with improved or worsened outcomes?

5. What are the future research directions for improving end-of-life care?

Three key questions evolved to evaluate progress in palliative and end-of-life care (see Figure 5-2).

The review of the scientific evidence for these key elements of palliative and end-of-life care illuminated both the strengths of the field and the research opportunities for oncology nurses. Evidence supported the association of satisfaction with care and quality of care with pain management, communication, practical support, and enhanced caregiving. The literature review identified evidence to support the effectiveness of interventions to improve satisfaction. These included amelioration of cancer pain, relief of depression, and fostering continuity in cancer care. Areas for future research to strengthen the evidence base for end-of-life care were identified. A summary statement on future directions for improving end-of-life care indicated that although the body of research covering a wide range of issues is growing, in many ways, the research is still in its infancy. This is especially evident in terms of rigorous testing and evaluation of models of care, patient and family outcomes, and resource utilization (Lorenz et al., 2004) (see Figure 5-3).

Figure 5-2. Key Questions to Evaluate Progress in the Field of Palliative and End-of-Life Care

1. What outcome variables are valid indicators of the quality of the end-of-life experience for the dying person and for the surviving loved ones?
   a) What individual outcome measures are most strongly associated with overall satisfaction with end-of-life care?
   b) What is the reliability and validity of specific instruments for measuring quality of life or quality of care at the end of life?
2. What patient, family, and healthcare system factors are associated with better or worse outcomes at end of life?
   a) What individual factors (e.g., age, gender, race/ethnicity, underlying illness, education, etc.) are associated with better to worse outcomes at the end of life?
   b) What family factors (e.g., relationship to the patient, race/ethnicity, etc.) are associated with better or worse outcomes at the end of life, including both outcomes reported by the family and how the family affects outcome experienced by patients?
   c) What healthcare system factors (e.g., site of care, type of provider, support services, etc.) are associated with better or worse outcomes?
3. What processes and interventions are associated with improved or worsened outcomes?
   a) What is the effectiveness of specific healthcare interventions for improving specific outcomes in patients at the end of life?
   b) Does effectiveness of specific interventions vary among different populations?

Note. From *National Institutes of Health State-of-the-Science Conference Statement on Improving End-of-Life Care. National Institutes of Health State-of-the-Science Conference Statement*, by National Institutes of Health Consensus Development Program, December 6–8, 2004. Retrieved May 24, 2007, from http://consensus.nih.gov/2004/2004EndOfLife CareSOS024html.htm

---

Figure 5-3. State-of-the-Science Conclusions in End-of-Life Care

- Circumstances surrounding end of life are poorly understood, leaving many Americans to struggle through this life event.
- The dramatic increase in the number of older adults facing the need for end-of-life care warrants development of a research infrastructure and resources to enhance that care for patients and their families.
- Ambiguity surrounding the definition of end of life hinders the development of science, delivery of care, and communications between patients and providers.
- Current end-of-life care includes some untested interventions that need to be validated.
- Subgroups of race, ethnicity, culture, gender, age, and disease states experience end-of-life care differently, and these differences remain poorly understood.
- Valid measures exist for some aspects of end of life; however, measures have not been used consistently or validated in diverse settings or with diverse groups.
- End-of-life care is often fragmented among providers and provider settings, leading to a lack of continuity of care and impeding the ability to provide high-quality, interdisciplinary care.
- Enhanced communication among patients, families, and providers is crucial to high-quality end-of-life care.
- The design of the current Medicare hospice benefit limits the availability of the full range of interventions needed by many persons at the end of life.

Note. From *National Institutes of Health State-of-the-Science Conference Statement on Improving End-of-Life Care. National Institutes of Health State-of-the-Science Conference Statement,* by National Institutes of Health Consensus Development Program, December 6–8, 2004. Retrieved May 24, 2007, from http://consensus.nih.gov/2004/2004EndOfLife CareSOS024html.htm

---

In 2005, the National Quality Forum initiated a project funded by the Robert Wood Johnson Foundation. The project was designed to endorse a national consensus framework for evaluating the quality of palliative care and hospice care across all health settings and professions, to achieve a consensus on a set of preferred practices for palliative care and hospice care based on the framework, and to identify areas for research in palliative care and hospice care (National Quality Forum, 2006). The framework consisted of eight domains of care important to palliative and end-of-life care: structure and process of care; physical; psychological and psychiatric; social; spiritual, religious, and existential; cultural; the imminently dying patient; and ethics and the law. This framework will be used later in the chapter to illustrate examples of nursing research in palliative and end-of-life care.

Attention also was given to cancer care quality measures, including those at end of life. AHRQ, through its Evidence-Based Practice Centers, sponsored the development of a technical evidence report (TEP) titled "Cancer Care Quality Measures: Symptoms and End-of-Life Care" (Lorenz et al., 2006). The TEP's purpose was to assist both public- and private-sector organizations in their quality improvement efforts. The TEP identified evidence-based quality measures to support quality assessment and improvement in the palliative care of patients with cancer in the areas of pain, dyspnea, depression, and advance care planning. Of the 537 articles that met the TEP criteria for review, only 25 contained quality measures—21 on advance care planning, 4 on depression, 2 on dyspnea, and 12 on pain—of which only a few had been specifically tested in a cancer population. It should be noted that oncology nurse scientists contributed both to the identified studies and the development of the evidence-based report.

These findings suggest that in spite of the prevalence of cancer and its enormous cost to the individual and to society on so many levels, little progress has occurred in systematization of quality-of-care assessments. In addition, although a large number of assessment measures are available, testing them in relevant populations still is urgently needed. Basic research that addresses measurement in populations with impaired ability to self-report also is lacking. Oncology nurse scientists can make a difference in these key research areas.

Research in Palliative Care and End-of-Life Care

Why Is It So Difficult?

Palliative care research is especially challenging given the vulnerability of this population, the changing nature of patients' illnesses, and the complexities of the phenomena to be studied. Longitudinal studies, although extremely important, are difficult to complete. Patients frequently are distressed by the multiple symptoms and cognitive impairment associated with both general organ failure and the numerous medications used to relieve symptoms. Family members are under pressure from changes in family dynamics, grief, accumulative losses, exhaustion (both emotional and physical), and a desire to protect their loved one from any added burden. As well, healthcare professionals may be protective of "their" patients, not wanting to add any additional "burden" of being a research participant (Ferrell & Grant, 2006; Watson, Lucas, Hoy, & Back, 2005) (see Figure 5-4).

Although difficulties in recruitment and high rates of subject attrition can be very discouraging to the researcher, strong arguments exist for conducting research with patients who are approaching the end of life and their families. It is an unavoidable imperative because evidence-based care leading to best practices at the end of life cannot be extrapolated from other populations. Despite the vulnerability of these patients and their families, and the stringent criteria for research design and ethical scrutiny that are necessary, patients who are terminally ill and their families should not be deprived of the opportunity to participate in research. Some patients and families genuinely want to participate so that future patients may benefit (Ferrell & Grant, 2006; Watson et al., 2005).

Figure 5-4. Difficulties in Palliative Care Research

Practical Considerations
- Attrition of patients from studies leads to difficulties in recruiting adequate numbers of patients, particularly for qualitative studies.
- Eligibility criteria for inclusion in studies, particularly if the patient is deteriorating, restrict the inclusion of adequate numbers.
- Measures of end points and outcomes often are complicated in the already complex clinical scenario.
- Compliance of deteriorating patients may be difficult to sustain.

Ethical and Emotional Considerations
- Patients often are considered to be too unwell with distressing symptoms to be asked to participate in research.
- Some professionals feel that patients with a short prognosis should not have extra burdens placed on them.
- Patients are vulnerable and may be exploited.
- The research may be of no benefit to the patient taking part.
- Questionnaires, if used, may be painful and intrusive either for patients, families, or in bereavement.
- Fully informed consent may be difficult to obtain; patients may try to please the researcher by agreeing to take part when they do not really want to; patients may feel their doctor will become less interested in them or transfer them to another's care if they refuse to participate; and patients are frequently cognitively impaired.
- Participating in any new protocol, even phase I, may encourage unrealistic expectations in patients. Their focus may be on the protocol and the illness rather than on how best to spend the short time left to them.

Note. From "Research in Palliative Care" (p. 32), by M.S. Watson, C.F. Lucas, A.M. Hoy, and I.N. Back (Eds.), *Oxford Handbook of Palliative Care,* 2005, New York: Oxford University Press. Copyright 2005 by Oxford University Press. Adapted with permission.

What About Methodology?

Although quantitative research and randomized controlled trials are considered the gold standard of evidence-based research, oncology nurses recognize that qualitative research methodology has a special place in palliative care and end-of-life research. Qualitative research and palliative care have common philosophical underpinnings. Both have an emphasis on understanding individual experiences that may not fit into established categories of knowledge. Both recognize that each person's perspective is unique, complex, and multifaceted. Personal experience is valued as one means of determining what is relevant to care and research. The varying ways people perceive and interpret their experiences as they construct meaning are respected (Kristjanson & Coyle, 2005).

Both palliative care and qualitative research recognize the need for a very flexible approach to accommodate the particular circumstances of this population of patients, families, and caregivers. These challenges offer opportunities for oncology nurse scientists to use qualitative methods that can circumvent some of the difficulties described. For example, use of a qualitative design may allow the researcher to examine variations within an illness trajectory more closely. The more personal and flexible approach afforded by qualitative methods can facilitate patient participation and decrease the magnitude of attrition. Most importantly, qualitative research methods allow patient and family participants to "give voice" to what is happening to them—they are the experts (Kristjanson & Coyle, 2005).

Oncology nurse scientists increasingly are using a mixed-method approach (combining different methods into a research strategy) in palliative care and end-of-life research. Pain as a multidimensional experience is an example well suited for this approach. A word of caution: Members of many institutional review boards are unfamiliar with the philosophical underpinnings, language, and methods of qualitative research and may present a particular challenge to qualitative nurse scientists.

How Well Is Research in Palliative and End-of-Life Care Represented in Oncology Nursing?

In 2000 and 2004, the Oncology Nursing Society (ONS) surveyed its general membership regarding research priorities (Cohen, Harle, Woll, Despa, & Munsell, 2004). Respondents ranked, by mean importance, their top 20 research priorities. Despite low general response rates, results from both surveys identified eight topics clearly related to palliative care and/or end-of-life care: (1) HRQOL, (2) participation in decision making about treatment in advanced disease, (3) pain, (4) palliative care, (5) fatigue/lack of energy, (6) cognitive impairment/mental changes, (7) hospice/end of life, and (8) ethical issues. Although these results indicated that the interest in palliative care and end-of-life research exists, the low response rate to the surveys presents a challenge as to how to "capture" the bedside oncology nurse's "voice" in identifying research priorities.

In 2006, Molassiotis et al. published a systematic review of worldwide cancer nursing research spanning 23 countries and covering years 1994–2003. The primary source for the review was the Cumulative Index of Nursing and Allied Health Literature. A total of 619 papers met the review criteria. Study populations included adult patients with cancer (49.8%). The setting, location, or source of information for the studies was 71% in a hospital or a cancer center and only 1.7% in a hospice setting. Symptoms were the most common study focus—predominantly pain and fatigue. Approximately 22% of the study participants had advanced disease, suggesting that patients with advanced cancer and at the end of life were underrepresented. Few studies addressed the needs of caregivers, a similarly underrepresented population.

Each year, ONS recognizes one oncology nurse scientist for his or her research program. A number of the ONS Distinguished Researchers (see

Chapter 2, Table 2-3) are known for their work in palliative care and end-of-life care, including Ruth McCorkle, Barbara A. Given, Betty R. Ferrell, Christine A. Miaskowski, Lesley F. Degner, and Carol E. Ferrans. Many other oncology nurses have contributed to the growing evidence base in these areas.

A few examples of oncology nursing research in palliative care and end-of-life care are illustrated in the following sections. These reflect a broad range of research interests, using both quantitative and qualitative research methods as well as multidisciplinary research. In general, the highlighted nurse scientists have a focused body of palliative care and end-of-life research spanning several decades. Some, however, are at the beginning of their research careers. The studies cited include cancer populations but may involve other patients with life-threatening illness as well. Research that focuses on specific symptoms, such as pain, dyspnea, and delirium, deliberately has been excluded as these were discussed in Chapter 4.

Caring for a Dying Family Member at Home and the Effect on the Family

Given et al. (2004) studied the patient and family caregiver variables that predicted caregiver burden and depression for family caregivers of patients with cancer at the end of life. This prospective, longitudinal study followed a cohort of patients and their family caregivers from time of diagnosis and treatment of cancer until the patients' deaths. Telephone interviews with patients were conducted at 6–8 weeks, 12–16 weeks, 24–30 weeks, and 52 weeks following diagnosis. The scientists examined the experiences of 152 family caregivers whose family members died during the course of the study. Although caregivers aged 45–54 reported the highest levels of depressive symptoms, caregivers aged 35–44 reported the strongest sense of abandonment. Depressive symptoms were high in caregivers who were employed and those who were the adult children of patients with cancer. Female, nonspouse, and adult children caregivers more often reported feeling abandoned. Adult children caregivers of patients with early-stage cancer and patients with multiple symptoms reported a high perception of disruption in their schedules. Caregivers whose family members died soon after diagnosis reported the highest depressive symptoms, burden, and impact on schedule.

McCorkle, Robinson, Nuamah, Lev, and Benoliel (1998) studied the effects of home nursing care for terminally ill patients with lung cancer on survivor psychological distress during bereavement. Randomly assigned to an oncology homecare (OHC) group, a standard homecare group, or an office-care control group, 46 patient-spousal dyads were entered into the study two months following a lung cancer diagnosis and were followed until the patients' deaths. Surviving spouses received follow-up for 25 months after the patients' deaths. Initially, psychological distress was significantly lower among spouses assigned to the OHC group compared with the other two groups. Subscales of depression and paranoid ideation indicated significant mean group differences, whereas subscales of hostility and psychoticism revealed marginal group differences. At 25 months, no significant differences were prevalent among the groups. The results of this analysis suggested that psychological distress associated with recent bereavement can be influenced positively, dependent upon how patients are cared for during the terminal phase (McCorkle et al.).

Noting the scarcity of empirical evidence that might help clinicians to identify family caregivers at risk of poor psychosocial functioning, Hudson, Hayman-White, Aranda, and Kristjanson (2006) performed a secondary analysis of baseline data from a larger study to ascertain if the psychological functioning of family members caring for a terminally ill patient with cancer was possible to predict. Data were obtained at the start of home-based palliative care services and five weeks later from 35 family caregivers. Caregivers completed instruments measuring caregiver preparedness, competence, mastery, social support, anxiety, and self-efficacy. Logistic and cluster analyses showed that self-reported anxiety and competence subscale total scores at the time home-based palliative care services began were associated with family caregivers being at risk for lower levels of psychosocial functioning after five weeks. The authors noted that their results need to be replicated in a larger sample before the use of this approach as a screening tool can be recommended (Hudson et al.).

Other studies by members of this group that looked at the vulnerabilities of families caring for the dying include the evaluation of a modified version of Parkes' (1993) Bereavement Risk Index (BRI) (Kristjanson, Cousins, Smith, & Lewin, 2005). The study aimed to test the validity, reliability, and feasibility of using a modified version of the BRI and a bereavement support protocol in a home hospice care setting. The study also explored what types of family members were likely to experience a more difficult bereavement. One hundred-fifty bereaved family members participated in this prospective, descriptive study. Based on BRI scores, bereaved family members were classified as high, medium, or low risk and received a structured bereaved support protocol according to their risk level. Results showed that a four-item version of the BRI was more internally consistent than the longer version; the shorter version demonstrated good predictive validity when correlated with outcome measures three months after the patient's death. The four items that were sufficient to assess risk of complicated bereavement were clinging or pining behavior, anger, self-reproach, and a general opinion of how well the bereaved person is likely to cope. The investigators concluded that the modified BRI demonstrated acceptable reliability and validity and was brief and easy to use (Kristjanson et al.).

A Greater Understanding of Death and Dying

Steeves and Kahn (2006) described their approach to end-of-life research as stepping back from the immediate demands of alleviating symptoms to a more distanced position as participant-observer: "We watch and interview and consider the dying of patients from as many points of view as possible: patient, family, and clinicians, as well as our own. The result of these observations is a text, the written account of what we have seen and have been told" (Steeves & Kahn, pp. 1209–1210). According to Steeves and Kahn, an analysis of these stories leads to a greater understanding of the experience of death, dying, and bereavement.

Using interpretive phenomenology, Coyle and Sculco (2004) examined the meanings and uses of an expressed desire for hastened death from the patients' perspectives. The findings were part of an exploratory qualitative study that examined the firsthand accounts of seven patients at an urban cancer research center who were living with advanced disease and had at least once expressed a desire for hastened death. A series of in-depth, semistructured interviews were audiotaped, transcribed, coded, and organized into themes. The expression of a desire for hastened death was found to have many meanings and uses, including (Coyle & Sculco)

- Manifestation of the will to live
- A dying process so difficult that an early death was preferred
- An intolerable immediate situation, even if not specifically identified by the patient, required immediate action
- A hastened death could extract a patient from an unendurable and specific situation
- A manifestation of the last control the dying person can exert
- A way of drawing attention to "me as a unique individual"
- A gesture of altruism
- An attempt at manipulation of the family in order to avoid abandonment
- A despairing cry depicting the misery of the current situation.

Coyle (2006), using a similar approach but asking a different question from the data, examined, from the patients' perspectives, the work of trying to live with advanced cancer while simultaneously facing the immediacy of death. Three subthemes emerged from the data, reflecting the hard work these patients undertook: orienting themselves to the disease and maintaining control, searching for and creating a system of support and safety, and struggling to find meaning and to create a legacy. These findings confirm that living with advanced cancer while facing one's own death is not easy and is not a passive enterprise.

Racial Differences in the Way Individuals Approach the End of Life

Important differences between African Americans and Caucasians regarding end-of-life decision making have been identified and provide a more "nuanced" way of understanding the experience of facing death. For example, in the Hopp and Duffy (2000) study, which looked at the differences between African Americans and Caucasians aged 70 years and older, Caucasians were found to be significantly more likely than African Americans to discuss treatment preferences before death, to complete a living will, and to designate a durable power of attorney. Although Caucasians were more likely to base treatment decisions on limiting care in certain situations and withholding treatment before death, African Americans were more likely to base treatment decisions on the desire to prolong life by providing all possible care. Study findings suggested that, even after controlling for sociodemographic factors, important differences exist between African Americans and Caucasians in approaching advance care planning and end-of-life decision making. Further studies are needed to elucidate the array of end-of-life preferences among racial and ethnic groups and why these differences exist (Hopp & Duffy). This is an important area for nursing research.

Psychosocial and Existential Distress at the End of Life

Lin and Bauer-Wu (2003) conducted an integrative literature review that identified 43 research investigations into the psychospiritual well-being of patients with advanced cancer. The studies were undertaken in 14 countries and were conducted by scientists from various disciplines, including nursing. Six major recurring themes appeared as critical components of psychospiritual well-being: self-awareness, coping and adjusting effectively with stress, relationships and connectedness with others, sense of faith, sense of empowerment and confidence, and living with meaning and hope (Lin & Bauer-Wu).

The concept of dignity is tied into these six major themes. Dignity therapy (an approach to address psychosocial and existential distress among the terminally ill) and advancing the science of spiritual care in terminal illness is a growing area of palliative care and end-of-life care research. Several studies were conducted that examined the notion of dignity and how it is understood and experienced by people as they approach death. In a multicenter investigation conducted in Canada, Australia, and the United States, Chochinov et al. (2005) studied the feasibility of dignity therapy and whether it had an effect on a variety of measures of psychosocial and existential distress. The study population included terminally ill inpatients and those receiving home-based palliative care. Patients completed pre- and postintervention measures of a sense of dignity, depression, suffering, and hopelessness, as well as a sense of purpose, a sense of meaning, the desire for death, the will to live, and suicidality (Chochinov et al.).

Postintervention patients reported the following (Chochinov et al., 2005).
- Satisfaction with dignity therapy (91%)
- A feeling that the therapy had been or would be of help to their family (81%)
- A heightened sense of dignity (76%)
- An increased sense of purpose (68%)
- A heightened sense of meaning (67%)
- An increased will to live (47%)

Significant improvement was noted in suffering and reduced depressive symptoms (Chochinov et al., 2005). The investigators concluded that dignity therapy shows promise for alleviating suffering and distress at the end of life. Linda Kristjanson, an established nurse scientist, was one of the lead investigators in this study.

Oncology nurse scientists also have been involved in intervention studies to increase hope and HRQOL. For example, Duggleby et al. (2007) evaluated the effectiveness of the "Living With Hope Program" (LWHP), a psychosocial supportive intervention intended to increase hope and HRQOL for terminally ill patients with cancer older than 60 years of age who were living at home. The LWHP comprises viewing a video on hope and choosing one of three hope activities to work on over a one-week period. This study, using a mixed-method concurrent nested experimental design, randomly assigned 60 terminally ill patients with cancer to either a treatment group or a control group. Findings indicated that patients in the treatment group had statistically significant higher hope scores and QOL scores at the second visit than patients in the control group. Specifically, 61.5% of those in the treatment group reported that the LWHP increased their hope. Although preliminary, this evaluation suggests that the LWHP may increase hope and QOL for older terminally ill patients with cancer at home (Duggleby et al.).

Betty R. Ferrell and Marcia Grant from City of Hope National Medical Center in California have built a program of extraordinarily well-funded HRQOL and palliative care research. Through both independent and collaborative work, they have focused not only on the needs of patients with advanced cancer but also on the needs of the families and the nurses who care for them. These nurse scientists have used both quantitative and qualitative research methods. Examples of their work include HRQOL in women with ovarian cancer (Grant et al., 1992); the symptom experience of women with ovarian cancer based on an analysis of data consisting of 21,806 letters, cards, and e-mails written by patients with ovarian cancer that were donated to the City of Hope investigators (Ferrell, Smith, Cullinane, & Melancon, 2003); a three-phase study (epidemiologic, qualitative, and quantitative) on decisions and outcomes of palliative surgery (McCahill et al., 2002, 2003); and research in palliative care and end-of-life care nursing education (Ferrell et al., 2005; Paice et al., 2006). The moral distress of nurses witnessing futile care also has been documented (Ferrell, 2006).

Quality Improvement in Palliative Care

Benchmarking Palliative Care

Twaddle et al. (2007) sought to benchmark the quality of palliative care services in 35 academic hospitals. This multidisciplinary team used a multicenter, cross-sectional, retrospective design and reviewed 1,596 patient records against 11 key performance measures (KPMs) (see Figure 5-5) derived from evidence-based practice standards. Results suggested wide variability in adherence among hospitals, ranging from 0%–100% (with 0 meaning no adherence and 100% meaning complete adherence). Greater improvement in KPMs indicated greater improvement in quality outcomes, cost, and length of stay. Institutions that benchmarked above 90% did so by incorporating KPMs into care processes and using systematized triggers, forms, and default pathways (Twaddle et al.). These results suggested that a "palliative care bundle" (i.e., selected KPMs) leads to improvement in areas of deficiency when all components of care are given to patients. For example, patients who had pain and other symptoms and who were assessed within 48 hours of admission were more likely to report relief of the symptoms within the same time frame than those patients who were not assessed. Nurses were coinvestigators in this research effort.

Figure 5-5. Key Performance Measures in a Palliative Care "Bundle"

1. Pain assessment within 48 hours of admission
2. Use of a quantitative pain rating scale
3. Reduction or relief of pain within 48 hours of admission
4. Bowel regimen ordered with opioid administration
5. Dyspnea assessment within 48 hours of admission
6. Reduction or relief of dyspnea within 48 hours of admission
7. Documentation of patient status (prognosis, psychosocial symptoms, functional status, overall symptom distress) within 48 hours of admission
8. Psychosocial assessment within the last year or four days after admission
9. Patient/family meeting to discuss patient treatment preferences or plans for discharge disposition within four days of admission
10. Documentation of discharge plan within four days of admission
11. Arrangement of services required for discharge

Note. Based on information from Twaddle et al., 2007.

Developing and Testing a Palliative Care Pathway for Advanced Disease

An urban institution identified the need to develop a systematic approach to the care of dying patients. A nurse-led multidisciplinary palliative care research team selected three hospital floors (oncology, geriatrics, and an inpatient palliative care/hospice unit) on which to develop and test the Palliative Care for Advanced Disease Pathway (PCAD). Two general medical units received the usual care. Four indices from a chart audit tool evaluated change over time in the mean number of (a) symptoms assessed, (b) problematic symptoms addressed, (c) interventions consistent with PCAD, and (d) consultations requested. Results showed that patients on PCAD were more likely to have do-not-resuscitate orders, more symptoms assessed, more problematic symptoms addressed, and more interventions consistent with state-of-the-science end-of-life care than the comparison units (Bookbinder et al., 2005). These results suggested that a clinical pathway may serve as an important treatment and educational tool to improve the care of the imminently dying inpatient.

Conclusion

This brief overview has emphasized the importance of palliative care and end-of-life care to oncology nursing and has underscored the contributions that nurse scientists have made and are making to the field. Only a very small part of their work has been highlighted in this chapter. Clearly, the scope of research needed in palliative care and end-of-life care remains huge and continues to be an extraordinarily rich and fruitful area for nursing research.

References

Bookbinder, M.B., Blank, A.E., Arney, E., Wollner, D., Lesage, P., McHugh, M., et al. (2005). Improving end-of-life care: Development and pilot-test of a clinical pathway. *Journal of Pain and Symptom Management, 29*(6), 529–543.

Chochinov, H.M., Hack, T., Hassard, T., Kristjanson, L.J., McClement, S., & Harlos, M. (2005). Dignity therapy: A novel psychotherapeutic intervention for patients near the end of life. *Journal of Clinical Oncology, 23*(24), 5520–5525.

Cohen, M.Z., Harle, M., Woll, A.M., Despa, S., & Munsell, M.F. (2004). Delphi survey of nursing research priorities. *Oncology Nursing Forum, 31*(5), 1011–1018.

Coyle, N. (2006). The hard work of living in the face of death. *Journal of Pain and Symptom Management, 32*(3), 266–274.

Coyle, N., & Sculco, L. (2004). Expressed desire for hastened death in seven patients living with advanced cancer: A phenomenologic inquiry. *Oncology Nursing Forum, 31*(4), 699–709.

Duggleby, W.D., Degner, L., Williams, A., Wright, K., Cooper, D., Popkin, D., et al. (2007). Living with hope: Initial evaluation of a psychosocial hope intervention for older palliative home care patients. *Journal of Pain and Symptom Management, 33*(3), 247–257.

Ferrell, B.R. (2006). Understanding the moral distress of nurses witnessing medically futile care. *Oncology Nursing Forum, 33*(5), 922–930.

Ferrell, B.R., & Grant, M. (2006). Nursing research. In B.R. Ferrell & N. Coyle (Eds.), *Textbook of palliative nursing* (2nd ed., p. 1093–1106). New York: Oxford University Press.

Ferrell, B.R., Smith, S., Cullinane, C., & Melancon, C. (2003). Symptom concerns of women with ovarian cancer. *Journal of Pain and Symptom Management, 25*(6), 528–538.

Ferrell, B.R., Virani, R., Grant, M., Rhome, A., Malloy, P., Bednash, G., et al. (2005). Evaluation of the End-of-Life Nursing Education Consortium undergraduate faculty training program. *Journal of Palliative Medicine, 8*(1), 107–114.

Ferris, F.D., Balfour, H.M., Bowen, K., Farley, J., Hardwick, M., Lamontagne, C., et al. (2002). A model to guide patient and family care: Based on nationally accepted principles and norms of practice. *Journal of Pain and Symptom Management, 24*(2), 106–123.

Given, B., Wyatt, G., Given, C., Sherwood, P., Gift, A., DeVoss, D., et al. (2004). Burden and depression among caregivers of patients with cancer at the end of life. *Oncology Nursing Forum, 31*(6), 1105–1117.

Grant, M., Ferrell, B.R., Schmidt, G.M., Fonbuena, P., Niland, J.C., & Forman, S.J. (1992). Measurement of quality of life of bone marrow transplantation survivors. *Quality of Life Research, 1*(6), 375–384.

Hopp, F.P., & Duffy, S.A. (2000). Racial variations in end-of-life care. *Journal of the American Geriatrics Society, 48*(6), 658–663.

Hudson, P.L., Hayman-White, K., Aranda, S., & Kristjanson, L.J. (2006). Predicting family caregiver psychosocial functioning in palliative care. *Journal of Palliative Care, 22*(3), 133–140.

Institute of Medicine. (1997). *Approaching death: Improving care at the end of life.* Washington, DC: National Academies Press.

Kristjanson, L., & Coyle, N. (2005). Qualitative research. In D. Doyle, G. Hanks, N. Cherny, & K. Calman (Eds.), *Oxford textbook of palliative medicine* (3rd ed., pp. 138–143). New York: Oxford University Press.

Kristjanson, L.J., Cousins, K., Smith, J., & Lewin, G. (2005). Evaluation of the Bereavement Risk Index (BRI): A community hospice care protocol. *International Journal of Palliative Nursing, 11*(12), 612–618.

Lin, H.R., & Bauer-Wu, S.M. (2003). Psycho-spiritual well-being in patients with advanced cancer: An integrative review of the literature. *Journal of Advanced Nursing, 44*(1), 69–80.

Lorenz, K., Lynn, J., Morton, S.C., Dy, S., Mularski, R., Shugarman, L., et al. (2004). *End-of-life care and outcomes. Evidence Report/Technology Assessment No. 110.* (Prepared by the Southern California Evidence-Based Practice Center under Contract No. 290-02-003.) [AHRQ Publication No. 05-E004-1]. Rockville, MD: Agency for Healthcare Research and Quality.

Lorenz, K., Lynn, K., Dy, S., Mularski, R., Shugarman, L., Sun, V., et al. (2006). *Cancer care quality measures: Symptoms and end-of-life care. Evidence Report/Technology Assessment No. 137.* (Prepared by the Southern California Evidence-Based Practice Center under Contract No. 290-02-003.) [AHRQ Publication No. 06-E001]. Rockville, MD: Agency for Healthcare Research and Quality.

McCahill, L.E., Krouse, R.S., Chu, D.Z., Juarez, G., Uman, G.C., Ferrell, B.R., et al. (2002). Decision making in palliative surgery. *Journal of the American College of Surgeons, 195*(3), 411–422.

McCahill, L.E., Smith, D.D., Borneman, T., Juarez, G., Cullinane, C., Chu, D.Z., et al. (2003). A prospective evaluation of palliative outcomes for surgery of advanced malignancies. *Annals of Surgical Oncology, 10*(6), 654–663.

McCarthy, E.P., Phillips, R.S., Zhong, Z., Drews, R.E., & Lynn, J. (2000). Dying with cancer: Patients' function, symptoms, and care preferences as death approaches. *Journal of the American Geriatrics Society, 48*(Suppl. 5), S110–S121.

McCorkle, R., Robinson, L., Nuamah, I., Lev, E., & Benoliel, J.Q. (1998). The effects of home nursing care for patients during terminal illness on the bereaved's psychological distress. *Nursing Research, 47*(1), 2–10.

Molassiotis, A., Gibson, F., Kelly, D., Richardson, A., Dabbour, R., Ahmad, A.M., et al. (2006). A systematic review of worldwide cancer nursing research: 1994 to 2003. *Cancer Nursing, 29*(6), 431–440.

National Comprehensive Cancer Network. (2008). *NCCN Clinical Practice Guidelines in Oncology™: Palliative care* [v.1.2008]. Retrieved May 24, 2008, from http://www.nccn.org/professionals/physician_gls/PDF/palliative.pdf

National Institutes of Health Consensus Development Program. (2004). *National Institutes of Health State-of-the-Science Conference Statement on Improving End-of-Life Care. National Institutes of Health state-of-the-science conference statement. December 6–8, 2004.* Retrieved May 24, 2007, from http://consensus.nih.gov/2004/2004EndOfLifeCareSOS024html.htm

National Quality Forum. (2006). *A national framework and preferred practices for palliative and hospice care quality.* Retrieved May 24, 2007, from http://www.qualityforum.org/publications/reports/palliative.asp

Paice, J.A., Ferrell, B.R., Virani, R., Grant, M., Malloy, P., & Rhome, A. (2006). Appraisal of the Graduate End-of-Life Nursing Education Consortium training program. *Journal of Palliative Medicine, 9*(2), 353–360.

Parkes, C.M. (1993). Bereavement. In D. Doyle, G.C.W. Hanks, & N. MacDonald (Eds.), *Oxford textbook of palliative medicine* (pp. 663–678). New York: Oxford University Press.

Steeves, R., & Kahn, D. (2006). Understanding a good death: James's story. In B.R. Ferrell & N. Coyle (Eds.), *Textbook of palliative nursing* (2nd ed., pp. 1209–1215). New York: Oxford University Press.

Teno, J.M. (1997). *TIME: Toolkit of instruments to measure end-of-life care.* Retrieved May 24, 2007, from http://www.chcr.brown.edu/pcoc/toolkit.htm

Twaddle, M.L., Maxwell, T.L., Cassel, J.B., Liao, S., Coyne, P.J., Usher, B.M., et al. (2007). Palliative care benchmarks from academic medical centers. *Journal of Palliative Medicine, 10*(1), 86–98.

Watson, M.S., Lucas, C.F., Hoy, A.M., & Back, I.N. (Eds.). (2005). Research in palliative care. *Oxford handbook of palliative care* (pp. 27–32). New York: Oxford University Press.

World Health Organization. (2002). *WHO definition of palliative care.* Retrieved May 24, 2007, from http://www.who.int/cancer/palliative/definition

SECTION III

LEADING CAUSES
OF CANCER

CHAPTER 6

Focus on Breast Cancer

Karen Meneses, PhD, RN, FAAN

Introduction

Breast cancer is the leading cause of cancer in women and is the second leading cause of female cancer death in the United States (American Cancer Society, 2007). Breast cancer survival rates have declined by 3.5% per year from 2001 to 2004. Breast cancer death rates also have declined since 1990. Survivors of breast cancer, defined as one from the moment of diagnosis to death, represent the largest group of cancer survivors. Their participation in oncology nursing research has contributed enormously to improving the knowledge and understanding of cancer. Oncology nurse scientists—past, present, and future—owe a debt of gratitude to survivors of breast cancer and their many contributions. With this in mind, the purposes of this chapter are to (a) highlight the significant contributions of oncology nursing research in breast cancer, (b) discuss the current state of the science in the understanding of research in breast cancer, (c) describe the gaps in the understanding of oncology nursing science, and (d) look to the future for further directions in oncology nursing research and breast cancer.

A Historic Review

From the early beginnings in the 1970s, oncology nursing research focused on individual case studies and nursing care of women with breast cancer (Brown & Kiss, 1979; Cox, 1979; Dixon, Moritz, & Baker, 1978; Dostal & Elder, 1979; Fitzpatrick, 1970a, 1970b; Giannola, 1979; Kay, 1979; Koyama, Wada, Nishizawa, Iwanaga, & Aoki, 1977; Krumm, 1979; Leo, Stanton, & Brus, 1979; Lewis & Bloom, 1978; Morris, Greer, & White, 1977; Warren, 1979). Much of the work centered on observations by nurses caring for women receiving treatment for breast cancer.

The 1980s saw a shift in breast cancer studies from care during treatment to the broader cancer continuum from screening and early detection to rehabilitation. Dow and Coleman (1996) reported on 88 breast cancer research studies conducted from 1980 to 1994. They grouped the review of breast cancer studies conducted by nurses into the following categories: prevention, risk factors, screening and early detection, diagnosis, treatment, and rehabilitation. During this time period, no published oncology nursing research studies existed on prevention, and only two studies had been done on breast cancer risk. The vast majority of studies reviewed were early-detection practices, specifically the Health Belief Model and its application to breast self-examination (BSE) practices. Two instrument-development studies on BSE and attitudes about BSE also were published during this time period.

The late 1980s saw the beginning of studies related to psychosocial issues and functional status in breast cancer during diagnosis and treatment. Within the context of standard breast cancer treatments during the late 1980s, comparisons between mastectomy and radiation therapy outcomes also began to appear. Early descriptions of other symptoms such as fatigue, pain, and skin changes that occurred during surgery, chemotherapy, and radiation therapy also were found in the literature (Dodd, 1984, 1988; Hassey, 1985, 1988; Janz, Becker, Anderson, & Marcoux, 1989; Lewis, Ellison, & Woods, 1985; Lewis, Woods, Hough, & Bensley, 1989; Lindsey, Dodd, & Kaempfer, 1987).

Arathuzik (1991) published one of the first symptom management studies for pain in advanced breast cancer. As the 1990s progressed, a plethora of focused symptom management studies began to appear. These studies examined common acute symptoms such as pain, nausea, vomiting, hair loss, anorexia, weight gain, and fatigue. From the mid-1990s to the present, quality of life, survivorship, genetics, and prevention and early-detection studies of breast cancer emerged in the literature.

The following section describes oncology nursing contributions to advancing nursing science through research in breast cancer. The work of several scientists with long-standing programs of research dedicated to breast cancer is highlighted. By no means is the following section an exhaustive description of the remarkable contributions made to advancing nursing science.

Oncology Nursing Contributions to Advancing Nursing Science

Oncology nurse scientists have made vital contributions in the area of breast cancer for nearly 40 years. The topical areas include breast cancer screening and early detection, hot flashes, lymphedema, sleep disturbance, sexuality and fertility, cognitive changes, and psychosocial adjustment and family relationships.

Screening and Early Detection

The first paper on the nurse's role in the early detection of breast cancer appeared in *Nursing Forum* in 1965 (Lewison, 1965). Thirteen years later, in 1978, Susan Hubbard published a paper dedicated to the same topic. Eight years later, in 1985, Victoria Champion published the first research describing the results of a study based on the Health Belief Model, a tool to determine the frequency of BSE using a convenience sample of more than 300 women. This paper was the beginning of a long research career trajectory describing adherence to screening and the early detection of breast cancer. Contributions by Champion and her research team have made significant strides in nurses' understanding of the Health Belief Model and BSE (Champion, 1985, 1987, 1988, 1992b) and adherence and compliance to mammography screening (Champion, 1988, 1994a, 1994b, 1994c; Champion & Huster, 1995; Champion & Menon, 1997; Champion & Miller, 1996).

In 1997, Champion refocused her research efforts on tailoring interventions to improve health behaviors in breast cancer screening (Champion, Foster, & Menon, 1997). This work shifted to a tailored approach based on individual data and beliefs about screening, thus beginning an odyssey into the use of tailored interventions to increase mammography screening in older women (Champion et al., 2003). Critical variables such as race and age were taken into consideration in her conceptual model (Champion, 1990, 1992a; Champion et al., 2003; Champion & Menon, 1997; Champion & Miller, 1996). Champion's program of research made significant strides in the understanding of telephone versus print tailoring for mammography adherence and the effectiveness of nurse-delivered interventions (Champion, 1995; Champion et al., 2006). She later developed a self-efficacy scale for mammography based on Bandura's theoretical framework (Champion, Skinner, & Menon, 2005). Therefore, her intervention research has had far-reaching implications beyond screening and early detection.

Another notable oncology nurse scientist who has made vast contributions to screening and early-detection practices in breast cancer is Elizabeth Ann Coleman (Coleman, 1991; Coleman, Coon, & Fitzgerald, 2001; Coleman, Coon, Fitzgerald, & Cantrell, 2001; Coleman, Coon, et al., 2003; Coleman & Feuer, 1992; Coleman et al., 2002, 2004; Coleman & Heard, 2001; Coleman, Lord, Bowie, & Worley, 1993; Coleman, Lord, et al., 2003; Coleman & O'Sullivan, 2001). Her work has improved the knowledge in this area, particularly in screening and early detection among rural African American women.

The study of factors and behaviors influencing screening and early detection in breast cancer has been a fruitful area of research and clinical interest among other oncology nurses (Ali, 1991; Black, Frisina, Hack, & Carpio, 2006; Brant, Fallsdown, & Iverson, 1999; Brown & Williams, 1994; Caplan & Coughlin, 1998; Coleman et al., 1993; Crooks & Jones, 1989; Culver & Alexander, 1989; Devine & Frank, 2000; Doogan, 1991; Elkind, 1980; Facione &

Katapodi, 2000; Ford et al., 1997; Gullatte, Phillips, & Gibson, 2006; Houfek, Waltman, & Kile, 1997; Judkins & Boutwell, 1991; Kochanczyk, 1982; Leight & Leslie, 1998; Leslie, 1995; Lillington, Gilbert, & Morales, 1991; Lillington, Padilla, Sayre, & Chlebowski, 1993; Mahon, 1993, 2003; Nettles-Carlson, 1989; Nielsen, 1989; Rudolph & McDermott, 1987; Smith, 1995; Stromborg, 1982; Wu & Bancroft, 2006; Yarbrough & Braden, 2001).

Hot Flashes

Hot flashes are a bothersome and troubling side effect of adjuvant therapy (Knobf, 1998, 2001, 2002; Schultz, Klein, Beck, Stava, & Sellin, 2005; Zibecchi, Greendale, & Ganz, 2003). Oncology nurse scientists Carpenter, Barton, and Knobf have contributed to improving knowledge about hot flashes and their management. Carpenter and her research team examined symptom distress and associated symptom clusters, impact on quality of life, hot flash management, and treatment with venlafaxine and magnetic therapy (Carpenter, 2000, 2001; Carpenter & Andrykowski, 1999; Carpenter et al., 1998, 2007; Carpenter, Elam, et al., 2004; Carpenter, Gautam, Freedman, & Andrykowski, 2001; Carpenter, Gilchrist, Chen, Gautam, & Freedman, 2004; Carpenter, Johnson, Wagner, & Andrykowski, 2002; Carpenter & Lambert, 2000; Carpenter, Wells, et al., 2002). Carpenter also published several studies examining the feasibility and psychometrics of an automated, ambulatory sternal skin conductance monitor to measure the frequency of hot flashes (Carpenter, Andrykowski, Freedman, & Munn, 1999; Carpenter, Azzouz, Monahan, Storniolo, & Ridner, 2005; Carpenter, Monahan, & Azzouz, 2004). Her team also developed a specific tool called the Hot Flash-Related Daily Interference Scale (Carpenter, 2001; Carpenter & Andrykowski; Carpenter et al., 2005; Carpenter, Monahan, et al.).

Barton and her research colleagues conducted pilot and intervention studies to examine the effectiveness of nonhormonal citalopram and alternative treatments such as vitamin E for hot flashes (Barton, Loprinzi, Quella, et al., 2002; Barton, Loprinzi, & Gostout, 2002; Barton, Loprinzi, & Wahner-Roedler, 2001; Barton et al., 1998, 2003).

Lymphedema

Lymphedema research gained increased attention in the early 2000s because more women are surviving longer and experiencing late effects of treatment. In the past, lymphedema outcomes generally were related to multifactorial problems such as lack of knowledge about lymphedema, lack of oncology provider attention to the problem, and lymphedema measurement problems. Advocacy organizations such as the National Lymphedema Network (2007) brought attention to the clinical problems with lymphedema. However, as a research topic, lymphedema was largely under-recognized.

Armer's research program has been instrumental in helping oncology nursing to focus attention on lymphedema and to improve understanding of the risk factors, measurement, co-occurring symptoms, and treatment of this problem (Armer, 2005; Armer & Fu, 2005; Armer, Fu, Wainstock, Zagar, & Jacobs, 2004; Armer & Heckathorn, 2005; Armer, Heppner, & Mallinkrodt, 2002; Armer, Radina, Porock, & Culbertson, 2003). Her program of research informed oncology nurses of the need to reexamine water displacement as the gold standard for measuring limb volume, to assess limb volume using a perometer, to develop better measurement strategies, and to consider age differences and treatment differences to improve patient outcomes.

Sleep Problems and Sleep Hygiene

Sleep research has been a fruitful area of study outside of oncology, and only recently have sleep problems and sleep habit interventions begun to receive more specific attention within oncology nursing research (Engstrom, Strohl, Rose, Lewandowski, & Stefanek, 1999; Gelinas & Fillion, 2004). Although previous research identified sleep problems from the perspective of symptom clusters (co-occurring with fatigue and pain) or symptom distress (Boehmke & Brown, 2005; Boehmke & Dickerson, 2005; Byar, Berger, Bakken, & Cetak, 2006; Cimprich, 1999; Cimprich, So, Ronis, & Trask, 2005; Dodd, Miaskowski, & Paul, 2001), Berger and her colleagues have thrust sleep problems and sleep hygiene into a more focused area of research (Berger & Farr, 1999; Berger & Higginbotham, 2000). A promising area for future study centers on Berger's individualized sleep promotion plan consisting of four components: sleep hygiene, relaxation therapy, stimulus control, and sleep reduction techniques. Adherence to the sleep hygiene intervention ranged from 77%–88% (Berger et al., 2002, 2003).

Sexuality and Fertility

Sexuality and sexual function as a research topic has been explored by a few scientists engaged in women's health issues related to gynecologic and breast cancers (Bruner & Boyd, 1999; Rogers & Kristjanson, 2002; Shell, 2002; Young-McCaughan, 1996). Despite the prevalence of sexual dysfunction in patients with breast and gynecologic cancers, the four papers cited are either literature reviews or qualitative descriptive studies. Surprisingly, no interventions on sexual functioning were located in the literature. Thus, the study of sexuality in cancer, a significant clinical problem, is deserving of additional research attention in the future.

Kaempfer first reported on fertility concerns in the early 1980s and drew oncology nurses' attention to the needs of younger patients with cancer and their fertility concerns (Kaempfer, 1981; Kaempfer, Wiley, Hoffman, & Rhodes, 1985). Although the initial focus of fertility was on young men and education about sperm-banking procedures, Dow subsequently reported about fertility concerns and pregnancy outcomes in young breast cancer survivors in the 1990s (Dow, 1990, 1994; Dow, Harris, & Roy, 1994). In a series of descriptive, qualitative, and mixed-methods designs, Dow described the psychosocial journey of young women with breast cancer whose quality of life was impeded as a result of concerns about fertility loss (Dow, 2000, 2004b; Dow & Kuhn, 2004; Dow & Lafferty, 2000). In 2004, she and her research team developed the Fertility and Breast Cancer Project, a Web-based psychoeducational support program dedicated to helping women to better understand the context of fertility and breast cancer (Dow, 2004a; Dow & McNees, 2006).

Cognitive Changes

Several multidisciplinary descriptive studies supported the hypothesis that adjuvant chemotherapy and hormonal therapy are associated with increased cognitive deficits, such as loss of concentration and memory, among a subset of women with breast cancer (Ahles & Saykin, 2002; Ahles et al., 2002; Freeman & Broshek, 2002; Hurria et al., 2006; Leyland-Jones & O'Shaughnessy, 2003; Olin, 2001; Rugo & Ahles, 2003; Schagen, Muller, Boogerd, Mellenbergh, & van Dam, 2006). Underlying mechanisms for cognitive deficits are not known, although genetic predisposition (Tannock, Ahles, Ganz, & Van Dam, 2004), older age (Ernst et al., 2002; Hurria et al.), and psychological factors (Ahles & Saykin) have been identified.

Oncology nurse scientists are involved in multidisciplinary teams examining differential types of cognitive deficits. The study of cognitive deficits is an exciting and yet embryonic area of research, and thus, the available papers in oncology nursing are either descriptive studies or case reports (Barton & Loprinzi, 2002; Bender, Paraska, Sereika, Ryan, & Berga, 2001; Bender et al., 2006; Paraska & Bender, 2003; Shilling & Jenkins, 2006).

Cimprich developed an intervention for attentional fatigue for women newly diagnosed with breast cancer (Cimprich, 1993; Cimprich & Ronis, 2003). Cimprich defined *attentional fatigue* as a reduced capacity to attend. The intervention involved regular exposure of 120 minutes per week to natural environment. She tested the intervention in 157 newly diagnosed women at 17 days before surgery and at 19 days after surgery. Results showed that the intervention group (n = 83) had higher recovery to direct attention from presurgery to postsurgery compared with the nonintervention group (n = 74). This study has interesting implications for possible interventions in women with cognitive deficits related to attention loss.

Psychosocial Adjustment and Family Relationships

The topic of psychosocial oncology is another vast area of concern and study in nursing research. This section will specifically focus on family research and breast cancer highlighting two oncology nurse scientists whose work has spanned more than 25 years in breast cancer research: Dr. Frances Marcus Lewis and Dr. Laurel Northouse.

In 1978, Lewis first reported on the psychosocial adjustment of women newly diagnosed with breast cancer (Lewis & Bloom, 1978). In the ensuing 30 years, Lewis and her research team conducted a series of descriptive, longitudinal, comparative, qualitative, mixed methods, and multisite longitudinal clinical trials centering on women with breast cancer and their families. Her and her research team's efforts have led oncology nurse scientists to better understand such areas as how to strengthen family supports, examine mother-child relationships from both the mother's and the child's perspectives, understand children's behavioral adjustment and change in self-esteem when their mother has breast cancer, examine how couples balance their lives in the face of recurrent breast cancer, and examine core concerns of couples living with early-stage breast cancer (Armsden & Lewis, 1994; Ersek, Issel, & Lewis, 1990; Kirsch, Brandt, & Lewis, 2003; Lewis, 1990; Lewis et al., 1985, 1989; Lewis & Hammond, 1992; Lewis, Zahlis, Shands, Sinsheimer, & Hammond, 1996; Shands, Lewis, Sinsheimer, & Cochrane, 2006; Shands, Lewis, & Zahlis, 2000; Stetz, Lewis, & Houck, 1994).

Lewis and others shifted the focus in oncology nursing research from the individual perspective to a family-centered approach by citing assumptions about family functions that need to be replaced by more informed, data-based views to develop programs and services (Lewis, 2004). Lewis's research team's intervention, the Enhancing Connections Program, reported on a cognitive-behavioral intervention for mothers and children with the aim of reducing psychosocial distress and morbidity (Lewis, Casey, Brandt, Shands, & Zahlis, 2006).

In 1981, Northouse reported on the experience of fear of recurrence among patients who have had a mastectomy. This paper was the first in nursing to report on the concept of fear of recurrence, which encouraged multidisciplinary behavioral oncology scientists to examine psychosocial distress after treatment. This initial study served as the basis for a productive program of research examining adjustment to recurrent breast cancer among patients and spouses (Northouse, 1981; Northouse, Dorris, & Charron-Moore, 1995; Northouse, Laten, & Reddy, 1995; Northouse, Mood, et al., 2002; Northouse, Templin, & Mood, 2001; Northouse, Walker, et al., 2002).

In 1988 and 1989, Northouse reported two studies that examined psychosocial adjustment of women with breast cancer and their spouses over time (Northouse, 1988, 1989). She compared 41 patients with mastectomy and their spouses at three time points corresponding to the immediate postoperative period, 30 days after surgery, and 18 months after surgery. Her results showed that mood and role functioning improved, but distress remained high. Her findings showed that psychosocial distress persists over time for both patients and spouses, thus sustaining her program of research focused on families and psychosocial adjustment.

From her carefully laid out program of research with families of patients with breast cancer, Northouse developed an intervention for women with recurrent breast cancer and their family caregivers (Northouse, Kershaw, Mood,

& Schafenacker, 2005; Northouse, Walker, et al., 2002). She used a randomized controlled trial (RCT) and enrolled 134 patient-caregiver dyads. The intervention focused on family involvement, optimism, coping, uncertainty reduction, and symptom management. Results showed that the dyads in the experimental intervention reported significantly less hopelessness and less negative appraisal compared with the controls. Her findings also showed that the family intervention effects were not sustained over time, leading to future considerations of intervention dose and duration of effects.

Multicultural Influences on Breast Cancer

A growing cadre of oncology scientists is examining the multicultural influences on breast cancer. Phillips and Wilbur (1995) examined adherence to breast cancer screening guidelines among 154 African American women. Their results showed that although a majority practiced BSE and had an annual professional breast examination, only 20% of subjects had annual recommended mammography. Findings emphasized the need to develop improved adherence to screening guidelines among African American women. In a follow-up study, Phillips, Cohen, and Moses (1999) further explored the beliefs, attitudes, and breast cancer screening practices among African American women using a focus-group method. Results showed that pain, fear, and fatalistic views were important factors that influenced screening behaviors. Findings indicated the need for tailored cancer-education interventions with African American women. In 2001, Phillips, Cohen, and Tarzian used a hermeneutic phenomenologic design to further understand the experiences of African American women with breast cancer screening. Results showed that the participants desired a holistic approach of minding the body, self, and spirit to promote screening. Gullatte et al. (2006) published an integrative review of the literature that summarized the knowledge to date about the influence of culture on breast cancer screening practices. Variables contributing to patient-controlled delays in screening were advancing age, low socioeconomic status, fear, shame, embarrassment, and faith-influenced delays.

Kagawa-Singer and colleagues have published several papers examining the cross-cultural experiences of Asian women and breast cancer. In 1997, Kagawa-Singer, Wellisch, and Durvasula published a pilot study examining the effect of breast cancer on Asian American women compared with Anglo Americans. Their results showed that Asian American women had lower breast-conserving surgery rates, lower professional help–seeking behaviors for psychosocial concerns, and different sources for social support compared with Anglo American women. Findings indicated further exploration of Asian American women's perspectives. In a follow-up study, Kagawa-Singer and Pourat (2000) first reported disaggregated national data for breast and cervical cancer screening in Asian Americans and Pacific Islanders. Results further confirmed the low rates of breast screening. Lack of insurance, low income, and lack of a primary care provider were the most consistent reasons for lower screening rates. In a 2006 paper, Kagawa-Singer et al. used participatory action research strategies to collect baseline survey data among non–English-speaking women. The approach was successfully conducted in eight communities with 1,825 surveys collected, which resulted in more than 99% participation.

Meade and Calvo (2001) conducted a literature review to evaluate strategies for community and academic partnerships to promote breast cancer education among rural and Hispanic farmworkers. Similar to Kagawa-Singer's outcomes, they found that community partnerships built on culturally competent staff and shared goals can achieve improved breast health education.

Summary

The programs of research by several oncology nurse scientists in the area of breast cancer have advanced oncology nursing science across the cancer continuum from screening and early detection through active treatment and survivorship and through symptom management studies.

Theoretical Approaches and Interventions in Breast Cancer Research

Several theoretical approaches have been applied in breast cancer, likely related to the availability and willingness of patients with breast cancer to participate and the desire of survivors to ease adjustment and transition for future women diagnosed with breast cancer. Specific theoretical and conceptual approaches have not necessarily been developed for breast cancer. However, the participants have made well-known theoretical or conceptual approaches, such as self-care, symptom distress, symptom clusters, and quality of life, more understandable. These theoretical approaches have been discussed elsewhere in the text.

With the 2006 publication of the Institute of Medicine report *From Cancer Patient to Cancer Survivor: Lost in Transition* (Hewitt, Greenfield, & Stoval, 2006), cancer survivorship as a conceptual framework is gaining wider acceptance and use. Self-care, symptom distress, symptom clusters, and quality of life can be positioned and tailored within a cancer survivorship framework. Thus, a tailored approach to interventions across the cancer continuum can be a potential avenue for conceptual and theoretical development in the future. The following section details a few notable examples of studies examining the effect of differential interventions in breast cancer survivorship.

Hoskins reported the results of her pilot study of phase-specific interventions based on time in treatment or survivorship (Hoskins, 2001; Hoskins et al., 2001). She used a patient-partner approach model and assigned 128 women and 121 partners to one of three interventions arms: standard education by videotape, telephone counseling, or a combination of the two interventions.

Pilot results showed that phase-specific educational counseling and interventions had a positive effect on adjustment.

Coleman et al. (2005) used a two-group experimental design to examine the differential effects of telephone social support and education on adaptation to breast cancer during the year following diagnosis. The experimental group received 13 months of telephone social support and education. Both groups received an educational resource kit. Results showed no significant differences between the group with the mailed educational resource kit alone and the group that received telephone social support.

Wilmoth, Tulman, Coleman, Stewart, and Samarel (2006) described 77 women's perceptions of emotional and interpersonal adaptation to breast cancer. Using content analysis, the investigators found that 54% of women receiving the telephone support interventions plus educational materials reported improvement, compared to 43% of those who received only educational materials. Forty-six percent of women in the intervention group reported improved relationships with their spouses, compared to 38% in the control group. The investigators concluded that telephone social support for one year improved patients' attitudes toward breast cancer and relationships with spouses.

Yates et al. (2005) evaluated the effectiveness of an individualized intervention consisting of three 10–20-minute education and support sessions on cancer-related fatigue (CRF) in 109 women with breast cancer. Study results showed that women in the control arm consistently experienced an increase in CRF by 50% more than women in the intervention arm. They concluded that the intervention can be effective in reducing CRF in women with breast cancer.

Mishel et al. (2005) conducted an RCT testing the efficacy of an uncertainty management intervention for older long-term survivors of breast cancer. The sample included 509 women with nonmetastatic disease who were five to nine years post-treatment. Participants were assigned to either the usual care or the intervention treatment arm. The intervention was delivered during four weekly telephone sessions where nurses supported the survivors in their use of audiotaped cognitive-behavioral strategies to manage uncertainty about recurrence and a self-help manual to help women to understand long-term treatment side effects.

Badger and colleagues compared a telephone interpersonal counseling intervention delivered over six weeks with a control group receiving the usual care attention among 48 women with breast cancer (Badger, Braden, & Mishel, 2001; Badger, Segrin, Meek, Lopez, & Bonham, 2004; Badger et al., 2005). Outcomes evaluated were symptoms (depression and fatigue) and quality of life (positive affect, negative affect, and stress).

Cimprich, Janz, et al. (2005) developed a program called "Taking Charge" that was designed to help to smooth the transition from treatment to survivorship for women with breast cancer. The intervention consisted of a combination of individual sessions (i.e., four intervention contacts), small group work, and two individualized telephone sessions delivered by nurse/health educators.

Schneider, Prince-Paul, Allen, Silverman, and Talaba (2004) reported on an innovative virtual reality intervention for distraction during chemotherapy among a sample of 20 women with breast cancer. The scientists used a crossover design where participants served as their own controls, receiving the virtual reality intervention during one chemotherapy session and no virtual reality during another chemotherapy session. Outcome variables of symptom distress, anxiety, and fatigue decreased with the virtual reality intervention.

Future Directions

Based on the historic review of the research literature in breast cancer conducted by oncology nurse scientists, their work and the research of many other oncology nurses clearly have contributed significantly to advancing oncology nursing science. Building on this review, future directions are discussed.

From a historic perspective, the largely quantitative descriptive, survey, and qualitative studies in the 1970s and 1980s were reasonable given the historical context and development of oncology nursing research and science. The 1990s saw the increased use of mixed methods, correlative approaches with the beginning of RCT designs, to evaluate nursing outcomes. By the mid-1990s, RCTs of behavioral, psychoeducational, and supportive care intervention studies increasingly were reported in the literature. RCTs are appropriate studies built on evidence of descriptive and correlative data, hypothesis testing, and large interdisciplinary research teams. Although descriptive work is still needed in developing research areas such as cognitive deficits, sexuality, sleep hygiene, and fertility, current and future efforts ideally should focus on further development of innovative pilot interventions and testing of interventions through RCTs.

Second, the approach to team science is vital for future research (Meneses, 2007). For example, Champion's leadership with the Behavioral Cooperative Oncology Group at the University of Indiana is an outstanding example of a multidisciplinary team science approach to research and cancer care. The program fosters collaboration between behavioral oncology scientists and community practitioners. Barton's work at the Mayo Clinic is another excellent example of team science with a multidisciplinary team examining the effectiveness of different agents in the management of hot flashes (Barton & Loprinzi, 2002; Barton, Loprinzi, & Gostout, 2002; Barton, Loprinzi, Quella, et al., 2002; Finck, Barton, Loprinzi, Quella, & Sloan, 1998; Loprinzi & Barton, 2000; Barton, Loprinzi, & Wahner-Roedler, 2001; Loprinzi et al., 2000, 2005; Molina, Barton, & Loprinzi, 2005; Pockaj et al., 2004, 2006; Quella et al., 2000; Rawl et al., 2002; Shanafelt, Barton, Adjei, & Loprinzi, 2002).

Third, strategies to improve research enterprise and productivity in the conduct of research are needed (Meneses & McNees, 2007). Applying new technology, developing new methods, and thinking outside of the box can streamline research processes and improve the effectiveness and efficiency of future oncology nurse scientists.

Finally, the tremendous contributions of oncology nurse scientists working in concert with patients and survivors of breast cancer over the past 30-plus years have resulted in significant advances in the knowledge and understanding of the continuum of cancer, symptom management and symptom clusters research, theoretical and conceptual frameworks, and instrument development. This knowledge should ideally be applied in other cancers to advance nursing science in the future.

Conclusion

From the first observations of patients with breast cancer—their response to the disease and illness and ways to manage symptoms during and after treatment—in the 1960s to the several innovative breast cancer clinical trials being conducted today among oncology nurse scientists, tremendous gains and outcomes in cancer care have occurred. The many contributions of oncology nurse scientists hold promise for current and future oncology nurse scientists to stand on the shoulders of such giants and forge incredible leaps forward in their knowledge and understanding of breast and other cancers.

References

Ahles, T.A., & Saykin, A.J. (2002). Breast cancer chemotherapy-related cognitive dysfunction. *Clinical Breast Cancer, 3*(Suppl. 3), S84–S90.

Ahles, T.A., Saykin, A.J., Furstenberg, C.T., Cole, B., Mott, L.A., Skalla, K., et al. (2002). Neuropsychologic impact of standard-dose systemic chemotherapy in long-term survivors of breast cancer and lymphoma. *Journal of Clinical Oncology, 20*(2), 485–493.

Ali, N.S. (1991). Teaching early breast cancer detection strategies. *Advancing Clinical Care, 6*(4), 21–23.

American Cancer Society. (2007). *Breast cancer facts and figures, 2007–2008.* Atlanta, GA: Author.

Arathuzik, D. (1991). Pain experience for metastatic breast cancer patients. Unraveling the mystery. *Cancer Nursing, 14*(1), 41–48.

Armer, J., & Fu, M.R. (2005). Age differences in post-breast cancer lymphedema signs and symptoms. *Cancer Nursing, 28*(3), 200–209.

Armer, J., Fu, M.R., Wainstock, J.M., Zagar, E., & Jacobs, L.K. (2004). Lymphedema following breast cancer treatment, including sentinel lymph node biopsy. *Lymphology, 37*(2), 73–91.

Armer, J.M. (2005). The problem of post-breast cancer lymphedema: Impact and measurement issues. *Cancer Investigation, 23*(1), 76–83.

Armer, J.M., & Heckathorn, P.W. (2005). Post-breast cancer lymphedema in aging women: Self-management and implications for nursing. *Journal of Gerontological Nursing, 31*(5), 29–39.

Armer, J.M., Heppner, P.P., & Mallinkrodt, B. (2002). Post breast cancer treatment lymphedema: The hidden epidemic. *Scope on Phlebology and Lymphology, 9*(1), 334–341.

Armer, J.M., Radina, M.E., Porock, D., & Culbertson, S.D. (2003). Predicting breast cancer-related lymphedema using self-reported symptoms. *Nursing Research, 52*(6), 370–379.

Armsden, G.C., & Lewis, F.M. (1994). Behavioral adjustment and self-esteem of school-age children of women with breast cancer. *Oncology Nursing Forum, 21*(1), 39–45.

Badger, T., Segrin, C., Meek, P., Lopez, A.M., & Bonham, E. (2004). A case study of telephone interpersonal counseling for women with breast cancer and their partners. *Oncology Nursing Forum, 31*(5), 997–1003.

Badger, T., Segrin, C., Meek, P., Lopez, A.M., Bonham, E., & Sieger, A. (2005). Telephone interpersonal counseling with women with breast cancer: Symptom management and quality of life. *Oncology Nursing Forum, 32*(2), 273–279.

Badger, T.A., Braden, C.J., & Mishel, M.H. (2001). Depression burden, self-help interventions, and side effect experience in women receiving treatment for breast cancer. *Oncology Nursing Forum, 28*(3), 567–574.

Barton, D., & Loprinzi, C. (2002). Novel approaches to preventing chemotherapy-induced cognitive dysfunction in breast cancer: The art of the possible. *Clinical Breast Cancer, 3*(Suppl. 3), S121–S127.

Barton, D., Loprinzi, C., Quella, S., Sloan, J., Pruthi, S., & Novotny, P. (2002). Depomedroxyprogesterone acetate for hot flashes. *Journal of Pain and Symptom Management, 24*(6), 603–607.

Barton, D., Loprinzi, C., & Wahner-Roedler, D. (2001). Hot flashes: Etiology and management. *Drugs and Aging, 18*(8), 597–606.

Barton, D.L., Loprinzi, C., & Gostout, B. (2002). Current management of menopausal symptoms in cancer patients. *Oncology (Williston Park), 16*(1), 67–72, 74.

Barton, D.L., Loprinzi, C.L., Novotny, P., Shanafelt, T., Sloan, J., Wahner-Roedler, D., et al. (2003). Pilot evaluation of citalopram for the relief of hot flashes. *Journal of Supportive Oncology, 1*(1), 47–51.

Barton, D.L., Loprinzi, C.L., Quella, S.K., Sloan, J.A., Veeder, M.H., Egner, J.R., et al. (1998). Prospective evaluation of vitamin E for hot flashes in breast cancer survivors. *Journal of Clinical Oncology, 16*(2), 495–500.

Bender, C.M., Paraska, K.K., Sereika, S.M., Ryan, C.M., & Berga, S.L. (2001). Cognitive function and reproductive hormones in adjuvant therapy for breast cancer: A critical review. *Journal of Pain and Symptom Management, 21*(5), 407–424.

Bender, C.M., Sereika, S.M., Berga, S.L., Vogel, V.G., Brufsky, A.M., Paraska, K.K., et al. (2006). Cognitive impairment associated with adjuvant therapy in breast cancer. *Psycho-Oncology, 15*(5), 422–430.

Berger, A.M., & Farr, L. (1999). The influence of daytime inactivity and nighttime restlessness on cancer-related fatigue. *Oncology Nursing Forum, 26*(10), 1663–1671.

Berger, A.M., & Higginbotham, P. (2000). Correlates of fatigue during and following adjuvant breast cancer chemotherapy: A pilot study. *Oncology Nursing Forum, 27*(9), 1443–1448.

Berger, A.M., VonEssen, S., Kuhn, B.R., Piper, B.F., Agrawal, S., Lynch, J.C., et al. (2003). Adherence, sleep, and fatigue outcomes after adjuvant breast cancer chemotherapy: Results of a feasibility intervention study. *Oncology Nursing Forum, 30*(3), 513–522.

Berger, A.M., VonEssen, S., Kuhn, B.R., Piper, B.F., Farr, L., Agrawal, S., et al. (2002). Feasibility of a sleep intervention during adjuvant breast cancer chemotherapy. *Oncology Nursing Forum, 29*(10), 1431–1441.

Black, M.E., Frisina, A., Hack, T., & Carpio, B. (2006). Improving early detection of breast and cervical cancer in Chinese and Vietnamese immigrant women. *Oncology Nursing Forum, 33*(5), 873–876.

Boehmke, M.M., & Brown, J.K. (2005). Predictors of symptom distress in women with breast cancer during the first chemotherapy cycle. *Canadian Oncology Nursing Journal, 15*(4), 215–227.

Boehmke, M.M., & Dickerson, S.S. (2005). Symptom, symptom experiences, and symptom distress encountered by women with breast cancer undergoing current treatment modalities. *Cancer Nursing, 28*(5), 382–389.

Brant, J.M., Fallsdown, D., & Iverson, M.L. (1999). The evolution of a breast health program for Plains Indian women. *Oncology Nursing Forum, 26*(4), 731–739.

Brown, J.H., & Kiss, M.E. (1979). Cancer audit: Nursing patient-care outcome audit. Criteria: Metastatic breast carcinoma. *Cancer Nursing, 2*(4), 309–312.

Brown, L.W., & Williams, R.D. (1994). Culturally sensitive breast cancer screening programs for older black women. *Nurse Practitioner, 19*(3), 21, 25–26, 31.

Bruner, D.W., & Boyd, C.P. (1999). Assessing women's sexuality after cancer therapy: Checking assumptions with the focus group technique. *Cancer Nursing, 22*(6), 438–447.

Byar, K.L., Berger, A.M., Bakken, S.L., & Cetak, M.A. (2006). Impact of adjuvant breast cancer chemotherapy on fatigue, other symptoms, and quality of life [Online exclusive]. *Oncology Nursing Forum, 33*(1), E18–E26. Retrieved June 4, 2008, from http://ons.metapress.com/content/um1281005428t806/fulltext.pdf

Caplan, L.S., & Coughlin, S.S. (1998). Worksite breast cancer screening programs: A review. *Journal of the American Association of Occupational Health Nurses, 46*(9), 443–451.

Carpenter, J.S. (2000). Hot flashes and their management in breast cancer. *Seminars in Oncology Nursing, 16*(3), 214–225.

Carpenter, J.S. (2001). The Hot Flash Related Daily Interference Scale: A tool for assessing the impact of hot flashes on quality of life following breast cancer. *Journal of Pain and Symptom Management, 22*(6), 979–989.

Carpenter, J.S., & Andrykowski, M.A. (1999). Menopausal symptoms in breast cancer survivors. *Oncology Nursing Forum, 26*(8), 1311–1317.

Carpenter, J.S., Andrykowski, M.A., Cordova, M., Cunningham, L., Studts, J., McGrath, P., et al. (1998). Hot flashes in postmenopausal women treated for breast carcinoma: Prevalence, severity, correlates, management, and relation to quality of life. *Cancer, 82*(9), 1682–1691.

Carpenter, J.S., Andrykowski, M.A., Freedman, R.R., & Munn, R. (1999). Feasibility and psychometrics of an ambulatory hot flash monitoring device. *Menopause, 6*(3), 209–215.

Carpenter, J.S., Azzouz, F., Monahan, P.O., Storniolo, A.M., & Ridner, S.H. (2005). Is sternal skin conductance monitoring a valid measure of hot flash intensity or distress? *Menopause, 12*(5), 512–519.

Carpenter, J.S., Elam, J.L., Ridner, S.H., Carney, P.H., Cherry, G.J., & Cucullu, H.L. (2004). Sleep, fatigue, and depressive symptoms in breast cancer survivors and matched healthy women experiencing hot flashes. *Oncology Nursing Forum, 31*(3), 591–598.

Carpenter, J.S., Gautam, S., Freedman, R.R., & Andrykowski, M. (2001). Circadian rhythm of objectively recorded hot flashes in postmenopausal breast cancer survivors. *Menopause, 8*(3), 181–188.

Carpenter, J.S., Gilchrist, J.M., Chen, K., Gautam, S., & Freedman, R.R. (2004). Hot flashes, core body temperature, and metabolic parameters in breast cancer survivors. *Menopause, 11*(4), 375–381.

Carpenter, J.S., Johnson, D., Wagner, L., & Andrykowski, M. (2002). Hot flashes and related outcomes in breast cancer survivors and matched comparison women [Online exclusive]. *Oncology Nursing Forum, 29*(3), E16–E25. Retrieved June 4, 2008, from http://ons.metapress.com/content/6616786818742847/fulltext.pdf

Carpenter, J.S., & Lambert, B. (2000). Managing hot flashes after breast cancer. *Oncology Nursing Forum, 27*(1), 23–25.

Carpenter, J.S., Monahan, P.O., & Azzouz, F. (2004). Accuracy of subjective hot flush reports compared with continuous sternal skin conductance monitoring. *Obstetrics and Gynecology, 104*(6), 1322–1326.

Carpenter, J.S., Storniolo, A.M., Johns, S., Monahan, P.O., Azzouz, F., Elam, J.L., et al. (2007). Randomized, double-blind, placebo-controlled crossover trials of venlafaxine for hot flashes after breast cancer. *Oncologist, 12*(1), 124–135.

Carpenter, J.S., Wells, N., Lambert, B., Watson, P., Slayton, T., Chak, B., et al. (2002). A pilot study of magnetic therapy for hot flashes after breast cancer. *Cancer Nursing, 25*(2), 104–109.

Champion, V.L. (1985). Use of the Health Belief Model in determining frequency of breast self-examination. *Research in Nursing and Health, 8*(4), 373–379.

Champion, V.L. (1987). The relationship of breast self-examination to Health Belief Model variables. *Research in Nursing and Health, 10*(6), 375–382.

Champion, V.L. (1988). Attitudinal variables related to intention, frequency and proficiency of breast self-examination in women 35 and over. *Research in Nursing and Health, 11*(5), 283–291.

Champion, V.L. (1990). Breast self-examination in women 35 and older: A prospective study. *Journal of Behavioral Medicine, 13*(6), 523–538.

Champion, V.L. (1992a). Relationship of age to factors influencing breast self-examination practice. *Health Care for Women International, 13*(1), 1–9.

Champion, V.L. (1992b). The role of breast self-examination in breast cancer screening. *Cancer, 69*(Suppl. 7), 1985–1991.

Champion, V.L. (1994a). Beliefs about breast cancer and mammography by behavioral stage. *Oncology Nursing Forum, 21*(6), 1009–1014.

Champion, V.L. (1994b). Relationship of age to mammography compliance. *Cancer, 74*(Suppl. 1), 329–335.

Champion, V.L. (1994c). Strategies to increase mammography utilization. *Medical Care, 32*(2), 118–129.

Champion, V.L. (1995). Results of a nurse-delivered intervention on proficiency and nodule detection with breast self-examination. *Oncology Nursing Forum, 22*(5), 819–824.

Champion, V.L., Foster, J.L., & Menon, U. (1997). Tailoring interventions for health behavior change in breast cancer screening. *Cancer Practice, 5*(5), 283–288.

Champion, V.L., & Huster, G. (1995). Effect of interventions on stage of mammography adoption. *Journal of Behavioral Medicine, 18*(2), 169–187.

Champion, V.L., Maraj, M., Hui, S., Perkins, A.J., Tierney, W., Menon, U., et al. (2003). Comparison of tailored interventions to increase mammography screening in nonadherent older women. *Preventive Medicine, 36*(2), 150–158.

Champion, V.L., & Menon, U. (1997). Predicting mammography and breast self-examination in African American women. *Cancer Nursing, 20*(5), 315–322.

Champion, V.L., & Miller, A.M. (1996). Recent mammography in women aged 35 and older: Predisposing variables. *Health Care for Women International, 17*(3), 233–245.

Champion, V.L., Skinner, C.S., Hui, S., Monahan, P., Juliar, B., Daggy, J., et al. (2006). The effect of telephone versus print tailoring for mammography adherence. *Patient Education and Counseling, 65*(3), 416–423.

Champion, V.L., Skinner, C.S., & Menon, U. (2005). Development of a self-efficacy scale for mammography. *Research in Nursing and Health, 28*(4), 329–336.

Cimprich, B. (1993). Development of an intervention to restore attention in cancer patients. *Cancer Nursing, 16*(2), 83–92.

Cimprich, B. (1999). Pretreatment symptom distress in women newly diagnosed with breast cancer. *Cancer Nursing, 22*(3), 185–194.

Cimprich, B., Janz, N.K., Northouse, L., Wren, P.A., Given, B., & Given, C.W. (2005). Taking charge: A self-management program for women following breast cancer treatment. *Psycho-Oncology, 14*(9), 704–717.

Cimprich, B., & Ronis, D.L. (2003). An environmental intervention to restore attention in women with newly diagnosed breast cancer. *Cancer Nursing, 26*(4), 284–292.

Cimprich, B., So, H., Ronis, D.L., & Trask, C. (2005). Pre-treatment factors related to cognitive functioning in women newly diagnosed with breast cancer. *Psycho-Oncology, 14*(1), 70–78.

Coleman, E.A. (1991). Practice and effectiveness of breast self examination: A selective review of the literature (1977–1989). *Journal of Cancer Education, 6*(2), 83–92.

Coleman, E.A., Coon, S., Mohrmann, C., Hardin, S., Stewart, B., Gibson, R.S., et al. (2003). Developing and testing lay literature about breast cancer screening for African American women. *Clinical Journal of Oncology Nursing, 7*(1), 66–71.

Coleman, E.A., Coon, S.K., & Fitzgerald, A.J. (2001). Breast cancer screening for primary care trainees: Comparison of two teaching methods. *Journal of Cancer Education, 16*(2), 72–74.

Coleman, E.A., Coon, S.K., Fitzgerald, A.J., & Cantrell, M.J. (2001). Breast cancer screening education: Comparing outcome skills of nurse practitioner students and medical residents. *Clinical Excellence for Nurse Practitioners, 5*(2), 102–107.

Coleman, E.A., & Feuer, E.J. (1992). Breast cancer screening among women from 65 to 74 years of age in 1987-88 and 1991. National Cancer Institute breast cancer screening consortium. *Annals of Internal Medicine, 117*(11), 961–966.

Coleman, E.A., Hardin, S.M., Lord, J.E., Heard, J.K., Cantrell, M.J., & Coon, S.K. (2002). General characteristics and experiences of specialized standardized patients: Breast teaching associate professionals. *Journal of Cancer Education, 17*(3), 121–123.

Coleman, E.A., & Heard, J.K. (2001). Clinical breast examination: An illustrated educational review and update. *Clinical Excellence for Nurse Practitioners, 5*(4), 197–204.

Coleman, E.A., Lord, J., Heard, J., Coon, S., Cantrell, M., Mohrmann, C., et al. (2003). The Delta Project: Increasing breast cancer screening among rural minority and older women by targeting rural healthcare providers. *Oncology Nursing Forum, 30*(4), 669–677.

Coleman, E.A., Lord, J.E., Bowie, M., & Worley, M.J. (1993). A statewide breast cancer screening project. *Cancer Nursing, 16*(5), 347–353.

Coleman, E.A., & O'Sullivan, P. (2001). Racial differences in breast cancer screening among women from 65 to 74 years of age: Trends from 1987–1993 and barriers to screening. *Journal of Women and Aging, 13*(3), 23–39.

Coleman, E.A., Stewart, C.B., Wilson, S., Cantrell, M.J., O'Sullivan, P., Carthron, D.O., et al. (2004). An evaluation of standardized patients in improving clinical breast examinations for military women. *Cancer Nursing, 27*(6), 474–482.

Coleman, E.A., Tulman, L., Samarel, N., Wilmoth, M.C., Rickel, L., Rickel, M., et al. (2005). The effect of telephone social support and education on adaptation to breast cancer during the year following diagnosis. *Oncology Nursing Forum, 32*(4), 822–829.

Cox, J. (1979). Nursing care study. Breast tumor: Taking the patient's point of view. *Nursing Mirror, 148*(12), 47–48.

Crooks, C.E., & Jones, S.D. (1989). Educating women about the importance of breast screenings: The nurse's role. *Cancer Nursing, 12*(3), 161–164.

Culver, J., & Alexander, E.J. (1989). Implementing the American Cancer Society breast cancer awareness program in the workplace. *Journal of the American Association of Occupational Health Nurses, 37*(5), 166–170.

Devine, S.K., & Frank, D.I. (2000). Nurses self-performing and teaching others breast self-examination: Implications for advanced practice nurses. *Clinical Excellence for Nurse Practitioners, 4*(4), 216–223.

Dixon, J.K., Moritz, D.A., & Baker, F.L. (1978). Breast cancer and weight gain: An unexpected finding. *Oncology Nursing Forum, 5*(3), 5–7.

Dodd, M.J. (1984). Self-care for patients with breast cancer to prevent side effects of chemotherapy: A concern for public health nursing. *Public Health Nursing, 1*(4), 202–209.

Dodd, M.J. (1988). Patterns of self-care in patients with breast cancer. *Western Journal of Nursing Research, 10*(1), 7–24.

Dodd, M.J., Miaskowski, C., & Paul, S.M. (2001). Symptom clusters and their effect on the functional status of patients with cancer. *Oncology Nursing Forum, 28*(3), 465–470.

Doogan, R.A. (1991). The role of mammography in the early detection of breast cancer. *Nurse Practitioner Forum, 2*(4), 217–224.

Dostal, E.R., & Elder, L.E. (1979). Breast cancer: Special nursing considerations. *Journal of Practical Nursing, 29*(4), 16–18, 45.

Dow, K.H. (1990). Breast cancer and fertility. *NAACOGS Clinical Issues in Perinatal and Women's Health Nursing, 1*(4), 444–452.

Dow, K.H. (1994). Having children after breast cancer. *Cancer Practice, 2*(6), 407–413.

Dow, K.H. (2000). Pregnancy and breast cancer. *Journal of Obstetric, Gynecologic, and Neonatal Nursing, 29*(6), 634–640.

Dow, K.H. (2004a, June). *Fertility after breast cancer: Web-based program.* Abstract and poster presentation presented at the 2004 Susan G. Komen Breast Cancer Mission Conference, New York.

Dow, K.H. (2004b). Psychosocial issues of fertility preservation in cancer survivors. In T. Tulandi & R.G. Gosden (Eds.), *Preservation of fertility* (pp. 237–246). New York: Taylor and Francis.

Dow, K.H., & Coleman, E.A. (1996). Breast cancer research: History and opportunities. In K.H. Dow (Ed.), *Contemporary issues in breast cancer* (Vol. 1, pp. 271–280). Sudbury, MA: Jones and Bartlett.

Dow, K.H., Harris, J., & Roy, C. (1994). Pregnancy after breast-conserving surgery and radiation therapy for breast cancer. *Journal of the National Cancer Institute Monographs, 16*, 131–137.

Dow, K.H., & Kuhn, D. (2004). Fertility options in young breast cancer survivors: A review of the literature [Online exclusive]. *Oncology Nursing Forum, 31*(3), E46–E53. Retrieved June 4, 2008, from http://ons.metapress.com/content/jmk637p88u75g14x/fulltext.pdf

Dow, K.H., & Lafferty, P. (2000). Quality of life, survivorship, and psychosocial adjustment of young women with breast cancer after breast-conserving surgery and radiation therapy. *Oncology Nursing Forum, 27*(10), 1555–1564.

Dow, K.H., & McNees, P. (2006). An electronic environment for conducting quality of life research: The fertility and breast cancer project. *Oncology Nursing Forum, 33*(22), Abstract 20.

Elkind, A.K. (1980). The nurse as health educator: The prevention and early detection of cancer. *Journal of Advanced Nursing, 5*(4), 417–426.

Engstrom, C.A., Strohl, R.A., Rose, L., Lewandowski, L., & Stefanek, M.E. (1999). Sleep alterations in cancer patients. *Cancer Nursing, 22*(2), 143–148.

Ernst, T., Chang, L., Cooray, D., Salvador, C., Jovicich, J., Walot, I., et al. (2002). The effects of tamoxifen and estrogen on brain metabolism in elderly women. *Journal of the National Cancer Institute, 94*(8), 592–597.

Ersek, M., Issel, L.M., & Lewis, F.M. (1990). How children cope with mother's breast cancer. *Oncology Nursing Forum, 17*(3), 5–13.

Facione, N.C., & Katapodi, M. (2000). Culture as an influence on breast cancer screening and early detection. *Seminars in Oncology Nursing, 16*(3), 238–247.

Finck, G., Barton, D.L., Loprinzi, C.L., Quella, S.K., & Sloan, J.A. (1998). Definitions of hot flashes in breast cancer survivors. *Journal of Pain and Symptom Management, 16*(5), 327–333.

Fitzpatrick, G. (1970a). Caring for the patient with cancer of the breast. I. *Bedside Nurse, 3*(2), 20–24.

Fitzpatrick, G. (1970b). Caring for the patient with cancer of the breast. II. *Bedside Nurse, 3*(3), 19–28.

Ford, M., Martin, R.D., Hilton, L.W., Ewert-Flannagan, T., Corrigan, G.K., Johnson, G., et al. (1997). Outcomes study of a course in breast-cancer screening. *Journal of Cancer Education, 12*(3), 179–184.

Freeman, J.R., & Broshek, D.K. (2002). Assessing cognitive dysfunction in breast cancer: What are the tools? *Clinical Breast Cancer, 3*(Suppl. 3), S91–S99.

Gelinas, C., & Fillion, L. (2004). Factors related to persistent fatigue following completion of breast cancer treatment. *Oncology Nursing Forum, 31*(2), 269–278.

Giannola, J. (1979). Caring for the cancer patient: The post-mastectomy patient. *Journal of Nursing Care, 12*(7), 26.

Gullatte, M.M., Phillips, J.M., & Gibson, L.M. (2006). Factors associated with delays in screening of self-detected breast changes in African-American women. *Journal of National Black Nurses Association, 17*(1), 45–50.

Hassey, K.M. (1985). Radiation therapy for breast cancer: A historic review. *Seminars in Oncology Nursing, 1*(3), 181–188.

Hassey, K.M. (1988). Pregnancy and parenthood after treatment for breast cancer. *Oncology Nursing Forum, 15*(4), 439–444.

Hewitt, M., Greenfield, S., & Stoval, E. (Eds.). (2006). *From cancer patient to cancer survivor: Lost in transition.* Washington, DC: National Academies Press.

Hoskins, C.N. (2001). Promoting adjustment among women with breast cancer and their partners: A program of research. *Journal of the New York State Nurses Association, 32*(2), 19–23.

Hoskins, C.N., Haber, J., Budin, W.C., Cartwright-Alcarese, F., Kowalski, M.O., Panke, J., et al. (2001). Breast cancer: Education, counseling, and adjustment—a pilot study. *Psychological Reports, 89*(3), 677–704.

Houfek, J.F., Waltman, N.L., & Kile, M.A. (1997). The nurse's role in promoting breast cancer screening. *Nebraska Nurse, 30*(3), 4–9.

Hubbard, S.M. (1978). Breast cancer: Nurse's role is vital in early detection. *Nursing Mirror, 147*(23), 31–37.

Hurria, A., Goldfarb, S., Rosen, C., Holland, J., Zuckerman, E., Lachs, M.S., et al. (2006). Effect of adjuvant breast cancer chemotherapy on cognitive function from the older patient's perspective. *Breast Cancer Research and Treatment, 98*(3), 343–348.

Janz, N.K., Becker, M.H., Anderson, L.A., & Marcoux, B.C. (1989). Interventions to enhance breast self-examination practice: A review. *Public Health Reviews, 17*(2–3), 89–163.

Judkins, A.F., & Boutwell, W.B. (1991). A model program for teaching nurses breast assessment and cancer screening. *Journal of Continuing Education in Nursing, 22*(6), 233–236.

Kaempfer, S.H. (1981). The effects of cancer chemotherapy on reproduction: A review of the literature. *Oncology Nursing Forum, 8*(1), 11–18.

Kaempfer, S.H., Wiley, F.M., Hoffman, D.J., & Rhodes, E.A. (1985). Fertility considerations and procreative alternatives in cancer care. *Seminars in Oncology Nursing, 1*(1), 25–34.

Kagawa-Singer, M., Park-Tanjasiri, S., Lee, S.W., Foo, M.A., Ngoc-Nguyen, T.U., Tran, J.H., et al. (2006). Breast and cervical cancer control among Pacific Islander and Southeast Asian women: Participatory action research strategies for baseline data collection in California. *Journal of Cancer Education, 21*(Suppl. 1), S53–S60.

Kagawa-Singer, M., & Pourat, N. (2000). Asian American and Pacific Islander breast and cervical carcinoma screening rates and Healthy People 2000 objectives. *Cancer, 89*(3), 696–705.

Kagawa-Singer, M., Wellisch, D.K., & Durvasula, R. (1997). Impact of breast cancer on Asian American and Anglo American women. *Culture, Medicine and Psychiatry, 21*(4), 449–480.

Kay, E. (1979). Cancer: I faced the facts—in my own time. *Nursing Mirror, 149*(17), 18–19.

Kirsch, S.E.D., Brandt, P.A., & Lewis, F.M. (2003). Making the most of the moment: When a child's mother has breast cancer. *Cancer Nursing, 26*(1), 47–54.

Knobf, M. (1998). Natural menopause and ovarian toxicity associated with breast cancer therapy. *Oncology Nursing Forum, 25*(9), 1519–1530.

Knobf, M.T. (2001). The menopausal symptom experience in young mid-life women with breast cancer. *Cancer Nursing, 24*(3), 201–210.

Knobf, M.T. (2002). Carrying on: The experience of premature menopause in women with early stage breast cancer. *Nursing Research, 51*(1), 9–17.

Kochanczyk, M.L. (1982). An education program which prepares nurses to teach breast self-examination. *Journal of Obstetric, Gynecologic, and Neonatal Nursing, 11*(4), 222–224.

Koyama, H., Wada, T., Nishizawa, Y., Iwanaga, T., & Aoki, Y. (1977). Cyclophosphamide-induced ovarian failure and its therapeutic significance in patients with breast cancer. *Cancer, 39*(4), 1403–1409.

Krumm, S. (1979). Cancer of the breast. Nursing care. *Major Problems in Clinical Surgery, 5,* 587–612.

Leight, S.B., & Leslie, N.S. (1998). Development of a competency-based curriculum for training women in breast self-examination skills. *Journal of the American Academy of Nurse Practitioners, 10*(7), 297–302.

Leo, J., Stanton, B., & Brus, H. (1979). Case history: Cancer of the breast. *Lamp, 36*(11), 26–29.

Leslie, N.S. (1995). Role of the nurse practitioner in breast and cervical cancer prevention. *Cancer Nursing, 18*(4), 251–257.

Lewis, F.M. (1990). Strengthening family supports. Cancer and the family. *Cancer, 65*(Suppl. 3), 752–759.

Lewis, F.M. (2004). Shifting perspectives: Family-focused oncology nursing research. *Oncology Nursing Forum, 31*(2), 288–292.

Lewis, F.M., & Bloom, J.R. (1978). Psychosocial adjustment to breast cancer: A review of selected literature. *International Journal of Psychiatry in Medicine, 9*(1), 1–17.

Lewis, F.M., Casey, S.M., Brandt, P.A., Shands, M.E., & Zahlis, E.H. (2006). The Enhancing Connections Program: Pilot study of a cognitive-behavioral intervention for mothers and children affected by breast cancer. *Psycho-Oncology, 15*(6), 486–497.

Lewis, F.M., Ellison, E.S., & Woods, N.F. (1985). The impact of breast cancer on the family. *Seminars in Oncology Nursing, 1*(3), 206–213.

Lewis, F.M., & Hammond, M.A. (1992). Psychosocial adjustment of the family to breast cancer: A longitudinal analysis. *Journal of the American Medical Women's Association, 47*(5), 194–200.

Lewis, F.M., Woods, N.F., Hough, E.E., & Bensley, L.S. (1989). The family's functioning with chronic illness in the mother: The spouse's perspective. *Social Science and Medicine, 29*(11), 1261–1269.

Lewis, F.M., Zahlis, E.H., Shands, M.E., Sinsheimer, J.A., & Hammond, M.A. (1996). The functioning of single women with breast cancer and their school-aged children. *Cancer Practice, 4*(1), 15–24.

Lewison, E.F. (1965). The nurse's role in early detection of cancer of the breast. *Nursing Forum, 4*(3), 82–86.

Leyland-Jones, B., & O'Shaughnessy, J.A. (2003). Erythropoietin as a critical component of breast cancer therapy: Survival, synergistic, and cognitive applications. *Seminars in Oncology, 30*(5, Suppl. 16), 174–184.

Lillington, L.B., Gilbert, O., & Morales, L. (1991). Nurses' practice of breast cancer screening and early detection: Results of a pilot survey. *Emphasis: Nursing, 4*(1), 34–47.

Lillington, L.B., Padilla, G.V., Sayre, J.W., & Chlebowski, R.T. (1993). Factors influencing nurses' breast cancer control activity. *Cancer Practice, 1*(4), 307–314.

Lindsey, A.M., Dodd, M., & Kaempfer, S.H. (1987). Endocrine mechanisms and obesity: Influences in breast cancer. *Oncology Nursing Forum, 14*(2), 47–51.

Loprinzi, C.L., & Barton, D. (2000). Estrogen deficiency: In search of symptom control and sexuality. *Journal of the National Cancer Institute, 92*(13), 1028–1029.

Loprinzi, C.L., Kugler, J.W., Sloan, J.A., Mailliard, J.A., LaVasseur, B.I., Barton, D.L., et al. (2000). Venlafaxine in management of hot flashes in survivors of breast cancer: A randomized controlled trial. *Lancet, 356*(9247), 2059–2063.

Loprinzi, C.L., Levitt, R., Barton, D.L., Sloan, J.A., Atherton, P.J., Smith, D.J., et al. (2005). Evaluation of shark cartilage in patients with advanced cancer: A North Central Cancer Treatment Group trial. *Cancer, 104*(1), 176–182.

Mahon, S.M. (1993). Early detection of breast cancer: Implications for nurses. *Missouri Nurse, 62*(4), 14–15.

Mahon, S.M. (2003). Evidence-based practice: Recommendations for the early detection of breast cancer. *Clinical Journal of Oncology Nursing, 7*(6), 693–696.

Meade, C.D., & Calvo, A. (2001). Developing community-academic partnerships to enhance breast health among rural and Hispanic migrant and seasonal farmworker women. *Oncology Nursing Forum, 28*(10), 1577–1584.

Meneses, K. (2007). From teamwork to team science. *Nursing Research, 56*(2), 71.

Meneses, K., & McNees, P. (2007). Transdisciplinary integration of electronic communication technology and nursing research. *Nursing Outlook, 55*(5), 242–249.

Mishel, M.H., Germino, B.B., Gil, K.M., Belyea, M., Laney, I.C., Stewart, J., et al. (2005). Benefits from an uncertainty management intervention for African-American and Caucasian older long-term breast cancer survivors. *Psycho-Oncology, 14*(11), 962–978.

Molina, J.R., Barton, D.L., & Loprinzi, C.L. (2005). Chemotherapy-induced ovarian failure: Manifestations and management. *Drug Safety, 28*(5), 401–416.

Morris, T., Greer, H.S., & White, P. (1977). Psychological and social adjustment to mastectomy: A two-year follow-up study. *Cancer, 40*(5), 2381–2387.

National Lymphedema Network. (2007). *Treatment of lyphedema.* Retrieved January 24, 2007, from http://www.lymphnet.org

Nettles-Carlson, B. (1989). Early detection of breast cancer. *Journal of Obstetric, Gynecologic, and Neonatal Nursing, 18*(5), 373–381.

Nielsen, B.B. (1989). The nurse's role in mammography screening. *Cancer Nursing, 12*(5), 271–275.

Northouse, L. (1988). Social support in patients' and husbands' adjustment to breast cancer. *Nursing Research, 37*(2), 91–95.

Northouse, L. (1989). A longitudinal study of the adjustment of patients and husbands to breast cancer. *Oncology Nursing Forum, 16*(4), 511–516.

Northouse, L., Kershaw, T., Mood, D., & Schafenacker, A. (2005). Effects of a family intervention on the quality of life of women with recurrent breast cancer and their family caregivers. *Psycho-Oncology, 14*(6), 478–491.

Northouse, L., Templin, T., & Mood, D. (2001). Couples' adjustment to breast disease during the first year following diagnosis. *Journal of Behavioral Medicine, 24*(2), 115–136.

Northouse, L.L. (1981). Mastectomy patients and the fear of cancer recurrence. *Cancer Nursing, 4*(3), 213–220.

Northouse, L.L., Dorris, G., & Charron-Moore, C. (1995). Factors affecting couple's adjustment to recurrent breast cancer. *Social Science and Medicine, 41*(1), 69–76.

Northouse, L.L., Laten, D., & Reddy, P. (1995). Adjustment of women and their husbands to recurrent breast cancer. *Research in Nursing and Health, 18*(6), 515–524.

Northouse, L.L., Mood, D., Kershaw, T., Schafenacker, A., Mellon, S., Walker, J., et al. (2002). Quality of life of women with recurrent breast cancer and their family members. *Journal of Clinical Oncology, 20*(19), 4050–4064.

Northouse, L.L., Walker, J., Schafenacker, A., Mood, D., Mellon, S., Galvin, E., et al. (2002). A family-based program of care for women with recurrent breast cancer and their family members. *Oncology Nursing Forum, 29*(10), 1411–1419.

Olin, J.J. (2001). Cognitive function after systemic therapy for breast cancer. *Oncology, 15*(5), 613–618.

Paraska, K., & Bender, C.M. (2003). Cognitive dysfunction following adjuvant chemotherapy for breast cancer: Two case studies. *Oncology Nursing Forum, 30*(3), 473–478.

Phillips, J.M., Cohen, M.Z., & Moses, G. (1999). Breast cancer and African American women: Fear, fatalism, and silence. *Oncology Nursing Forum, 26*(3), 561–571.

Phillips, J.M., Cohen, M.Z., & Tarzian, A. (2001). African American women's experiences with breast cancer screening. *Journal of Nursing Scholarship, 33*(2), 135–140.

Phillips, J.M., & Wilbur, J. (1995). Adherence to breast cancer screening guidelines among African-American women of differing employment status. *Cancer Nursing, 18*(4), 258–269.

Pockaj, B.A., Gallagher, J.G., Loprinzi, C.L., Stella, P.J., Barton, D.L., Sloan, J.A., et al. (2006). Phase III double-blind, randomized, placebo-controlled crossover trial of black cohosh in the management of hot flashes: NCCTG trial n01cc1. *Journal of Clinical Oncology, 24*(18), 2836–2841.

Pockaj, B.A., Loprinzi, C.L., Sloan, J.A., Novotny, P.J., Barton, D.L., Hagenmaier, A., et al. (2004). Pilot evaluation of black cohosh for the treatment of hot flashes in women. *Cancer Investigation, 22*(4), 515–521.

Quella, S.K., Loprinzi, C.L., Barton, D.L., Knost, J.A., Sloan, J.A., LaVasseur, B.I., et al. (2000). Evaluation of soy phytoestrogens for the treatment of hot flashes in breast cancer survivors: A North Central Cancer Treatment Group trial. *Journal of Clinical Oncology, 18*(5), 1068–1074.

Rawl, S.M., Given, B.A., Given, C.W., Champion, V.L., Kozachik, S.L., Kozachik, S.L., et al. (2002). Intervention to improve psychological functioning for newly diagnosed patients with cancer. *Oncology Nursing Forum, 29*(6), 967–975.

Rogers, M., & Kristjanson, L.J. (2002). The impact on sexual functioning of chemotherapy-induced menopause in women with breast cancer. *Cancer Nursing, 25*(1), 57–65.

Rudolph, A., & McDermott, R.J. (1987). The breast physical examination. Its value in early cancer detection. *Cancer Nursing, 10*(2), 100–106.

Rugo, H.S., & Ahles, T. (2003). The impact of adjuvant therapy for breast cancer on cognitive function: Current evidence and directions for research. *Seminars in Oncology, 30*(6), 749–762.

Schagen, S.B., Muller, M.J., Boogerd, W., Mellenbergh, G.J., & van Dam, F.S. (2006). Change in cognitive function after chemotherapy: A prospective longitudinal study in breast cancer patients. *Journal of the National Cancer Institute, 98*(23), 1742–1745.

Schneider, S.M., Prince-Paul, M., Allen, M.J., Silverman, P., & Talaba, D. (2004). Virtual reality as a distraction intervention for women receiving chemotherapy. *Oncology Nursing Forum, 31*(1), 81–88.

Schultz, P.N., Klein, M.J., Beck, M.L., Stava, C., & Sellin, R.V. (2005). Breast cancer: Relationship between menopausal symptoms, physiologic health effects of cancer treatment and physical constraints on quality of life in long-term survivors. *Journal of Clinical Nursing, 14*(2), 204–211.

Shanafelt, T.D., Barton, D.L., Adjei, A.A., & Loprinzi, C.L. (2002). Pathophysiology and treatment of hot flashes. *Mayo Clinic Proceedings, 77*(11), 1207–1218.

Shands, M.E., Lewis, F.M., Sinsheimer, J., & Cochrane, B.B. (2006). Core concerns of couples living with early stage breast cancer. *Psycho-Oncology, 15*(12), 1055–1064.

Shands, M.E., Lewis, F.M., & Zahlis, E.H. (2000). Mother and child interactions about the mother's breast cancer: An interview study. *Oncology Nursing Forum, 27*(1), 77–85.

Shell, J.A. (2002). Evidence-based practice for symptom management in adults with cancer: Sexual dysfunction. *Oncology Nursing Forum, 29*(1), 53–66.

Shilling, V., & Jenkins, V. (2006). Self-reported cognitive problems in women receiving adjuvant therapy for breast cancer. *European Journal of Oncology Nursing, 1*(1), 6–15.

Smith, M.K. (1995). Implementing annual cancer screenings for elderly women. *Journal of Gerontological Nursing, 21*(7), 12–17.

Stetz, K.M., Lewis, F.M., & Houck, G.M. (1994). Family goals as indicants of adaptation during chronic illness. *Public Health Nursing, 11*(6), 385–391.

Stromborg, M. (1982). Early detection of cancer in the elderly: Problems and solutions. *International Journal of Nursing Studies, 19*(3), 139–156.

Tannock, I.F., Ahles, T.A., Ganz, P.A., & Van Dam, F.S. (2004). Cognitive impairment associated with chemotherapy for cancer: Report of a workshop. *Journal of Clinical Oncology, 22*(11), 2233–2239.

Warren, B. (1979). Adjuvant chemotherapy for breast disease: The nurse's role. *Cancer Nursing, 2*(1), 32–37.

Wilmoth, M.C., Tulman, L., Coleman, E.A., Stewart, C.B., & Samarel, N. (2006). Women's perceptions of the effectiveness of telephone support and education on their adjustment to breast cancer. *Oncology Nursing Forum, 33*(1), 138–144.

Wu, T.-Y., & Bancroft, J. (2006). Filipino American women's perceptions and experiences with breast cancer screening [Online exclusive]. *Oncology Nursing Forum, 33*(4), E71–E78. Retrieved June 4, 2008, from http://ons.metapress.com/content/e81vt241817p2p50/fulltext.pdf

Yarbrough, S.S., & Braden, C.J. (2001). Utility of Health Belief Model as a guide for explaining or predicting breast cancer screening behaviors. *Journal of Advanced Nursing, 33*(5), 677–688.

Yates, P., Aranda, S., Hargraves, M., Mirolo, B., Clavarino, A., McLachlan, S., et al. (2005). Randomized controlled trial of an educational intervention for managing fatigue in women receiving adjuvant chemotherapy for early-stage breast cancer. *Journal of Clinical Oncology, 23*(25), 6027–6036.

Young-McCaughan, S. (1996). Sexual functioning in women with breast cancer after treatment with adjuvant therapy. *Cancer Nursing, 19*(4), 308–319.
Zibecchi, L., Greendale, G.A., & Ganz, P.A. (2003). Continuing education: Comprehensive menopausal assessment: An approach to managing vasomotor and urogenital symptoms in breast cancer survivors. *Oncology Nursing Forum, 30*(3), 393–407.

CHAPTER 7

Focus on Lung Cancer

Cynthia Chernecky, PhD, RN, AOCN®, FAAN

Introduction

Lung cancer often is spoken of as one disease entity. However, *lung cancer* refers to many different types of diseases with several different stages and treatment regimens. Lung cancer results from multiple mutations and is the leading cause of cancer death in both men and women worldwide, with the highest prevalence in Japan (Shibuya, Mathers, Boschi-Pinto, Lopez, & Murray, 2002). Although no racial or ethnic barriers exist in the development of lung cancer (Parker, Sussman, Crippens, Elder, & Scholl, 1998), the death rate is rising significantly in African American women in the United States and women in Asia and Africa (Patel, Bach, & Kris, 2004), France, Spain, and Hungary (Didkowska, Manczuk, McNeill, Powles, & Zatonski, 2005). In the United States, lung cancer accounts for 26%–31% of all cancer deaths (American Cancer Society, 2008; Jemal et al., 2007) and is the leading cause of cancer deaths in African Americans (Green & Davis, 2004). Also, the death rates from lung cancer exceeded the combined death rates for breast, prostate, and colon cancers, resulting in approximately 18 deaths from lung cancer every hour (Jemal et al.). The annual percent of change of incidence has decreased for males by 1.7% (except for Native Americans and Alaskan Natives) and increased for females by 0.5% (Jemal et al.). The lung cancer incidence rates are highest for males in the states of Kentucky, Nevada, Louisiana, and Arkansas and for females in Kentucky, Nevada, West Virginia, and Delaware (Jemal et al.).

The development of lung cancer takes approximately 20 years (Manser et al., 2008), with the lifetime probability of developing lung cancer being 1:13 for men and 1:17 for women (Vogel, Wilson, & Melvin, 2003). Recent evidence indicates that the relatives of African Americans who are diagnosed with lung cancer are at a statistically significant increased risk for developing lung cancer compared to the relatives of Caucasians (Cote, Kardia, Wenzlaff, Ruckdeschel, & Schwartz, 2005).

Smoking has long been established as the major risk factor for lung cancer (Doll & Hill, 1952). Approximately 50 million former smokers in the United States are at increased risk for developing lung cancer (Didkowska et al., 2005; U.S. Department of Health and Human Services, 2000), as are all current smokers. Smoking accounts for greater than 50% and as many as 90% of lung cancers (Flannery, 2005; Sarna, Cooley, & Danao, 2003; Strauss, Gleason, & Sugarbaker, 1995; Tolley, Crane, & Shipley, 1991). The prevalence of current smoking varies inversely with education, with high school dropouts having the highest prevalence at 35% (U.S. Centers for Disease Control and Prevention [CDC], 2007). However, quitting smoking is very difficult, with estimates that of the 70% of adult smokers who want to quit, fewer than 5% succeed (National Institutes of Health, 2006). Mortality rates for lung cancer decline with reduction in per capita tobacco consumption (Tovar-Guzman, Lopez-Antunano, & Rodriguez-Salgado, 2005), and the rate increases the most for males with stage IV large cell carcinoma who are older than age 70 and have decreased performance status (Black et al., 2006). Secondhand smoke is another primary risk factor in developing lung cancer (Fidanza, Franco, Malamani, & Moscato, 1986; Husgafvel-Pursiainen, 2004; Sarna et al., 2004) and needs to be addressed on a global basis.

People with lung cancer have higher symptom distress than people with breast cancer (Degner & Sloan, 1995), multiple symptoms (Beckles, Spiro, Colice, & Rudd, 2003; Chernecky & Sarna, 2000; Chernecky, Sarna, Waller, & Brecht, 2004; Cooley, 2000; Corner, Hopkinson, Fitzsimmons, Barclay, & Muers, 2005; Gift, Stommel, Jablonski, & Given, 2003; Miaskowski, Dodd, & Lee, 2004; Sarna, 1994; Thomas & von Gunten, 2002), symptom clusters (Dodd, Miaskowski, & Paul, 2001; Gift et al., 2003; Given, Given, Azzouz, Kozachik, & Stommel, 2001; Miaskowski & Lee, 1999; Sarna & Brecht, 1997; Sarna et al., 2006; Sarna, Cooley, Brown, Chernecky, & Elashoff, 2007), multiple sequelae (Chernecky & Sarna; Collins, 1998; Reiser & Visovsky, 1998; Timmerman, 1998), and multiple negative influences on their quality of life (QOL) (Barlesi et al., 2006). Routinely, lung cancer is diagnosed in late stage, leading to an overall five-year survival rate of 15%. However, if lung cancer can be diagnosed at the earliest stage, stage 1A, the five-year survival rate is 70% (Petersen & Harpole, 2006). Although treatment is similar for males and females, the type and severity of symptoms (Brown, Sarna, Cooley, & Chernecky, 2007; Sarna, 1993a, 1993b; Sarna & McCorkle, 1996), meaning of illness (Ferrell, Dow, Leigh, Ly, & Gulasekaram, 1995; Sarna et al., 2007), QOL (Sarna et al., 2002; Sarna, Brown, et al., 2005; Sprangers et al., 1998;), and recovery (Zang & Wynder, 1996) may be different by sex, age, and race.

In summary, lung cancer comprises a complex number of diseases with a high death rate, primarily resulting from tobacco use and late-stage diagnosis.

Current State of the Science

Eight major areas of nursing science are related to lung cancer: prevention, screening, diagnosis, symptom management, treatment, recovery, oncologic emergencies, and end-of-life care. The top 20 research priorities of the Oncology Nursing Society (ONS, 2007) include the areas of prevention, screening, diagnosis, evidence-based practice, and end-of-life care. Therefore, ONS supports all the major areas of nursing science related to lung cancer.

Prevention

Only a few strategies are known to help to prevent lung cancer, including not ever smoking; quitting smoking; and avoiding secondhand smoke, pollution, industrial-related carcinogens, radon, and asbestos. Cigarette smoking is the predominant cause of lung cancer; hence, the largest impact can be made through policies and programs that prevent smoking and aid in smoking cessation and include long-term follow-up. Because one in five Americans (CDC, 2002a) and 27%–29% of high school students (CDC, 2002b) continue to smoke, cessation programs must be directed toward those groups, as well as toward prevention programs for younger groups. This approach is essential to long-term health because even after quitting, long-term smokers remain at high risk for lung cancer for more than a decade even though their risk of coronary artery disease drops promptly. Globally, the majority of new smokers are in developing and poor countries, and implementing smoking prevention is critical now to avoid a large health burden in the future.

Further research reveals that a history of eczema (Castaing et al., 2005) or hay fever (Gorlova et al., 2006) decreases one's risk of lung cancer, and a diet rich in fruits and vegetables reduces the incidence of lung cancer by approximately 25% (Fabricius & Lange, 2003; Sorensen et al., 2006). Research also has determined that supplementation with vitamins A, C, E, and beta-carotene offers no protection against the development of lung cancer, and in the case of beta-carotene, its use will actually increase mortality (ATBC Cancer Prevention Study Group, 1994).

Several organizations have called for global action in preventing tobacco use (e.g., American Society of Clinical Oncology, ONS, International Society of Nurses in Cancer Care, World Health Organization Framework Convention on Tobacco Control), and their implementation of actions is essential in the prevention of unnecessary death and human suffering. Nurses have taken a lead in this area of strategic development of nursing research for tobacco dependence (Sarna & Bialous, 2006), and the focus includes the individual as well as a public health context for changing policy.

Screening

Population-based screening for lung cancer has not been adopted in most countries, partly because of the lack of technology and the evidence that frequent screening using chest x-rays is associated with an 11% relative increase in mortality (Manser et al., 2008) and that sputum cytology and urine analysis are not effective. However, the good news is that the compliance rate is high at approximately 63%–75% (Manser et al.) for screening. Low-dose helical computed tomography (CT) is sensitive as a screening tool, but the prevalence of lung cancer detected is low at 0.4%–3.2% (Black et al., 2006). Currently, evidence is insufficient to support screening for lung cancer based on technology, and no studies to date have shown that early detection and treatment significantly alter the cure rate and disease outcomes. Comorbidities do not lead to lung cancer overdiagnosis (Read et al., 2004); therefore, their effect should be negligible for screening.

Although public policy has recommended against screening, the time has come when nurses and other healthcare professionals need to assume responsibility for identifying high-risk individuals and informing them of available screening options, such as CT and positron emission tomography (PET) scans. High-risk individuals include those who smoke or use tobacco products (Gritz, Dresler, & Sarna, 2005; Talaska et al., 2006), have a positive family history (Cote et al., 2005), have an allergy to penicillin (Chernecky, 2003; Rusznak & Davies, 1998), and have had frequent chest x-rays (Flehinger, Kimmel, Polyak, & Melamed, 1993; Kubik, Parkin, & Zatloukal, 2000). Another risk factor is carcinogen exposure, such as secondhand smoke (Hackshaw, Law, & Wald, 1997), traffic emissions (Nerriere et al., 2005), asbestos and radon (ATBC Cancer Prevention Study Group, 1994), agent orange (Mahan, Bullman, Kang, & Selvin, 1997), and pesticides and dry cleaning products (Brownson, Alavanja, & Chang, 1993). Individuals who also are at risk include mining and construction workers (Keller & Howe, 1993; Tsuda et al., 2002), female RNs (Keller & Howe), and females with short menstrual cycles or late-stage menopause (Shimizu, Tominaga, Nishimura, & Urata, 1984). Other risk factors include increased plasma fibrinogen and serum C-reactive protein (Jones, McGonigle, McAnespie, Cran, & Graham, 2006), as well as the genetic risk factors of *TP53* tumor gene (Tammemagi et al., 2000), *p63* protein expression (Narahashi et al., 2006), low expression of the *ERCC* gene (Simon, Sharma, Cantor, Smith, & Bepler, 2005), and cyclin A1 overexpression (Cho et al., 2006). This responsibility is echoed in the Como International Conference on lung cancer screening in 2003 and by the American Cancer Society (Oncology News International, 2005).

Rates of smoking cessation are higher after CT scanning than the rates for cessation counseling alone (Mulshine & Sullivan, 2005), and smokers who participate in screening are more motivated to participate in tobacco dependence treatment (Hahn, Rayens, Hopenhayn, & Christian, 2006). Hence, screening alone may be a motivator that leads to actual participation in treatment.

The identification of susceptibility differences in genes, epigenetic mechanisms, such as methylation, and the discovery of a family linkage for lung cancer on chromosome 6q23-25 (Bailey-Wilson et al., 2004) suggest that future research in genetics will better define high-risk populations and aid in the advancement of multiple biomarkers. However, whether specific genes are responsible for enhanced risk of lung cancer still is unknown.

Diagnosis

Lung cancer is being diagnosed in late stages, with common symptoms including pain, dyspnea, and fatigue (Kitely & Fitch, 2006). Early diagnosis could lead to increased survival and improvement in QOL; however, no valid method currently exists for early diagnosis. Advances in genetics (Schwartz, Prysak, Bock, & Cote, 2007), molecular and protein markers, and imaging techniques show promise for detecting and diagnosing lung cancer at early stages, where the prognosis is best. Epidermal growth factor receptor (EGFR) mutations were associated with improved response rates, whereas K-ras mutations led to poorer clinical outcomes in non-small cell lung cancer (NSCLC). Nurses' involvement in cancer diagnosis is associated with roles as clinical research managers, data collectors, and clinical nurses. Educational changes need to be implemented in nursing curricula to include early assessment for lung cancer symptoms so that nurses can help to improve early diagnosis. The symptom education should extend to public health nurses who can further add to the effect of early diagnosis.

Symptom Management

Patients with lung cancer may experience a wide variety of symptoms at diagnosis and during surgical/adjuvant treatment. Historically, respiratory symptoms have been identified as common at the time of diagnosis (Chute et al., 1985), along with other symptoms such as fatigue, pain, weight loss, and depression. More than 90% of patients are symptomatic at presentation, and they experience symptoms for four months before reporting them to a healthcare worker (Kelly, 2006). This lag time between symptom onset and report to a healthcare provider is sufficient to influence the stage at diagnosis and outcomes. Therefore, healthcare workers must acknowledge that patients experience symptoms of lung cancer but may recognize them as normal health changes and attribute them to everyday fluctuations in bodily functions. Patients also can misinterpret the symptoms, associate the symptoms with other comorbidities, or fail to associate the symptoms and their severity with a disease as serious as lung cancer. Early symptoms include cough and dyspnea, whereas later symptoms include anorexia, weight loss, pain, and fatigue. Fatigue and pain are the most distressing symptoms, and symptom distress decreases during the first three months after diagnosis and then increases from three to six months (Cooley, Short, & Moriarty, 2003). Effective treatments are available for cancer-related pain (Abrahm, 1998; Ferrell, Jacox, Miaskowski, Paice, & Hester, 1994) and fatigue (Nail, 2002). Evidence exists that stage is related to total symptom distress; therefore, clinical nurses need to know the stage of the patients' disease in order to properly anticipate symptom distress for assessment and interventions. Comorbid conditions and chemotherapy also have been reported as predictors of symptoms (Gift, Jablonski, Stommel, & Given, 2004) and should be information that is imparted during nurse-to-nurse reports. Very little research exists to explain symptoms, severity of symptoms, and management of symptoms based on caregiver demographics or needs (Lobchuk, Degner, Chateau, & Hewitt, 2006), and very limited nursing research exists on developing rehabilitation for lung cancer and its effect on symptom number and severity or QOL. Initial research exists on noninvasive nursing interventions that have a positive effect on symptom distress and emotional functioning (Sola, Thompson, Subirana, Lopez, & Pascual, 2008), with one study concluding that nursing interventions can relieve breathlessness (Thompson, Sola, & Subirana, 2005). Evidence has demonstrated that physical exercise reduces fatigue, but this knowledge has not been translated into mainstream clinical nursing care. Symptoms need to be defined more thoroughly and aligned with treatment, stage, time, and QOL.

Treatment

Video-assisted thoracic surgery has replaced conventional open thoracotomy as a standard procedure for surgical treatment of lung cancer (Luh & Liu, 2006). For NSCLC, radical surgery and resection with complete mediastinal lymph node dissection remains the only treatment with curative potential for those with early-stage, operable disease. Although adjuvant chemotherapy and concurrent chemoradiotherapy as standards of care are still a matter of debate, insufficient evidence is available to support the use of prophylactic cranial radiation in efforts to negate the high incidence of brain metastases. The use of postoperative radiotherapy in patients with early-stage disease should not be implemented because it reduces overall survival. The role of second-line chemotherapy for those in relapse remains under investigation because the number of patients and randomized trials are limited, but initial reports indicated minimal effectiveness, with an increased survival rate in small cell cancer of approximately 5.2 months (Froeschl, Nicholas, Gallant, & Laurie, 2008). The use of gemcitabine chemotherapy, although somewhat effective, is responsible for dyspnea and therefore needs to be assessed by staff nurses in the clinical setting. Current research shows that treatments with single agents that target EGFRs are promising as a treatment modality for NSCLC.

For small cell lung cancer (SCLC), the mainstay of treatment is *combination chemotherapy*, which is defined as the use of two or more chemotherapeutic agents (Fong, Morgensztern, & Govindan, 2008), and chest radiotherapy for limited-stage disease and surgery with combination chemotherapy for extensive disease. Although SCLC accounts for only 20% of all lung cancers, it has high mortality and low survival rates. Relapsed or refractory SCLC has a very poor prognosis. When treating lung cancer with combination therapies, treatment-related side effects are highly prevalent, as well as symptoms of disease progression that highlight the need for high-quality palliative, supportive, and caregiver care. Forty-four percent of patients with lung cancer use complementary and alternative medicines (Wells et al., 2007) at an average monthly cost of 142 euros or 184 USD (Molassiotis et al., 2006).

In summary, effective treatments for lung cancer are on the horizon, but clinical trials are lacking to support definitive therapies.

Recovery

Recovery begins at diagnosis, with the premier issue involving QOL. Although health-related QOL measures frequently are included as part of clinical trials for advanced lung cancer, limited information is available about the relationship to symptom burden and degree of effect on psychological distress, loss of physical functioning, and specific aspects of QOL. A number of sociodemographic variables, including spirituality (Meraviglia, 2004), may affect the experience of symptoms and appraisal of QOL during recovery from lung cancer. Therefore, a clear understanding of the symptoms that adults with lung cancer experience over time, including those from various cancer treatments, is essential to develop empirically based clinical interventions. The time needed for full recovery and effective interventions to gain maximum QOL has not been determined. Little is known about recovery based on treatment modalities, mental health, and roles within the family. Limited information is available about the healthcare provider's or caregiver's impact during the recovery process. In general, as the stage of disease and the number of treatment modalities increase, the length of the recovery phase also increases. Specialized homecare interventions by advanced practice nurses significantly improve the survival rates of late-stage postsurgical patients with cancer, and symptom distress in patients with lung cancer can be forestalled with nursing interventions (McCorkle et al., 1989, 2000). These studies lend support for future nursing research's effect on patient care and survival. The use of specific pre- and postoperative rehabilitation programs have shown to be beneficial in the areas of lowering the risk for postoperative complications and increasing respiratory function, particularly for forced expiratory volume in one second and maximum oxygen consumption (Lovin, Bouille, Orliaguet, & Veale, 2006), as well as for exercise capacity and QOL (Schultz et al., 2006). Although pulmonary rehabilitation is effective in patients with lung cancer, its use is limited, its value is not accepted readily, and its translation into clinical practice is negligible. Research on how symptoms and their severity affect distress and QOL currently is focused at the descriptive level, where valid, brief, and clinically useful tools are available (Chang, Hwang, Kasimis, & Thaler, 2004; Hollen & Gralla, 1996).

Oncologic Emergencies

Several oncologic emergencies in patients with lung cancer have been identified (Chernecky & Berger, 1998; Chernecky & Murphy-Ende, 2008;

Chernecky & Sarna, 2000), including but not limited to superior vena cava syndrome, pleural and cardiac effusions, syndrome of inappropriate secretion of antidiuretic hormone, and hypercalcemia. Approximately 7% of the Oncology Certified Nurse (OCN®) examination covers oncologic emergencies (McMillan, Heusinkveld, Chai, Murphy, & Huany, 2002); therefore, this domain remains important to cancer care. Besides occurrence rates, no specific nursing research on oncologic emergencies has been conducted. Therefore, the profession needs evidence in the areas of preventing, diagnosing, and treating emergencies in patients with lung cancer. Although the medical literature also is sparse in these areas, evidence supports that the use of surgical sealants does not prevent postoperative air leaks and that the treatment of choice for malignant pleural effusions is systemic chemotherapy with pleurodesis used in chemotherapy failure (American Thoracic Society, 2000). Although critical care oncology has been a subspecialty in oncology nursing for more than 20 years, much remains to be accomplished by nurses in the realm of education and evidence-based care.

End-of-Life Care

The issue of hydration for terminal patients has persisted for many years. In patients with lung cancer, the application of routine IV hydration often causes fluid retention, adding to respiratory compromise. Hence, the overall reduction of fluid volume by 20%–70% is recommended (Morita, Shima, Miyashita, Kimura, & Adachi, 2004).

Nurses have begun to investigate interventions to moderate symptom severity of dyspnea at the end of life by use of agents such as nebulized furosemide (Shimoyama & Shimoyama, 2002), fentanyl (Coyne, Viswanathan, & Smith, 2002), and morphine (Spector, Klein, & Rice-Wyllie, 2000); however, insufficient evidence is available to warrant their usage in practice. The ONS Putting Evidence Into Practice® card on dyspnea is an excellent reference on the state of the science and application for practice (Disalvo, Joyce, Culkin, Tyson, & Mackay, 2007).

Although not specific to lung neoplasms, pain control is an area of nursing research where great strides have been made. Medicine has added strong evidence that higher doses of palliative radiotherapy should not be utilized because it increases acute toxicities, especially esophagitis, and also does not increase survival. More than a decade has passed since the identification of nine as the median number of symptoms experienced by adults with advanced lung cancer (Krech, Davis, Walsh, & Curtis, 1992), yet despite the multitude of symptoms, little research has focused on interventional change.

Caregivers and bereavement associated with patients with lung cancer is another area with minimal research. One study showed that psychological distress initially was lower among spouses of terminally ill patients with cancer who received homecare interventions (McCorkle, Robinson, Nuamah, Lev,

& Benoliel, 1998). This leads the way into further exploration regarding the development of interventions and their long-term effects.

Research Tools in Lung Cancer

Many tools are available for measuring symptoms, QOL, and outcomes in patients with cancer in general. A few tools were developed or utilized specifically for screening and assessing major symptoms in patients with lung cancer and are described as follows.

- The Risk Factor Screening Tool for Lung Cancer is a 14-item yes/no questionnaire that includes handheld spirometry (Chernecky, 2006).
- The Lung Cancer Cough Questionnaire is an eight-item self-report tool that features scoring ranges from 0–36, with higher scores indicating more cough ($r = 0.98$, $p < 0.001$) (Chernecky et al., 2004).
- The Lung Cancer Wheezing Questionnaire is a seven-item self-report tool that features scoring ranges from 0–21, with higher scores indicating more wheezing ($r = 0.97$, $p < 0.001$) (Chernecky et al., 2004).
- The Cancer Dyspnea Scale is a 12-item scale that measures dyspnea ($r = 0.66$, $p < .005$) (Tanaka et al., 2000).
- The Lung Cancer Symptoms Scale (LCSS) (version 2) is a nine-item tool that measures six symptoms (loss of appetite, fatigue, cough, dyspnea, hemoptysis, and pain) and overall QOL (Hollen & Gralla, 1996; Hollen, Gralla, Kris, & Potanovich, 1993). The LCSS is suitable for patients with different levels of symptom burden undergoing different treatments and is sensitive to detecting change over time (Hollen & Gralla). The further validation and use of these tools and the development of tools specific for lung cancer symptoms or symptom clusters might aid clinicians in efficiently assessing and interpreting treatment outcomes.
- The Piper Fatigue Scale (Piper et al., 1998), a 22-item scale with four subscales, and the Functional Assessment of Cancer Therapy–Fatigue Instrument (Yellen, Cella, Webster, Blendowski, & Kaplan, 1997), a 13-item subscale, are self-report scales that measure fatigue.
- A visual analog scale for pain measurement and the Brief Pain Inventory (Cleeland & Ryan, 1994) measure pain.
- The Center for Epidemiologic Studies—Depression Scale (Radloff, 1977) is a Likert-type self-report scale that measures depression.

The development of specific tools for use in lung cancer research will aid in the measurement of outcomes in the areas of diagnosis, treatment, and recovery.

Emerging Issues in Science

Screening is recognized as a method of diagnosing lung cancer early, but only one screening tool is in development (Chernecky, 2006; Chernecky,

Chang, Stachura, & Khasanshina, 2007) and technologic tools for diagnosis are not yet sensitive or cost-effective (Shimizu et al., 2005). Problems abound with many individuals who are diagnosed with lung cancer stating that they did not recognize signs or symptoms or no specific avenue was available for screening for lung cancer, even though patients were at high risk. The current state of the science now deems it reasonable for an individual at risk to choose to undergo testing for lung cancer. Those at greatest risk include individuals with a history of smoking or exposure to secondhand smoke, a family history of lung cancer, and a genetic susceptibility. Testing involves several issues related to screening, cost, implementation, and navigation into healthcare systems. Many attempts have been made to develop lung cancer screening technology that is efficient, effective, and not cost prohibitive, but none exists to date. Although current trials of spiral CT scans show initial evidence of effectiveness, conclusion of the trials is necessary before effectiveness and risks are known. The possibility of synergistic effects of screening technology on tobacco-related carcinogens needs to be considered because these effects seem to be present in cases of frequent chest x-rays and radon exposure. Because smokers who participate in screening are more motivated to participate in tobacco dependence treatment, perhaps both screening and cessation interventions should be offered concurrently in research trials and practice.

Multiple studies have been conducted on the risk factors associated with smoking, but fewer have been performed on comorbidities, stressors, and chemical exposures. Evidence is beginning to emerge regarding the risk factors for nonsmokers and never-smokers. The risk factors for bronchoalveolar carcinoma include exposure to residential radon, exposure to secondhand smoke (Vogel et al., 2003), and being female (Kazerouni, Alverson, Redd, Mott, & Mannino, 2004).

The development of a predictive model based on gene expression has shown promise in predicting recurrence in 93% of patients with early-stage NSCLC, including major histologic subtypes, and hence can be used for treatment decisions such as adjuvant chemotherapy (Potti et al., 2006). Carriers of genetic susceptibility for some lung cancers can be identified and include high-risk individuals who have had small amounts of tobacco exposure, thereby laying the groundwork for screening programs and prevention trials for families with a genetic susceptibility (Schwartz & Ruckdeschel, 2006). The ultimate goal is to identify genetic and/or molecular predictors of people at risk and predictors for prognoses that will assist in chemoprevention and targeted therapies.

Treatments that increase survival are supported by some evidence, but further exploration is required for maintaining best care, including treatments of traditional medicine, as well as complementary and alternative treatments (Wells et al., 2007). In NSCLC, research supports that increased survival occurs in females with early-stage disease who have had complete resection by lobectomy (Fernandes et al., 2003), and three-dimensional conformal radiation therapy increases survival in patients with unresectable NSCLC (Wolski et al., 2005). Research is severely lacking in SCLC, but treatment with monoclonal antibodies (mAb 17-1A) shows promise (Brezicka, 2005). Little research is available on the effects of treatments on patients' mental and social functions. However, one recent study (Wilkie, Rhodes, Stewart, Rankin, & Ried, 2007) showed that cognitive impairment following chemotherapy for lung cancer influences differential selection, thereby rendering a negative effect on decision-making abilities.

Genetic scientists have found an increase in K-ras abnormalities, downregulation of tumor suppressor gene *TP53*, and aberrant expression of epidermal growth factor in NSCLC adenocarcinoma. This opens the door to genotypes and phenotypes as possible genetic mechanisms in relation to lung cancer (Griese et al., 1998; McWilliams, Sanderson, Harris, Richert-Boe, & Henner, 1995). Nurse scientists have discovered that carriers of the tumor necrosis factor-alpha minor allele have less fatigue and fewer sleep disturbances than individuals who do not carry the minor allele (Aouizerat et al., 2007). This opens the possibility of genotyping for symptom management and in the development of intervention strategies.

Developing and testing nursing interventions for symptom management in newly diagnosed patients and throughout the patients' life span is in the very early stages. Nursing interventions that are effective for managing symptoms and their severity need to be developed and should include both the science and art of nursing. Nurse scientists need to monitor symptoms from the time of diagnosis and over time in order to develop effective care strategies.

QOL has been an area of research interest for more than a decade. Evidence is developing regarding factors that negatively influence QOL in people with lung cancer, such as living alone (Barlesi et al., 2006). Further factors need to be assessed regarding both positive and negative influences as single items of influence and clusters of influence for patients and caregivers (Juarez, Ferrell, & Uman, 2007).

The use of pre- and postoperative pulmonary rehabilitation is not well accepted and hence not implemented widely, although its usefulness has been scientifically noted.

Metastatic patterns of lung cancer (Yurdakul, Halilcolar, Ozturk, Tatar, & Karakaya, 2006) are known (e.g., brain, liver, adrenal glands, bone), but their relationship to disease subtype, genetic makeup, comorbidity types, or specificity and severity of symptoms is unknown.

Oncologic emergencies have been recognized, but specific clinical protocols for patient care are either underdeveloped or undeveloped. These emergencies include airway obstruction, hypercalcemia, syndrome of inappropriate secretion of antidiuretic hormone, spinal cord compression, acute pain, effusions (pleural and pericardial), paraneoplastic syndromes, disseminated intravascular coagulation, Lambert-Eaton syndrome, and carcinoid syndrome.

Oncology nurse scientists have made numerous contributions in multiple areas of lung cancer research (see Table 7-1). The next step is to expand knowledge and fill in the gaps, and then use the knowledge to develop effective interventions for specific populations, paying close attention to factors of diversity, environment, and health.

Table 7-1. Oncology Nurse Scientists' Contributions to Lung Cancer Research

Research Problem Area	Nurse Scientists
Allergies	Chernecky, 2003
Animal models	Beckett, 2007
Genetics	Aouizerat et al., 2007; Dodd et al., 2001; Miaskowski et al., 2004; Schwartz & Ruckdeschel, 2006
Meaning of illness	Ferrell et al., 1995; Sarna, Brown, et al., 2005
Nursing education	McMillan et al., 2002; Sarna, Bialous, Wewers, et al., 2005
Nursing interventions	Abrahm, 1998; Coyne et al., 2002; Ferrell et al., 1995; Given et al., 2004; Jantarakupt & Porock, 2005; John, 2007; McCorkle et al., 1998; Nail, 2002; Sola et al., 2008; Spector et al., 2000; Thompson et al., 2005
Oncologic emergencies	Chernecky & Berger, 1998; Chernecky & Murphy-Ende, 2008; Chernecky & Sarna, 2000; Reiser & Visovsky, 1998; Timmerman, 1998
Quality of life	Ferrell et al., 1995; Juarez et al., 2007; Pud et al., 2007; Sarna, 1993a; Sarna, Brown, et al., 2005; Sarna et al., 2002, 2004, 2006; Vena et al., 2006
Risk factors	Chernecky, 2005, 2006; Chernecky et al., 2007; Vogel et al., 2003
Screening	Chernecky, 2005, 2006; Chernecky et al., 2007; Hahn et al., 2006
Spirituality	Meraviglia, 2004
Symptoms and symptom clusters	Abrahm, 1998; Bialous et al., 2004; Brown et al., 2007; Chan et al., 2007; Chernecky, 2004; Cooley, 2000; Cooley & Xiarhos, 2007; Corner et al., 2005; Degner & Sloan, 1995; Dodd et al., 2001; Fox & Lyon, 2006; Gift et al., 2003, 2004; Given et al., 2001; Green & Davis, 2004; Hoffman et al., 2007; Keehne-Miron et al., 2007; Kelly, 2006; Kim et al., 2007; Kitely & Fitch, 2006; Krech et al., 1992; Lobchuk et al., 2006; McCorkle et al., 1989; Miaskowski et al., 2004; Nail, 2002; Piper et al., 1998; Reiser & Visovsky, 1998; Sarna, 1993a; Sarna et al., 2004; Sarna & Brecht, 1997; Sarna & McCorkle, 1996; Wilkie et al., 2007
Tobacco use and cessation	Bialous et al., 2004; Cooley & Xiarhos, 2007; Cooley et al., 2003, 2007; Flannery, 2005; Gritz et al., 2005; Sarna & Bialous, 2005, 2006; Sarna, Bialous, Wewers, et al., 2005; Sarna et al., 2003; Wewers et al., 2006
Treatments: Accepted and alternative	Chan et al., 2007; Daehler et al., 2007; Jantarakupt & Porock, 2005; Wells et al., 2007

Future Directions

Implementation of effective and efficient lung cancer–specific screening and intervention strategies for smoking cessation and controlling symptoms and symptom clusters are of the highest priorities (Miaskowski et al., 2004). The validation of a screening tool for public use is necessary for a global health initiative. Only randomized controlled studies that examine mortality can truly inform the healthcare community about the benefits and risks of screening. Evidence-based symptom control practices are needed across the healthcare continuum along with the validation of tools to measure symptoms. This will assist in differentiating symptoms, clusters, and severity based on genetics, stage, and disease subtype and in evaluating treatment-related side effects based on the treatment regimens employed. The development of lung cancer–specific tools will help clinicians in assessing and interpreting treatment outcomes. The adaptation of these tools to computer and telehealth (the ability to evaluate patients remotely) methods can aid in efficiency. The use of animal models for the testing of targeted symptom-specific interventions also should be acknowledged (Beckett, 2007), as well as the need for clinical trials that include geriatric assessment in the search for best treatment approaches. The use of genotyping for symptoms for use in developing the type and number of intervention strategies is an exciting new direction. Further qualitative and quantitative research data are needed on the effects of a lung cancer diagnosis on QOL, as well as physical, emotional, social, and spiritual components along with differences that may exist because of gender, race, culture, and economic status. Limited attention has been given to insurance providers' effect on decision making, preferences, and patient outcomes. No research has been performed in the areas of organizational theory and the health services model as they relate to the outcomes of care for patients with lung cancer. Gaps still exist in identifying differences and diversity among patients, caregivers, and providers and the establishment of systems that meet best practice and realistic outcomes. Also, further work is needed in determining the clinical significance of symptoms, their severity, and the associated distress that affects patient preferences, functioning, and QOL. The effect of certain factors on survival requires more research, particularly in the areas of gene expression, depression, age, sex, the use of complementary and alternative medications and treatments, and pre- and postoperative pulmonary rehabilitation.

Research is needed in tracing individuals who have worked in industries where workers are exposed to carcinogens as well as in ways of preventing smoking through both biologic and behavioral means. Medical technologies need to be developed in the areas of diagnosis, chemoprevention, and treatment to aid in care and cure. The development of biomarkers for cancer prevention, disease progression, and targeted therapies is another area that requires continued research. Although a strong beginning regarding the positive effects of interventions on patients and caregivers is present, further research will require the combined efforts of research from both oncology and critical care nurses who are working with interdisciplinary teams. Several smoking cessation strategies have been developed, but few studies are available that determine relapse rates over time or in severity, which render the outcomes of these studies to be of minimal value. Nurse scientists also need to address the high levels of nicotine addiction and low readiness to quit among smokers (Cooley & Xiarhos, 2007). The financial impact of lung cancer must not be forgotten, which can be devastating because the diagnosis commonly occurs prior to the patient's eligibility for Medicare; therefore, access to care may directly and indirectly affect QOL during recovery and rehabilitation. The overall goal of nursing in lung cancer care should be to develop, implement, and evaluate models of care based on best practice and outcomes.

Challenges and Opportunities

Currently, caring for patients with lung cancer is challenging because of the lack of evidence-based interventions in both the science and art of nursing. This challenge is compounded by insufficient research tool development to assess lung cancer symptoms, clusters, and severity. Long-term survival is very low because of the lack of valid and cost-effective tools for screening general populations and for diagnosing lung cancers. For example, evidence that CT screening reduces mortality is lacking; analysis of sputum cytology is not effective; and frequent chest x-rays actually increase mortality. These research opportunities are numerous from patient bedside care to national policy with expansion into global initiatives. Nurse scientists are in the early stages of identifying symptoms and clusters, validating them, and beginning the exploration of evidence-based interventions that may be of benefit to patients and caregivers, including the effects on QOL. These scientists also are beginning to develop a model and framework that will assist in creating and evaluating interventions that will help patients from a clinical perspective (such as smoking cessation), physically, psychologically, socially, spiritually, economically, and globally. Exercise to decrease fatigue and pulmonary rehabilitation to aid in respiratory function are known effective interventions, yet they are not translated into standards of care in healthcare settings. Nurse scientists are beginning to look at differences based on genetics, gender, age, race, and economic status in clinical trials and nursing research. Exploration of genetics in the area of chemoprevention is just beginning and holds great promise for future clinical applications. Because lung cancer is the leading killer, national and international teams of dedicated scientists and clinicians are needed to develop and test aims in order to make an effective contribution to mankind (Ruckdeschel, Spitz, & Saxman, 2001). Oncology nurse scientists and clinicians must work together at the national and international levels and participate in multisite studies that are supported and fostered by professional organizations and research initiatives so that evidence-based nursing practice can be enhanced (see Table 7-2).

Encouraging more nurses to enter the field of oncology nursing research is imperative because the profession will suffer and care will be negated without

Table 7-2. Areas of Research Needs in Lung Cancer	
Area	**Examples of Research Needs**
Diagnosis	• Development and validation of quantitative methods that include symptoms, clusters, genetics, and biomarkers • Correlation of quantitative methods to stage, disease type, and quality of life
End of life	• Symptom management interventions based on severity • Caregiver education needs, including culture, spirituality, and ethnicity
Oncologic emergencies	• Validation of interventions and care maps for specific emergencies • Strategies for nursing education rooted in evidence-based interventions
Prevention	• Political and societal interventions for negating smoking and encouraging tobacco cessation • Translational research in smoking cessation to include relapse rates, severity of addiction, readiness to quit, comorbidities, stress, anxiety, depression, income, and losses in diverse and special populations • Role of industry and pollution in development of lung cancer • Implementation of qualitative research methods to discover factors associated with prevention
Recovery	• Impact of health-service models and quality of life as outcomes • Roles and needs of caregivers • Impact of psychological health and spirituality
Screening	• Development and validation of global screening tool • Randomized controlled trials on mortality
Symptom management	• Randomized controlled trials on symptom and cluster management, including accepted and alternative approaches • Use of animal models to test interventions • Identification of disparities by age, race, sex, ethnicity, and culture
Treatment	• Types and dosages of medications based on age, physiologic variables, finances, race, and sex • Issues of insurance versus care versus disparity • Impact of treatment on quality of life and symptoms and their severity • Impact of genetics on chemoprevention

new talent. Also, an effective research environment will be realized only if funding for lung cancer increases above the current level.

Conclusion

Factors that increase and decrease the risk of lung cancer, symptoms (see Table 7-3), and symptom clusters (see Table 7-4) have been identified, and

Table 7-3. Lung Cancer Symptoms Research	
Symptoms	References
Appetite loss	Brown et al., 2007; Mystakidou et al., 2006
Cough	Beckles et al., 2003
Depression	Brown et al., 2007; Given et al., 2004; Nakaya et al., 2006
Dyspnea or shortness of breath	Chernecky, 2004; Wickham, 2002
Fatigue	Aouizerat et al., 2007; Brown et al., 2007; Miaskowski et al., 2004
Hemoptysis	Herth et al., 2001; Sarna et al., 2002
Insomnia	Aouizerat et al., 2007; Hoffman et al., 2007; Pud et al., 2007; Vena et al., 2006
Pain	Brown et al., 2007; Keehne-Miron et al., 2007
Sputum production	Epstein et al., 1993; Selim et al., 1997
Weight loss	Gift et al., 2003; Sarna et al., 1993
Wheezing	Chernecky et al., 2004; Martins & Pereira, 1999

programs for educating the public, including nurses themselves, have been developed (Bialous, Sarna, Wewers, Froelicher, & Danao, 2004; Sarna, Bialous, Wewers, Froelicher, & Danao, 2005) on such issues such as secondhand smoke (Sarna & Bialous, 2005) and the need for smoking cessation (Sarna & Bialous, 2006; Wewers, Sarna, & Rice, 2006). Although information on smoking cessation is abundant, a recent study found that 81% of smokers did not receive assistance in cessation (Ferketich, Khan, & Wewers, 2006). Some nursing intervention strategies are available regarding effective smoking cessation interventions for pregnant women, and long-term smoking cessation programs and interventions for patients who relapse are emerging (Cooley, Powell, Hoskinson, & Garvey, 2007). The predictors for continued smoking include the type of diagnosis, type of treatment, number of smokers in the patient's social network, level of nicotine dependence, and readiness to quit smoking (Cooley & Xiarhos, 2007). The first screening tool to measure risk factors for lung cancer is in development (Chernecky, 2005, 2006), and the first tools specific to patients with lung cancer that measure the major respiratory symptoms of coughing, wheezing (Chernecky et al., 2004), and dyspnea (Tanaka, Akechi, Okuyama, Nishiwaki, & Uchitomi, 2000) have been developed. Interventions to relieve symptoms have been initiated in palliative care, such as nebulized morphine for dyspnea (Jantarakupt & Porock, 2005) and

Table 7-4. Lung Cancer Symptom Clusters Research	
Symptom Clusters	**References**
Breathlessness, fatigue, and anxiety	Chan et al., 2007
Cough, dyspnea, and wheezing	Sarna & Brecht, 1997
Fatigue and depression	Miaskowski et al., 2004
Fatigue, cough, pain, and comorbidities	Sarna et al., 2007
Fatigue, depression, and pain	Fox & Lyon, 2006
Fatigue, dyspnea, and cough	Brown et al., 2007
Fatigue, insomnia, and depression	Hoffman et al., 2007; Kim et al., 2007
Fatigue, insomnia, and poor sleep quality	Daehler et al., 2007
Fatigue, shortness of breath, cough, pain, and anorexia	Brown et al., 2007
Pain, fatigue, insomnia, and anxiety	Hoffman et al., 2007
Weight loss and fatigue	Gift et al., 2003, 2004

psychoeducation for the cluster of breathlessness, fatigue, and anxiety (Chan, Chang, Leung, & Mak, 2007), but little data exist for patients with early- or middle-stage disease (John, 2007). Cost-effective, sensitive technology for diagnosing lung cancer has not been developed. Sputum, urine, and chest radiographs have not been effective in diagnosis, but spiral CT and PET scans and molecular imaging may hold promise. Specific research tools are limited for clinical use in screening, assessing symptoms and symptom clusters, and evaluating interventions for patients with lung cancer. Currently, nurse scientists are in the middle of discovery and are developing lung cancer nursing care models. These professionals need to intensely move toward numerous rigorous multisite intervention studies in all areas of nursing care.

References

Abrahm, J.L. (1998). Promoting symptom control in palliative care. *Seminars in Oncology Nursing, 14*(2), 95–109.

American Cancer Society. (2008). *Cancer facts and figures, 2008.* Atlanta, GA: Author.

American Thoracic Society. (2000). Management of malignant pleural effusions. *American Journal of Respiratory and Critical Care Medicine, 162*(5), 1987–2001.

Aouizerat, B., Miaskowski, C., Dodd, M., Lee, K., West, C., Paul, S., et al. (2007). Evidence of genetic association of a cytokine gene variation with sleep disturbance and fatigue in oncology patients and their family caregivers (FCs) [Abstract 8]. *Oncology Nursing Forum, 34*(1), 171–172.

ATBC Cancer Prevention Study Group. (1994). The Alpha-Tocopherol, Beta-Carotene Lung Cancer Prevention Study: Design, methods, participant characteristics, and compliance. *Annals of Epidemiology, 4*(1), 1–10.

Bailey-Wilson, J.E., Amos, C.I., Pinney, S.M., Petersen, G.M., de Andrade, M., Wiest, J.S., et al. (2004). A major lung cancer susceptibility locus maps to chromosome 6q23-25. *American Journal of Human Genetics, 75*(3), 460–474.

Barlesi, F., Doddoli, C., Loundou, A., Pillet, E., Thomas, P., & Auquier, P. (2006). Preoperative Psychological Global Well Being Index (PGWBI) predicts postoperative QOL for patients with non-small cell lung cancer managed with thoracic surgery. *European Journal of Cardio-Thoracic Surgery, 30*(3), 548–553.

Beckett, D.M. (2007). Animal models of cancer or treatment-related symptoms [Abstract 6]. *Oncology Nursing Forum, 34*(1), 170.

Beckles, M.A., Spiro, S.G., Colice, G.L., & Rudd, R.M. (2003). Initial evaluation of the patient with lung cancer: Symptoms, signs, laboratory tests, and paraneoplastic syndromes. *Chest, 123*(Suppl. 1), 97S–105S.

Bialous, S.A., Sarna, L., Wewers, M.E., Froelicher, E.S., & Danao, L. (2004). Nurses' perspectives of smoking initiation, addiction, and cessation. *Nursing Research, 53*(6), 387–395.

Black, C., Bagust, A., Boland, A., Walker, S., McLeod, C., DeVerteuil, R., et al. (2006). 4-year mortality in patients with non-small-cell lung cancer: Development and validation of a prognostic index. *Lancet Oncology, 7*(10), 829–836.

Brezicka, T. (2005). Expression of epithelial-cell adhesion molecule (Ep-CAM) in small cell lung cancer as defined by monoclonal antibodies 17-1A and BerEP4. *Acta Oncologica, 44*(7), 723–727.

Brown, J., Sarna, L., Cooley, M., & Chernecky, C. (2007). Analysis of symptom clusters in women with lung cancer [Abstract 63]. *Oncology Nursing Forum, 34*(1), 192–193.

Brownson, R.C., Alavanja, M.C., & Chang, J.C. (1993). Occupational risk factors for lung cancer among nonsmoking women: A case-control study in Missouri (United States). *Cancer Causes and Control, 4*(5), 449–454.

Castaing, M., Youngson, J., Zaridze, D., Szeszenia-Dabrowska, N., Rudnai, P., Lissowska, J., et al. (2005). Is the risk of lung cancer reduced among eczema patients? *American Journal of Epidemiology, 162*(6), 542–547.

Chan, C., Chang, A., Leung, S.F., & Mak, S.S. (2007). A randomized clinical trial of the effectiveness of a psychoeducational intervention in combating a symptom cluster in patients with advanced lung cancer [Abstract 129]. *Oncology Nursing Forum, 34*(1), 217–218.

Chang, V.T., Hwang, S.S., Kasimis, B., & Thaler, H.T. (2004). Shorter symptom assessment instruments: The Condensed Memorial Symptom Assessment Scale (CMSAS). *Cancer Investigation, 22*(4), 526–536.

Chernecky, C. (2003). Documented allergies of patients with cancer. *European Journal of Cancer Care, 14*(4), 369–371.

Chernecky, C. (2004). Respiratory/dyspnea. In C.G. Varricchio (Ed.), *A cancer source book for nurses* (8th ed., pp. 407–414). Sudbury, MA: Jones and Bartlett.

Chernecky, C. (2005). Risk factor screening tool for lung cancer (RFST-LC) revised: Pilot data [Abstract 32]. *Oncology Nursing Forum, 32*(2), 431.

Chernecky, C. (2006). Reliability of the risk factor screening tool for lung cancer (RFST-LC) [Abstract]. *14th International Conference on Cancer Nursing,* Toronto, Canada, p. 210.

Chernecky, C., Chang, A., Stachura, M.E., & Khasanshina, E.V. (2007). Risk factor screening tool for lung cancer (RFST-LC): Technology and potential [Abstract]. *2007 CDC Cancer Conference,* Atlanta, GA, p. 125.

Chernecky, C., & Sarna, L. (2000). Pulmonary toxicities. *Critical Care Nursing Clinics of North America, 12*(3), 281–295.

Chernecky, C., Sarna, L., Waller, J.L., & Brecht, M.L. (2004). Assessing coughing and wheezing in lung cancer: A pilot study. *Oncology Nursing Forum, 31*(6), 1095–1101.

Chernecky, C.C., & Berger, B.J. (1998). *Advanced and critical care oncology: Managing primary complications.* Philadelphia: Saunders.

Chernecky, C.C., & Murphy-Ende, K. (2008). *Acute care oncology nursing* (2nd ed.). St. Louis, MO: Elsevier Saunders.

Cho, N.H., Choi, Y.P., Moon, D.S., Kim, H., Kang, S., Ding, O., et al. (2006). Induction of cell apoptosis in non-small cell lung cancer cells by cyclin A1 small interfering RNA. *Cancer Science, 97*(10), 1082–1092.

Chute, C.G., Greenber, E.R., Baron, J., Korson, R., Baker, J., & Yates, J. (1985). Presenting conditions of 1,539 population-based lung cancer patients by cell type and stage in New Hampshire and Vermont. *Cancer, 56*(8), 2107–2111.

Cleeland, C.S., & Ryan, K.M. (1994). Pain assessment: Global use of the Brief Pain Inventory. *Annals of the Academy of Medicine, Singapore, 23*(2), 129–138.

Collins, P.M. (1998). Malignant pleural effusions. In C.C. Chernecky & B.J. Berger (Eds.), *Advanced and critical care oncology nursing: Managing primary complications* (pp. 444–460). Philadelphia: Saunders.

Cooley, M., Powell, M., Hoskinson, R., & Garvey, A. (2007). Age-related differences in smoking relapse among women [Abstract 51]. *Oncology Nursing Forum, 34*(1), 188.

Cooley, M., & Xiarhos, B. (2007). Smoking cessation interventions in cancer care: Missed opportunities [Abstract 159]. *Oncology Nursing Forum, 34*(1), 228–229.

Cooley, M.E. (2000). Symptoms in adults with lung cancer: A systematic research review. *Journal of Pain and Symptom Management, 19*(2), 137–153.

Cooley, M.E., Short, T.H., & Moriarty, H.J. (2003). Symptom prevalence, distress, and change over time in adults receiving treatment for lung cancer. *Psycho-Oncology, 12*(7), 694–708.

Corner, J., Hopkinson, J., Fitzsimmons, D., Barclay, S., & Muers, M. (2005). Is late diagnosis of lung cancer inevitable? Interview study of patients' recollections of symptoms before diagnosis. *Thorax, 60*(4), 314–319.

Cote, M.L., Kardia, S.L.R., Wenzlaff, A.S., Ruckdeschel, J.C., & Schwartz, A.G. (2005). Risk of lung cancer among white and black relatives of individuals with early-onset lung cancer. *JAMA, 293*(24), 3036–3042.

Coyne, P.J., Viswanathan, R., & Smith, T.J. (2002). Nebulized fentanyl citrate improves patients' perception of breathing, respiratory rate, and oxygen saturation in dyspnea. *Journal of Pain and Symptom Management, 23*(2), 157–160.

Daehler, M., Levin, R., Grutsch, J., Jardinico, J., & Hrushesky, W. (2007). Circadian function in patients with advanced non-small cell lung cancer [Abstract 118]. *Oncology Nursing Forum, 34*(1), 213–214.

Degner, L.F., & Sloan, J.A. (1995). Symptom distress in newly diagnosed ambulatory cancer patients and as a predictor of survival in lung cancer. *Journal of Pain and Symptom Management, 10*(6), 423–431.

Didkowska, J., Manczuk, M., McNeill, A., Powles, J., & Zatonski, W. (2005). Lung cancer mortality at ages 35–54 in the European Union: Ecological study of evolving tobacco epidemics. *BMJ (Clinical Research Edition), 331*(7510), 189–191.

Disalvo, W.M., Joyce, M.M., Culkin, A.E., Tyson, L.B., & Mackay, K. (2007). *Putting evidence into practice: Dyspnea.* Pittsburgh, PA: Oncology Nursing Society.

Dodd, M.J., Miaskowski, C., & Paul, S.M. (2001). Symptom clusters and their effect on the functional status of patients with cancer. *Oncology Nursing Forum, 28*(3), 465–470.

Doll, R., & Hill, A.B. (1952). A study of the aetiology of carcinoma of the lung. *BMJ, 2*(4797), 1271–1286.

Epstein, S.K, Faling, L.J., Daly, B.D., & Celli, B.R. (1993). Predicting complications after pulmonary resection: Preoperative exercise testing vs. a multifactorial cardiopulmonary risk index. *Chest, 104*(3), 694–700.

Fabricius, P.G., & Lange, P. (2003). Diet and lung cancer (Danish). *Ugeskrift for Laeger, 165*(34), 3234–3237.

Ferketich, A.K., Khan, Y., & Wewers, M.E. (2006). Are physicians asking about tobacco use and assisting with cessation? Results from the 2001–2004 National Ambulatory Medical Care Survey (NAMCS). *Preventive Medicine, 43*(6), 472–476.

Fernandes, O.J., Almgren, S.O., Thaning, L., Filbey, D., Helsing, M., Karlsson, M., et al. (2003). Prognostic factors for the survival of surgically treated patients for non-small cell lung cancer. *Acta Oncologica, 42*(4), 338–341.

Ferrell, B.R., Dow, K.H., Leigh, S., Ly, J., & Gulasekaram, P. (1995). Quality of life in long-term cancer survivors. *Oncology Nursing Forum, 22*(6), 915–922.

Ferrell, B.R., Jacox, A., Miaskowski, C., Paice, J.A., & Hester, N.O. (1994). Cancer pain guidelines: Now that we have them, what do we do? *Oncology Nursing Forum, 21*(7), 1229–1231.

Fidanza, L., Franco, G., Malamani, T., & Moscato, G. (1986). Passive smoking: A risk factor in the home environment [Italian]. *Giornale Italiano di Medicina del Lavoro, 8*(5–6), 233–240.

Flannery, M. (2005). Nursing care of the client with lung cancer. In J.K. Itano & K.N. Taoka (Eds.), *Core curriculum for oncology nursing* (4th ed., pp. 512–523). Philadelphia: Elsevier Saunders.

Flehinger, B.J., Kimmel, M., Polyak, T., & Melamed, M.R. (1993). Screening for lung cancer: The Mayo Lung Project revisited. *Cancer, 72*(5), 1573–1580.

Fong, T., Morgensztern, D., & Govindan, R. (2008). EGFR inhibitors as first-line therapy in advanced non-small cell lung cancer. *Journal of Thoracic Oncology, 3*(3), 303–310.

Fox, S.W., & Lyon, D.E. (2006). Symptom clusters and quality of life in survivors of lung cancer. *Oncology Nursing Forum, 33*(5), 931–936.

Froeschl, S., Nicholas, G., Gallant, V., & Laurie, S. (2008). Outcomes of second-line chemotherapy in patients with relapsed extensive small cell lung cancer. *Journal of Thoracic Oncology, 3*(2), 163–169.

Gift, A.G., Jablonski, A., Stommel, M., & Given, C.W. (2004). Symptom clusters in elderly patients with lung cancer. *Oncology Nursing Forum, 31*(2), 202–212.

Gift, A.G., Stommel, M., Jablonski, A., & Given, W. (2003). A cluster of symptoms over time in patients with lung cancer. *Nursing Research, 52*(6), 393–400.

Given, C., Given, B., Rahbar, M., Jeon, S., McCorkle, R., Cimprich, B., et al. (2004). Does a symptom management intervention affect depression among cancer patients? Results from a clinical trial. *Psycho-Oncology, 13*(11), 818–830.

Given, C.W., Given, B., Azzouz, F., Kozachik, S., & Stommel, M. (2001). Predictors of pain and fatigue in the year following diagnosis among elderly cancer patients. *Journal of Pain and Symptom Management, 21*(6), 456–466.

Gorlova, O.Y., Zhang, Y., Schabath, M.B., Lei, L., Zhang, Q., Amos, C.I., et al. (2006). Never smokers and lung cancer risk: A case-control study of epidemiological factors. *International Journal of Cancer, 118*(7), 1798–1804.

Green, P.M., & Davis, M.A. (2004). Lung cancer in African-Americans. *Journal of National Black Nurses Association, 15*(2), 54–60.

Griese, E.U., Zanger, U.M., Brudermanns, U., Gaedigk, A., Mikus, G., Morike, K., et al. (1998). Assessment of the predictive power of genotypes for the in-vivo catalytic function of CYP2D6 in a German population. *Pharmacogenetics, 8*(1), 15–26.

Gritz, E.R., Dresler, C., & Sarna, L. (2005). Smoking, the missing drug interaction in clinical trials: Ignoring the obvious. *Cancer Epidemiology, Biomarkers and Prevention, 14*(10), 2287–2293.

Hackshaw, A.K., Law, M.R., & Wald, N.J. (1997). The accumulated evidence on lung cancer and environmental tobacco smoke. *BMJ, 315*(7114), 980–988.

Hahn, E.J., Rayens, M.K., Hopenhayn, C., & Christian, W.J. (2006). Perceived risk and interest in screening for lung cancer among current and former smokers. *Research in Nursing and Health, 29*(4), 359–370.

Herth, F., Ernst, A., & Becker, H.D. (2001). Long-term outcome and lung cancer incidence in patients with hemoptysis of unknown origin. *Chest, 120*(5), 1592–1594.

Hoffman, A., Given, B., Given, C., von Eye, A., & Gift, A. (2007). How do physical and psychological symptoms relate to each other in patients with different cancer diagnoses? [Abstract 41]. *Oncology Nursing Forum, 34*(1), 184.

Hollen, P.J., & Gralla, R.J. (1996). Comparison of instruments for measuring quality of life in patients with lung cancer. *Seminars in Oncology, 23*(2, Suppl. 5), 31–40.

Hollen, P.J., Gralla, R.J., Kris, M.G., & Potanovich, L.M. (1993). Quality of life assessment in individuals with lung cancer: Testing the Lung Cancer Symptom Scale (LCSS). *European Journal of Cancer, 29A*(Suppl. 1), S51–S58.

Husgafvel-Pursiainen, K. (2004). Genotoxicity of environmental tobacco smoke: A review. *Mutation Research, 567*(2–3), 427–445.

Jantarakupt, P., & Porock, D. (2005). Dyspnea management in lung cancer: Applying the evidence from chronic obstructive pulmonary disease. *Oncology Nursing Forum, 32*(4), 785–797.

Jemal, A., Siegel, R., Ward, E., Murray, T., Xu, J., & Thun, M.J. (2007). Cancer statistics, 2007. *CA: A Cancer Journal for Clinicians, 57*(1), 43–66.

John, L. (2007). Pilot study of a seated exercise intervention of lung cancer patients: Clinical significance [Abstract 56]. *Oncology Nursing Forum, 34*(1), 190.

Jones, J.M., McGonigle, N.C., McAnespie, M., Cran, G.W., & Graham, A.N. (2006). Plasma fibrinogen and serum C-reactive protein are associated with non-small cell lung cancer. *Lung Cancer, 53*(1), 97–101.

Juarez, G., Ferrell, B., & Uman, G. (2007). Distress and quality of life concerns of family caregivers of patients undergoing palliative surgery [Abstract 142]. *Oncology Nursing Forum, 34*(1), 222.

Kazerouni, N., Alverson, C.J., Redd, S.C., Mott, J.A., & Mannino, D.M. (2004). Sex differences in COPD and lung cancer mortality trends—United States, 1968–1999. *Journal of Women's Health, 13*(1), 17–23.

Keehne-Miron, J., Sikorskii, A., Given, C., & Given, B. (2007). The association of pain and fatigue with each other and their impact on physical functioning among adult chemotherapy patients [Abstract 36]. *Oncology Nursing Forum, 34*(1), 182.

Keller, J.E., & Howe, H.L. (1993). Risk factors for lung cancer among nonsmoking Illinois residents. *Environmental Research, 60*(1), 1–11.

Kelly, D. (2006). Delays in diagnosis of lung cancer occurred because patients failed to recognize symptoms as serious and warranting medical attention. *Evidence-Based Nursing, 9*(4), 127.

Kim, J.-E.E., Miaskowski, C., Dodd, M., Lee, K., West, C., & Cooper, B. (2007). The use of responses to a single item versus multiple items in a cluster analysis to identify subgroups of patients with different symptom experiences [Abstract 62]. *Oncology Nursing Forum, 34*(1), 192.

Kitely, C.A., & Fitch, M.I. (2006). Understanding the symptoms experienced by individuals with lung cancer. *Canadian Oncology Nursing Journal, 16*(1), 25–30.

Krech, R.L., Davis, J., Walsh, D., & Curtis, E.B. (1992). Symptoms of lung cancer. *Palliative Medicine, 6*(3), 309–315.

Kubik, A.K., Parkin, D.M., & Zatloukal, P. (2000). Czech Study on Lung Cancer Screening: Post-trial follow-up of lung cancer deaths up to year 15 since enrollment. *Cancer, 89*(Suppl. 11), 2363–2368.

Lobchuk, M.M., Degner, L.F., Chateau, D., & Hewitt, D. (2006). Promoting enhanced patient and family caregiver congruence on lung cancer symptom experiences. *Oncology Nursing Forum, 33*(2), 273–282.

Lovin, S., Bouille, S., Orliaguet, O., & Veale, D. (2006). Preoperative rehabilitation in the surgical treatment of lung cancer [Romanian]. *Pneumologia (Bucharest, Romania), 55*(3), 109–112.

Luh, S.P., & Liu, H.P. (2006). Video-assisted thoracic surgery—The past, present status and the future. *Journal of Zhejiang University Science B, 7*(2), 118–128.

Mahan, C.M., Bullman, T.A., Kang, H.K., & Selvin, S. (1997). A case-control study of lung cancer among Vietnam veterans. *Journal of Occupational and Environmental Medicine, 9*(8), 740–747.

Manser, R.L., Irving, L.B., Stone, C., Byrnes, G., Abramson, M., & Campbell, D. (2008). Screening for lung cancer. *Cochrane Database of Systemic Reviews 2008,* Issue 2. Art. No.: CD001991 DOI: 10.1002/14651858.CD001991.pub2.

Martins, S.J., & Pereira, J.R. (1999). Clinical factors and prognosis in non-small cell lung cancer. *American Journal of Clinical Oncology, 22*(5), 453–457.

McCorkle, R., Benoliel, J.Q., Donaldson, G., Georgiadou, F., Moinpour, C., & Goodell, B. (1989). A randomized clinical trial of home nursing care for lung cancer patients. *Cancer, 64*(6), 1375–1382.

McCorkle, R., Robinson, L., Nuamah, I., Lev, E., & Benoliel, J.Q. (1998). The effects of home nursing care for patients during terminal illness on the bereaved's psychological distress. *Nursing Research, 47*(1), 2–10.

McCorkle, R., Strumpf, N.E., Nuamah, I.F., Adler, D.C., Cooley, M.E., Jepson, C., et al. (2000). A specialized home care intervention improves survival among older post-surgical cancer patients. *Journal of the American Geriatrics Society, 48*(12), 1707–1713.

McMillan, S.C., Heusinkveld, K., Chai, S., Murphy, C.M., & Huany, C.Y. (2002). Revising the blueprint for the Oncology Certified Nurse (OCN®) examination: A role delineation study [Online exclusive]. *Oncology Nursing Forum, 29*(9), E110–E117.

McWilliams, J.E., Sanderson, B.J., Harris, E.L., Richert-Boe, K.E., & Henner, W.D. (1995). Glutathione S-transferase M1 (GSTM1) deficiency and lung cancer risk. *Cancer Epidemiology, Biomarkers and Prevention, 4*(60), 589–594.

Meraviglia, M.G. (2004). The effects of spirituality on well-being of people with lung cancer. *Oncology Nursing Forum, 31*(1), 89–94.

Miaskowski, C., Dodd, M., & Lee, K. (2004). Symptom clusters: The new frontier in symptom management research. *Journal of the National Cancer Institute Monographs, 32*, 17–21.

Miaskowski, C., & Lee, K.A. (1999). Pain, fatigue, and sleep disturbances in oncology outpatients receiving radiation therapy for bone metastasis: A pilot study. *Journal of Pain and Symptom Management, 17*(5), 320–332.

Molassiotis, A., Panteli, V., Patiraki, E., Ozden, G., Platin, N., Madsen, E., et al. (2006). Complementary and alternative medicine use in lung cancer patients in eight European countries. *Complementary Therapies in Clinical Practice, 12*(1), 34–39.

Morita, T., Shima, Y., Miyashita, M., Kimura, R., & Adachi, I. (2004). Physician- and nurse-reported effects of intravenous hydration therapy on symptoms of terminally ill patients with cancer. *Journal of Palliative Medicine, 7*(5), 683–693.

Mulshine, J.L., & Sullivan, D.C. (2005). Lung cancer screening. *New England Journal of Medicine, 353*(26), 2714–2720.

Mystakidou, K., Parpa, E., Katsouda, E., Galanos, A., & Vlahos, L. (2006). The role of physical and psychological symptoms in desire for death: A study of terminally ill cancer patients. *Psycho-Oncology, 15*(4), 355–360.

Nail, L.M. (2002). Fatigue in patients with cancer. *Oncology Nursing Forum, 29*(3), 537–544.

Nakaya, N., Saito-Nakaya, K., Akizuki, N., Yoshikawa, E., Kobayakawa, M., Fujimori, M., et al. (2006). Depression and survival in patients with non-small cell lung cancer after curative resection: A preliminary study. *Cancer Science, 97*(3), 199–205.

Narahashi, T., Niki, T., Wang, T., Goto, A., Matsubara, D., Funata, N., et al. (2006). Cytoplasmic localization of p63 is associated with poor patient survival in lung adenocarcinoma. *Histopathology, 49*(4), 349–357.

National Institutes of Health. (2006). *State-of-the-science conference statement on tobacco use: Prevention, cessation, and control.* Retrieved February 26, 2007, from http://consensus.nih.gov/2006/2006TobaccoSOS029html.htm

Nerriere, E., Zmirou-Navier, D., Desqueyroux, P., Leclerc, N., Momas, I., & Czernichow, P. (2005). Lung cancer risk assessment in relation with personal exposure to airborne particles in four French metropolitan areas. *Journal of Occupational and Environmental Medicine, 47*(12), 1211–1217.

Oncology News International. (2005). ACS urges comprehensive approach to lung cancer screening. *Oncology News International, 14*(6), 13.

Oncology Nursing Society. (2007). *Top 20 research priorities.* Retrieved June 23, 2007, from http://www.ons.org/research/information/agenda.shtml

Parker, V., Sussman, S., Crippens, D., Elder, P., & Scholl, D. (1998). The relation of ethnic identification with cigarette smoking among US urban African American and Latino youth: A pilot study. *Ethnicity and Health, 3*(1–2), 135–143.

Patel, J.D., Bach, P.B., & Kris, M.G. (2004). Lung cancer in US women: A contemporary epidemic. *JAMA, 291*(14), 1763–1768.

Petersen, R.P., & Harpole, D.H., Jr. (2006). Computerized tomography screening for the early detection of lung cancer. *Journal of the National Comprehensive Cancer Network, 4*(6), 591–594.

Piper, B.F., Dibble, S.L., Dodd, M.J., Weiss, M.C., Slaughter, R.E., & Paul, S.M. (1998). The Revised Piper Fatigue Scale: Psychometric evaluation in women with breast cancer. *Oncology Nursing Forum, 25*(4), 677–684.

Potti, A., Mukherjee, S., Peterson, R., Dressman, H., Bild, A., Koontz, J., et al. (2006). A genomic strategy to refine prognosis in early-stage non-small-cell lung cancer. *New England Journal of Medicine, 355*(6), 570–580.

Pud, D., Ben-Ami, S., Yaffe, A., & Miaskowski, C. (2007). The symptom experiences of oncology outpatients have a negative impact on quality of life outcomes: The results of a cluster analysis multi-site replication study [Abstract 42]. *Oncology Nursing Forum, 34*(1), 184.

Radloff, L.S. (1977). The CES-D Scale: A self-report depression scale for research in the general population. *Applied Psychological Measurement, 1*(3), 385–401.

Read, W., Tierney, R., Page, N.C., Costas, I., Govindan, R., Spitznagel, E.L., et al. (2004). Differential impact of comorbidity. *Journal of Clinical Oncology, 22*(15), 3099–3103.

Reiser, M., & Visovsky, C. (1998). Airway obstruction. In C.C. Chernecky & B.J. Berger (Eds.), *Advanced and critical care oncology nursing: Managing primary complications* (pp. 56–66). Philadelphia: Saunders.

Ruckdeschel, J.C., Spitz, M.R., & Saxman, S. (2001). *Report of the Lung Cancer Progress Review Group* [NIH Publication No. 01-5025]. Retrieved August 1, 2001, from http://osp.nci .nih.gov/prg_assess/prg/lungprg/lung_rpt.htm

Rusznak, C., & Davies, R.J. (1998). ABC of allergies: Diagnosing allergy. *BMJ, 316*(7132), 686–689.

Sarna, L. (1993a). Correlates of symptom distress in women with lung cancer. *Cancer Practice, 1*(1), 21–28.

Sarna, L. (1993b). Women with lung cancer: Impact on quality of life. *Quality of Life Research, 2*(1), 13–22.

Sarna, L. (1994). Functional status in women with lung cancer. *Cancer Nursing, 17*(2), 87–93.

Sarna, L., & Bialous, S. (2005). Tobacco control in the 21st century: A critical issue for the nursing profession. *Research and Theory for Nursing Practice, 19*(1), 15–24.

Sarna, L., & Bialous, S.A. (2006). Strategic directions for nursing research in tobacco dependence. *Nursing Research, 55*(Suppl. 4), S1–S9.

Sarna, L., Bialous, S.A., Wewers, M.E., Froelicher, E.S., & Danao, L. (2005). Nurses, smoking, and the workplace. *Research in Nursing and Health, 28*(1), 79–90.

Sarna, L., & Brecht, M.L. (1997). Dimensions of symptom distress in women with advanced lung cancer: A factor analysis. *Heart and Lung, 26*(1), 23–30.

Sarna, L., Brown, J.K., Cooley, M.E., Williams, R.D., Chernecky, C., Padilla, G., et al. (2005). Quality of life and meaning of illness of women with lung cancer [Online exclusive]. *Oncology Nursing Forum, 32*(1), E9–E19. Retrieved November 25, 2006, from http://ons .metapress.com/content/k41211340546kw09/fulltext.pdf

Sarna, L., Cooley, M.E., Brown, J.K., Chernecky, C., & Elashoff, D. (2007). Symptom patterns after thoracotomy for lung cancer [Abstract 44]. *Oncology Nursing Forum, 34*(1), 185.

Sarna, L., Cooley, M.E., Brown, J.K., Williams, R.D., Chernecky, C., Padilla, G., et al. (2006). Quality of life and health status of dyads of women with lung cancer and family members. *Oncology Nursing Forum, 33*(6), 1109–1116.

Sarna, L., Cooley, M.E., & Danao, L. (2003). The global epidemic of tobacco and cancer. *Seminars in Oncology Nursing, 19*(4), 233–243.

Sarna, L., Evangelista, L., Tashkin, D., Padilla, G., Holmes, C., Brecht, M.L., et al. (2004). Impact of respiratory symptoms and pulmonary function on quality of life of long-term survivors of non-small cell lung cancer. *Chest 125*(2), 439–445.

Sarna, L., Lindsey, A.M., Dean, H., Brecht, M.L., & McCorkle, R. (1993). Nutritional intake, weight change, symptom distress, and functional status over time in adults with lung cancer. *Oncology Nursing Forum, 20*(3), 481–489.

Sarna, L., & McCorkle, R. (1996). Burden of care and lung cancer. *Cancer Practice, 4*(5), 245–251.

Sarna, L., Padilla, G., Holmes, C., Tashkin, D., Brecht, M.L., & Evangelista, L. (2002). Quality of life of long-term survivors of non-small-cell lung cancer. *Journal of Clinical Oncology, 20*(13), 2920–2929.

Schultz, K., Bergmann, K.C., Kenn, K., Petro, W., Heitmann, R.H., Fischer, R., et al. (2006). Effectiveness of impatient pulmonary rehabilitation (AHB): Results of a multicenter prospective observation study (German). *Deutsche Medizinische Wochenschrift, 131*(33), 1793–1798.

Schwartz, A.G., Prysak, G.M., Bock, C.H., & Cote, M.L. (2007). The molecular epidemiology of lung cancer. *Carcinogenesis, 28*(3), 507–518.

Schwartz, A.G., & Ruckdeschel, J.C. (2006). Familial lung cancer: Genetic susceptibility and relationship to chronic obstructive pulmonary disease. *American Journal of Respiratory and Critical Care Medicine, 173*(1), 16–22.

Selim, A.J., Xinhua, S.R., Fincke, G., Rogers, W., Lee, A., & Kazis, L. (1997). A symptom-based measure of the severity of chronic lung disease: Results from the Veterans Health Study. *Chest, 111*(6), 1607–1614.

Shibuya, K., Mathers, C.D., Boschi-Pinto, C., Lopez, A.D., & Murray, C.J. (2002). Global and regional estimates of cancer mortality and incidence by site: II. Results for the global burden of disease 2000. *BMC Cancer, 2*, 37.

Shimizu, H., Tominaga, S., Nishimura, M., & Urata, A. (1984). Comparison of clinico-epidemiological features of lung cancer patients with and without a history of smoking. *Japanese Journal of Clinical Oncology, 14*(4), 595–600.

Shimizu, K., Yamada, K., Saito, H., Noda, K., Nakayama, H., Kameda, Y., et al. (2005). Surgically curable peripheral lung carcinoma: Correlation of thin-section CT findings with histologic prognostic factors and survival. *Chest, 127*(3), 871–878.

Shimoyama, N., & Shimoyama, M. (2002). Nebulized furosemide as a novel treatment for dyspnea in terminal cancer patients. *Journal of Pain and Symptom Management, 23*(1), 73–76.

Simon, G.R., Sharma, S., Cantor, A., Smith, P., & Bepler, G. (2005). ERCC1 expression is a predictor of survival in resected patients with non-small cell lung cancer. *Chest, 127*(3), 978–983.

Sola, I., Thompson, E., Subirana, M., Lopez, C., & Pascual, A. (2008). Non-invasive interventions for improving well-being and quality of life in patients with lung cancer. *Cochrane Database of Systematic Reviews 2008,* Issue 2. Art. No: CD004282. DOI: 10.1002/14651858 .CD004282.pub2.

Sorensen, M., Raaschou-Nielsen, O., Hansen, R.D., Tjonneland, A., Overvad, K., & Vogel, U. (2006). Interactions between the OGG1 Ser326Cys polymorphism and intake of fruit and vegetables in relation to lung cancer. *Free Radical Research, 40*(8), 885–891.

Spector, N., Klein, D., & Rice-Wyllie, L. (2000). Advanced practice. Terminally ill patients breathe easier with nebulized morphine. *Nursing Spectrum (Greater Chicago/NE Illinois and NW Indiana Edition), 13*(24), 16–17.

Sprangers, M.A., Cull, A., Groenvold, M., Bjordal, K., Blazeby, J., & Aaronson, N.K. (1998). The European Organization for Research and Treatment of Cancer approach to developing questionnaire modules: An update and overview. EORTC Quality of Life Study Group. *Quality of Life Research, 7*(4), 291–300.

Strauss, G.M., Gleason, R.E., & Sugarbaker, D.J. (1995). Chest x-ray screening improves outcome in lung cancer: A reappraisal of randomized trials on lung cancer screening. *Chest, 107*(Suppl. 6), 270S–279S.

Talaska, G., Al-Zoughool, M., Malaveille, C., Fiorini, L., Schumann, B., Vietas, J., et al. (2006). Randomized controlled trial: Effects of diet on DNA damage in heavy smokers. *Mutagenesis, 21*(3), 179–183.

Tammemagi, M.C., McLaughlin, J.R., Mullen, J.B., Bull, S.B., Johnston, M.R., Tsao, M.S., et al. (2000). A study of smoking, *p53* tumor suppressor gene alterations and non-small cell lung cancer. *Annals of Epidemiology, 10*(3), 176–185.

Tanaka, K., Akechi, T., Okuyama, T., Nishiwaki, Y., & Uchitomi, Y. (2000). Development and validation of the Cancer Dyspnea Scale: A multidimensional, brief, self-rating scale. *British Journal of Cancer, 82*(4), 800–805.

Thomas, J.R., & von Gunten, C.F. (2002). Treatment of dyspnea in cancer patients. *Oncology, 16*(6), 745–758.

Thompson, E., Sola, I., & Subirana, M. (2005). Non-invasive interventions for improving well-being and quality of life in patients with lung cancer—A systematic review of the evidence. *Lung Cancer, 50*(2), 163–176.

Timmerman, P. (1998). Pulmonary fibrosis. In C.C. Chernecky & B.J. Berger (Eds.), *Advanced and critical care oncology nursing: Managing primary complications* (pp. 512–535). Philadelphia: Saunders.

Tolley, H.D., Crane, L., & Shipley, N. (1991). Smoking prevalence and lung cancer death rates. In *Strategies to control tobacco use in the United States: A blueprint for public health action in the 1990s. Smoking and Tobacco Control Monograph No. 1* [NIH Publication No. 92-3316]. Bethesda, MD: U.S. Public Health Service, National Institutes of Health, National Cancer Institute.

Tovar-Guzman, V.J., Lopez-Antunano, F.J., & Rodriguez-Salgado, N. (2005). Trends in mortality from lung cancer in Mexico, 1980–2000 [Spanish, English Abstract]. *Pan American Journal of Public Health, 17*(4), 254–262.

Tsuda, T., Mino, Y., Babazono, A., Shigemi, J., Otsu, T., Yamamoto, E., et al. (2002). A case-control study of lung cancer in relation to silica exposure and silicosis in a rural area in Japan. *Annals of Epidemiology, 12*(5), 288–294.

U.S. Centers for Disease Control and Prevention. (2002a). Cigarette smoking among adults—United States, 2000. *Morbidity and Mortality Weekly Report, 51*(29), 642–645.

U.S. Centers for Disease Control and Prevention. (2002b). Trends in cigarette smoking among high school students—United States, 1991–2001. *Morbidity and Mortality Weekly Report, 51*(19), 409–412.

U.S. Centers for Disease Control and Prevention. (2007). *Fact sheet: Adult cigarette smoking in the United States: Current estimates.* Retrieved June 4, 2008, from http://www.cdc.gov/tobacco/data_statistics/factsheets/adult_cig_smoking.htm

U.S. Department of Health and Human Services. (2000). *Healthy people 2010.* Washington, DC: Author.

Vena, C., Parker, K., Allen, R., Bliwise, D., Jain, S., & Kimble, L. (2006). Sleep-wake disturbances and quality of life in patients with advanced lung cancer. *Oncology Nursing Forum, 33*(4), 761–769.

Vogel, W.H., Wilson, M.A., & Melvin, M.S. (2003). Lung cancer. In W.H. Vogel, M.A. Wilson, & M.S. Melvin (Eds.), *Advanced practice oncology and palliative care guidelines* (pp. 170–179). Philadelphia: Lippincott Williams and Wilkins.

Wells, M., Sarna, L., Cooley, M.E., Brown, J.K., Williams, R., Chernecky, C., et al. (2007). Use of complementary and alternative medicine therapies to control symptoms in women living with lung cancer. *Cancer Nursing, 30*(1), 45–57.

Wewers, M.E., Sarna, L., & Rice, V.H. (2006). Nursing research and treatment of tobacco dependence: State of the science. *Nursing Research, 55*(Suppl. 4), 11–15.

Wickham, R. (2002). Dyspnea: Recognizing and managing an invisible problem. *Oncology Nursing Forum, 29*(6), 925–933.

Wilkie, E., Rhodes, S., Stewart, M., Rankin, E., & Ried, I. (2007). Cognitive function prior to and following chemotherapy treatment in patients with lung cancer [Abstract 108]. *Oncology Nursing Forum, 34*(1), 210.

Wolski, M.J., Bhatnagar, A., Flickinger, J.C., Belani, C.P., Ramalingam, S., & Greenberger, J.S. (2005). Multivariate analysis of survival, local control, and time to distant metastases in patients with unresectable non-small-cell lung carcinoma treated with 3-dimensional conformal radiation therapy with or without concurrent chemotherapy. *Clinical Lung Cancer, 7*(2), 100–106.

Yellen, S.B., Cella, D.F., Webster, K., Blendowski, C., & Kaplan, E. (1997). Measuring fatigue and other anemia-related symptoms with the Functional Assessment of Cancer Therapy (FACT) measurement system. *Journal of Pain and Symptom Management, 13*(2), 63–74.

Yurdakul, A.S., Halilcolar, H., Ozturk, C., Tatar, D., & Karakaya, J. (2006). Factors affecting the prognosis in patients with primary lung cancer and brain metastases [Turkish, English Abstract]. *Tuberkuloz ve Toraks, 54*(3), 235–242.

Zang, E.A., & Wynder, E.L. (1996). Differences in lung cancer risk between men and women: Examination of the evidence. *Journal of the National Cancer Institute, 88*(3–4), 183–192.

CHAPTER 8

Focus on Prostate Cancer

Shanita D. Williams-Brown, PhD, MPH, APRN, and
Maureen E. O'Rourke, RN, PhD

Introduction

Prostate cancer is the most common non-skin cancer in men in the United States and accounts for a full third of all new cancer cases diagnosed in men each year. In 2008, an estimated 186,320 men will have been diagnosed with prostate cancer, and approximately 28,660 will die from the disease, making prostate cancer the leading cause of new cancer cases and the second leading cause of cancer-related deaths in men in the United States (American Cancer Society [ACS], 2008).

Oncology nurse scientists have participated actively in the recent development of a substantive body of knowledge related to prostate cancer. The oncology nursing research literature has contributed a great deal to the understanding of prostate cancer's impact on men and their families. Oncology nurses use the novel findings generated by oncology nurse scientists to inform nursing practice (Cunningham, 2006; Harrison, Dowswell, & Wright, 2002).

This chapter will present a summary of how oncology nurse scientists have advanced prostate cancer science over the past two decades. Specifically, this chapter will first highlight the evolution of oncology nursing science that focuses on prostate cancer, identify research studies that have informed nursing practice across the prostate cancer continuum, and conclude with a discussion of future directions for advancing prostate-related oncology nursing science.

Evolution of Nurse Scientists' Role in Prostate Cancer Research

Much of what is known about prostate cancer has been discovered through research and clinical practice over the past 50 years. Yet, most of the oncology nursing research related to prostate cancer has taken place in the past two decades. Research conducted by biomedical scientists, medical oncologists, and epidemiologists has focused primarily on the biologic and morphologic characteristics of prostate cancer, patterning and rates of disease, and appropriate drug therapies and treatment regimens. Consequently, much of the initial focus of oncology nursing research related to prostate cancer focused on improving prostate cancer care outcomes (Heinrich-Rynning, 1987; Held, Osborne, Volpe, & Waldman, 1994; Robinson et al., 1999; Rose, Shrader-Bogen, Korlath, Priem, & Larson, 1996; Walker, Nail, Larsen, Magill, & Schwartz, 1996).

As nursing practice domains continually extended beyond the traditional clinical setting in the past 20 years, oncology nursing science also has evolved. In addition to maintaining a clinical practice–based focus, oncology nurse scientists have extended their scientific base to include detection, diagnosis, and equitable treatment of prostate cancer disease. In addition, oncology nurses explored psychosocial, interpersonal, economic, and environmental factors that are affected by a prostate cancer diagnosis and have begun to develop appropriate nursing interventions.

Advances in prostate cancer nursing research have been achieved primarily by oncology nurse scientists through conducting individual and collaborative research, developing and testing cancer care models (Johnson, Fieler, Wlasowicz, Mitchell, & Jones, 1997; Walton & Sullivan, 2004), and applying research findings in clinical practice (Cunningham, 2006). Oncology nurse scientists have guided the understanding of prostate cancer by expanding knowledge in the areas of prevention (Greco & Kulawiak, 1994), screening and early detection (Meade, Calvo, Rivera, & Baer, 2003; Zimmerman, 1997), appropriate management (Held et al., 1994; Moore & Estey, 1999; Rose et al., 1996), patient and family decision making (O'Rourke, 1999; O'Rourke & Germino, 1998), quality of life (QOL) (Fossa et al., 1989; Galbraith, Arechiga, Ramirez, & Pedro, 2005; Lev et al., 2004; Mellon, 2002), survivorship concerns (Waxman, 1993), and ensuring quality cancer care across the continuum (Williams-Brown, Phillips, & Rust, 2005).

Contributions of Oncology Nurse Scientists to Prostate Cancer Research

Major contributions by oncology nurse scientists to prostate cancer research have evolved in essentially three interwoven phases over the past 20 years. During the mid- to late 20th century, especially during the 1960s through the 1980s, the emphasis across disciplines was the treatment of symptomatic or advanced-stage prostate cancers. The majority of prostate cancer care took place within inpatient hospital settings. During this period, oncology nursing practice primarily was concerned with the nurse clinician's ability to effectively manage patient symptoms and treatment-related side effects. Much of the initial oncology nursing research in the late 1980s through the 1990s involved studies that investigated oncology nurses' abilities to effectively deliver postoperative care, which included the ability to adequately identify patients' postsurgical concerns and to effectively manage their symptoms after treatment (Abel et al., 1999; Rose et al., 1996; Walker et al., 1996). Several nursing research studies also involved treatment comparisons and clinical outcomes of various treatment regimens (Fossa et al., 1989; Held et al., 1994; Moore & Estey, 1999; Moul & Lipo, 1999; Waxman, 1993).

The second phase of oncology nursing research reflected a shift from the effective management and treatment of advanced-stage prostate cancers among symptomatic patients to a focus on the early detection and screening of prostate cancer among asymptomatic men. This shift coincided with the development of prostate-specific antigen (PSA) testing leading to investigations by nurses of men with early-stage disease and different needs. This second phase, which began in the early 1990s and continues today, is marked by the development of an extensive body of cross-disciplinary research that establishes associations between early detection and appropriate/timely treatment of prostate cancer emphasizing decreasing morbidity and mortality. Contributions of oncology nurse scientists have included the development of assessment tools designed to examine the perceptions of risk and risk behaviors related to prostate cancer (Gelmann, 1985; Johnson & Smolenski, 2007).

In addition to risk awareness and assessment, the importance of screening behaviors also has been a major focus of oncology nursing research. Several population-based oncology nursing research studies tested the hypothesis that the lack of awareness about prostate cancer and the lack of understanding of the importance of screening and early detection contributed to decreased prostate cancer screening rates (Clarke-Tasker & Wade, 2002; Lang, 1991; Plowden, 1999; Tingen, Weinrich, Heyd, Boyd, & Weinrich, 1998; Weinrich, Weinrich, Boyd, & Atkinson, 1998). Findings indicated that lack of knowledge was related significantly to low levels of screening participation.

A logical extension of the prostate cancer screening and early detection literature was the new focus by oncology nurse scientists on disenfranchised populations, such as racial and ethnic minorities and the uninsured. Bruner, Jones, Buchanan, and Russo (2006) have been instrumental in increasing racial and ethnic minority participation in cancer clinical trials, and the extensive work of Dr. Sally P. Weinrich has led to the identification of specific barriers and promoters of screening among African American men and the development of effective strategies to increase their participation in prostate cancer screening (Weinrich, Greiner, Reis-Starr, Yoon, & Weinrich,1998; Weinrich, Reynolds, Tingen, & Starr, 2000). Disparities between African Americans and Caucasians in prostate cancer screening and clinical outcomes also were highlighted by other oncology nurse scientists, and their collective findings suggested that knowledge, attitudes, and lack of access to care were barriers to screening participation (Abbott, Taylor, & Barber, 1998; Jones & Wenzel, 2005; Woods, Montgomery, & Herring, 2004). Oncology nurse scientists have been at the forefront in the identification of factors that both inhibit and promote prostate cancer screening among all men in general and African American men in particular (Clarke-Tasker & Wade, 2002; Kleier, 2003, 2004; Woods et al., 2004; Woods, Montgomery, Herring, Gardner, & Stokols, 2006). The work of Dr. Weinrich influenced the many nurse scientists' direction and led to the development of an extensive scientific knowledge base with respect to prostate cancer screening and African American men (see Table 8-1).

Table 8-1. Select Research Contributions of Dr. Sally P. Weinrich to Prostate Cancer and African American Men, 1997–2006

Citation by Publication Date	Title	Journal
Tingen et al. (1997)	Prostate Cancer Screening: Predictors of Participation	*Journal of the American Academy of Nurse Practitioners*
Reis-Starr et al. (1998)	The Association Between Family History and Participation in Free Prostate Cancer Screening	*American Journal of Health Studies*
Tingen et al. (1998)	Perceived Benefits: A Predictor of Participation in Prostate Cancer Screening	*Cancer Nursing*
Weinrich, Atwood, et al. (1998)	Cost for Prostate Cancer Educational Programs in Work and Church Sites	*American Journal of Health Behavior*
Weinrich, Boyd, Bradford, et al. (1998)	Recruitment of African-American Men Into Prostate Cancer Screening	*Cancer Practice*
Weinrich, Greiner, et al. (1998)	Predictors of Participation in Prostate Cancer Screening at Work Sites	*Journal of Community Health Nursing*
Weinrich, Holdford, et al. (1998)	Prostate Cancer Screening in African American Churches	*Public Health Nursing*
Weinrich, Jacobsen, et al. (1998)	Reference Ranges for Serum Prostate-Specific Antigen in Black and White Men Without Cancer	*Urology*
Weinrich et al. (1999)	Contrasting Costs of Prostate Cancer Educational Programs by Race and Educational Method	*American Journal of Health Behavior*
Weinrich, Weinrich, Boyd, et al. (1998)	The Impact of Prostate Cancer Knowledge on Cancer Screening	*Oncology Nursing Forum*
Weinrich, Boyd, Weinrich, et al. (1998)	Increasing Prostate Cancer Screening in African American Men With Peer-Educator and Client-Navigator Interventions	*Journal of Cancer Education*

(Continued on next page)

Table 8-1. Select Research Contributions of Dr. Sally P. Weinrich to Prostate Cancer and African American Men, 1997–2006 *(Continued)*

Citation by Publication Date	Title	Journal
Weinrich, Weinrich, Mettlin, et al. (1998)	Urinary Symptoms as a Predictor for Participation in Prostate Cancer Screening Among African American Men	*Prostate*
Shelton & Weinrich (1999)	Barriers to Prostate Cancer Screening in African American Men	*Journal of National Black Nurses Association*
Weinrich, Ellison, et al. (2000)	Participation in Prostate Cancer Screening Among Low-Income Men	*Psychology, Health, and Medicine*
Weinrich, Reynolds, et al. (2000)	Barriers to Prostate Screening	*Cancer Nursing*
Weinrich, Weinrich, et al. (2000)	Contrasting Cost of a Prostate Cancer Educational Program By Income	*American Journal of Health Behavior*
Boyd et al. (2001)	Obstacles to Prostate Cancer Screening in African-American Men	*Journal of National Black Nurses Association*
Ellison et al. (2001)	Psychosocial Stress and Prostate Cancer: A Theoretical Model	*Ethnicity and Disease*
Weinrich, Faison-Smith, et al. (2002)	Stability of Self-Reported Family History of Prostate Cancer Among African American Men	*Journal of Nursing Measurement*
Weinrich, Royal, et al. (2002)	Interest in Genetic Prostate Cancer Susceptibility Testing Among African American Men	*Cancer Nursing*
Weinrich et al. (2003)	Self-Reported Reasons Men Decide Not to Participate in Free Prostate Cancer Screening	*Oncology Nursing Forum*
Giesler et al. (2005)	Improving the Quality of Life of Prostate Cancer Patients: A Randomized Trial Testing the Efficacy of a Nurse-Driven Intervention	*Cancer*
Weinrich (2006)	Prostate Cancer Screening in High-Risk Men: African American Hereditary Prostate Cancer Study Network	*Cancer*

The sentinel work of Dr. Sally P. Weinrich and colleagues has made a tremendous contribution to the body of research on prostate cancer and the inequities in cancer screening and quality cancer care experienced by men of color, and most specifically, African American men.

The third overlapping phase of oncology nursing research was marked by growth in multidisciplinary collaboration, which has led to an expansion of research into genetic and biologic studies. One exemplar in this area is Dr. Sally P. Weinrich, who has been a key team member of the African American Hereditary Prostate Cancer Study Network (Weinrich, 2006) and has collaborated on multiple projects examining genetic and familial contributions to prostate cancer risk in African American men (Gilligan et al., 2004; Panguluri et al., 2004).

Contemporary oncology nurse scientists are now involved in prostate cancer research at every level: basic science, including genetic and biologic studies, and population-based epidemiologic studies, as well as studies focused on screening and early-detection methods, treatment, and examination of the impact of prostate cancer on every aspect of QOL.

Oncology Nursing Research Across the Prostate Cancer Care Continuum

The continuum of cancer care begins with prevention and extends to palliation. Oncology nursing research spans this same trajectory.

Prevention

The exact cause of prostate cancer remains unknown; however, age, race, ethnicity, and family history are well-established risk factors. A consensus exists that genetic and constitutional factors play an etiologic role. Although numerous genetic factors have been associated with prostate cancer, no single genetic factor has been identified as demonstrating the same strength of association with prostate cancer as the *APC* gene in colon cancer or the *BRCA1* gene in female breast cancer. A distinct paucity of oncology nursing research exists in primary prevention of prostate cancer, which may be directly related to the current state of science regarding preventive strategies. Oncology nurse scientists have devoted significant energy and resources toward developing a body of knowledge upon which to base interventions in the area of secondary prevention of prostate cancer.

Early Detection and Diagnosis

Disease stage at initial diagnosis is a key determinant of prostate cancer survival among men. The best survival rates are observed among men diagnosed in the earliest stages of prostate cancer. Survival rates steadily decline as the stage at diagnosis progresses. The five-year relative survival rate for localized/regional prostate cancer is approximately 100%; however, for men with distant metastases, survival rates decline precipitously to approximately 32% (Surveillance, Epidemiology and End Results Program [SEER], 2007).

Numerous cross-disciplinary studies show consistent significant associations between late/advanced-stage prostate cancer diagnoses and underutilization or delay in prostate cancer screening. Urban, rural, racial/ethnic minority, and impoverished men are least likely to participate in timely routine prostate cancer screening and consequently are most likely to present with advanced-stage prostate disease (ACS, 2007; SEER, 2007).

Nurses assume key roles in the early detection of prostate cancer through their involvement with cancer screening. Numerous oncology nursing research studies have targeted the design and evaluation of effective strategies to increase both the access to and the effectiveness of prostate cancer screening. Multiple factors associated with the underutilization of prostate cancer screening have been identified, including lack of access to state-of-the-art cancer screening services, low levels of cancer knowledge, lack of provider recommendation for cancer screening, cultural and language barriers on the part of both providers and patients, and misconceptions about cancer and cancer screening (Weinrich, Ellison, et al., 2000; Weinrich, Greiner, et al., 1998; Weinrich, Reynolds, et al., 2000; Weinrich, Weinrich, Boyd, et al., 1998). Oncology nurse scientists also have described factors that promote access to screening and reduce racial disparities in screening rates and have identified the supportive role of women and female significant others in promoting prostate cancer screening and follow-up care in men (Riechers, 2004; Weinrich, Greiner, et al., 1998, Weinrich, Holdford, et al.; Woods et al., 2006).

PSA testing in combination with digital rectal examination (DRE) are currently the best screening tools available for the early detection of prostate cancer. However, PSA testing is unable to specifically differentiate those cancers that are clinically significant from those that are not. Elevated serum PSA levels may potentiate an involved diagnostic process resulting in unnecessary treatment, which may have deleterious effects on QOL, such as impotence, incontinence, and bowel dysfunction. This is the source of great controversy within the scientific community and highlights the importance of informed decision making.

Nurses routinely are expected to assist families in making informed choices regarding the utility of PSA testing and interpreting the implications of a positive or negative test. Davison and her colleagues in Canada have made significant contributions to the literature in this area by investigating decision-making preferences and by developing and testing innovative strategies and decisional aids to assist men with their decision making (Colella & DeLuca, 2004; Davison, Degner, & Morgan, 1995; Davison et al., 2002; Davison, Goldenberg, Wiens, & Gleave, 2007; Oliffe, 2006).

Management and Supportive Care

Controversy with respect to prostate cancer extends to the realm of treatment decisions. As the empiric basis for treatment recommendations for early-stage prostate cancer is being developed, men and their families face treatment decisions fraught with uncertainty. Treatment recommendations for early-stage prostate cancer include three-dimensional conformal external beam radiation therapy, brachytherapy, radical prostatectomy, and watchful waiting (National Comprehensive Cancer Network, 2008). Oncology nurses have been at the forefront of the exploration of men's decision-making process (Berry et al., 2003; Gwede et al., 2005; O'Rourke, 1999; O'Rourke & Germino, 1998). Involvement of spouses and significant others as well as the influence of emotion, anecdote, and biases for and against surgery were found to be significant factors in the treatment decision-making process. These findings suggested that interventions to assist men in their decision making should include significant others and should include attention to both emotive and cognitive factors.

The pervasiveness of uncertainty among patients with cancer was described extensively by Mishel (1990) as she developed and tested her theory of uncertainty in illness. More recently, she has worked with colleagues Germino and Bailey to apply the theory to build and test interventions aimed at uncertainty experienced by men with prostate cancer (Bailey, Mishel, Belyea, Stewart, & Mohler, 2004; Mishel et al., 2002, 2003). Psychoeducational interventions were found to improve uncertainty management using cognitive reframing and problem solving. Bailey reported that men choosing watchful waiting who received an uncertainty intervention reported less confusion and believed their QOL in the future would be better (Bailey et al.). Wallace also utilized the uncertainty in illness theory as she examined QOL among men with prostate cancer (Bailey & Wallace, 2007; Wallace, 2003).

Oncology nurse scientists have extensively studied QOL among patients with prostate cancer, beginning with the work of Yarbro in 1998. Data suggested that QOL is affected negatively by each treatment option and that virtually all domains are affected. Men opting for surgical treatment are bothered by incontinence and impotence, whereas those treated with radiation therapy experience a high rate of bowel symptoms. Even men who forgo active treatment and elect watchful waiting may experience bothersome symptoms caused by the prostate cancer itself or related to dealing with conditions of near-constant uncertainty (Fossa et al., 1989; Galbraith et al., 2005; Galbraith, Ramirez, & Pedro, 2001; Lev et al., 2004; Mellon, 2002; Yarbro, 1998). Symptom management and uncertainty interventions developed by oncology nurses may attenuate the negative effects of treatment and assist men in coping with their anxiety and fears regarding potential disease recurrence or progression.

Oncology nurse scientists also examined how men and their spouses make sense of the prostate cancer diagnosis and cope with treatment side effects such as incontinence and impotence (Maliski, Heilemann, & McCorkle, 2001, 2002). In an integrative review of spousal response to prostate cancer, Resendes and McCorkle (2006) concluded that the literature shows that overall, spouses are significantly more distressed than the patients themselves. Specific sources of distress were identified as lack of information, fear of both the unknown and what the future might bring, and treatment-related side effects. They were able to identify only a single study that attempted to address these concerns, suggesting an area for future research.

Racial Disparities in Prostate Cancer Care

Scientists in other disciplines have begun to examine racial disparities in prostate cancer treatment. Shavers and colleagues noted that African American males are more likely than Caucasian males to go untreated for their prostate cancer and less likely than Caucasians to receive definitive treatment (Shavers & Brown, 2002; Shavers et al., 2004). Shavers reported that in her review, African American and Hispanic/Latino patients with prostate cancer who chose watchful waiting received less medical monitoring than Caucasians. Additionally, African American and Hispanic/Latino men experienced longer median time intervals from the date of diagnosis to receipt of medical monitoring, diagnostic procedures, or definitive treatment compared to Caucasians (Shavers & Brown; Shavers et al.). Shavers' research suggested that racial disparities with respect to prostate cancer are not limited to screening. No nursing studies were located on this high-priority topic. This is an area in desperate need of attention from oncology nurse scientists.

Palliative Care

Nursing research addressing palliative care of men with advanced prostate cancer is lacking. One study by Berry et al. (2006) examined two chemotherapy protocols. The study compared docetaxel and estramustine to mitoxantrone and prednisone in terms of QOL and pain. Although one arm of the trial (docetaxel and estramustine) had superior clinical efficacy, QOL and pain palliation were similar in both arms.

Lindqvist, Widmark, and Rasmussen (2006) used the phenomenologic hermeneutic approach to guide interviews of 18 men living with advanced prostate cancer. Findings indicated that the meaning of living with bodily problems centered on a cycle of experiencing wellness and experiencing illness. New or changed bodily problems meant losing the feeling of wellness for these men. The scientists noted that pain and fatigue are the most prominent problems experienced. They suggested that nurses may obstruct the patient's possibility of experiencing wellness by focusing on symptoms and disease but offered no suggestions as to how to alter this focus while meeting the patient's needs in terms of pain and symptom management.

One final study by Esper, Hampton, Smith, and Pienta (1999) was located. They compared the QOL of 33 men who were receiving therapy for advanced prostate cancer. Not surprisingly, findings indicated that patients who demonstrated a response to therapy based on declining PSA levels demonstrated a significant increase in their QOL scores as compared to those patients who were not responding to treatment.

These studies suggest an acute need for the expansion of research in this area. As the population ages, more men will be living with prostate cancer who may experience symptoms caused by advanced disease. Building a scientific basis for nursing care that addresses the unique needs of these men and their families is crucial.

Conclusion

The growth and development of more doctoral-based, research-intensive training programs and postdoctoral opportunities, aligned with the strong financial support of the Oncology Nursing Society (ONS), the ONS Foundation, ACS, and the National Institute of Nursing Research, has contributed to the exponential growth in the area of prostate cancer–related nursing research. Oncology nurse scientists have taken a strategic position in advancing prostate cancer research across the cancer continuum over the past 20 years. Understanding of the complex factors that affect prostate cancer risk and outcomes is continually evolving. These complex factors include cancer biology and genetics, stage at diagnosis, and the often-elusive behavioral and environmental determinants of prostate cancer.

Oncology nurse scientists are in a unique position to contribute to the body of knowledge in the area of prostate cancer prevention on multiple fronts. Given the scant amount of nursing research dealing with the primary prevention of prostate cancer, aspiring oncology nurse scientists would be well served to initiate work in this area. Examination of lifestyle modifications, such as diet and exercise, are warranted. Research into the use of dietary supplements taken by men to prevent prostate cancer is another area in need of further investigation. Future oncology nurse scientists must continue to develop cross-disciplinary collaborative relationships as they work to identify genetic, biologic, and molecular risk factors for prostate disease.

Secondary prevention of prostate cancer consists of annual DRE and PSA testing. This review highlighted the tremendous amount of work in the area of PSA screening; however, application of these findings and investigation of barriers to and promoters of participation in screening must be extended to other populations, particularly Hispanic/Latino men.

Although scientists have initiated work in the area of treatment decision making, they are challenged to use these descriptive and exploratory findings to develop interventions to assist men and their families as they struggle to decide which treatment is best for them. As new information emerges from the medical literature, nurses must be prepared to respond to potential changes in treatment recommendations and the effects this may have on men who have already received treatment. Decision making regarding the need for additional treatment in the face of rising PSA levels also is an underexplored area.

Evidence exists that suggests that men of color are treated more conservatively and are less likely to receive innovative but costly therapies. Additionally, research has suggested that they are diagnosed later and have longer time-to-treatment intervals. The development and testing of strategic initiatives to overcome these disparities is desperately needed.

Expansion of the symptom management research and the testing of novel interventions to assist men in dealing with incontinence and impotence are warranted. Further development and testing of psychoeducational interventions for uncertainty would benefit both men and their partners. Additionally, studies investigating symptom management utilizing complementary and alternative modalities are needed.

Finally, although the palliative care literature is extensive, nurse scientists have only begun to develop a scientific basis for palliative care of men with advanced prostate cancer, thus suggesting another area for the expansion of nursing research.

Although much has been accomplished in nursing science regarding prostate cancer, much work remains. Given the past achievements and future potential of oncology nurse scientists in the field of prostate cancer, the future of prostate cancer nursing research is promising indeed.

References

Abbott, R.R., Taylor, D.K., & Barber, K.A. (1998). A comparison of prostate knowledge of African-American and Caucasian men: Changes from prescreening baseline to postintervention. *Cancer Journal From Scientific American, 4*(3), 175–177.

Abel, L.J., Blatt, H.J., Stipetich, R.L., Fuscardo, J.A., Zeroski, D., Miller, S.E., et al. (1999). Nursing management of patients receiving brachytherapy for early stage prostate cancer. *Clinical Journal of Oncology Nursing, 3*(1), 7–15.

American Cancer Society. (2007). *Cancer facts and figures, 2007.* Retrieved December 10, 2007, from http://www.cancer.org/downloads/STT/CAFF2007PWSecured.pdf

American Cancer Society. (2008). *Cancer facts and figures, 2008.* Retrieved May 13, 2008, from http://www.cancer.org/downloads/STT/2008CAFFfinalsecured.pdf

Bailey, D.E., Jr., Mishel, M.H., Belyea, M., Stewart, J.L., & Mohler, J. (2004). Uncertainty intervention for watchful waiting in prostate cancer. *Cancer Nursing, 27*(5), 339–346.

Bailey, D.E., Jr., & Wallace, M. (2007). Critical review: Is watchful waiting a viable management option for older men with prostate cancer? *American Journal of Men's Health, 1*(1), 18–28.

Berry, D.L., Ellis, W.J., Woods, N.F., Scwien, C., Mullen, K.H., & Yang, C. (2003). Treatment decision-making by men with localized prostate cancer: The influence of personal factors. *Urologic Oncology, 21*(2), 93–100.

Berry, D.L., Moinpour, C.M., Jiang, C.S., Ankerst, D.P., Petrylak, D.P., Vinson, L.V., et al. (2006). Quality of life and pain in advanced stage prostate cancer: Results of a Southwest Oncology Group randomized trial comparing docetaxel and estramustine to mitoxantrone and prednisone. *Journal of Clinical Oncology, 24*(18), 2828–2835.

Boyd, M., Weinrich, S., Weinrich, M., & Norton, A. (2001). Obstacles to prostate cancer screening in African-American men. *Journal of National Black Nurses Association, 12*(2), 1–5.

Bruner, D.W., Jones, M., Buchanan, D., & Russo, D. (2006). Reducing cancer disparities for minorities: A multidisciplinary research agenda to improve patient access to health systems, clinical trials, and effective cancer therapy. *Journal of Clinical Oncology, 24*(14), 2209–2215.

Clarke-Tasker, V.A., & Wade, R. (2002). What we thought we knew: African American males' perceptions of prostate cancer and screening methods. *ABNF Journal, 13*(3), 56–60.

Colella, K.M., & DeLuca, G. (2004). Shared decision making in patients with newly diagnosed prostate cancer: A model for treatment education and support. *Urologic Nursing,* 24(3), 187–191, 195–196.

Cunningham, R.S. (2006). Clinical practice guideline use by oncology advanced practice nurses. *Applied Nursing Research, 19*(3), 126–133.

Davison, B.J., Degner, L.F., & Morgan, T.R. (1995). Information and decision-making preferences of men with prostate cancer. *Oncology Nursing Forum, 22*(9), 1401–1408.

Davison, B.J., Gleave, M.E., Goldenberg, S.L., Degner, L.F., Hoffart, D., & Berkowitz, J. (2002). Assessing information and decision preferences of men with prostate cancer and their partners. *Cancer Nursing, 25*(1), 42–49.

Davison, B.J., Goldenberg, S.L., Wiens, K.P., & Gleave, M.E. (2007). Comparing a generic and individualized information decision support intervention for men newly diagnosed with localized prostate cancer. *Cancer Nursing, 30*(5), E7–E15.

Ellison, G.L., Coker, A.L., Hebert, J.R., Sanderson, M., Royal, C.D., & Weinrich, S.P. (2001). Psychosocial stress and prostate cancer: A theoretical model. *Ethnicity and Disease, 11*(3), 484–495.

Esper, P., Hampton, J.N., Smith, P.C., & Pienta, K.J. (1999). Quality of life evaluation in patients receiving treatment for advanced prostate cancer. *Oncology Nursing Forum, 26*(1), 107–112.

Fossa, S.D., Aaronson, N., Calais Da Silva, F., Denis, L., Newling, D., Hosbach, G., et al. (1989). Quality of life in patients with muscle-infiltrating bladder cancer and hormone-resistant prostatic cancer. *European Urology, 16*(5), 335–339.

Galbraith, M.E., Arechiga, A., Ramirez, J., & Pedro, L.W. (2005). Prostate cancer survivors' and partners' self-reports of health-related quality of life, treatment symptoms, and marital satisfaction 2.5–5.5 years after treatment [Online exclusive]. *Oncology Nursing Forum, 32*(2), E30–E41. Retrieved June 9, 2008, from http://ons.metapress.com/content/ t128147q6u1684t8/fulltext.pdf

Galbraith, M.E., Ramirez, J.M., & Pedro, L.W. (2001). Quality of life, health outcomes, and identity for patients with prostate cancer in five different treatment groups. *Oncology Nursing Forum, 28*(3), 551–560.

Gelmann, G.R. (1985). The predictive value of diagnostic procedures. *Nurse Practitioner, 10*(3), 25, 28–30, 32.

Giesler, R.B., Given, B., Given, C.W., Rawl, S., Monahan, P., Burns, D., et al. (2005). Improving the quality of life of prostate cancer patients: A randomized trial testing the efficacy of a nurse-driven intervention. *Cancer, 104*(4), 752–762.

Gilligan, T., Manola, J., Weinrich, S.P., Moul, J., Sartor, O., & Kantoff, P. (2004). Absence of a correlation of CAG repeat length and prostate cancer risk in an African American population. *Clinical Prostate Cancer, 3*(2), 98–103.

Greco, K.E., & Kulawiak, L. (1994). Prostate cancer prevention: Risk reduction through life-style, diet, and chemoprevention. *Oncology Nursing Forum, 21*(9), 1504–1511.

Gwede, C.K., Pow-Sang, J., Seigne, J., Heysek, R., Helal, M., Shade, K., et al. (2005). Treatment decision-making strategies and influences in patients with localized prostate carcinoma. *Cancer, 104*(7), 1381–1390.

Harrison, S., Dowswell, G., & Wright, J. (2002). Practice nurses and clinical guidelines in a changing primary care context: An empirical study. *Journal of Advanced Nursing, 39*(3), 299–307.

Heinrich-Rynning, T. (1987). Prostate cancer treatments and their effects on sexual functioning. *Oncology Nursing Forum, 14*(6), 37–41.

Held, J.L., Osborne, D.M., Volpe, H., & Waldman, A.R. (1994). Cancer of the prostate: Treatment and nursing implications. *Oncology Nursing Forum, 21*(9), 1517–1529.

Johnson, C.M., & Smolenski, D. (2007). Risk assessment models to estimate cancer probabilities. *Current Oncology Reports, 9*(6), 503–508.

Johnson, J.E., Fieler, V.K., Wlasowicz, G.S., Mitchell, M.L., & Jones, L.S. (1997). The effects of nursing care guided by Self-Regulation Theory on coping with radiation therapy. *Oncology Nursing Forum, 24*(6), 1041–1050.

Jones, R.A., & Wenzel, J. (2005). Prostate cancer among African-American males: Understanding the current issues. *Journal of National Black Nurses Association, 16*(1), 55–62.

Kleier, J. (2003). Prostate cancer in black men of African-Caribbean descent. *Journal of Cultural Diversity, 10*(2), 56–61.

Kleier, J. (2004). Using the Health Belief Model to reveal the perceptions of Jamaican and Haitian men regarding prostate cancer. *Journal of Multicultural Nursing and Health, 10*(3), 41–48.

Lang, B.A. (1991). Implementation of a screening program for carcinoma of the prostate. *Urologic Nursing, 11*(4), 24–27.

Lev, E.L., Eller, L.S., Gejerman, G., Lane, P., Owen, S.V., White, M., et al. (2004). Quality of life of men treated with brachytherapies for prostate cancer. *Health and Quality of Life Outcomes, 2*(28). Retrieved January 14, 2008, from http://www.hqlo.com/content/2/1/28

Lindqvist, O., Widmark, A., & Rasmussen, B.H. (2006). Reclaiming wellness—living with bodily problems, as narrated by men with advanced prostate cancer. *Cancer Nursing, 29*(4), 327–337.

Maliski, S.L., Heilemann, M.V., & McCorkle, R. (2001). Mastery of postprostatectomy incontinence and impotence: His work, her work, our work. *Oncology Nursing Forum, 28*(6), 985–992.

Maliski, S.L., Heilemann, M.V., & McCorkle, R. (2002). From "death sentence" to "good cancer." Couples transformation of a prostate cancer diagnosis. *Nursing Research, 51*(6), 391–397.

Meade, C.D., Calvo, A., Rivera, M.A., & Baer, R.D. (2003). Focus groups in the design of prostate cancer screening information for Hispanic farmworkers and African American men. *Oncology Nursing Forum, 30*(6), 967–975.

Mellon, S. (2002). Comparisons between cancer survivors and family members on meaning of the illness and family quality of life. *Oncology Nursing Forum, 29*(7), 1117–1125.

Mishel, M. (1990). Reconceptualization of uncertainty in illness theory. *Image: The Journal of Nursing Scholarship, 22*(4), 256–262.

Mishel, M.H., Belyea, M., Germino, B.B., Stewart, J.L., Bailey, D.E., Jr., Robertson, C., et al. (2002). Helping patients with localized prostate carcinoma manage uncertainty and treatment side effects: Nurse-delivered psychoeducational intervention over the phone. *Cancer, 94*(6), 1854–1866.

Mishel, M.H., Germino, B.B., Belyea, M., Stewart, J.L., Bailey, D.E., Jr., Mohler, J., et al. (2003). Moderators of an uncertainty management intervention. *Nursing Research, 52*(2), 89–97.

Moore, K.N., & Estey, A. (1999). The early post-operative concerns of men after radical prostatectomy. *Journal of Advanced Nursing, 29*(5), 1121–1129.

Moul, J.W., & Lipo, D.R. (1999). Prostate cancer in the late 1990s: Hormone refractory disease options. *Urologic Nursing, 19*(2), 125, 131.

National Comprehensive Cancer Network. (2008). *NCCN Clinical Practice Guidelines in Oncology™: Prostate cancer* [v.1.2008]. Retrieved January 10, 2008, from http://www.nccn.org/professionals/physician_gls/PDF/prostate.pdf

Oliffe, J. (2006). Being screened for prostate cancer: A simple blood test or a commitment to treatment? *Cancer Nursing, 29*(1), 1–8.

O'Rourke, M.E. (1999). Narrowing the options: The process of deciding on prostate cancer treatment. *Cancer Investigation, 17*(5), 349–359.

O'Rourke, M.E., & Germino, B.B. (1998). Prostate cancer treatment decisions: A focus group exploration. *Oncology Nursing Forum, 25*(1), 97–104.

Panguluri, R., Long, L., Chen, W., Wang, S., Coulibaly, A., Ukoli, F., et al. (2004). COX-2 gene promoter haplotypes and prostate cancer risk. *Carcinogenesis, 25*(6), 961–966.

Plowden, K.O. (1999). Using the Health Belief Model in understanding prostate cancer in African American men. *ABNF Journal, 10*(1), 4–8.

Reis-Starr, C., Weinrich, S., Creanga, D., & Weinrich, M. (1998). The association between family history and participation in free prostate cancer screening. *American Journal of Health Studies, 14*(2), 95–104.

Resendes, L.A., & McCorkle, R. (2006). Spousal response to prostate cancer: An integrative review. *Cancer Investigation, 24*(2), 192–198.

Riechers, E.A. (2004). Including partners into the diagnosis of prostate cancer: A review of the literature to provide a model of care. *Urologic Nursing, 24*(1), 22, 29, 38.

Robinson, L., Hughes, L.C., Adler, D.C., Strumpf, N., Grobe, S.J., & McCorkle, R. (1999). Describing the work of nursing: The case of postsurgical nursing interventions for men with prostate cancer. *Research in Nursing and Health, 22*(4), 321–328.

Rose, M.A., Shrader-Bogen, C.L., Korlath, G., Priem, J., & Larson, L.R. (1996). Identifying patient symptoms after radiotherapy using a nurse-managed telephone interview. *Oncology Nursing Forum, 23*(1), 99–102.

Shavers, V.L., & Brown, M. (2002). Racial and ethnic disparities in the receipt of cancer treatment. *Journal of the National Cancer Institute, 94*(5), 334–357.

Shavers, V.L., Brown, M., Klabunde, C.N., Potosky, A.L., Davis, W., Moul, J., et al. (2004). Race/ethnicity and the intensity of medical monitoring under "watchful waiting" for prostate cancer. *Medical Care, 42*(3), 239–250.

Shelton, P., & Weinrich, S. (1999). Barriers to prostate cancer screening in African American men. *Journal of National Black Nurses Association, 10*(2), 14–28.

Surveillance, Epidemiology and End Results Program. (2007). *Cancer stat fact sheets: Cancer of the prostate*. Retrieved January 14, 2008, from http://www.seer.cancer.gov/statfacts/html/prost.html

Tingen, M., Weinrich, S., Heyd, D., Boyd, M., & Weinrich, M. (1998). Perceived benefits: A predictor of participation in prostate cancer screening. *Cancer Nursing, 21*(5), 349–357.

Tingen, M.S., Weinrich, S.P., Boyd, M.D., & Weinrich, M.C. (1997). Prostate cancer screening: Predictors of participation. *Journal of the American Academy of Nurse Practitioners, 9*(12), 557–567.

Walker, B.L., Nail, L.M., Larsen, L., Magill, J., & Schwartz, A. (1996). Concerns, affect, and cognitive disruption following completion of radiation treatment for localized breast or prostate cancer. *Oncology Nursing Forum, 23*(8), 1181–1187.

Wallace, M. (2003). Uncertainty and quality of life of older men who undergo watchful waiting for prostate cancer. *Oncology Nursing Forum, 30*(2), 303–309.

Walton, J., & Sullivan, N. (2004). Men of prayer: Spirituality of men with prostate cancer: A grounded theory study. *Journal of Holistic Nursing, 22*(2), 133–151.

Waxman, E.S. (1993). Sexual dysfunction following treatment for prostate cancer: Nursing assessment and interventions. *Oncology Nursing Forum, 20*(10), 1567–1571.

Weinrich, M.C., Jacobsen, S.J., Weinrich, S.P., Moul, J.W., Oesterling, J.E., Jacobson, D., et al. (1998). Reference ranges for serum prostate-specific antigen in black and white men without cancer. *Urology, 52*(6), 967–973.

Weinrich, S.P. (2006). Prostate cancer screening in high-risk men: African American Hereditary Prostate Cancer Study Network. *Cancer, 106*(4), 796–803.

Weinrich, S.P., Atwood, J., Cobb, M., Ellison, G., Deets, J., & Weinrich, M. (1998). Cost for prostate cancer educational programs in work and church sites. *American Journal of Health Behavior, 22*(6), 421–433.

Weinrich, S.P., Boyd, M.D., Bradford, D., Mossa, M.S., & Weinrich, M.C. (1998). Recruitment of African-American men into prostate cancer screening. *Cancer Practice, 6*(1), 23–30.

Weinrich, S.P., Boyd, M.D., Weinrich, M., Greene, F., Reynolds, W.A., Jr., & Metlin, C. (1998). Increasing prostate cancer screening in African American men with peer-educator and client-navigator interventions. *Journal of Cancer Education, 13*(4), 213–219.

Weinrich, S.P., Ellison, G.L., Boyd, M., Hudson, J., Bradford, B., & Weinrich, M.C. (2000). Participation in prostate cancer screening among low-income men. *Psychology, Health, and Medicine, 5*(4), 439–450.

Weinrich, S.P., Faison-Smith, L., Hudson-Priest, J., Royal, C., & Powell, I. (2002). Stability of self-reported family history of prostate cancer among African American men. *Journal of Nursing Measurement, 10*(1), 39–46.

Weinrich, S.P., Greiner, E., Reis-Starr, C., Yoon, S., & Weinrich, M. (1998). Predictors of participation in prostate cancer screening at work sites. *Journal of Community Health Nursing, 15*(2), 113–129.

Weinrich, S.P., Holdford, D., Boyd, M., Creanga, D., Cover, K., Johnson, A., et al. (1998). Prostate cancer screening in African American churches. *Public Health Nursing, 15*(3), 188–195.

Weinrich, S.P., Reynolds, W.A., Jr., Tingen, M.S., & Starr, C.R. (2000). Barriers to prostate cancer screening. *Cancer Nursing, 23*(2), 117–121.

Weinrich, S.P., Royal, C., Pettaway, C.A., Dunston, G., Faison-Smith, L., Hudson, J., et al. (2002). Interest in genetic prostate cancer susceptibility testing among African American men. *Cancer Nursing, 25*(1), 28–34.

Weinrich, S.P., Weinrich, M., Atwood, J., & Cobb, M. (1999). Contrasting costs of prostate cancer educational programs by race and educational method. *American Journal of Health Behavior, 23*(2), 144–156.

Weinrich, S.P., Weinrich, M., Ellison, G., Hudson, J., Reeder, G., & Weissbecker, I. (2000). Contrasting cost of a prostate cancer educational program by income. *American Journal of Health Behavior, 24*(6), 422–433.

Weinrich, S.P., Weinrich, M., Mettlin, C., Reynolds, W.A., Jr., & Wofford, J.E. (1998). Urinary symptoms as a predictor for participation in prostate cancer screening among African American men. *Prostate, 37*(4), 215–222.

Weinrich, S.P., Weinrich, M.C., Boyd, M.D., & Atkinson, C. (1998). The impact of prostate cancer knowledge on cancer screening. *Oncology Nursing Forum, 25*(3), 527–534.

Weinrich, S.P., Weinrich, M.C., Priest, J., & Fodi, C. (2003). Self-reported reasons men decide not to participate in free prostate cancer screening [Online exclusive]. *Oncology Nursing Forum, 30*(1), E12–E16. Retrieved June 9, 2008, from http://ons.metapress.com/content/b743120318h46670/fulltext.pdf

Williams-Brown, S., Phillips, J.M., & Rust, G. (2005). Ensuring consistent quality care to address disparities in cancer screening. *Journal of Nursing Care Quality, 20*(2), 99–102.

Woods, V.D., Montgomery, S.B., & Herring, R.P. (2004). Recruiting Black/African American men for research on prostate cancer prevention. *Cancer, 100*(5), 1017–1025.

Woods, V.D., Montgomery, S.B., Herring, R.P., Gardner, R.W., & Stokols, D. (2006). Social ecological predictors of prostate-specific antigen blood test and digital rectal examination in black American men. *Journal of the National Medical Association, 98*(4), 492–504.

Yarbro, C.H. (1998). Quality of life of patients with prostate cancer treated with surgery or radiation therapy. *Oncology Nursing Forum, 25*(4), 685–693.

Zimmerman, S.M. (1997). Factors influencing Hispanic participation in prostate cancer screening. *Oncology Nursing Forum, 24*(3), 499–504.

CHAPTER 9

Focus on Colorectal Cancer

Susan M. Rawl, PhD, RN

Introduction

In the United States, colorectal cancer (CRC) is the second most common cause of cancer deaths affecting both men and women, second only to lung cancer. In 2008, 148,810 people are expected to be diagnosed, and 49,960 are expected to die from this disease (Jemal et al., 2008). CRC deaths can be prevented, but unless preventive action is taken, approximately 6% of Americans will develop CRC during their lifetime. Currently, the five-year survival rate is 90% when CRC is diagnosed at an early stage. Unfortunately, only 39% of CRC cases are diagnosed while still localized (Jemal et al.).

CRC exacts a substantial toll on society in terms of healthcare costs, morbidity, and mortality. Fortunately, screening can significantly reduce this burden. The natural development of most CRCs from adenomatous polyps allows for early identification and removal of precancerous polyps via endoscopic screening. If current screening recommendations were employed, an estimated 50% of deaths from CRC could be prevented (Progress Review Group, 2000).

CRC incidence and mortality rates began to decline in 1985, and a significant decline in the death rate occurred from 2003 to 2004. Over one year, the number of deaths from all cancers decreased by 1,160 among men and 1,854 among women. The majority of the reduction in cancer death rates was attributed to fewer deaths from CRC; 1,110 fewer men and 1,094 fewer women died from CRC (Jemal et al., 2008). The reductions in CRC incidence and mortality primarily are thought to be the result of greater utilization of endoscopic screening.

Both CRC incidence and mortality rates are higher among African Americans than among Caucasians (American Cancer Society [ACS], 2007; Rex, Rawl, Rabeneck, Rex, & Hamilton, 2004). Although the reasons for these disparities are not well understood, differences in screening rates may contribute to the unequal burden of CRC on African Americans (Chen et al., 1997; Cooper & Koroukian, 2004; Marcella & Miller, 2001; Ward et al., 2004; Weir et al., 2003).

Colorectal Cancer Risk Factors

Approximately 75% of all CRC occurs in people who are considered to be at "average" risk, that is, those who have no known risk factors other than being 50 years of age or older (Winawer et al., 1997). Advancing age is the most common risk factor, with men and women aged 70 and older having the highest probability of developing CRC (Jemal et al., 2008). Other risk factors include having a personal or family history of adenomatous polyps or inflammatory bowel disease.

Behavioral risk factors implicated in the development of CRC include red meat consumption, a diet high in animal fat, obesity, a sedentary lifestyle, smoking, and chronic alcohol consumption. Protective dietary and lifestyle factors include vegetable consumption, nonsteroidal anti-inflammatory drugs, and regular exercise (Cuzick, 1999; Potter, 1999). Inherited genetic syndromes such as familial adenomatous polyposis (FAP) and hereditary nonpolyposis CRC increase the risk of developing CRC. Individuals with FAP have almost a 100% chance of developing the disease. Gene-environment interactions are believed to play an important role in the development of CRC (Cuzick; Potter).

Effectiveness of Screening

Randomized clinical trials have demonstrated a 15%–33% mortality benefit from annual screening with fecal occult blood testing (FOBT) (Hardcastle et al., 1996; Kronborg, Fenger, Olsen, Jorgensen, & Sondergaard, 1996; Mandel et al., 1993). Recent evidence from a randomized trial of different CRC screening strategies indicated that the detection rate for advanced neoplasia was three times higher with flexible sigmoidoscopy compared to FOBT (Segnan et al., 2005). A mortality reduction of two-thirds was reported for cancers within reach of the sigmoidoscope, as well as a lower incidence of CRC for patients with a history of screening sigmoidoscopy (Kavanagh, Giovannucci, Fuchs, & Colditz, 1998; Newcomb, Norfleet, Storer, Surawicz, & Marcus, 1992; Selby, Friedman, Quesenberry, & Weiss, 1993). Annual FOBT *combined with* sigmoidoscopy has been found to increase the benefits of screening compared to either test alone. Mortality was reduced for participants of all age groups who were screened with FOBT and sigmoidoscopy from 0.63 per thousand per year for the control group to 0.36 per thousand for the study group (Winawer, Flehinger, Schottenfeld, & Miller, 1993). In one randomized trial, screening sigmoidoscopy, followed by colonoscopy when polyps were detected, resulted in an 80% reduction in CRC incidence (Thiis-Evensen et al., 1999). Another study among U.S. military veterans suggested that flexible sigmoidoscopy, followed by colonoscopy if a polyp was found, would have identified 70%–80% of patients with advanced proximal neoplasia (Lieberman et al., 2000).

Screening Participation

Although screening can both prevent CRC and find it early, screening rates among the general population remain low. Recent data from the National Health Interview Survey indicated that men were significantly more likely to have had any CRC screening test: 46.5% of screening-eligible men versus 43% of women received FOBT, sigmoidoscopy, or colonoscopy in the recommended time frames (Meissner, Breen, Klabunde, & Vernon, 2006). For individual tests, 16% of men and 15% of women had an FOBT in the preceding year, 7.6% of men and 6% of women had a sigmoidoscopy within the preceding 5 years, and 32% of men and 30% of women had a colonoscopy in the past 10 years. Increased rates of screening were attributed to greater use of colonoscopy among people older than age 65. Coverage for screening colonoscopy for Medicare beneficiaries was instituted in 2000, resulting in significantly higher rates of any screening test among people 65 or older compared to those aged 50–64 years (Meissner et al.). The subsequent increase in use of colonoscopy among Medicare beneficiaries resulted in higher rates of early-stage diagnoses, which will reduce CRC morbidity and mortality for this group (Gross et al., 2006).

In a recent study, investigators used data from the 2002 Nationwide Inpatient Sample of the Healthcare Cost and Utilization Project to examine predictors and healthcare costs associated with emergency CRC resections (Diggs, Xu, Diaz, Cooper, & Koroukain, 2007). Of 26,269 people discharged with CRC after undergoing surgical resection, 2,753 (9.5%) had the procedure performed as an emergency because of bowel perforation, peritonitis, or obstruction. Those most at risk for emergency CRC resection were uninsured or receiving Medicaid. Emergency resection was associated with a threefold increase in hospital mortality, almost 55,000 excess hospital days, and more than $250 million in hospital charges. The burden of emergency resection for CRC was considered a "failure to screen" that was both significant and preventable (Diggs et al.).

As the Medicare example illustrates, interventions at the *public policy level* can increase screening utilization through legislation and reimbursement. Promoting the uptake of CRC screening also can occur by motivating changes in knowledge, attitudes, and behaviors at the *individual level* among individuals in the community as well as patients in healthcare systems. Other interventions to promote screening have focused on changes at the *healthcare provider or healthcare systems level*. The remainder of this chapter will focus on studies that have been conducted by nurse scientists as well as randomized trials of interventions designed to increase CRC screening participation.

Screening Guidelines: Test Recommendations Based on Risk Assessment

Clinical practice guidelines for CRC screening were updated in 2008 by ACS, the U.S. Multisociety Task Force on Colorectal Cancer, and the American College of Radiology (Levin et al., 2008). In these guidelines, screening tests were categorized into two groups: (a) tests that primarily detect cancer early and (b) tests that detect cancer and adenomatous polyps.

Previous guidelines had suggested that "screening programs should begin by classifying the individual patient's level of risk based on personal, family, and medical history, which will determine the appropriate screening" (Winawer et al., 2003, p. 545). An individual is considered to be at average risk for developing CRC if he or she has no known risk other than age. For asymptomatic, average-risk individuals, screening should begin at age 50. The seven screening test options and their schedules are as follows.

- Tests that detect cancer and adenomatous polyps:
  – Flexible sigmoidoscopy every five years or
  – Colonoscopy every 10 years or
  – Double-contrast barium enema every five years or
  – Computed tomographic colonography every five years
- Tests that primarily detect cancer:
  – Annual guaiac-based FOBT or
  – Annual fecal immunochemical test or
  – Stool DNA test, interval undetermined

For people at increased risk for CRC, including those with a family history of CRC or adenomatous polyps, or inflammatory bowel disease or high-risk genetic syndromes, recommendations for surveillance and screening are individualized based on risk factors present (Chen et al., 1997; Hardcastle et al., 1996; Kronborg et al., 1996). For example, ACS and the Multisociety Task Force recommended that people who have a single first-degree relative diagnosed with CRC *after* age 60 should be offered the same five testing options as average-risk people, but those who have a single first-degree relative diagnosed *before* age 60 should receive colonoscopy starting at age 40 or 10 years earlier than the age of the youngest affected relative.

Factors Related to Participation in Colorectal Cancer Screening

As shown in Table 9-1, most of the studies conducted by nurses have used descriptive, correlational designs and were guided by the Health Belief Model. One of the strengths of nursing research is that investigators often focus on special populations or those at increased risk for CRC. Several studies have been conducted with African Americans (Busch, 2003; Green & Kelly, 2004; Powe, 2001, 2002; Powe, Ntekop, & Barron, 2004; Powe & Weinrich, 1999), one with Korean Americans (Kim, Yu, Chen, Kim, & Brintnall, 1998), one with lesbians (Dibble & Roberts, 2003), and one with older female caregivers (Sarna & Chang, 2000). Several studies have focused on first-degree relatives of CRC survivors (Jacobs, 2002; Rawl et al., 2001, 2005; Rawl, Menon, Champion, Foster, & Skinner, 2000).

Qualitative studies using focus group methods have yielded important insights about people's perceptions of CRC and screening (Busch, 2003; Holmes-Rovner et al., 2002; Rawl et al., 2000). Psychometric studies have established valid and reliable measures of constructs related to CRC screening behaviors in English and other languages (Ozsoy, Ardahan, & Ozmen, 2007; Rawl et al., 2001). Other investigators have used a single group, post-test–only design to evaluate an educational program (Greenwald, 2006) and a case-control design to examine CRC risk factors (Kinney, Harrell, Slattery, Martin, & Sandler, 2006). Because cost can be a significant barrier to screening, studies have focused on samples for which cost should not be an issue. Examples of these were conducted with members of health maintenance organizations and patients seen in federally funded primary care centers (Menon, Belue, Skinner, Rothwell, & Champion, 2007; Powe, Finnie, & Ko, 2006).

Much of the research examining factors associated with CRC screening has focused on FOBT and flexible sigmoidoscopy. Because colonoscopy only recently has been considered a mass-screening test, knowledge of predictors of colonoscopy utilization is limited. Predictors of adherence to FOBT include being younger than age 70, being female, having more education, and having a higher income. In contrast to FOBT, men are more likely than women to be screened with flexible sigmoidoscopy, with authors of one study suggesting a gender bias against women for undergoing sigmoidoscopy (McCaffery, Wardle, Nadel, & Atkin, 2002; Myers et al., 1994; Polednak, 1990). Predictors of ever having had any endoscopic screening (e.g., sigmoidoscopy, colonoscopy) were being male, being older, having insurance, and having a strong family history of CRC (Codori, Petersen, Miglioretti, & Boyd, 2001; Dolan et al., 2004). Additionally, studies consistently show the importance of physician recommendation for CRC screening participation (Breen, Wagener, Brown, Davis, & Ballard-Barbash, 2001; Codori et al.; Herold, Hanlon, Movsas, & Hanks, 1998; Janz, Wren, Schottenfeld, & Guire, 2003; McCaffery et al.; Myers et al., 1994; Polednak; Rawl et al., 2000; Richards & Reker, 2002).

Health beliefs have been examined in several studies in relation to participation in CRC screening. Among African Americans, *cancer fatalism*—the belief

Table 9-1. Colorectal Cancer Screening Studies Conducted by Nurse Scientists

Authors (Year)	Design	Sample	Theory	Results
Busch (2003)	Qualitative/ focus groups	13 African American women; 39% of participants were younger than age 50.	Health Belief Model	Knowledge of colorectal cancer (CRC) and the need for screening was very low. Perceived risk was low, and only 23% had ever been screened.
Dibble & Roberts (2003)	Single group, pre-/post-test	22 lesbian participants aged 50–81	None	At six months post-intervention, 10% of women had flexible sigmoidoscopy; 55% (n = 12) were compliant with CRC screening at baseline.
Green & Kelly (2004)	Descriptive, correlational	100 African American men and women aged 50–90	Health Belief Model	Educational level was inversely related to perceived threat of CRC and perceived barriers. CRC knowledge was positively related to education and income; males had higher knowledge scores than females (p = .008).
Greenwald (2006)	Single group, post-test only	20 female employees in an accounting firm; 65% of participants were younger than age 50	Health Belief Model	Perceived risk for CRC, intent to discuss screening with their provider, and intent to share information with others were increased by the 15-minute educational program.
Holmes-Rovner et al. (2002)	Qualitative/ focus groups	21 screening-eligible men and women from one rural community health center	None	Barriers to screening included concerns about efficacy of screening tests, treatment effectiveness, access to quality care, distrust of the healthcare system, and racism.
Jacobs (2002)	Descriptive, correlational	90 first-degree relatives of patients with CRC	Health Belief Model	Perceived barriers, perceived seriousness, and level of education were associated with health maintenance visits.

(Continued on next page)

Table 9-1. Colorectal Cancer Screening Studies Conducted by Nurse Scientists (Continued)

Authors (Year)	Design	Sample	Theory	Results
Kim et al. (1998)	Descriptive, correlational	263 Korean American men and women in the Midwest	None	Fecal occult blood testing (FOBT) participation for both men and women was only 10%; lack of awareness of CRC and need for screening contributed to low participation rates.
Kinney et al. (2006)	Case-control	558 cases with colon cancer, 952 controls	None	Living in a rural area was associated with a higher risk for CRC (OR = 1.4, 95% CI = 1.1–1.8). This association was no longer significant after controlling for recent CRC screening. Rural residents reported lower screening rates than their urban counterparts.
Menon et al. (2007)	Descriptive, correlational	169 male and female members of a health maintenance organization who were eligible for CRC screening	Health Belief Model and Transtheoretical Model	Differences in health beliefs were observed by stages of change. For FOBT, those in precontemplation had the lowest perceived risk, lower perceived benefits, and higher barriers. Those in precontemplation for sigmoidoscopy had lower perceived risk, lower self-efficacy, and higher barriers than those in other stages.
Menon et al. (2003)	Descriptive, correlational	220 men and women employed by a pharmaceutical company	PRECEDE-PROCEED Model and Health Belief Model	Predictors of colonoscopy screening participation were higher perceived benefits, higher self-efficacy, higher knowledge of CRC, and healthcare provider recommendation. Barriers and perceived risk were not associated with colonoscopy use.
Ozsoy et al. (2007)	Instrument development, psychometric analyses	470 members of the general population in Turkey	Health Belief Model	Turkish-language version of the Champion Health Belief Model Scale as modified by Jacobs (2002) for CRC testing. Construct validity using factor analyses yielded five factors; Cronbach alphas for the five subscales ranged from 0.54 to 0.88.
Powe (2001)	Descriptive, correlational	204 female African Americans attending senior citizen centers	None	Women with high cancer fatalism scores were older and had less education, less knowledge of CRC, and lower incomes.

(Continued on next page)

Table 9-1. Colorectal Cancer Screening Studies Conducted by Nurse Scientists *(Continued)*

Authors (Year)	Design	Sample	Theory	Results
Powe (2002)	Clustered randomized trial	106 African American women in senior citizen centers	None	Those in the cultural and self-empowerment group had higher rates of FOBT completion (63%) compared to 34% of women in a modified cultural intervention group and 7% in the traditional intervention group. Predictors of FOBT completion were family history of CRC and a higher number of healthcare visits.
Powe et al. (2006)	Descriptive, correlational	354 patients being seen in a federally funded primary care center	Patient/Provider/System Model	CRC knowledge scores were low and did not differ across three age groups (20–39, 40–49, 50–74 years). Screening was viewed as unnecessary in the absence of symptoms.
Powe et al. (2004)	Clustered randomized trial	134 attendees from 15 senior citizen centers	Powe Fatalism Model	Gains in CRC knowledge scores were higher for those who received the cultural and self-empowerment intervention compared to the modified cultural intervention and traditional intervention ($p > .001$); 61% of the cultural and self-empowerment group completed FOBT compared to 46% in the modified group and 15% in the traditional group.
Powe & Weinrich (1999)	Randomized trial	70 attendees at senior citizen centers in rural South Carolina	None	Overall, 63% returned completed FOBTs; the difference in completion between experimental and control groups was not significant (68% versus 60%). Greater decrease in fatalism scores ($p = .003$) and increase in CRC knowledge occurred in the experimental group ($p = .04$).
Rawl et al. (2001)	Instrument development, psychometric analyses	225 first-degree relatives of survivors of CRC and 190 people with polyps	Health Belief Model	Six scales measuring perceived benefits and barriers to FOBT, sigmoidoscopy, and colonoscopy demonstrated good reliability, with Cronbach alphas ranging from 0.65 to 0.77. Construct validity was supported by factor analyses and known-groups comparison.

(Continued on next page)

Table 9-1. Colorectal Cancer Screening Studies Conducted by Nurse Scientists *(Continued)*

Authors (Year)	Design	Sample	Theory	Results
Rawl et al. (2008)	Randomized trial	177 first-degree relatives of survivors of CRC	Transtheoretical Model and Health Belief Model	Tailored and nontailored print interventions were equally effective at increasing screening. Baseline stage of adoption and income moderated intervention efficacy, with the tailored print intervention being more effective with precontemplators and those with higher incomes.
Rawl et al. (2000)	Qualitative/ focus groups	22 first-degree relatives of patients with CRC seen at two midwestern cancer centers	Health Belief Model	Benefits of screening were finding CRC early, decreasing chances of dying from CRC, and freedom from worry about CRC. Main barriers included lack of public awareness, concerns about the efficacy of some tests, fear of finding CRC, and embarrassment.
Rawl et al. (2005)	Descriptive, correlational	257 first-degree relatives of patients with CRC	Transtheoretical Model and Health Belief Model	Most first-degree relatives were in precontemplation for all three tests: 66% for FOBT, 61% for sigmoidoscopy, and 64% for colonoscopy. Older age was related to being in action for FOBT and sigmoidoscopy but not colonoscopy. Those in precontemplation endorsed more barriers to and fewer benefits of screening than those in other stages.
Sarna & Chang (2000)	Descriptive, correlational	52 older female caregivers	None	Participation in CRC screening was higher than the general population: 47% had undergone a sigmoidoscopy in the past five years, 28% had FOBT in past year, and 36% had both annual FOBT and sigmoidoscopy in the recommended time frame. Caregiving burden was not associated with CRC screening.
Weinrich et al. (1998)	Clustered randomized trial	211 low-income older adults in congregate meal sites	None	Overall, 65% of participants completed FOBT. Predictors of completion were being male, aged 65–75 years old, and able to travel without assistance and having had FOBT in the past.

that death is inevitable when cancer is present—has negatively affected FOBT participation (Powe, 1995; Powe & Finnie, 2003). Having knowledge about cancer and knowing someone who had CRC are related to adherence to both FOBT (Farrands, Hardcastle, Chamberlain, & Moss, 1984; Myers et al., 1990) and flexible sigmoidoscopy (Brown, Potosky, Thompson, & Kessler, 1990). Barriers to participation in FOBT include conflicts with work or family, inconvenience, being too busy, lack of interest, cost, not having any health problems or symptoms of CRC, embarrassment or the unpleasantness of the test, not wanting to know about health problems, and being anxious or worried about test results (Janz et al., 2003; Powe, 1995; Powe & Finnie; Rawl et al., 2000, 2005; Richards & Reker, 2002). Barriers to participation in flexible sigmoidoscopy include the reasons previously listed, with the most frequently cited reason being the lack of current health problems or CRC symptoms. In addition, concerns about pain, discomfort, or injury were barriers to flexible sigmoidoscopy (Vernon, 1997). Consistent with Health Belief Model predictions, studies have demonstrated consistently the positive relationships between CRC screening and its perceived benefits and the negative relationships between screening and perceived barriers (Menon et al., 2003; Rawl et al., 2000, 2005; Vernon).

Although understanding the CRC-related health beliefs and attitudes of studied populations is necessary, the body of literature on factors that predict, or are associated with, CRC screening is now quite robust. Nurse scientists' developing, rigorously testing, and translating effective interventions is critical to increase CRC screening in both clinical and community settings. Nurses are positioned to redesign and evaluate healthcare system interventions to promote greater use of CRC screening in order to reduce morbidity and mortality from this preventable disease. The remainder of this chapter will present an overview of the intervention research conducted in the past decade by nurse scientists and others.

Systematic Reviews of Colorectal Cancer Screening Interventions

Vernon (1997) published an extensive review of literature on adherence to CRC screening with FOBT and sigmoidoscopy. The review included 18 intervention studies designed to increase participation in screening with FOBT and four intervention studies focusing on sigmoidoscopy. Intervention strategies ranged from mailed letters of invitation from one's personal physician that included FOBT kits to intensive follow-up with in-person or telephone counseling. Such interventions increased participation up to 50%, and mailed follow-up reminders increased participation in all studies that used them. Limitations of CRC screening intervention studies included the lack of theoretically driven studies (only five investigators used theory-based interventions), the use of volunteers who may already have been motivated to screen as study participants, and the lack of attention to repeat adherence to screening. Readers are referred to Vernon's work for a detailed discussion of these studies, all of which were published prior to 1997.

Peterson and Vernon (2000) subsequently reviewed the literature that focused on interventions directed at increasing physicians' adherence to CRC screening guidelines. Of the 18 studies reviewed, most interventions consisted of some type of screening reminder system. Computer-generated reminder systems generally outperformed manual reminder systems in increasing physician adherence to CRC screening guidelines, with postintervention adherence rates increasing 31%–90% for FOBT and 40%–64% for sigmoidoscopy (Peterson & Vernon).

One of the most commonly used and effective strategies to increase the use of CRC screening and other preventive services in primary care settings is the clinical reminder system. Shea, DuMouchel, and Bahamonde (1996) conducted a meta-analysis of 16 randomized trials to evaluate the effectiveness of these reminder systems and concluded that

1. Use of a manual reminder system significantly increased use of CRC screening (OR = 1.86, 95% CI = 1.39–2.47).
2. Use of a computerized reminder system more than doubled the odds of CRC screening (OR = 2.25, 95% CI = 1.74–2.91).
3. Combining manual and computerized reminders increased CRC screening almost threefold (OR = 2.71, 95% CI =2.01–3.66).

Stone et al. (2002) conducted a meta-analysis of interventions designed to increase use of breast, cervical, and CRC screening. Studies included interventions targeting patients, providers, organizations, and communities that focused on provision of education, provider feedback, patient financial incentives, reminder systems, organizational change, and/or mass media. Of 19 studies designed to increase FOBT participation, organizational change was consistently shown to be the most effective intervention component (OR = 17.6, 95% CI = 12.3–25.2) (Stone et al.). Specific organizational changes found to be effective included the establishment of separate clinics devoted to prevention and screening, the use of planned preventive care visits, the use of continuous quality improvement techniques, and delegation of prevention responsibilities to healthcare professionals who are not physicians (Stone et al.). Other interventions found to be effective at increasing FOBT uptake were, in decreasing order, provider education (OR = 3.01, 95% CI = 1.98–4.56), patient reminders (OR = 2.75, 95% CI = 1.90–3.97), patient financial incentives, such as reducing or eliminating copayments (OR = 1.82, 95% CI = 1.35–2.46), and provider reminder systems (OR = 1.46, 95% CI = 1.15–1.85).

Randomized Trials of Effective Screening Interventions

A systematic search of randomized trials conducted in the past decade whose outcomes included participation in CRC screening was performed via searches of the MEDLINE® (searchable via PubMed at www.ncbi.nlm.nih.gov/sites/entrez) and PsycINFO (www.apa.org/psycinfo) electronic databases. Of the trials identified, 21 provided evidence of positive effects on CRC screening participation. Of these, 10 were directed at individuals to be screened (Cole, Young, Byrne, Guy, & Morcom, 2002; Courtier et al., 2002; Denberg et al., 2006; Goldberg et al., 2004; Hart et al., 1997; Miller, Kimberly, Case, & Wofford, 2005; Pignone, Harris, & Kinsinger, 2000; Tu et al., 2006; Wolf & Schorling, 2000; Zapka et al., 2004), and eight were conducted with community-based samples or at worksites (Braun, Fong, Kaanoi, Kamaka, & Gotay, 2005; Campbell et al., 2004; Church et al., 2004; Lipkus et al., 2005; Marcus et al., 1999, 2005; Powe & Weinrich, 1999; Tilley et al., 1999; Weinrich, Weinrich, Atwood, Boyd, & Greene, 1998). Three studies were directed at providers (Hillman et al., 1998; Schroy et al., 1999; Zubarik et al., 2000). Randomized trials that provided evidence of effective interventions and may have potential for translation or dissemination are described in the following sections.

Individual-Level Interventions

Hart et al. (1997) conducted a randomized trial to test the effect of an educational brochure with 1,571 residents of a suburban/rural area in Britain. All were patients of a large group practice staffed by 10 physicians. The educational leaflet contained information on CRC incidence, screening with FOBT, and common reasons for not getting screened. All participants were sent a letter signed by the senior partner of the practice inviting them to receive a free FOBT. Half were randomly assigned to receive the educational leaflet. Those who accepted screening were then sent an FOBT kit with instructions to return it to the hospital lab for processing. Results indicated that gender was a moderator of intervention effectiveness. Among men aged 61–65, compliance increased 9% (36% versus 27%, p > .05), whereas for men aged 66–70, compliance rates increased 16% (39% versus 23%, p > .01). However, no intervention effect resulted for women of either age group (38% versus 36% and 31% versus 31%, respectively). A significantly greater proportion of women in the control group returned completed FOBT cards than men (33% versus 25%, p <.02).

To test the effects of physician endorsement of a mailed invitation to be screened with FOBT, Cole et al. (2002) tested three different letter formats with 1,800 Australians. Group 1 received a letter from a central screening service with no reference to the primary care provider, group 2 received a letter from the central screening service that included a statement that the patient's group practice supported the invitation, and group 3 received a letter from their primary care provider on relevant letterhead that was personally signed by that physician. Each letter was accompanied by a CRC information sheet, an FOBT collection card, and a brief questionnaire. Higher participation rates occurred with greater involvement of the provider in the invitation, with the highest found in the group that received the invitation letter from their physician (40% versus 32%, p = .002).

Scientists in Spain found that two brief home visits from a trained layperson increased FOBT participation to 58% among attendees in a primary health-care center (Courtier et al., 2002). In this randomized trial, the home visits were compared to mailed invitation letters with FOBT collection kits. In advance of the interventions, both groups received an informative letter about benefits of CRC screening and advance notification that FOBT kits would be forthcoming. Two visits were made to those randomized to this group—the first to drop off a stool kit and explain the sample collection procedure and the second to collect the specimens on an agreed-upon date. The participation rates were 36.5% for those who received a mailed FOBT kit and 57.7% for those who received home visits. The cost of the home visits was estimated at 4.96 euros (7.71 USD) per subject.

Tu et al. (2006) provided evidence for the effectiveness of a comprehensive, culturally targeted intervention to increase FOBT participation among Chinese patients seen in two primary care clinics in Seattle, Washington. The scientists randomly assigned 210 patients to usual care or to a clinic-based intervention. The intervention group received in-person CRC education from a health educator, a motivational video on CRC screening produced in Cantonese and dubbed into Mandarin, a motivational pamphlet developed for the study, a CRC pamphlet produced by the Federation of Chinese American and Chinese Canadian Medical Societies, and an FOBT instruction sheet with testing cards. All written materials were available in both Chinese and English. Results indicated a strong intervention effect, with 69.5% of the intervention group completing FOBT compared to 27.6% of the control group. The odds of completing FOBT within six months was more than six times greater for those who received this comprehensive clinic-based intervention (OR = 6.38, 95% CI = 3.44,11.85).

In another study, the effect of mailing FOBT cards to low-income African American patients in advance of a primary care visit was examined (Goldberg et al., 2004). Scientists randomly assigned 119 patients to usual care or to the intervention, which consisted of FOBT cards, standard instructions, and an introductory letter signed by the clinic director and staff of the Colon Cancer Screening Program. The letter, instructions, and specimen collection cards were mailed 10–14 days prior to a scheduled clinic visit. The effects were significant, with 35.6% of intervention patients returning completed FOBT cards at the index clinic visit compared to 3.3% of patients who received usual care (p < .001).

Denberg et al. (2006) tested the effect of a mailed informational brochure as a reminder to schedule a colonoscopy. Patients (N = 781) who were referred for screening colonoscopy by their primary care providers were randomly assigned to receive either a mailed informational brochure that was personalized with the name of the patient's primary care provider or usual care. The brochure was mailed within 10 days of referral from the primary physician and included information about CRC, risk factors, the concept of prevention, benefits of screening, descriptions of screening tests, and instructions for scheduling a colonoscopy. Results supported the effectiveness of this minimal prompt intervention, with 71% of the intervention group completing a colonoscopy compared to 59% of the usual care group (p = .001).

A multimedia computer program demonstrated the same effectiveness as individual nurse counseling at increasing FOBT participation rates in a community-based primary care practice (Miller et al., 2005). Miller et al. randomized 204 patients to receive FOBT kits along with either one-on-one counseling from a nurse on how to complete FOBT or a multimedia computer program that provided the same information about completing FOBT with a two-minute introductory segment on the incidence of CRC and the rationale for screening. Both interventions were delivered in the office after the patient had received a recommendation for FOBT from his or her provider. Results indicated that both interventions were strong and were equally effective—63% of patients who received nurse counseling completed FOBT within 30 days of their office visit, and 62% of those who used the computer program did so.

Zapka et al. (2004) tested the effect of a mailed educational video on CRC screening participation by randomizing 938 patients in five primary care practices in Massachusetts to the video intervention or to usual care. The 15-minute theory-based video was designed to encourage and prepare patients to discuss CRC screening, specifically sigmoidoscopy, with their provider at their upcoming appointment. Narrated by a nationally known actress who had CRC, the video addressed benefits and barriers to sigmoidoscopy, the importance of screening, footage of patients undergoing sigmoidoscopy, and patients discussing their sigmoidoscopy experiences. The video was mailed to patients' homes before their scheduled physician appointment accompanied by a letter signed by their primary provider encouraging them to view the video. A higher percentage of intervention patients who viewed most or all of the video reported having had a discussion with their provider about sigmoidoscopy (74%) compared to patients who received the video but did not view it (57%), versus 59% of the control group (p < .001). Higher sigmoidoscopy participation occurred among those who viewed the video (39%) compared to those who received it but did not view it (17%) or the control group (21%). Patients who viewed most or all of the video were 2.8 times more likely to have a sigmoidoscopy compared to the controls (OR = 2.81, 95% CI =1.85–4.26).

A trial involving 249 patients being seen in three community primary care practices in North Carolina tested a videotape decision aid (Pignone et al., 2000). Patients were randomly assigned to view either an 11-minute educational video about colon cancer screening or a video on automobile safety (control condition). Intervention patients then were asked to choose one of three color-coded informational brochures to indicate their stage of readiness to be screened; choosing the green brochure indicated readiness to be screened, the yellow brochure indicated interest in screening but need for additional information, and the red brochure indicated no interest in screening at this time. A color-coded card corresponding to the patients' selected stage of readiness was attached to the patients' chart before they went in to see their provider. Results showed higher rates of FOBT among the intervention group, 28.5% versus 20.2% of controls, and higher rates of sigmoidoscopy uptake (17.6% versus 4.8%, respectively). Examining any test completed, the rate of screening for the intervention group was 14.2% higher than the controls (36.8% versus 22.6%). Patients who received the intervention were 1.8 times more likely to be screened than controls (95% CI = 1.2–2.6).

Community-Based and Workplace Interventions

In a 2005 review, Bowie et al. concluded that although effective community-based breast and cervical cancer screening intervention studies have been conducted, "there is an urgent need for amplification of CRC screening" (p. 58). Weinrich et al. (1998) tested four educational interventions designed to increase participation in FOBT among 211 socioeconomically disadvantaged older adults. Fourteen congregate meal sites in South Carolina were randomly selected and assigned to receive one of four types of educational interventions. The traditional educational intervention consisted of a nurse presenting an ACS slide-tape program on CRC screening. The second intervention involved older-adult educators, matched by age and education for each meal site, who provided testimony regarding the advantages of FOBT and demonstrated the test procedure using peanut butter. In the third intervention, titled Adaptation for Aging Changes, the traditional presentation was modified to accommodate normal aging changes and provided opportunities for participants to practice the FOBT test procedure with peanut butter. The fourth intervention combined the older-adult educator and the Adaptation for Aging Changes interventions. Following all interventions, participants were given free FOBT kits with dietary restriction instructions and told to return completed tests to the meal site. Results indicated a high level of compliance overall, with 65% of participants completing FOBT. The investigator reported significant intervention effects for the Adaptation for Aging Changes intervention (p = .01) and the combined intervention group (p = .04).

Powe and Weinrich (1999) randomized 70 attendees (42 intervention, 28 controls) at senior citizen centers to receive a videotaped intervention designed to decrease cancer fatalism and increase CRC screening among African Americans. The intervention video was a 20-minute tape designed to model CRC screening behaviors specifically targeted to African Americans. The control group viewed the 13-minute ACS video titled *Colorectal Cancer: The Cancer No One Talks About*. Although the rates of completion of FOBT were not significantly different, rates were high for both groups; 60% of the intervention group and 68% of controls completed FOBT (p = .48).

Powe tested the effect of a multiphase, culturally relevant intervention delivered over one year on CRC knowledge and FOBT participation (Powe, 2002; Powe et al., 2004). This investigator randomized 15 senior citizen centers in one southeastern state to receive either the multiphase, yearlong intervention, a modified cultural intervention, or no intervention (control). The multiphase intervention, called the "cultural and self-empowerment group," received a 20-minute culturally targeted video titled *Telling the Story . . . To Live Is God's Will,* a 12-month educational calendar with information about CRC, an educational poster that reinforced getting checked with FOBT, an informational trifold brochure about CRC screening, and a one-page flyer depicting the steps for completing FOBT. The "modified cultural intervention group" received only the 20-minute video. Results showed that participants in the "cultural and self-empowerment group" had a greater increase in CRC knowledge than the other groups (p < .001). Predictors of participation in FOBT were group membership and CRC knowledge scores.

Rawl and colleagues conducted a randomized trial of two print interventions, a computer-tailored educational booklet versus a nontailored (generic) brochure, mailed to 177 first-degree relatives of CRC survivors (Rawl et al., 2008). The tailored print intervention was a 10-page color booklet that contained graphics and messages that were individualized based on assessment of each participant's demographic profile, CRC risk factors, perceptions of CRC risk, and perceived barriers to screening. The nontailored intervention was the ACS brochure titled *Colon Testing Can Save Your Life.* The two interventions were equally effective at increasing screening rates at the three-month follow-up. Intervention efficacy was moderated by baseline stage of adoption and income. The tailored intervention was more likely to move precontemplators (OR = 2.98, 95% CI = 1.01–8.85) and those with higher incomes forward in stage of adoption for FOBT (OR = 6.54, 95% CI = 1.32–32.4).

Campbell et al. (2004) used a 2 × 2 factorial design to compare the effects of two different theory-based interventions, alone and in combination, on participation in CRC prevention behaviors among members of 12 rural African American churches. Specific outcomes measured were fruit and vegetable consumption, recreational physical activity, and CRC screening. One intervention included four tailored print newsletters and four targeted videotapes delivered over nine months; this was compared to, and combined with, a lay health adviser intervention. Among the 287 participants who were age 50 or older, FOBT participation rates increased by 87% in the group who received the tailored print and video intervention, compared to 59% in the combined intervention group and 42% in the lay health adviser–only group. A 29% decrease in FOBT participation occurred in the control group. These differences were only borderline significant (p = .08).

In a large randomized trial conducted with more than 4,000 callers to the National Cancer Institute's Cancer Information Service, Marcus and colleagues tested the effects of four different interventions to promote CRC screening (Marcus et al., 2005). Participants were randomized to one of four experimental conditions: Group 1, the control group, received a single nontailored mailing of the National Cancer Institute publication *What You Need to Know About Cancer of the Colon and Rectum.* Groups 2, 3, and 4 initially received a tailored 16-page booklet with information on CRC screening tests, guidelines, efficacy of screening, and the need to visit a physician. The booklet also included tailored messages based on each participant's stage of change, CRC risk, and self-reported barriers. Group 2 received a single mailing of this tailored booklet, and group 3 received four tailored mailings—at baseline, 6 months, 9 months, and 12 months. Participants in group 4 received tailored print materials in the mail at the same time points as group 3, with retailoring done based on responses to the six-month interview. Results indicated that group 1, who received the single nontailored mailing, more than doubled their CRC screening rate, from 20% at baseline to 42% at 14 months. An overall significant trend developed across groups with increased tailoring and intensity of the intervention being associated with higher rates of screening (p = .05). At six months, the rates of screening among the experimental groups were not significantly different.

Another community-based study focused on increasing FOBT uptake among native Hawaiians by comparing two experimental conditions that varied in intensity and degree of cultural targeting (Braun et al., 2005). Sixteen Hawaiian civic clubs were randomized to one of two intervention groups. Group 1 (n = 52) received a culturally targeted presentation on CRC and its effect on native Hawaiians delivered by a non-Hawaiian nurse, a culturally targeted brochure on CRC, free FOBT cards, and instructions from the nurse on completing the test. At 30 days, nonresponders in this group received one reminder phone call and replacement FOBT cards if requested. Group 2 (n = 69) received a CRC presentation delivered by a native Hawaiian physician and a native Hawaiian survivor of CRC whose cancer had been found through screening. Scientists incorporated several strategies based on the Social Learning Theory to increase mastery of FOBT use, model the desired behavior, increase self-efficacy, and reinforce screening. Strategies included FOBT demonstration and return demonstration, challenging participants to engage a family member in free screening, and multiple telephone calls over 4–16 weeks for those who did not complete FOBT. Results indicated that the more intensive Social Learning Theory–based intervention was less effective than the culturally targeted intervention delivered by a non-Hawaiian nurse (OR = 0.364, 95% CI = 0.14–0.97).

The effectiveness of direct mailings of FOBT kits to a community-based sample, with and without reminders, was tested with 1,943 residents in one Minnesota county (Church et al., 2004). The sample was randomly divided into three groups: Group 1 served as a control group and received no mailing; group 2 received a mailed FOBT kit with a pamphlet explaining the test; and group 3 received mailed FOBT kits and the pamphlet, with nonresponders in this group receiving a reminder letter one month later, a second FOBT kit with a reminder letter two months later, and a reminder phone call three months later. Changes in rates of self-reported adherence to FOBT one year later increased by 1.5% in the control group, 16.9% in group 2 (no reminders), and 23.2% in group 3 (intensive reminders). The difference between groups 2 and 3 was not significant. Intervention effects were strongest for men older than age 65.

Two studies tested CRC screening intervention in worksites. The Next Step Trial was designed to increase screening participation and dietary change among 5,042 employees involved in the pattern- and model-making areas of the automotive industry—a group at risk for developing CRC caused by occupational exposure to potential carcinogens (Tilley et al., 1999). Interventions were tested at 15 worksites, with 13 worksites randomized to usual care. Usual care for these high-risk employees included a long-standing worksite CRC-screening program offered by the employer on work time. Intervention worksites included 2,240 employees who, in addition to a standard screening program already in place, received a tailored educational intervention based on behavior change theories. The intervention consisted of a mailed invitation to receive screening and a personally tailored educational booklet that included information about the employees' screening history and individualized screening recommendations. The mailing was followed by a five- to seven-minute telephone counseling session in which an interviewer highlighted messages from the booklet, answered questions, and encouraged scheduling of a screening appointment. Intervention worksite employees also received a quarterly newsletter that included nutrition and screening information and interviews with coworkers who had been screened.

After adjusting for baseline and worksite characteristics, intervention effects were modest but significant for both screening compliance (OR = 1.46, 95% CI = 1.1–2.0) and coverage (OR = 1.33, 95% CI = 1.1–1.6) (Tilley et al., 1999). Compliance was defined as having had all recommended CRC tests during the two-year study period, whereas coverage was defined as having had at least one of the recommended screening tests during the trial period.

Lipkus and colleagues used a 2 × 2 factorial design to test four interventions that varied the amount and intensity of CRC risk factor information given to 860 members of the carpentry trade (Lipkus et al., 2005). These investigators aimed to increase participation in annual FOBT among this group, which is at increased risk for CRC caused by occupational exposure to potential carcinogens. Group 1 received a four-page brochure with nontailored basic information about three CRC risk factors (age, family history, and polyps), as well as general information about CRC incidence, lifetime risk, colon function, and screening tests. Group 2 received nontailored comprehensive information similar in format to the basic information, except that it included information on a more comprehensive list of lifestyle (e.g., diet, exercise, smoking, alcohol use) and occupational (e.g., asbestos, wood dust, solvent exposure) risk factors. Group 3 received tailored basic information in the same print format as the other groups. This group differed from the nontailored group in two ways:
- The risk factor section was individually tailored, indicating which risk factors increased the individual's personal risk for CRC
- Group 3 participants received a phone call from a trained counselor two weeks after receiving the print materials to discuss their risk factors and the importance of getting screened.

Participants in group 4 received comprehensive tailored information in a section that addressed all of their personal risk factors, including age, family history, polyps, lifestyle, and occupational risks. This group also received tailored phone counseling with additional discussions about the influence of lifestyle and occupational factors on their individual CRC risk. All interventions were delivered annually for three years, with slight modification (updating) of the information provided in years two and three.

Results indicated that all four interventions were successful in facilitating screening. The investigators' hypothesis that carpenters who received comprehensive tailored intervention would have the highest screening rates was supported in year one only. Among those participants (group 4), 74% completed FOBT in the first year, compared to 68% in group 2, 60% in group 3, and 60% in group 1. In year three, however, participants who had received the nontailored comprehensive information had higher yearly FOBT participation rates (59%) than the other groups.

Provider-Directed Interventions

In one randomized trial, regular performance feedback and financial incentives were tested as interventions to increase physician adherence to cancer screening guidelines, including CRC, in a managed care organization (Hillman et al., 1998). Fifty-two sites with 100 physicians were randomly assigned to the intervention or to usual care. Providers in the intervention group received semiannual feedback regarding their adherence to screening guidelines and financial rewards for those who were adherent. Physicians received bonuses based on aggregate compliance scores and improvement in scores over time. Baseline compliance scores for all types of cancer screening were low, with the mean compliance score for CRC screening being the lowest of all cancer screenings. Repeated measured analyses demonstrated significant change over time, with CRC screening compliance rates increasing from 14.9% at baseline to 43.7% in the intervention group and from 10.8% at baseline to 37.4% among the controls. However, no significant intervention effect was observed. Investigators credited the changes in practice to the increased emphasis on preventive care that was occurring on a national level. The investigators acknowledged that, although screening compliance improved dramatically during the study, they remained suboptimal, with approximately 60% of eligible people not receiving annual CRC screening.

One study directed an intervention at both patients and providers in two primary care clinics at a Veterans Affairs Medical Center (Ferreira et al., 2005). Providers in the intervention clinic received a two-hour educational workshop on rationale and guidelines for CRC screening and improving communication with patients with low health literacy. In addition, intervention providers attended one-hour feedback sessions, during which they received feedback on the clinic's rates for CRC screening recommendations and patient adherence to screening. Small group discussions and role-playing sessions were intended to assist providers to effectively discuss screening in the limited time available in busy clinics. Intervention providers also received confidential information on their own performance, specifically their screening recommendation rates and patient adherence rates. Additionally, 204 patients of providers in the intervention group viewed an educational video about CRC screening and received an informational brochure. All FOBT kits in the intervention clinic contained simplified instructions for completing the test. Results showed that, over the 18 months after index clinic visits, screening recommendation rates were higher in the intervention clinic: 76% versus 69.4% for the control clinic (p = .02). Patient screening adherence rates also were higher in the intervention clinic; 41.3% of intervention patients completed FOBT, sigmoidoscopy, or colonoscopy compared to 32.4% of the control patients (p = 0.003). The investigators acknowledged that because the patient-directed component of the intervention was not fully implemented as designed, their ability to assess its effect was compromised. Additional analyses suggested that most of the improvement in screening recommendation and adherence rates could be attributed to the provider intervention.

Conclusion

Currently, CRC screening participation rates are unacceptably low, providing both challenges and opportunities for behavioral scientists. Investigators of CRC screening behaviors are beginning to apply the knowledge gained from intervention work on mammography screening. Tailored interventions that are theoretically based increase screening (Champion et al., 2002; Saywell et al., 1999; Tilley et al., 1999). In the studies reviewed to date, CRC screening interventions have been directed at individuals, providers, and communities using in-person delivery, telephone delivery, and mailed print interventions. Unfortunately, multiple intervention modalities often were combined in a single study, making it difficult to determine which parts of the intervention were most effective. Surprisingly, several studies included individuals who were already up-to-date with screening at baseline, resulting in inefficient delivery of interventions to people who did not need them. Few theoretically based intervention strategies have been tested, although that number is growing. Only one trial addressed the issue of cost-effectiveness. Much work is needed to identify cost-effective methods for delivering interventions to appropriate populations.

Several studies showed that technology holds great promise for tailoring interventions that can be delivered via interactive computer programs or the Internet. Scientists need to increase screening among at-risk populations, such as people with a family history of polyps or CRC, and focus their efforts appropriately. They need to focus their research efforts on reducing serious racial and geographic disparities in screening among African Americans, Hispanics/Latinos, and other minority groups. Intervention research to increase

CRC screening is an important frontier for oncology nursing that holds great potential for decreasing CRC morbidity and mortality.

Directions for Future Research

Although investigators are beginning to demonstrate efficacy of a variety of CRC screening interventions, effect sizes rarely exceed 50%. Research has already demonstrated that many of the theoretical variables important in mammography also are associated with CRC screening (Peterson & Vernon, 2000; Rawl et al., 2000; Vernon, 1997).

Progress in intervention research is dependent on reliable and valid measures of both mediators and outcomes. Recognizing the need for standardization of outcomes in CRC research, Vernon et al. (2004) developed and tested a core set of self-report measures for use in behavioral, health-services, and epidemiologic research. To overcome the measurement challenges and enable comparisons across studies, future scientists should include these core measures to assess initial, past, recent, periodic, and on-schedule screening.

Measures of theoretical constructs such as benefits, barriers, and self-efficacy related to screening have not been standardized, but attempts are under way. The National Cancer Institute's Division of Cancer Control and Population Sciences recently established a comprehensive and useful Web site on health behavior constructs, theories, and measurement (http://dccps.cancer.gov/brp/constructs/index.html). This resource will be invaluable for investigators in public health, health communications, nursing, and psychology whose goal is to understand and change health behaviors. Opportunities for collaboration and comparisons across studies will expand with the use of common measures of important behavioral constructs. Psychometric testing of behavioral measures specific to CRC screening also have been conducted (Menon, 2000; Rawl et al., 2001).

Because the available CRC screening modalities differ greatly in their barriers to use, healthcare providers must carefully address each modality separately. For instance, barriers to FOBT may include the unpleasantness and inconvenience of obtaining three separate stool samples, whereas significant barriers to colonoscopy include the bowel preparation and, for many people younger than age 65, the cost. Before interventions can be developed, nurse scientists must carefully identify issues specific to each screening behavior.

At the same time, acknowledging the interdependence of CRC screening tests is equally important. A narrow focus on FOBT and flexible sigmoidoscopy has limited past research. Since 2000, colonoscopy increasingly has been used for screening rather than diagnostic purposes. Efficacy studies that are currently under way will guide refinement of CRC screening recommendations and ultimately will influence intervention research. Until then, screening behaviors for FOBT, flexible sigmoidoscopy, and colonoscopy must be examined in relation to one another. Individuals who have a colonoscopy no longer need annual FOBT. Vernon (1997) first addressed this interdependency issue by suggesting the measurement of both CRC screening compliance (e.g., participation in the appropriate screening tests in the correct time frame) and coverage (e.g., participation in at least one screening test). More work is needed to clarify the measurement of CRC screening participation and to examine the processes and constructs that may mediate intervention effectiveness.

Figure 9-1 presents research questions that still need to be answered. Studies are needed that examine the interplay between individual factors, healthcare provider factors, health system factors, and public policy. New theoretical frameworks that move beyond the individual hold promise to further explain CRC screening behavior. Interdependence theory and couple communal coping frameworks propose that examining behavior change, such as CRC screening, from a dyadic perspective may be useful (Lewis et al., 2006). Understanding which interventions work for whom and under what conditions will enable healthcare professionals to efficiently and effectively improve early detection of CRC, thereby reducing morbidity and mortality from this preventable disease.

Figure 9-1. Future Research Questions in Colorectal Cancer Screening

1. What variables are critical to use in tailoring interventions to promote colorectal cancer (CRC) screening?
2. How can stage-related theories be used to promote CRC screening?
3. How does patient-provider communication influence CRC screening outcomes?
4. What types of messages are most effective for motivating CRC screening among different sociocultural groups?
5. How important are patient preferences and shared decision making in the context of colorectal cancer screening?
6. What healthcare system factors or designs facilitate or hinder implementation of new approaches to increasing CRC screening in clinical practice?
7. Are interventions that are delivered within or outside of the healthcare system more effective at increasing uptake of appropriate CRC screening tests?
8. Are interventions that are directed at changing patient behavior, provider behavior, or both most effective?
9. Does combining interventions to address early detection for multiple cancers simultaneously (e.g., breast, colorectal, cervical) result in better outcomes?
10. What are the barriers to and facilitators of effective follow-up care after positive screening results?

References

American Cancer Society. (2007). *Cancer facts and figures for African Americans, 2007–2008.* Atlanta, GA: Author.
Bowie, J.V., Curbow, B.A., Garza, M.A., Dreyling, E.K., Scott, L.A., & McDonnell, K.A. (2005). A review of breast, cervical, and colorectal cancer screening interventions in older women. *Cancer Control, 12*(Suppl. 2), 58–69.

Braun, K.L., Fong, M., Kaanoi, M.E., Kamaka, M.L., & Gotay, C.C. (2005). Testing a culturally appropriate, theory-based intervention to improve colorectal cancer screening among Native Hawaiians. *Preventive Medicine, 40*(6), 619–627.

Breen, N., Wagener, D.K., Brown, M.L., Davis, W.W., & Ballard-Barbash, R. (2001). Progress in cancer screening over a decade: Results of cancer screening from the 1987, 1992, and 1998 National Health Interview Surveys. *Journal of the National Cancer Institute, 93*(22), 1704–1713.

Brown, M.L., Potosky, A.L., Thompson, G.B., & Kessler, L.G. (1990). The knowledge and use of screening tests for colorectal and prostate cancer: Data from the 1987 National Health Interview Survey. *Preventive Medicine, 19*(5), 562–574.

Busch, S. (2003). Elderly African American women's knowledge and belief about colorectal cancer. *ABNF Journal, 14*(5), 99–103.

Campbell, M.K., James, A., Hudson, M.A., Carr, C., Jackson, E., Oates, V., et al. (2004). Improving multiple behaviors for colorectal cancer prevention among African American church members. *Health Psychology, 23*(5), 492–502.

Champion, V.L., Skinner, C.S., Menon, U., Seshadri, R., Anzalone, D., & Rawl, S.M. (2002). Comparisons of tailored mammography interventions at two months postintervention. *Annals of Behavioral Medicine, 24*(3), 211–218.

Chen, V.W., Fenoglio-Preiser, C.M., Wu, X.C., Coates, R.J., Reynolds, P., Wickerham, D.L., et al. (1997). Aggressiveness of colon carcinoma in blacks and whites. National Cancer Institute Black/White Cancer Survival Study Group. *Cancer Epidemiology, Biomarkers and Prevention, 6*(12), 1087–1093.

Church, T.R., Yeazel, M.W., Jones, R.M., Kochevar, L.K., Watt, G.D., Mongin, S.J., et al. (2004). A randomized trial of direct mailing of fecal occult blood tests to increase colorectal cancer screening. *Journal of the National Cancer Institute, 96*(10), 770–780.

Codori, A.M., Petersen, G.M., Miglioretti, D.L., & Boyd, P. (2001). Health beliefs and endoscopic screening for colorectal cancer: Potential for cancer prevention. *Preventive Medicine, 33*(2, Pt. 1), 128–136.

Cole, S.R., Young, G.P., Byrne, D., Guy, J.R., & Morcom, J. (2002). Participation in screening for colorectal cancer based on a faecal occult blood test is improved by endorsement by the primary care practitioner. *Journal of Medical Screening, 9*(4), 147–152.

Cooper, G.S., & Koroukian, S.M. (2004). Racial disparities in the use of and indications for colorectal procedures in Medicare beneficiaries. *Cancer, 100*(2), 418–424.

Courtier, R., Casamitjana, M., Macia, F., Panades, A., Castells, X., Gil, M.J., et al. (2002). Participation in a colorectal cancer screening programme: Influence of the method of contacting the target population. *European Journal of Cancer Prevention, 11*(3), 209–213.

Cuzick, J. (1999). Colorectal cancer. In B.S. Kramer, J.K. Gohagan, & P.C. Prorok (Eds.), *Cancer screening: Theory and practice* (pp. 219–266). New York: Marcel Dekker.

Denberg, T.D., Coombes, J.M., Byers, T.E., Marcus, A.C., Feinberg, L.E., Steiner, J.F., et al. (2006). Effect of a mailed brochure on appointment-keeping for screening colonoscopy: A randomized trial. *Annals of Internal Medicine, 145*(12), 895–900.

Dibble, S.L., & Roberts, S.A. (2003). Improving cancer screening among lesbians over 50: Results of a pilot study [Online exclusive]. *Oncology Nursing Forum, 30*(4), E71–E79. Retrieved August 6, 2005, from http://ons.metapress.com/content/mh3437h32672246h/fulltext.pdf

Diggs, J.C., Xu, F., Diaz, M., Cooper, G.S., & Koroukian, S.M. (2007). Failure to screen: Predictors and burden of emergency colorectal cancer resection. *American Journal of Managed Care, 13*(3), 157–164.

Dolan, N.C., Ferreira, M.R., Davis, T.C., Fitzgibbon, M.L., Rademaker, A., Liu, D., et al. (2004). Colorectal cancer screening knowledge, attitudes, and beliefs among veterans: Does literacy make a difference? *Journal of Clinical Oncology, 22*(13), 2617–2622.

Farrands, P.A., Hardcastle, J.D., Chamberlain, J., & Moss, S. (1984). Factors affecting compliance with screening for colorectal cancer. *Community Medicine, 6*(1), 12–19.

Ferreira, M.R., Dolan, N.C., Fitzgibbon, M.L., Davis, T.C., Gorby, N., Ladewski, L., et al. (2005). Health care provider-directed intervention to increase colorectal cancer screening among veterans: Results of a randomized controlled trial. *Journal of Clinical Oncology, 23*(7), 1548–1554.

Goldberg, D., Schiff, G.D., McNutt, R., Furumoto-Dawson, A., Hammerman, M., & Hoffman, A. (2004). Mailings timed to patients' appointments: A controlled trial of fecal occult blood test cards. *American Journal of Preventive Medicine, 26*(5), 431–435.

Green, P.M., & Kelly, B.A. (2004). Colorectal cancer knowledge, perceptions, and behaviors in African Americans. *Cancer Nursing, 27*(3), 206–215.

Greenwald, B. (2006). Promoting community awareness of the need for colorectal cancer screening: A pilot study. *Cancer Nursing, 29*(2), 134–141.

Gross, C.P., Andersen, M.S., Krumholz, H.M., McAvay, G.J., Proctor, D., & Tinetti, M.E. (2006). Relation between Medicare screening reimbursement and stage at diagnosis for older patients with colon cancer. *JAMA, 296*(23), 2815–2822.

Hardcastle, J.D., Chamberlain, J.O., Robinson, M.H., Moss, S.M., Amar, S.S., Balfour, T.W., et al. (1996). Randomised controlled trial of faecal-occult-blood screening for colorectal cancer. *Lancet, 348*(9040), 1472–1477.

Hart, A.R., Barone, T.L., Gay, S.P., Inglis, A., Griffin, L., Tallon, C.A., et al. (1997). The effect on compliance of a health education leaflet in colorectal cancer screening in general practice in central England. *Journal of Epidemiology and Community Health, 51*(2), 187–191.

Herold, D.M., Hanlon, A.L., Movsas, B., & Hanks, G.E. (1998). Age-related prostate cancer metastases. *Urology, 51*(6), 985–990.

Hillman, A.L., Ripley, K., Goldfarb, N., Nuamah, I., Weiner, J., & Lusk, E. (1998). Physician financial incentives and feedback: Failure to increase cancer screening in Medicaid managed care. *American Journal of Public Health, 88*(11), 1699–1701.

Holmes-Rovner, M., Williams, G.A., Hoppough, S., Quillan, L., Butler, R., & Given, C.W. (2002). Colorectal cancer screening barriers in persons with low income. *Cancer Practice, 10*(5), 240–247.

Jacobs, L.A. (2002). Health beliefs of first-degree relatives of individuals with colorectal cancer and participation in health maintenance visits: A population-based survey. *Cancer Nursing, 25*(4), 251–265.

Janz, N.K., Wren, P.A., Schottenfeld, D., & Guire, K.E. (2003). Colorectal cancer screening attitudes and behavior: A population-based study. *Preventive Medicine, 37*(6, Pt. 1), 627–634.

Jemal, A., Siegel, R., Ward, E., Hao, Y., Xu, J., Murray, T., et al. (2008). Cancer statistics, 2008. *CA: A Cancer Journal for Clinicians, 58*(2), 71–96.

Kavanagh, A.M., Giovannucci, E.L., Fuchs, C.S., & Colditz, G.A. (1998). Screening endoscopy and risk of colorectal cancer in United States men. *Cancer Causes and Control, 9*(4), 455–462.

Kim, K., Yu, E.S., Chen, E.H., Kim, J., & Brintnall, R.A. (1998). Colorectal cancer screening. Knowledge and practices among Korean Americans. *Cancer Practice, 6*(3), 167–175.

Kinney, A.Y., Harrell, J., Slattery, M., Martin, C., & Sandler, R.S. (2006). Rural-urban differences in colon cancer risk in Blacks and Whites: The North Carolina Colon Cancer Study. *Journal of Rural Health, 22*(2), 124–130.

Kronborg, O., Fenger, C., Olsen, J., Jorgensen, O.D., & Sondergaard, O. (1996). Randomised study of screening for colorectal cancer with faecal-occult-blood test. *Lancet, 348*(9040), 1467–1471.

Levin, B., Lieberman, D.A., McFarland, B., Smith, R.A., Brooks, D., Andrews, K.S., et al. (2008). Screening and surveillance for the early detection of colorectal cancer and adenomatous polyps, 2008: A joint guideline from the American Cancer Society, the U.S. Multi-Society Task Force on Colorectal Cancer, and the American College of Radiology. *CA: A Cancer Journal for Clinicians, 58*(3), 130–160.

Lewis, M.A., McBride, C.M., Pollak, K.I., Puleo, E., Butterfield, R.M., & Emmons, K.M. (2006). Understanding health behavior change among couples: An interdependence and communal coping approach. *Social Science and Medicine, 62*(6), 1369–1380.

Lieberman, D.A., Weiss, D.G., Bond, J.H., Ahnen, D.J., Garewal, H., Chejfec, G., et al. (2000). Use of colonoscopy to screen asymptomatic adults for colorectal cancer: Veterans Affairs Cooperative Study Group 380. *New England Journal of Medicine, 343*(3), 162–168.

Lipkus, I.M., Skinner, C.S., Dement, J., Pompeii, L., Moser, B., Samsa, G.P., et al. (2005). Increasing colorectal cancer screening among individuals in the carpentry trade: Test of risk communication interventions. *Preventive Medicine, 40*(5), 489–501.

Mandel, J.S., Bond, J.H., Church, T.R., Snover, D.C., Bradley, G.M., Schuman, L.M., et al. (1993). Reducing mortality from colorectal cancer by screening for fecal occult blood. Minnesota Colon Cancer Control Study. *New England Journal of Medicine, 328*(19), 1365–1371.

Marcella, S., & Miller, J.E. (2001). Racial differences in colorectal cancer mortality. The importance of stage and socioeconomic status. *Journal of Clinical Epidemiology, 54*(4), 359–366.

Marcus, A.C., Ahnen, D., Cutter, G., Calonge, N., Russell, S., Sedlacek, S.M., et al. (1999). Promoting cancer screening among the first-degree relatives of breast and colorectal cancer patients: The design of two randomized trials. *Preventive Medicine, 28*(3), 229–242.

Marcus, A.C., Mason, M., Wolfe, P., Rimer, B.K., Lipkus, I., Strecher, V., et al. (2005). The efficacy of tailored print materials in promoting colorectal cancer screening: Results from a randomized trial involving callers to the National Cancer Institute's Cancer Information Service. *Journal of Health Communication, 10*(Suppl. 1), 83–104.

McCaffery, K., Wardle, J., Nadel, M., & Atkin, W. (2002). Socioeconomic variation in participation in colorectal cancer screening. *Journal of Medical Screening, 9*(3), 104–108.

Meissner, H.I., Breen, N., Klabunde, C.N., & Vernon, S.W. (2006). Patterns of colorectal cancer screening uptake among men and women in the United States. *Cancer Epidemiology, Biomarkers and Prevention, 15*(2), 389–394.

Menon, U. (2000). *Factors associated with colorectal cancer screening in an average-risk population.* Unpublished dissertation, Indiana University School of Nursing, Indianapolis.

Menon, U., Belue, R., Skinner, C., Rothwell, B.E., & Champion, V. (2007). Perceptions of colon cancer screening by stage of screening test adoption. *Cancer Nursing, 30*(3), 178–185.

Menon, U., Champion, V.L., Larkin, G.N., Zollinger, T.W., Gerde, P.M., & Vernon, S.W. (2003). Beliefs associated with fecal occult blood test and colonoscopy use at a worksite colon cancer screening program. *Journal of Occupational and Environmental Medicine, 45*(8), 891–898.

Miller, D.P., Jr., Kimberly, J.R., Jr., Case, L.D., & Wofford, J.L. (2005). Using a computer to teach patients about fecal occult blood screening: A randomized trial. *Journal of General Internal Medicine, 20*(11), 984–988.

Myers, R.E., Ross, E., Jepson, C., Wolf, T., Balshem, A., Millner, L., et al. (1994). Modeling adherence to colorectal cancer screening. *Preventive Medicine, 23*(2), 142–151.

Myers, R.E., Trock, B.J., Lerman, C., Wolf, T., Ross, E., & Engstrom, P.F. (1990). Adherence to colorectal cancer screening in an HMO population. *Preventive Medicine, 19*(5), 502–514.

Newcomb, P.A., Norfleet, R.G., Storer, B.E., Surawicz, T.S., & Marcus, P.M. (1992). Screening sigmoidoscopy and colorectal cancer mortality. *Journal of the National Cancer Institute, 84*(20), 1572–1575.

Ozsoy, S.A., Ardahan, M., & Ozmen, D. (2007). Reliability and validity of the colorectal cancer screening belief scale in Turkey. *Cancer Nursing, 30*(2), 139–145.

Peterson, S., & Vernon, S. (2000). A review of patient and physician adherence to colorectal cancer screening guidelines. *Seminars in Colon and Rectal Surgery, 11*(1), 1–17.

Pignone, M., Harris, R., & Kinsinger, L. (2000). Videotape-based decision aid for colon cancer screening: A randomized, controlled trial. *Annals of Internal Medicine, 133*(10), 761–769.

Polednak, A.P. (1990). Knowledge of colorectal cancer and use of screening tests in persons 40–74 years of age. *Preventive Medicine, 19*(2), 213–226.

Potter, J.D. (1999). Colorectal cancer: Molecules and populations. *Journal of the National Cancer Institute, 91*(11), 916–932.

Powe, B.D. (1995). Cancer fatalism among elderly Caucasians and African Americans. *Oncology Nursing Forum, 22*(9), 1355–1359.

Powe, B.D. (2001). Cancer fatalism among elderly African American women: Predictors of the intensity of the perceptions. *Journal of Psychosocial Oncology, 19*(3/4), 85–95.

Powe, B.D. (2002). Promoting fecal occult blood testing in rural African American women. *Cancer Practice, 10*(3), 139–146.

Powe, B.D., & Finnie, R. (2003). Cancer fatalism: The state of the science. *Cancer Nursing, 26*(6), 454–465.

Powe, B.D., Finnie, R., & Ko, J. (2006). Enhancing knowledge of colorectal cancer among African Americans: Why are we waiting until age 50? *Gastroenterology Nursing, 29*(1), 42–49.

Powe, B.D., Ntekop, E., & Barron, M. (2004). An intervention study to increase colorectal cancer knowledge and screening among community elders. *Public Health Nursing, 21*(5), 435–442.

Powe, B.D., & Weinrich, S. (1999). An intervention to decrease cancer fatalism among rural elders. *Oncology Nursing Forum, 26*(3), 583–588.

Progress Review Group. (2000). *Conquering colorectal cancer: A blueprint for the future.* Bethesda, MD: National Cancer Institute.

Rawl, S., Champion, V., Menon, U., Loehrer, P., Vance, G., & Skinner, C. (2001). Validation of scales to measure benefits and barriers to colorectal cancer screening. *Journal of Psychosocial Oncology, 19*(3/4), 47–63.

Rawl, S.M., Champion, V.L., Scott, L.L., Zhou, H., Monahan, P., Ding, Y., et al. (2008). A randomized trial of two print interventions to increase colon cancer screening among first-degree relatives. *Patient Education and Counseling, 71*(2), 215–227.

Rawl, S.M., Menon, U., Champion, V.L., Foster, J.L., & Skinner, C.S. (2000). Colorectal cancer screening beliefs. Focus groups with first-degree relatives. *Cancer Practice, 8*(1), 32–35.

Rawl, S.M., Menon, U., Champion, V.L., May, F.E., Loehrer, P., Sr., Hunter, C., et al. (2005). Do benefits and barriers differ by stage of adoption for colorectal cancer screening? *Health Education Research, 20*(2), 137–148.

Rex, D.K., Rawl, S.M., Rabeneck, L., Rex, E.K., & Hamilton, F. (2004). Colorectal cancer in African Americans. *Reviews in Gastroenterological Disorders, 4*(2), 60–65.

Richards, R.J., & Reker, D.M. (2002). Racial differences in use of colonoscopy, sigmoidoscopy, and barium enema in Medicare beneficiaries. *Digestive Diseases and Sciences, 47*(12), 2715–2719.

Sarna, L., & Chang, B.L. (2000). Colon cancer screening among older women caregivers. *Cancer Nursing, 23*(2), 109–116.

Saywell, R.M., Jr., Champion, V.L., Skinner, C.S., McQuillen, D., Martin, D., & Maraj, M. (1999). Cost-effectiveness comparison of five interventions to increase mammography screening. *Preventive Medicine, 29*(5), 374–382.

Schroy, P.C., Heeren, T., Bliss, C.M., Pincus, J., Wilson, S., & Prout, M. (1999). Implementation of on-site screening sigmoidoscopy positively influences utilization by primary care providers. *Gastroenterology, 117*(2), 304–311.

Segnan, N., Senore, C., Andreoni, B., Arrigoni, A., Bisanti, L., Cardelli, A., et al. (2005). Randomized trial of different screening strategies for colorectal cancer: Patient response and detection rates. *Journal of the National Cancer Institute, 97*(5), 347–357.

Selby, J.V., Friedman, G.D., Quesenberry, C.P., Jr., & Weiss, N.S. (1993). Effect of fecal occult blood testing on mortality from colorectal cancer: A case-control study. *Annals of Internal Medicine, 118*(1), 1–6.

Shea, S., DuMouchel, W., & Bahamonde, L. (1996). A meta-analysis of 16 randomized controlled trials to evaluate computer-based clinical reminder systems for preventive care in the ambulatory setting. *Journal of the American Medical Informatics Association, 3*(6), 399–409.

Stone, E.G., Morton, S.C., Hulscher, M.E., Maglione, M.A., Roth, E.A., Grimshaw, J.M., et al. (2002). Interventions that increase use of adult immunization and cancer screening services: A meta-analysis. *Annals of Internal Medicine, 136*(9), 641–651.

Thiis-Evensen, E., Hoff, G.S., Sauar, J., Langmark, F., Majak, B.M., & Vatn, M.H. (1999). Population-based surveillance by colonoscopy: Effect on the incidence of colorectal cancer: Telemark Polyp Study I. *Scandinavian Journal of Gastroenterology, 34*(4), 414–420.

Tilley, B.C., Vernon, S.W., Myers, R., Glanz, K., Lu, M., Hirst, K., et al. (1999). The Next Step Trial: Impact of a worksite colorectal cancer screening promotion program. *Preventive Medicine, 28*(3), 276–283.

Tu, S.P., Taylor, V., Yasui, Y., Chun, A., Yip, M.P., Acorda, E., et al. (2006). Promoting culturally appropriate colorectal cancer screening through a health educator: A randomized controlled trial. *Cancer, 107*(5), 959–966.

Vernon, S.W. (1997). Participation in colorectal cancer screening: A review. *Journal of the National Cancer Institute, 89*(19), 1406–1422.

Vernon, S.W., Meissner, H., Klabunde, C., Rimer, B.K., Ahnen, D.J., Bastani, R., et al. (2004). Measures for ascertaining use of colorectal cancer screening in behavioral, health services, and epidemiologic research. *Cancer Epidemiology, Biomarkers and Prevention, 13*(6), 898–905.

Ward, E., Jemal, A., Cokkinides, V., Singh, G.K., Cardinez, C., Ghafoor, A., et al. (2004). Cancer disparities by race/ethnicity and socioeconomic status. *CA: A Cancer Journal for Clinicians, 54*(2), 78–93.

Weinrich, S.P., Weinrich, M.C., Atwood, J., Boyd, M., & Greene, F. (1998). Predictors of fecal occult blood screening among older socioeconomically disadvantaged Americans: A replication study. *Patient Education and Counseling, 34*(2), 103–114.

Weir, H.K., Thun, M.J., Hankey, B.F., Ries, L.A., Howe, H.L., Wingo, P.A., et al. (2003). Annual report to the nation on the status of cancer, 1975–2000, featuring the uses of surveillance data for cancer prevention and control. *Journal of the National Cancer Institute, 95*(17), 1276–1299.

Winawer, S., Fletcher, R., Rex, D., Bond, J., Burt, R., Ferrucci, J., et al. (2003). Colorectal cancer screening and surveillance: Clinical guidelines and rationale—Update based on new evidence. *Gastroenterology, 124*(2), 544–560.

Winawer, S.J., Flehinger, B.J., Schottenfeld, D., & Miller, D.G. (1993). Screening with colorectal cancer with fecal occult blood testing and sigmoidoscopy. *Journal of the National Cancer Institute, 85*(16), 1311–1318.

Winawer, S.J., Fletcher, R.H., Miller, L., Godlee, F., Stolar, M.H., Mulrow, C.D., et al. (1997). Colorectal cancer screening: Clinical guidelines and rationale. *Gastroenterology, 112*(2), 594–642.

Wolf, A.M.D., & Schorling, J.B. (2000). Does informed consent alter elderly patients' preferences for colorectal cancer screening? *Journal of General Internal Medicine, 15*(1), 24–30.

Zapka, J.G., Lemon, S.C., Puleo, E., Estabrook, B., Luckmann, R., & Erban, S. (2004). Patient education for colon cancer screening: A randomized trial of a video mailed before a physical examination. *Annals of Internal Medicine, 141*(9), 683–692.

Zubarik, R., Eisen, G., Zubarik, J., Teal, C., Benjamin, S., Glaser, M., et al. (2000). Education improves colorectal cancer screening by flexible sigmoidoscopy in an inner city population. *American Journal of Gastroenterology, 95*(2), 509–512.

SECTION IV

CURRENT AND EMERGING ISSUES IN ONCOLOGY RESEARCH

CHAPTER 10

Nursing Research: Cancer-Related Disparities

Sandra Underwood, PhD, RN, FAAN,
Mary K. Canales, PhD, RN, Barbara D. Powe, PhD, RN,
Randy A. Jones, PhD, RN, and Patricia K. Bradley, PhD, RN

Introduction

According to reports published by the American Cancer Society (ACS), an estimated 1,437,180 new cases of invasive cancer will be diagnosed in the United States in 2008, and 565,650 deaths from cancer will occur (ACS, 2008). Although cancer is exceeded by cardiovascular disease as the leading cause of disease and mortality in the United States, it is responsible for more estimated years of life lost than any other cause of death (National Center for Health Statistics, 2008). Cancer confers an undue burden on all population groups. However, research has shown that the burden of cancer is not borne equally among population groups within the United States.

The validity of using the racial and ethnic categories defined in the Statistical Policy on Race and Ethnic Standards for Federal Statistics and Administrative Reporting (U.S. Department of Commerce, 1978; U.S. Office of Management and Budget, 1994) to make distinctions among population groups within the United States has been the focus of much debate (Burchard et al., 2003; Collins, 2004; Freeman, 1998; Williams, Lavizzo-Mourey, & Warren, 1994). However, data collected, analyzed, and reported by the National Cancer Institute (NCI) using these standards revealed significant variations in cancer incidence and mortality among racial and ethnic population groups within the United States.

The NCI Surveillance, Epidemiology and End Results (SEER) Program reported that African Americans, Native Americans and Alaskan Natives, Asians/

Pacific Islanders, and Hispanics generally experience higher cancer incidence, higher cancer mortality, and lower five-year relative cancer survival rates when compared to the non-Hispanic Caucasian population (Clegg, Li, Hankey, Chu, & Edwards, 2002; Ries et al., 2006). Variations in cancer incidence and mortality also have been observed among racial and ethnic subpopulation groups for many site-specific cancers (Miller et al., 1996) (see Tables 10-1 and 10-2). For example, when compared with other racial and ethnic population groups in the United States, African American populations experience the highest overall cancer incidence and the highest overall cancer mortality, and Native American and Alaskan Native populations experience the lowest cancer five-year relative survival.

According to reports of the NCI SEER program, the incidence rates of stomach and liver cancers among Asians/Pacific Islanders, cervical cancer among Hispanics, uterine cancer among Native Hawaiians, and prostate cancer among African Americans are substantially higher than those reported in any other racial and ethnic population group in the United States (Ries et al., 2006). In addition, the mortality rates of stomach cancer among Asians/Pacific Islanders, cervical cancer among African Americans, and prostate cancer among African Americans are substantially higher than for any other racial and ethnic population group in the United States. Finally, the five-year relative cancer survival rates of lung and bronchial cancers among Native American and Alaskan Native men and women, colon and rectal cancers among African American men and Native American and Alaskan Native women, prostate cancer among Native American and Alaskan Native men, and breast cancer among African American women are substantially lower than those reported in any other racial and ethnic population group in the United States (Clegg et al., 2002).

Subgroup analysis of trends in cancer incidence and mortality among Hispanic and Asian/Pacific Islander population groups revealed similar variations (Miller et al., 1996). In general, the rate of cancer incidence and cancer mortality among Hispanics is lower than the cancer incidence and mortality rates of non-Hispanics. However, Hispanics, especially first-generation migrants, experience a heavy burden of stomach, liver, and cervical cancers (Canto & Chu, 2000). For example, data revealed that Hispanic American women have twice the incidence of cervical cancer compared to non-Hispanic American women. Cervical cancer incidence is higher in Mexican American and Puerto Rican American women than in non-Hispanic Caucasian women. With the exception of those living in the Southeast, the incidence rates of stomach cancer are at least 1.5 times higher among Hispanics compared to non-Hispanic Caucasians. Hispanics experienced a 60% higher mortality rate from stomach cancer and liver cancer compared with non-Hispanic populations. Finally, the mortality rate from cervical cancer is 40% higher among Hispanic women than non-Hispanic American women (Canto & Chu; Miller et al.).

Within the Asian/Pacific Islander population in the United States, Filipino Americans and Korean Americans have the lowest cancer incidence and lowest

Table 10-1. Age-Adjusted Surveillance, Epidemiology and End Results Program Cancer Incidence Rates, 2000–2003*										
	Non-Hispanic Caucasian		Black		Asian/Pacific Islander		Native American/ Alaskan Native		Hispanic	
Cancer Site	Male	Female	Male	Female	Male	Female	Male	Female	Male	Female
All sites	574.0	438.8	666.4	395.4	361.8	285.5	359.9	305.0	419.1	310.9
Brain and nervous system	8.8	6.1	4.9	3.5	4.0	2.9	4.7	3.1	5.9	4.8
Female breast (in-situ)	n/a	32.7	n/a	25.0	n/a	25.5	n/a	18.1	n/a	17.6
Female breast	n/a	140.6	n/a	118.0	n/a	88.6	n/a	74.4	n/a	89.1
Uterine cervix	n/a	7.3	n/a	11.5	n/a	8.2	n/a	7.2	n/a	14.2
Colon and rectum	62.7	45.7	72.9	56.1	51.2	35.7	52.7	41.9	47.3	32.7
Uterine corpus	n/a	25.4	n/a	19.5	n/a	15.8	n/a	15.6	n/a	17.0
Esophagus	8.1	2.1	10.8	3.3	4.0	1.2	9.5	–	5.2	1.2
Hodgkin lymphoma	3.5	2.9	2.8	2.0	1.4	1.0	–	–	2.9	1.6
Kidney and renal pelvis	17.9	8.8	20.1	9.7	8.8	4.4	20.9	10.0	16.0	9.0
Larynx	6.6	1.5	11.7	2.0	3.1	0.3	–	–	5.3	0.7
Leukemia	16.8	9.8	12.9	8.0	9.2	5.9	8.6	5.7	11.7	7.8
Liver and intrahepatic bile duct	6.9	2.5	12.1	3.5	20.9	8.0	14.5	6.5	14.1	5.6
Lung and bronchus	81.9	56.8	112.2	53.1	55.7	27.3	55.5	33.8	44.7	24.0

(Continued on next page)

Table 10-1. Age-Adjusted Surveillance, Epidemiology and End Results Program Cancer Incidence Rates, 2000–2003* (Continued)

Cancer Site	Non-Hispanic Caucasian		Black		Asian/Pacific Islander		Native American/ Alaskan Native		Hispanic	
	Male	Female	Male	Female	Male	Female	Male	Female	Male	Female
Melanoma	30.2	19.8	1.1	0.9	1.6	1.2	–	–	4.4	4.4
Multiple myeloma	6.4	3.9	13.7	9.1	3.7	3.0	6.2	6.2	6.8	4.6
Non-Hodgkin lymphoma	24.4	17.1	17.6	11.7	15.7	11.3	15.0	10.1	18.9	13.9
Oral cavity and pharynx	16.5	6.5	18.0	5.8	11.0	5.4	11.4	5.4	9.2	3.7
Ovary	n/a	14.9	n/a	10.1	n/a	9.7	n/a	13.1	n/a	11.4
Pancreas	13.1	9.8	16.2	13.7	9.9	8.3	10.8	10.8	10.8	9.9
Prostate	167.9	n/a	258.3	n/a	96.8	n/a	70.7	n/a	141.1	n/a
Stomach	9.5	4.1	17.7	9.3	18.9	11.0	21.6	12.3	15.9	9.6
Testis	7.1	n/a	1.5	n/a	1.7	n/a	3.7	n/a	3.8	n/a
Thyroid	4.9	13.4	2.4	7.1	3.8	12.5	2.5	10.0	3.2	11.2
Urinary bladder	42.6	10.6	19.8	7.4	16.4	3.9	12.5	–	19.9	5.5

*Incidence data used in calculating the rates are from the 17 Surveillance, Epidemiology and End Results Program areas (San Francisco [SF], Connecticut, Detroit, Hawaii, Iowa, New Mexico, Seattle, Utah, Atlanta, San Jose-Monterey [SJM], Los Angeles [LA], Alaska Native Registry, rural Georgia, California excluding SF/SJM/LA, Kentucky, Louisiana, and New Jersey).

Note. Based on information from Ries et al., 2006.

Table 10-2. Age-Adjusted U.S. Cancer Mortality Rates, 2000–2003*

Cancer Site	Caucasian		Black		Asian/Pacific Islander		Native American/ Alaskan Native		Hispanic	
	Male	Female	Male	Female	Male	Female	Male	Female	Male	Female
All sites	241.7	155.3	326.8	191.1	143.3	98.0	150.0	111.1	165.1	108.1
Brain and nervous system	6.0	4.0	3.3	2.2	2.5	1.5	2.5	1.6	3.5	2.4
Female breast (invasive)	n/a	25.8	n/a	34.3	n/a	12.6	n/a	13.4	n/a	16.2
Uterine cervix (invasive)	n/a	2.3	n/a	5.0	n/a	2.5	n/a	2.8	n/a	3.4
Colon and rectum	23.8	16.5	33.4	23.4	15.4	10.5	15.6	11.0	17.3	11.3
Uterine corpus (invasive)	n/a	3.9	n/a	7.1	n/a	2.4	n/a	2.3	n/a	3.2
Esophagus	7.9	1.7	10.5	3.0	3.0	0.8	5.0	1.2	4.2	1.0
Hodgkin lymphoma	0.6	0.4	0.5	0.3	0.3	0.2	–	–	0.6	0.3
Kidney and renal pelvis	6.3	2.8	6.2	2.8	2.6	1.2	6.4	3.2	5.3	2.4
Larynx	2.3	0.5	5.1	0.9	0.8	0.1	1.7	0.5	1.9	0.2
Leukemia	10.5	5.9	8.7	5.3	4.9	3.1	4.4	3.5	6.5	4.2
Liver and intrahepatic bile duct	6.1	2.6	9.8	3.8	15.6	6.8	8.1	3.9	10.7	5.0
Lung and bronchus	76.2	44.3	97.2	39.8	38.6	18.6	41.4	26.8	36.6	14.7

(Continued on next page)

Table 10-2. Age-Adjusted U.S. Cancer Mortality Rates, 2000–2003* *(Continued)*

Cancer Site	Caucasian		Black		Asian/Pacific Islander		Native American/ Alaskan Native		Hispanic	
	Male	Female	Male	Female	Male	Female	Male	Female	Male	Female
Melanoma	4.6	2.1	0.5	0.4	0.5	0.3	0.9	0.6	1.0	0.6
Multiple myeloma	4.4	2.9	8.5	6.3	1.8	1.5	3.0	3.0	3.8	2.7
Non-Hodgkin lymphoma	10.3	6.6	6.6	4.3	5.9	4.0	4.8	4.0	7.1	4.9
Oral cavity and pharynx	3.9	1.5	6.8	1.7	3.6	1.4	3.2	1.4	2.8	0.8
Ovary	n/a	9.5	n/a	7.4	n/a	4.9	n/a	5.5	n/a	6.1
Pancreas	12.2	9.1	15.4	12.5	7.7	6.9	6.1	5.8	9.0	7.6
Prostate	26.2	n/a	64.0	n/a	11.3	n/a	18.1	n/a	21.8	n/a
Stomach	5.0	2.4	12.1	6.0	10.8	6.5	6.8	39	9.1	5.1
Testis	0.3	n/a	0.2	n/a	0.1	n/a	–	n/a	0.2	n/a
Thyroid	0.5	0.4	0.4	0.5	0.4	0.7	–	–	0.5	0.6
Urinary bladder	8.0	2.3	5.4	2.8	2.9	1.0	2.6	1.2	4.1	1.4

*Mortality data calculated from data provided by the National Center for Health Statistics.

Note. Based on information from Ries et al., 2006.

cancer mortality rates (Miller et al., 1996). However, Native Hawaiians have the highest overall cancer incidence rates and the highest overall cancer mortality rates. Japanese Americans have the highest incidence rate for stomach and colorectal cancers. Chinese Americans have the highest incidence rates of nasopharyngeal and liver cancers, and Filipino Americans have the highest incidence rates of thyroid cancer. Vietnamese American women have the highest incidence rates of liver and intrahepatic bile duct cancers (Miller et al.).

These data demonstrate the disproportionate cancer burden experienced by racial and ethnic minority populations in the United States. Although the specific causative factors that contribute to these disproportionate cancer experiences are unclear, knowledge of the factors and mechanisms associated with the genesis of cancer is increasing.

Nurse Scientists Pioneer Cancer Disparities Research

The variations in cancer incidence and mortality among minority population groups in the United States have been shown to result from complex interactions of environmental conditions, lifestyle choices, and social and cultural factors. The influence of many of these factors on the cancer experience of minority population groups has long been recognized by leaders within the oncology nursing community. Well before the U.S. Department of Health and Human Services (2000) declared eliminating health-related disparities a national health priority, nurse scientists were undertaking efforts to study the influence of these factors on the cancer prevention, cancer control, and cancer care experiences of ethnically and racially defined populations and to propose the design of theory-based and evidence-based interventions to enhance and/or improve their cancer care.

In the late 1980s and early 1990s, several reports published in the nursing literature highlighted outcomes of comparative, exploratory, and descriptive studies aimed to describe the cancer care needs and concerns of Hispanic, Asian/Pacific Islander, Native American/Alaskan Native, and African American populations (Antle, 1987; Brant & Vanderhoof, 1994; Guillory, 1987; Gutoski, 1995; Kagawa-Singer, 1987; Lu, 1995; Millon-Underwood & Sanders, 1990; Millon-Underwood, Sanders, & Davis, 1993; O'Hare, Malone, Lusk, & McCorkle, 1993; Phillips & Wilbur, 1995; Sugarek, Deyo, & Holmes, 1988); the outcomes of exploratory and descriptive studies that aimed to identify factors contributing to the health promotion and cancer prevention behaviors of minority men and women (Burnett, Steakley, & Tefft, 1995; Douglass, Bartolucci, Waterbor, & Sirles, 1995; Gelfand, Parzuchowski, Cort, & Powell, 1995; Mickley & Soeken, 1993; Millon-Underwood & Sanders, 1991; Nemcek, 1989; Underwood, 1991); the outcomes of exploratory studies that aimed to propose and/or construct theories, models, and frameworks that are useful for explaining or predicting the cancer beliefs and behaviors of ethnically/

racially specific population groups (Powe, 1994, 1995a, 1995b; Underwood, 1991, 1992); and the outcomes of descriptive and intervention studies that proposed the design and evaluation of culturally tailored, multidisciplinary, community-based nursing interventions to improve cancer screening among minority men and women (Lacey et al., 1989; Lovejoy, Jenkins, Wu, Shankland, & Wilson, 1989; Manfredi, Lacey, & Warnecke, 1990; Nielsen, 1989; Willis, Davis, Cairns, & Janiszewski, 1989).

Reports that summarize and analyze the focus, methods, and outcomes of studies conducted by nurse scientists addressing cancer prevention and control among ethnic/racial minority population groups, published from 1986 to 2002 (Underwood, Powe, Canales, Meade, & Im, 2004), attest to the significance of this body of science. The same holds true of this chapter, which includes the additional review of the focus, methods, and outcomes of studies published from 2002 to 2006 that were conducted by nurse scientists and designed to address cancer prevention and control among ethnic/racial minority population groups (see Table 10-3). These nurse scientists' efforts have contributed much to understanding the challenges faced by minority men and women related to cancer prevention, early detection, and cancer control; the identification of individual, familial, cultural, and economic factors associated with the excess cancer morbidity and mortality of minority population groups; the identification of cancer care concerns and needs of population groups considered to be at risk for being medically underserved; and the proposition of nursing interventions to improve the cancer care of minority men and women. However, upon critical analysis of the breadth of this body of science, the need to expand cancer nursing research related to racial and ethnic populations becomes strikingly apparent.

Examining Past Efforts Before Forging Ahead

The cancer-related disparities reported in U.S. racial and ethnic minority populations, measured in terms of overall cancer incidence, mortality, and five-year relative survival, are profound. Data reported by the NCI SEER program indicate that racial and ethnic minority men and women generally experience significantly higher cancer incidence, higher cancer mortality, and lower five-year relative cancer survival rates when compared to the non-Hispanic Caucasian population. The most common types of cancer experienced by racial and ethnic minority men are cancers of the prostate, lung, bronchus, colon, and rectum. The most common types of cancer experienced by racial and ethnic minority women are cancers of the breast, lung, bronchus, colon, and rectum (Ries et al., 2006).

Outcomes of several studies conducted by nurse scientists over the past two decades in an effort to address the racial and ethnic cancer disparities have been reported in the nursing literature. Included among them are reports of studies that focused on issues and concerns related to breast, colon,

Table 10-3. Nursing Research Designed to Address the Elimination of Cancer-Related Disparities in U.S. Racial and Ethnic Population Groups, 2002–2006

Citation	Purpose	Sample, Characteristics, and Setting	Design and Instrumentation	Theory Framework	Findings
Breast Cancer					
Adams et al. (2004) The Role of Emotion in Mammography Screening of African-American Women	Identify emotions related to breast cancer screening behavior of African American women.	Volunteer sample of 37 African American women 40 years of age and older from central and north Texas (27 had at least one mammogram and 10 never had a mammogram)	Descriptive State-Trait Anxiety Inventory, Breast Cancer Early Detection Questionnaire, Mammography Feeling Scale	Health Belief Model	Fear of getting breast cancer, fear of dying from breast cancer, and fear that breast cancer was incurable were the most common themes identified by the study participants. Women who had had a previous mammogram expressed fear of losing a breast and fear that if they lost a breast their husbands would not find them attractive. Women who had not had a previous mammogram expressed a fear of radiation and a fear of pain from the mammogram procedure.
Baldwin & Williams-Brown (2005) Uncovering Homeless African-American Women's Knowledge of Breast Cancer and Their Use of Breast Cancer Screening Services	Explore the knowledge related to breast cancer and breast cancer screening services among homeless African American women.	Volunteer sample of 25 African American women recruited from a transient women's shelter located in a large city in the southeastern part of the United States	Exploratory Interview guide	—	Fear, death, familial cancer, and loss were the primary themes that emerged from the data. Although most of the women reported that they performed breast self-examination, they had limited knowledge of the self-examination procedure. Homelessness, unemployment, and lack of adequate health insurance were cited as barriers to mammography screening.

(Continued on next page)

Table 10-3. Nursing Research Designed to Address the Elimination of Cancer-Related Disparities in U.S. Racial and Ethnic Population Groups, 2002–2006 *(Continued)*

Citation	Purpose	Sample, Characteristics, and Setting	Design and Instrumentation	Theory Framework	Findings
Bradley (2005) The Delay and Worry Experience of African American Women With Breast Cancer	Examine the delay in seeking treatment and worry experiences of African American women with breast cancer symptoms.	Volunteer sample of 60 premenopausal and postmenopausal African American women who were receiving or completed breast cancer treatment	Descriptive Illness-Related Information Sheet, Self-Reported Delay, Ware Health Perceptions Questionnaire, Worry Measure, medical record	Attribution Theory	African American women in the study sample reported minimal patient/provider delay in seeking treatment. Women who expressed a higher degree of worry had delay scores similar to women expressing lower degree of worry. No relationship was found between the worry experiences of the women and patient/provider delay.
Bradley et al. (2006) Getting Ready: Developing an Educational Intervention to Prepare African American Women for Breast Biopsy	Evaluate an educational intervention designed to prepare African American women for breast biopsy.	Purposive sample of 20 African American women with history of breast biopsy recruited from a breast cancer support group and by word of mouth	Exploratory Focus group guide	Self-Regulation Theory	The focus group methodology proved to be an effective method for obtaining feedback regarding the study intervention. In addition to identifying strengths related to the content, illustrations, layout, and design, text recommendations were offered by the focus group participants about the graphics, the design and size of the booklet, and the tone and language used to tailor the intervention for the targeted group of African American women.

(Continued on next page)

Table 10-3. Nursing Research Designed to Address the Elimination of Cancer-Related Disparities in U.S. Racial and Ethnic Population Groups, 2002–2006 *(Continued)*

Citation	Purpose	Sample, Characteristics, and Setting	Design and Instrumentation	Theory Framework	Findings
Canales & Rakowski (2006) Development of a Culturally Specific Instrument for Mammography Screening: An Example With American Indian Women in Vermont	Design a culturally specific mammography screening instrument for American Indian women.	Purposive sample of 20 women self-identified as American Indian from Vermont with a history of consistent annual mammograms, who were underusers or nonusers of mammography, and who were breast cancer survivors	Exploratory Focused interview guide	Transtheoretical Model of Behavior Change	Investigational process and data analysis resulted in the development of a 31-item quantitative mammography screening instrument for American Indian women designed to measure the influence of traditionality on mammography screening behaviors. Included within the instrument are 8 items reflective of the pros of screening, 7 items reflective of the cons of screening, 16 items reflective of the processes of change, 4 items reflective of information sharing, 4 items that address the degree to which women think beyond self, 4 items reflective of the degree to which women approach/avoid the healthcare system, and 12 items reflective of the sense of traditionality.

(Continued on next page)

Table 10-3. Nursing Research Designed to Address the Elimination of Cancer-Related Disparities in U.S. Racial and Ethnic Population Groups, 2002–2006 (Continued)

Citation	Purpose	Sample, Characteristics, and Setting	Design and Instrumentation	Theory Framework	Findings
Chen & Bakken (2004) Breast Cancer Knowledge Assessment in Female Chinese Immigrants in New York	Examine the relationships between acculturation level and perceptions of health access, health beliefs, health practices, and knowledge of breast cancer risk in female Chinese immigrants.	Convenience sample of 135 Chinese immigrant women recruited from churches, temples, and health education classes in the New York City metropolitan area	Descriptive correlational Acculturation, access to medical care, attitudes toward health care and cancer, breast cancer screening practices tool	Acculturation Framework	No significant relationships were noted between acculturation and health access, health beliefs, health practices, and breast cancer risk knowledge. However, data indicated that years of education, marital status, and household income were predictors of knowledge of breast cancer risk.
Coleman et al. (2003) The Delta Project: Increasing Breast Cancer Screening Among Rural Minority and Older Women by Targeting Rural Healthcare Providers	Test multimethod educational approach designed for rural healthcare providers to increase breast cancer screening among rural low-income African American and older adult women.	Volunteer sample of 224 nurses, physicians, and mammography technicians recruited from primary care clinics in 27 counties in the Arkansas Delta	Experimental Delayed Control Group Pretest/ Post-test Standardized Patients; Professional Education, Knowledge, Attitudes and Behaviors Survey; Clinical Breast Examination, Proficiency Instrument; Medical Record	PRECEDE-PROCEED Model	Breast cancer screening practices of the healthcare providers improved after participating in the intervention. No differences were found in the performance of clinical breast examination between the intervention group and the control group prior to the delayed intervention. Data revealed that, when compared with the comparison group, a higher number of African American and older adult women in the intervention group received mammography.

(Continued on next page)

Table 10-3. Nursing Research Designed to Address the Elimination of Cancer-Related Disparities in U.S. Racial and Ethnic Population Groups, 2002–2006 *(Continued)*

Citation	Purpose	Sample, Characteristics, and Setting	Design and Instrumentation	Theory Framework	Findings
Dirksen & Erickson (2002) Well-Being in Hispanic and Non-Hispanic White Survivors of Breast Cancer	Test the conceptual model of well-being among Hispanic and non-Hispanic Caucasian breast cancer survivors.	Convenience sample of 50 Hispanic and 50 non-Hispanic Caucasian women 30–83 years of age who had completed primary treatment for breast cancer and were deemed to be disease-free	Descriptive correlational Short Acculturation Scale, Healthcare Orientation Subscale of the Psychosocial Adjustment to Illness Scale, Mishel Uncertainty to Illness Scale, Personal Resource Questionnaire, Self-Control Schedule, Self-Esteem Index, Index of Well-Being	Well-Being Among Survivors of Breast Cancer	Data demonstrated the strength of healthcare orientation, uncertainty, social support, resourcefulness, and self-esteem in predicting well-being in both Hispanic and non-Hispanic Caucasian survivors of breast cancer. Social support was found to be a significant predictor of resourcefulness for Hispanic women; social support and resourcefulness were found to be significant predictors of self-esteem for Hispanic and non-Hispanic Caucasian women; and self-esteem and healthcare orientation were found to be significant predictors of well-being for Hispanic and non-Hispanic Caucasian women.
Eversley et al. (2005) Post-Treatment Symptoms Among Ethnic Minority Breast Cancer Survivors	Examine relationship among surgical treatments, adjuvant therapies, and post-treatment symptoms.	Women aged 18–60 years diagnosed and treated for breast cancer within past two years and working at least 20 hours, recruited from programs offering advocacy and support for survivors and support programs at a public hospital	Descriptive Piper Fatigue Scale, Brief Pain Inventory, CES-D (Center for Epidemiologic Studies—Depression) Scale	—	Latinas reported higher rates of depression and fatigue. Latinas and African Americans reported higher levels of pain. Social and economic factors play a role in women being able to access post-treatment rehabilitation care.

(Continued on next page)

Table 10-3. Nursing Research Designed to Address the Elimination of Cancer-Related Disparities in U.S. Racial and Ethnic Population Groups, 2002–2006 *(Continued)*

Citation	Purpose	Sample, Characteristics, and Setting	Design and Instrumentation	Theory Framework	Findings
Ford et al. (2002) Modifying a Breast Cancer Risk Factor Survey for African American Women	Evaluate a breast cancer risk factor survey for use with African American women.	Randomly selected group of 11 African American women 18–50 years of age and 9 African American women 51 years of age and older who were listed in the Henry Ford Health System administrative database who had made at least one visit to the health system during the first six months of 1998	Structured interview guide	–	Multiple suggestions were made by the study participants to modify the survey to make it more appropriate for use among African American women. Included among them were suggestions regarding the language and the terms used in the survey, coding the sections of the survey by color to make them more distinct, inclusion of culturally appropriate options reflective of health/risk behaviors, and the inclusion of pictures and names of devices referenced in the survey.
Fowler (2006) Claiming Health: Mammography Screening Decision Making of African American Women	Develop theory to explain how African American women of diverse socioeconomic status make decisions about mammography.	Volunteer sample of 30 African American women 52–72 years of age with no prior history of breast cancer who had not had a mammogram within the past two years recruited by word of mouth and from two large Baptist churches in a large city in Ohio	Exploratory Semistructured interview guide	–	Claiming health emerged as the theory that explained decision making about mammography. Claiming health was noted to involve sisterhood and fellowship relationships and was different based on age and socioeconomic status.

(Continued on next page)

Table 10-3. Nursing Research Designed to Address the Elimination of Cancer-Related Disparities in U.S. Racial and Ethnic Population Groups, 2002–2006 *(Continued)*

Citation	Purpose	Sample, Characteristics, and Setting	Design and Instrumentation	Theory Framework	Findings
Fowler et al. (2005) Collaborative Breast Health Intervention for African American Women of Lower Socioeconomic Status	Describe the phases of collaborative breast health intervention delivered by paraprofessionals or specially trained community health advisers designed to increase mammography screening among African American women.	Volunteer sample of 90 African American women 50–65 years of age recruited from two inner-city communities in Montgomery County, Ohio	Breast health knowledge and mammography screening questionnaire	–	Although the collaborative breast health intervention resulted in increased knowledge related to breast health and increased mammography screening, attrition was significant (22%) among the group of African American women recruited to the study. Included among the reasons for the attrition were the length of the intervention, issues specific to the use of the telephone, and healthcare system delays.
Gill et al. (2004) Triggers of Uncertainty About Recurrence and Physical Symptoms Linked to Long-Term Treatment Side Effects in Older African American and Caucasian Long-term Survivors of Breast Cancer	Examine sources of uncertainty and physical symptoms linked to long-term treatment side effects in older African American and Caucasian long-term survivors of breast cancer.	Volunteer sample of 171 Caucasian and 73 African American women 49–87 years of age who participated in study of women surviving breast cancer recruited through cancer registries at 15 hospitals and medical centers in North Carolina	Descriptive Triggers of uncertainty Symptoms	–	No significant difference occurred in the number of triggers reported by the African American and Caucasian women. The most frequent trigger of uncertainty identified was hearing about someone else's cancer; new aches, pains, or physical symptoms; sights, sounds, and smells associated with the breast cancer experience; information from television, radio, the Internet, and

(Continued on next page)

Table 10-3. Nursing Research Designed to Address the Elimination of Cancer-Related Disparities in U.S. Racial and Ethnic Population Groups, 2002–2006 (Continued)

Citation	Purpose	Sample, Characteristics, and Setting	Design and Instrumentation	Theory Framework	Findings
					magazines; and doctors appointments for annual checkups. The most frequent trigger for African American women was new symptoms; for Caucasian women, it was hearing about someone else's cancer. The most common and frequent symptoms reported were fatigue, joint stiffness, and pain. No significant difference was noted in the occurrence and frequency of symptoms.
Graham et al. (2002) Health Beliefs and Self Breast Examination in Black Women	Examine the influence of demographic attributes and health beliefs on the breast self-examination among African American women.	Convenience sample of 179 African American women recruited from a teaching hospital, churches, and health fairs in New York City	Descriptive correlational Champion's Health Belief Survey	Health Belief Model	Breast self-examination frequency was observed to be directly related to perceived seriousness of breast cancer, perceived risk of developing breast cancer, perceived benefit of breast self-examination, regularity of health examinations, and age among the African American women involved in the study.

(Continued on next page)

Table 10-3. Nursing Research Designed to Address the Elimination of Cancer-Related Disparities in U.S. Racial and Ethnic Population Groups, 2002–2006 (Continued)

Citation	Purpose	Sample, Characteristics, and Setting	Design and Instrumentation	Theory Framework	Findings
Grindel et al. (2004) The Effect of Breast Cancer Screening Messages on Knowledge, Attitudes, Perceived Risk, and Mammography Screening of African American Women in the Rural South	Determine effect of positive/upbeat, cognitive/neutral, and negative/fearful video breast cancer screening messages on knowledge, attitudes, perceived risk, and mammography screening behavior among rural African American women.	Volunteer sample of 450 African American women 45–65 years of age who had not had a screening mammogram in the past 12 months recruited from three counties in the South	Repeated measures experimental design Breast Cancer Awareness Survey, Perceived Breast Cancer Risk, Visual Analog Scale, self-reported mammogram	Persuasive Health Message Framework	Affective tone of the breast cancer screening messages had no effect on the breast cancer knowledge, attitudes, and screening behaviors of rural African American women. The number of women getting mammography screening increased after the intervention among each of the study groups. However, researchers were unable to correlate the increased screening with the video messages.
Hall et al. (2005) Teaching Breast Cancer Screening to African American Women in the Arkansas Mississippi River Delta	Determine the effectiveness of a multifaceted, culturally sensitive breast cancer educational program for African American women in the Arkansas Mississippi River Delta.	Volunteer sample of 53 African American women 40 years of age and older from the northeastern counties of the Arkansas Mississippi River Delta recruited from African American churches and county Extension Homemakers Club	Experimental posttest-only control group design Breast Cancer Knowledge Test, Breast Cancer Screening Belief Scales, Client Satisfaction Questionnaire	Health Belief Model	Mean scores for the breast cancer knowledge test, breast cancer susceptibility, and confidence in breast cancer screening for the experimental group were significantly higher than in the control group. Because of a poor return rate of study instruments for the three-month follow-up, the impact of the intervention on breast cancer screening could not be assessed.

(Continued on next page)

Table 10-3. Nursing Research Designed to Address the Elimination of Cancer-Related Disparities in U.S. Racial and Ethnic Population Groups, 2002–2006 (Continued)

Citation	Purpose	Sample, Characteristics, and Setting	Design and Instrumentation	Theory Framework	Findings
Hamilton & Sandelowski (2004) Types of Social Support in African American Americans With Cancer	Determine types of social support African Americans use to cope with cancer.	Purposively selected group of 13 African American men 61–79 years of age treated for prostate cancer and 15 African American women 42–87 years of age treated for breast cancer who had participated in three National Institutes of Health–funded studies in southeastern United States	Exploratory Interview guide	–	Three types of social support were identified by the study participants: emotional support (e.g., presence of others, encouraging words, distracting activities, protection, monitoring), instrumental support (e.g., prayer, assistance in maintaining social roles, assistance in the home), and information support (e.g., advice and information about the disease, treatment, symptoms, and follow-up).
Henderson & Fogel (2003) Support Networks Used by African American Breast Cancer Support Group Participants	Explore the support networks used by African American cancer support group participants to cope with the physical and psychological consequences of breast cancer.	Convenience sample of 43 African American women from the southeastern United States who were participants in an African American breast cancer support group	Descriptive Ways of Coping Questionnaire	–	African American women noted that they most often relied on the support group, God, family, and friends for support. Healthcare professionals and the Internet were noted as being less likely to be used as a source of support.

(Continued on next page)

Table 10-3. Nursing Research Designed to Address the Elimination of Cancer-Related Disparities in U.S. Racial and Ethnic Population Groups, 2002–2006 *(Continued)*

Citation	Purpose	Sample, Characteristics, and Setting	Design and Instrumentation	Theory Framework	Findings
Henderson et al. (2003) African American Women Coping With Breast Cancer: A Qualitative Analysis	Gain a deeper understanding of coping strategies used by African American women diagnosed with breast cancer.	Purposive sample of 66 African American women 35–76 years of age diagnosed with breast cancer recruited from churches, breast cancer support groups, community centers, physician's offices, and sororities in southeastern United States	Exploratory Focus group guide	–	The most common coping strategies reported by the African American female survivors of breast cancer were prayer and spirituality, seeking social support, and participating in breast cancer support groups. Avoiding negativity, maintaining positive attitudes, and maintaining the will to live also were identified as being helpful.
Ho et al. (2005) Predictors of Breast and Cervical Screening in Vietnamese Women in Harris County, Houston, Texas	Characterize the demographic factors, beliefs, and barriers to cervical and breast cancer screening in Vietnamese women; and, evaluate the effect of demographic factors, beliefs, and barriers to cervical and breast cancer screening on	Nonprobability sample of 209 Vietnamese immigrant women 20–88 years of age identified from the telephone directory or the membership lists of all temples and churches in Harris County, Texas	Descriptive cross-sectional Breast and Cervical Cancer Questionnaire	Health Belief Model	The most significant predictors of Pap test, breast self-examination, clinical breast examination, and mammography use among the Vietnamese American women were marital status (being married), high school education, lack of barriers, a family history of cancer, older age, and increased perception of seriousness.

(Continued on next page)

Table 10-3. Nursing Research Designed to Address the Elimination of Cancer-Related Disparities in U.S. Racial and Ethnic Population Groups, 2002–2006 (Continued)

Citation	Purpose	Sample, Characteristics, and Setting	Design and Instrumentation	Theory Framework	Findings
	Pap test, breast self-examination, clinical breast examination, and mammography use in Vietnamese women.				
Katapodi et al. (2002) The Influence of Social Support on Breast Cancer Screening in a Multicultural Community Sample	Examine the relationship between social support and women's adherence to breast cancer screening guidelines and examine whether women who reported having more social support followed recommended screening guidelines more frequently	Convenience sample of 838 mostly low-income African American, Caucasian, and Latina women recruited from the San Francisco Bay area	Cross-sectional community survey Instrument measuring social support, adherence to breast self-examination, clinical breast examination, and mammography screening guidelines, and demographics Acculturation Scale	Breast Cancer Screening Behavior	Social support was found to be associated with adherence to breast cancer screening. Women who reported never performing breast self-examination had significantly lower social support scores in comparison to those who "rarely" or "regularly" performed breast self-examination. Women who followed the recommended guidelines for clinical breast examination had significantly higher social support scores. No significant difference was found in the mammography screening among women with higher or lower social support scores.

(Continued on next page)

Table 10-3. Nursing Research Designed to Address the Elimination of Cancer-Related Disparities in U.S. Racial and Ethnic Population Groups, 2002–2006 (Continued)

Citation	Purpose	Sample, Characteristics, and Setting	Design and Instrumentation	Theory Framework	Findings
Kim et al. (2006) Breast Cancer Among Asian Americans: Is Acculturation Related to Health-Related Quality of Life?	Explore association of acculturation with health-related quality of life (HRQOL); examine association of demographic, medical, and socioecologic characteristics with HRQOL.	Volunteer sample of 206 Chinese, Filipino, Korean, and Japanese women, 40–75 years of age, with-in five years of breast cancer diagnosis recruited from hospitals, community agencies, and a state cancer surveillance program in California	Cross-sectional; Functional Assessment of Cancer Therapy for Breast Cancer, Breast Cancer Subscale, Acculturation Scale, Urban Life Stressor Scale, Social Support Scale	–	Chinese and Korean Americans were less likely to be acculturated; Korean Americans showed lower HRQOL.
Kim & Sarna (2004) An Intervention to Increase Mammography Use by Korean American Women	Test effectiveness of a community-based intervention to increase mammography screening among Korean American women.	Convenience sample of 141 Korean American women 40–75 years of age who had not received a screening mammogram in the previous 12 months, recruited from two randomly selected Korean churches in southern California	Quasi-experimental pre-/post-test, three-group design; Champion's Attitudes Scales, Powe's Fatalism Inventory, Miller and Champion's Knowledge Scale, Acculturation Scale	PRECEDE-PROCEED Model	The Let's Talk intervention was shown to be an effective approach for improving the breast cancer knowledge and breast cancer screening attitudes among the Korean American women. However, the mammography screening rates of women in the Let's Talk intervention group were not significantly different than those of women in the group that was provided access to low-cost mammography service alone.

(Continued on next page)

Table 10-3. Nursing Research Designed to Address the Elimination of Cancer-Related Disparities in U.S. Racial and Ethnic Population Groups, 2002–2006 (Continued)

Citation	Purpose	Sample, Characteristics, and Setting	Design and Instrumentation	Theory Framework	Findings
Kinney et al. (2002) Screening Behaviors Among African American Women at High Risk for Breast Cancer: Do Beliefs About God Matter?	Examine the relationship between beliefs about God as a controlling force in health and breast cancer screening behavior in female family members of a large African American family with a *BRCA1* mutation.	Purposive sample of 52 females who were members of a large kindred with a *BRCA1* mutation	Cross-sectional cohort survey Self-reported adherence to Cancer Genetics Study Consortium screening recommendations, God Health Locus of Control Scale (GHLC)	Transactional Model of Stress and Coping	When compared to women in the kindred with low GHLC scores, women in the kindred scoring high on the GHLC were found to be less likely to adhere to clinical breast examination and mammography screening recommendations. However, GHLC was not found to be associated significantly with adherence to breast self-examination recommendations. The presence of primary care providers had significant influence on breast cancer screening adherence.
Morgan et al. (2006) African American Women With Breast Cancer and Their Spouses' Perception of Care Received From Physicians	Assess the perceptions of breast cancer care and patient/provider communication patterns among African American women with breast cancer and their spouses.	Purposive sample of 12 African American couples from the mid-Atlantic United States coping with a first-time diagnosis of breast cancer	Exploratory Interview guide	–	Couples perceived that the care they received was compassionate, competent, comprehensive, and comparable to the care received by other women of different ethnicities. The breadth of information provided by physicians was viewed positively and perceived to be adequate.

(Continued on next page)

Table 10-3. Nursing Research Designed to Address the Elimination of Cancer-Related Disparities in U.S. Racial and Ethnic Population Groups, 2002–2006 (Continued)

Citation	Purpose	Sample, Characteristics, and Setting	Design and Instrumentation	Theory Framework	Findings
Morgan et al. (2005) African American Couples Merging Strengths to Successfully Cope With Breast Cancer	Explore process of coping with breast cancer among African American women and their spouses.	Purposive sample of 12 African American couples coping with a first-time diagnosis of breast cancer recruited from breast cancer support groups, African American churches, and patient referrals in the mid-Atlantic region of the United States	Exploratory Focus group interview guide	–	Six core values were identified as assisting the couples to merge their strengths in the effort to cope, survive, live through, and live beyond the diagnosis of breast cancer: walking together, praying together, seeking together, trusting together, adjusting together, and being together.
Robertson et al. (2006) African American Community Breast Health Education: A Pilot Project	Examine effectiveness of a Train the Trainer breast health education and screening program for African American, older adult, and underserved women in Tennessee.	Volunteer sample of 63 African American and Hispanic women from greater Nashville participating in a breast health education program	Descriptive Retrospective pre-/post-test program evaluation	–	Data suggested that prior to the program, although recognizing the importance of breast cancer screening, women had limited knowledge of breast cancer signs and symptoms warranting medical attention and breast cancer screening resources available in their community. Following participation in programs facilitated by community trainers, participants' knowledge of breast cancer, breast cancer signs and symptoms, and local breast cancer resources significantly increased.

(Continued on next page)

Table 10-3. Nursing Research Designed to Address the Elimination of Cancer-Related Disparities in U.S. Racial and Ethnic Population Groups, 2002–2006 (Continued)

Citation	Purpose	Sample, Characteristics, and Setting	Design and Instrumentation	Theory Framework	Findings
Russell et al. (2003) Development of Cultural Belief Scales for Mammography Screening	Develop instruments to measure culturally related variables that may influence mammography screening behaviors in African American women.	Purposive sample of 111 African American and 64 Caucasian women 40–97 years of age recruited from churches, community service organizations, a social club, sororities, and public housing projects in Indianapolis, Indiana	Psychometric evaluation Personal space, temporal health orientation, personal control scale	Giger & Davidhizer's Cultural Assessment Model for Health	Internal consistency, reliability, and construct validity of the personal space, temporal health orientation, and personal control scales were confirmed. The cultural constructs of interpersonal space preference, health temporal orientation, and perceived internal control scales were predictive of mammography screening adherence in the African American and Caucasian women.
Russell, Champion, et al. (2006) Psychosocial Factors Related to Repeat Mammography Screening Over 5 Years in African American Women	Measure demographic, knowledge, and health belief predictors of repeat mammography screening in African American women.	Volunteer sample of 602 African American women from three primary care health centers in the Midwest with no history of breast cancer, who had at least one reported screening mammogram in the past 5 years but had no screening mammogram in the past 15 months who were participants in a randomized controlled trial of tailored mammography screening interventions	Descriptive Mammography knowledge, beliefs, and practices instrument	Health Belief Model	Frequency of mammography screening in African American women was associated with education, total annual income, knowledge of screening guidelines, and provider recommendations.

(Continued on next page)

Table 10-3. Nursing Research Designed to Address the Elimination of Cancer-Related Disparities in U.S. Racial and Ethnic Population Groups, 2002–2006 (Continued)

Citation	Purpose	Sample, Characteristics, and Setting	Design and Instrumentation	Theory Framework	Findings
Russell, Perkins, et al. (2006) Sociocultural Context of Mammography Screening Use	Differences in cultural beliefs and health beliefs between African Americans and Caucasians; identify beliefs that predict mammography adherence.	Convenience sample of 111 African American and 64 Caucasian women, 40–97 years of age, with no history of breast cancer, recruited from community organizations and public housing	Descriptive, cross-sectional Health Temporal Orientation Scale, Personal, Internal, and External Control Scale, Fatalism Scale, Susceptibility Scale, Benefits and Barriers Scale, Self-Efficacy Scale, Mammography Screening Adherence	Combination of Cultural Assessment Model for Health and the Health Belief Model	Women who were more oriented to finding health problems early were more likely to adhere to screening guidelines. Internal control was related inversely to screening. Higher sensitivity to space was related to higher screening (when controlling other factors); African American women held more fatalistic beliefs; barriers were the only health belief related to screening.
Sanders et al. (2004) Overcoming: Breast Cancer and Its Effect on Intimacy in Middle Aged African-American Women	Identify how middle-aged African American women diagnosed with breast cancer coped with changes in their personal/intimate relationships.	Purposive sample of 16 African American women, 41–80 years of age and six months postdiagnosis, recruited from community groups and a large church in southeastern United States	Exploratory Interview guide	–	Adjusting to living with breast cancer, or overcoming breast cancer, within the context of intimacy was identified as being influenced by participants' belief in a higher power, the support of their social network, and information provided to them by their physicians.

(Continued on next page)

Table 10-3. Nursing Research Designed to Address the Elimination of Cancer-Related Disparities in U.S. Racial and Ethnic Population Groups, 2002–2006 (Continued)

Citation	Purpose	Sample, Characteristics, and Setting	Design and Instrumentation	Theory Framework	Findings
Spurlock & Cullins (2006) Cancer Fatalism and Breast Cancer Screening in African American Women	Examine the relationships between cancer fatalism and breast cancer screening in African American women.	Convenience sample of 71 African American women who had no history of breast cancer recruited from low-income housing developments, senior citizen housing sites, churches, community centers, and a university campus	Descriptive correlational Powe Fatalism Inventory	Powe Fatalism Model	Cancer fatalism was found to influence the breast cancer screening practices of study participants. Women with higher cancer fatalism scores were less likely to practice breast self-examination, less likely to have obtained a clinical breast examination, and more likely to have obtained a mammogram.
Thomas (2004) African American Women's Breast Memories, Cancer Beliefs, and Feelings About Screening Behaviors	Examine associations between African American women's memories and feelings concerning their breasts and breast cancer screening behaviors.	Purposive sample of 12 professional African American women 42–64 years of age with no history of breast cancer recruited by word of mouth in a large urban Midwestern city	Exploratory Narrative analysis, participant journal, interview guide	–	Barriers to breast cancer screening identified by the study participants included fear of finding a lump, lack of knowledge about breast cancer screening recommendations, limited perceptions of risk, and distrust of the healthcare system. The breast cancer screening behaviors of the study participants were described as being associated with feelings about breast development and feelings about changes in the breast that occurred during early adolescence, puberty, pregnancy, and aging.

(Continued on next page)

Table 10-3. Nursing Research Designed to Address the Elimination of Cancer-Related Disparities in U.S. Racial and Ethnic Population Groups, 2002–2006 (Continued)

Citation	Purpose	Sample, Characteristics, and Setting	Design and Instrumentation	Theory Framework	Findings
Thompson et al. (2006) Post-Treatment Breast Cancer Surveillance and Follow-Up Care Experiences of African American and African Caribbean Survivors of Breast Cancer Survivors of African Descent: An Exploratory Qualitative Study	Explore the post-treatment breast cancer surveillance and follow-up care experiences of African American and African Caribbean survivors of breast cancer.	Volunteer sample of 10 female breast cancer survivors self-identified as black or of African descent who resided in the New York City area	Exploratory Semistructured interview guide	Behavioral Model for Health Services Utilization Afrocentric Model	Participants indicated that following treatment for their breast cancer, although they were encouraged to increase the number of physician visits over the course of the year, most were not given specific recommendations regarding breast care and breast cancer surveillance. The most common follow-up reported by the women were visits to oncology specialists. Factors identified as motivating the women to secure follow-up care included the desire to maintain good health, concern about recurrence, provider recommendation, familial support, support received from other breast cancer survivors, and religious/spiritual faith. Factors identified as barriers to care included fear of recurrence, mixed support from family and friends, lack of information about post-treatment follow-up care, and medical health-care costs.

(Continued on next page)

Table 10-3. Nursing Research Designed to Address the Elimination of Cancer-Related Disparities in U.S. Racial and Ethnic Population Groups, 2002–2006 *(Continued)*

Citation	Purpose	Sample, Characteristics, and Setting	Design and Instrumentation	Theory Framework	Findings
Underwood (2004) Promoting Breast Health Among African American Women in Community-Based Settings: Identifying Good, Better and Best Practices	Assess the potential impact of breast cancer education and outreach programs designed to reach African American women in faith-based institutions, hair salons, beauty salons, and community-oriented social service centers.	A volunteer sample of 644 African American women engaged in forums, meetings, programs, and activities at multiple community-based social service institutions within a large urban community in the Midwest	Descriptive Investigator-designed instrument	–	Data analysis revealed the study participants to be more receptive to receiving breast health programming within faith-based institutions than in hair salons, beauty salons, and social service community centers. Although supportive of the involvement of spiritual leaders, proprietors of hair salons and beauty salons, and directors of social service centers in the facilitation of breast health programs, study participants expressed a preference for the involvement of healthcare professionals in the program presentation.

(Continued on next page)

Table 10-3. Nursing Research Designed to Address the Elimination of Cancer-Related Disparities in U.S. Racial and Ethnic Population Groups, 2002–2006 (Continued)

Citation	Purpose	Sample, Characteristics, and Setting	Design and Instrumentation	Theory Framework	Findings
Wood et al. (2002) The Effect of an Educational Intervention on Promoting Breast Self-Examination in Older African American and Caucasian Women	Test the effects of innovative age- and ethnicity-sensitive, self-monitored video breast health kits to increase knowledge about breast cancer risk and screening and breast self-examination proficiency in a sample of older African American and Caucasian women.	Volunteer sample of 328 African American and Caucasian women 60 years of age and older recruited from senior centers, churches, housing projects for older adults, health fairs, beauty salons, and social or service clubs in Massachusetts and Georgia	Nonequivalent control group, quasi-experimental Breast Self-Examination Proficiency Rating Instrument, Mini-Mental State Examination	Social Learning Theory	The use of the video breast health kits was effective in increasing knowledge about breast cancer risk, knowledge about breast cancer screening, and breast self-examination proficiency in the sample of older African American and Caucasian women.
Wu & Bancroft, (2006) Filipino American Women's Perceptions and Experiences With Breast Cancer Screening	Examine views about breast cancer and screening practices of Filipino American women in the midwestern region of the United States.	Purposive sample of 11 Filipino American women 45–80 years of age recruited from the metropolitan area of southeastern Michigan through community organizations and word of mouth	Exploratory Unstructured interview guide	—	Avoidance was a main theme to deal with cancer. Facilitators for screening were family support, provider recommendation, health insurance reinforcement, and personal attributes such as family history or symptoms. Barriers were attitudes and unpleasant experiences with the healthcare system.

(Continued on next page)

Table 10-3. Nursing Research Designed to Address the Elimination of Cancer-Related Disparities in U.S. Racial and Ethnic Population Groups, 2002–2006 (Continued)

Citation	Purpose	Sample, Characteristics, and Setting	Design and Instrumentation	Theory Framework	Findings
Wu & Yu (2003) Reliability and Validity of the Mammography Screening Beliefs Questionnaire Among Chinese American Women	Describe the reliability and validity of a questionnaire designed for measuring Chinese women's beliefs related to breast cancer and mammogram screening.	Consecutive nonprobability sample of 220 Asian American women identified from a mailing list of Chinese women aged 40–85 years of age residing in a suburban midwestern county	Psychometric analysis Chinese Mammogram Screening Beliefs Questionnaire	Health Belief Model	Psychometric analysis demonstrated satisfactory internal consistency and validity of the Chinese Mammogram Screening Beliefs Questionnaire
Yu et al. (2005) Cultural Affiliation and Mammography Screening of Chinese Women in an Urban County of Michigan	Explore the effects of culturally based attitudes on breast cancer screening behaviors of Chinese women residing in the United States.	Consecutive nonprobability sample of 220 Asian American women identified from a mailing list of Chinese women 40–85 years of age residing in an urban county of Michigan	Cross-sectional, correlational Affiliation Scale Factors Affecting Breast Cancer Screening Among Women of Asian Descent Survey	Behavior Model of Health Services Strength of Cultural Affiliation	Data analyses revealed that cultural affiliation and cultural beliefs were related to the breast cancer screening behavior of immigrant Chinese women.

(Continued on next page)

Table 10-3. Nursing Research Designed to Address the Elimination of Cancer-Related Disparities in U.S. Racial and Ethnic Population Groups, 2002–2006 (Continued)

Citation	Purpose	Sample, Characteristics, and Setting	Design and Instrumentation	Theory Framework	Findings
Colorectal Cancer					
Busch (2003) Elderly African American Women's Knowledge and Belief About Colorectal Cancer	Identify older African American women's colorectal cancer knowledge, beliefs, and behaviors.	Convenience sample of 16 African American women 45–69 years of age recruited from a moderately large church on the southeast side of Chicago	Exploratory Focus group guide	—	African American women study participants had limited knowledge about colon cancer and colon cancer screening. Their level of knowledge, beliefs regarding colorectal cancer screening, and perceived barriers to screening resulted in a low level of participation in colorectal cancer screening.
Frank et al. (2004) Colon Cancer Screening in African American Women	Examine colorectal cancer knowledge, attitudes, beliefs, and practices in African American women.	Volunteer sample of 69 African American women 50 years of age and older recruited from the directories of four primarily African American churches in north Florida	Descriptive Health Belief Model Scale	Health Belief Model	Findings revealed a positive association between health beliefs and colorectal cancer screening. Study participants reporting higher perceptions of colorectal cancer susceptibility, benefit of colorectal cancer screening, confidence in colorectal screening, and fewer barriers had higher frequency of colorectal cancer screening.

(Continued on next page)

Table 10-3. Nursing Research Designed to Address the Elimination of Cancer-Related Disparities in U.S. Racial and Ethnic Population Groups, 2002–2006 (Continued)

Citation	Purpose	Sample, Characteristics, and Setting	Design and Instrumentation	Theory Framework	Findings
Green & Kelly (2004) Colorectal Cancer Knowledge, Perceptions, and Behaviors in African Americans	Determine the colorectal cancer knowledge, perceptions, and screening behaviors of low-income older African American men and women; examine the differences between men and women in colorectal cancer knowledge, perceptions, screening behaviors, and factors influencing colorectal cancer screening behaviors.	Convenience sample of 58 African American women and 42 African American men recruited from a low-income senior citizen housing residence in an urban setting	Descriptive, correlational Colorectal Cancer Knowledge, Perceptions, and Screening Survey	Health Belief Model	Data analysis revealed limited knowledge about colorectal cancer among the older low-income African American men and women in the study sample. When compared with women, men had higher levels of knowledge about colorectal cancer and perceived themselves to be at greater risk for developing colorectal cancer. History of colorectal cancer screening was noted to exert a significant influence on colorectal cancer screening behavior.

(Continued on next page)

Table 10-3. Nursing Research Designed to Address the Elimination of Cancer-Related Disparities in U.S. Racial and Ethnic Population Groups, 2002–2006 (Continued)

Citation	Purpose	Sample, Characteristics, and Setting	Design and Instrumentation	Theory Framework	Findings
Oral Cancer					
Powe & Finnie (2004) Knowledge of Oral Cancer Risk Factors Among African Americans: Do Nurses Have a Role?	Assess knowledge of oral cancer risk factors.	Volunteer sample of 141 African American men and women, 18–69 years of age, recruited from federally qualified primary care centers in the southeastern United States	Descriptive Oral Cancer Risk Factor Questionnaire	Patient/Provider/System Model for Cancer Screening	The majority of the study participants recognized tobacco as a risk factor but were less familiar with the roles of alcohol, sun, and diet. Many identified nonrisk factors such as spicy foods as enhancing risk. Those with higher incomes and annual dental visits had more knowledge.
Prostate Cancer					
Clarke-Tasker & Dutta (2005) African-American Men and Their Reflections and Thoughts on Prostate Cancer	Assess African American men's knowledge, attitudes, and beliefs regarding prostate cancer and early-detection methods.	Volunteer sample of 67 African American men, 42–88 years of age, recruited from churches in the greater Washington, DC, area.	Exploratory Prostate Cancer Knowledge Questionnaire	—	African American men involved in the study expressed a belief in the benefits of prostate cancer screening and a belief that early detection of prostate cancer was beneficial. Most did not perceive the screening for prostate cancer to be embarrassing or uncomfortable or fear that they would be diagnosed with prostate cancer.

(Continued on next page)

Table 10-3. Nursing Research Designed to Address the Elimination of Cancer-Related Disparities in U.S. Racial and Ethnic Population Groups, 2002–2006 (Continued)

Citation	Purpose	Sample, Characteristics, and Setting	Design and Instrumentation	Theory Framework	Findings
Clarke-Tasker & Wade (2002) What We Thought We Knew: African American Males' Perceptions of Prostate Cancer and Screening Methods	Assess African American males' knowledge, attitudes, and behaviors regarding prostate cancer and prostate cancer early-detection methods (e.g., digital rectal examination [DRE], prostate-specific antigen [PSA] test).	Purposive sample of 12 African American men 38–80 years of age	Exploratory	Health Belief Model	On average, study participants were not aware of the risk factors associated with prostate cancer, did not perceive themselves as being susceptible to prostate cancer, had much anxiety about the DRE yet believed in the efficacy of prostate cancer screening early-detection methods, and felt that physicians either did not screen or did not suggest that men be screened for prostate cancer.
Kleier (2004) Using the Health Belief Model to Reveal the Perceptions of Jamaican and Haitian Men Regarding Prostate Cancer	Determine the knowledge and perceptions of Jamaican and Haitian men regarding prostate cancer.	Convenience sample of 10 Jamaican men and 10 Haitian men from south Florida	Exploratory Focus group guide	Health Belief Model	Among the study participants, Jamaican men were more knowledgeable than the Haitian men about prostate cancer. Haitian men had more misconceptions, were less optimistic that prostate cancer could be controlled, and were less likely to have been screened than the Jamaican men involved in the study. Language and cultural variables were believed to influence the differences observed among the study participants.

(Continued on next page)

Table 10-3. Nursing Research Designed to Address the Elimination of Cancer-Related Disparities in U.S. Racial and Ethnic Population Groups, 2002–2006 (Continued)

Citation	Purpose	Sample, Characteristics, and Setting	Design and Instrumentation	Theory Framework	Findings
Lambert et al. (2002) A Comparative Study of Prostate Screening Health Beliefs and Practices Between African American and Caucasian Men	Investigate the prostate cancer screening health beliefs and practices of African American and Caucasian men older than age 45.	Volunteer sample of 55 African American men and 49 Caucasian men older than age 45 recruited from fraternal organizations, health fairs, and churches within a midwestern community	Descriptive Investigator-designed questionnaire	Health Promotion Model	African American men were more likely than Caucasian men to express a belief that a healthy diet and exercise decreased the risk of prostate cancer and that prostate cancer and prostate cancer treatment would adversely affect sexual function. African American men were more likely than Caucasian men to rely on faith to stay healthy. Caucasian men were more likely than African American men to believe that family history of prostate cancer increased their risk and that maintaining good health reduces prostate cancer risk. African American men were less likely to have had the DRE than Caucasian men, although Caucasian men were less likely to have had a PSA test. Significantly more Caucasian men than African American men expressed a belief that that they were likely to develop prostate cancer.

(Continued on next page)

Table 10-3. Nursing Research Designed to Address the Elimination of Cancer-Related Disparities in U.S. Racial and Ethnic Population Groups, 2002–2006 (Continued)

Citation	Purpose	Sample, Characteristics, and Setting	Design and Instrumentation	Theory Framework	Findings
Weinrich, Royal, et al. (2002) Interest in Genetic Prostate Cancer Susceptibility Testing Among African American Men	Identify demographic predictors for interest in prostate cancer susceptibility testing among African American men.	Volunteer sample of 320 men, 21–98 years of age, from the African American Hereditary Prostate Cancer Study and the South Carolina Prostate Cancer Education and Screening Study	Descriptive, correlational Interest in prostate cancer susceptibility testing, family history, and demographic questionnaire	–	The greater majority of the men involved in the study expressed an interest in prostate cancer susceptibility testing; however, most were unable to differentiate between prostate cancer screening and genetic susceptibility testing.
Weinrich, Faison-Smith, et al. (2002) Stability of Self-Reported Family History of Prostate Cancer Among African American Men	Examine the reliability of self-reported family history of prostate cancer among African American men.	Targeted sample of 96 African American men, 40–70 years of age, who participated in the South Carolina Prostate Cancer Study	Correlational Telephone interview	–	Significant differences were observed in self-report of family history of prostate cancer. African American men who were unmarried, who reported low incomes, and who had not participated in free prostate cancer screening were noted to be the least consistent in reporting their family history of prostate cancer.
Weinrich et al. (2004) Knowledge of the Limitations and Benefits of Prostate Cancer Screening Among Low-Income Men	Measure knowledge of the limitations and benefits of prostate cancer screening among African American and Caucasian men.	Volunteer sample of 81 low-income Caucasian and African American men, 40–70 years of age, with no history of prostate cancer, recruited from Jefferson County, Kentucky	Descriptive Knowledge About Prostate Cancer Screening Questionnaire	–	Married men, men with low incomes, and Caucasian men had significantly less total knowledge about prostate cancer screening than unmarried men, men with higher incomes, and African American men.

(Continued on next page)

Table 10-3. Nursing Research Designed to Address the Elimination of Cancer-Related Disparities in U.S. Racial and Ethnic Population Groups, 2002–2006 (Continued)

Citation	Purpose	Sample, Characteristics, and Setting	Design and Instrumentation	Theory Framework	Findings
Weinrich et al. (2003) Self-Reported Reasons Men Decide Not to Participate in Free Prostate Cancer Screening	Determine reasons men do not participate in a free prostate cancer screening.	Volunteer sample of 190 African American men and 51 white men 40–68 years of age who chose not to participate in a free prostate cancer screening following an educational program	Descriptive, correlational Telephone survey	–	Time was noted to be the primary reason African American men reported for not participating in free prostate cancer screening following an educational program. Losing the screening voucher, physicians' refusal to invoice for payment, and the lack of a physician also were cited as reasons for not participating.
Not Specific					
Clarke-Tasker (2003) Socioeconomic Status and African Americans' Perceptions of Cancer	Examine the relationship of socioeconomic status and perceptions regarding cancer susceptibility, risks, prevention, early detection, and screening.	Convenience sample of 139 urban African American men and women 26–74 years of age recruited from a local church	Descriptive Cancer Awareness Inventory	Health Belief Model	Socioeconomic status was found to predict perceptions regarding cancer detection, risk, prevention, susceptibility, and screening.

(Continued on next page)

Table 10-3. Nursing Research Designed to Address the Elimination of Cancer-Related Disparities in U.S. Racial and Ethnic Population Groups, 2002–2006 (Continued)

Citation	Purpose	Sample, Characteristics, and Setting	Design and Instrumentation	Theory Framework	Findings
Swinney (2002) African Americans With Cancer: The Relationships Among Self-Esteem, Locus of Control, and Health Perception	Examine the relationships among self-esteem, locus of control, and perceived health status in African Americans with cancer.	Convenience sample of 95 African American patients recruited from oncology outpatient units of two large medical centers in southern Louisiana and southern Texas	Descriptive Tennessee Self-Concept Scale, Multi-Dimensional Health Locus of Control, Cantril Ladder Visual Analog Scale	–	A positive relationship was found between self-esteem and perceived health status. Study participants with higher levels of self-esteem tended to perceive their health more positively. A modest relationship was found between chance health locus of control and self-esteem. Study participants with higher levels of self-esteem tended to score lower on the chance health locus of control subscale.
Taylor (2003) Spiritual Needs of Patients With Cancer and Family Caregivers	Identify the spiritual needs experienced living with cancer from the perspective of patients with cancer and family members.	Purposive sample of 21 male and female African American and European American patients and 7 female family caregivers recruited from inpatient units and outpatient chemotherapy clinics in a county hospital and a comprehensive cancer center in a large southwestern metropolitan area	Descriptive, cross-sectional Semistructured interview guide	–	No substantial differences were noted in the needs of patients and caregivers. Participants identified spiritual needs including needs associated with relating to an Ultimate Other, need for positivity, hope, and gratitude; the need to give and receive love; the need to review beliefs; the need to have meaning; and needs related to religiosity and preparation for death. African American participants were more likely than

(Continued on next page)

Table 10-3. Nursing Research Designed to Address the Elimination of Cancer-Related Disparities in U.S. Racial and Ethnic Population Groups, 2002–2006 (Continued)

Citation	Purpose	Sample, Characteristics, and Setting	Design and Instrumentation	Theory Framework	Findings
					European American participants to believe that a causal relationship exists between having cancer and sin and that God could cure their cancers if they maintained enough faith and prayed.
Underwood & Powell (2006) Religion and Spirituality: Influence on Health/ Risk Behavior and Cancer Screening Behavior of African Americans	Examine the influence of religion and spirituality on the health/ risk behavior and cancer screening practices of African American congregants.	Purposive sample of 471 African American congregants from six churches within a large urban community in the Midwest	Descriptive Religious intensity/ religiousness, spiritual intensity/spirituality, religious practices, religious problem solving, health-promoting behavior, health risk behavior, cancer risk behavior, healthcare tool	Multidimensional religion, spirituality, and health framework	Religion/spirituality of the participants did not exert a significant influence on exercise, weight management, or participation in prostate, breast, cervical, or colorectal cancer screening among the congregants. However, data revealed that communication with healthcare providers, personal health assessment, and dietary behaviors of the study participants were influenced by religious/spiritual intensity.

and prostate cancer. However, analysis of the summative review of nursing science on racial and ethnic cancer disparities published from 1986 to 2002 (Underwood et al., 2004) and the subsequent review of nursing science published from 2002 to 2006 (see Table 10-3) suggest that significant gaps and limitations in this body of science exist. The mechanisms prescribed by Cooper (1982) were used to review reports of the outcomes of empirical research that addressed cancer prevention and control among ethnic/racial population groups published in *Advances in Nursing Science, Cancer Nursing, Cultural Diversity, Hispanic Health Care International, Image: The Journal of Nursing Scholarship, Journal of the Association of Black Nursing Faculty, Journal of Chi Eta Phi Sorority, Journal of Community Health Nursing, Journal of National Black Nurses Association, Journal of Nursing Measurement, Journal of Pediatric Oncology Nursing, Multicultural Nursing and Health, Nursing Outlook, Oncology Nursing Forum, Nursing Research, Research in Nursing and Health, Seminars in Oncology Nursing,* and *Transcultural Nursing.*

Analysis of the breadth of this body of science by the study subjects' race and ethnicity reveals that the overwhelming majority of studies were designed to examine the cancer experiences of African Americans. Analysis by gender reveals that the overwhelming majority of the studies appear to have been designed to examine the cancer experiences of women. Further analysis by cancer type reveals that the overwhelming majority of the studies were designed to examine issues and concerns associated with breast cancer. Comparatively few of these studies were designed to examine the cancer experiences of minority men. In addition, studies that focused on the cancer care needs and concerns of Asian, Hispanic, and Native American populations were limited.

In spite of national efforts to improve access to health care for all, minority Americans, more often than not, do not have access to quality cancer care. The continuum of cancer care includes cancer prevention, risk management, screening, diagnosis, treatment, symptom management, survivorship, and rehabilitation. If cancer cannot be controlled, the spectrum of care also includes palliative and end-of-life care. Studies designed by nurse scientists to address the manner in which cancer care is provided to racial and ethnic minority populations have focused primarily on breast and prostate cancer screening. Although a few studies have addressed cancer risk management, none have been reported that address palliative or end-of-life care.

Exploration of Culture, Cancer, and Nursing Care

Culture is presumed to influence an individual's attitudes, beliefs, and behaviors associated with cancer prevention, cancer risk management, and cancer care. Several theoretical and conceptual models that describe cultural phenomena that influence health perceptions and behaviors have been proposed (Andrews & Boyle, 2008; Campinha-Bacote, 2002; Giger & Davidhizar,

2008; Leininger, 1985; Leininger & McFarland, 2002; Orque, Bloch, & Monrroy, 1983; Purnell & Paulanka, 2003; Spector, 2004). Increasing numbers of instructional modules, texts, and scholarly reports are being published that posit the associations among culture, cultural phenomena, cancer morbidity, cancer mortality, and cancer care (Frank-Stromborg & Olsen, 2001; Itano & Taoka, 2005; Oncology Nursing Society, 1999, 2001; Otto, 2001; Varricchio, Ades, Hinds, & Pierce, 2004). However, a review of the scientific literature reveals that nurse scientists are making a limited effort to undertake studies that evaluate (and/or validate) the mediating influence of culture and cultural phenomena on cancer prevention and control in ethnic/racial minority population groups.

The cultural phenomena purported to be associated most closely with the trends in cancer morbidity and mortality among racial and ethnic minority groups are ethnic identity, cultural affiliation, cultural heritage, acculturation, social organization, communication, religion and spirituality, and perceptions regarding health. Studies undertaken by nurse scientists to examine the influence of culture and cultural phenomena on cancer prevention and control in ethnic/racial minority population groups have focused primarily on the exploration of phenomena specific to social support, religion and spirituality, cultural affiliation, and acculturation (Canales & Rakowski, 2006; Chen & Bakken, 2004; Hamilton & Sandelowski, 2004; Henderson & Fogel, 2003; Henderson, Gore, Davis, & Condon, 2003; Katapodi, Facione, Miaskowski, Dodd, & Waters, 2002; Kinney, Emery, Dudley, & Croyle, 2002; Taylor, 2003; Underwood & Powell, 2006; Yu, Wu, & Mood, 2005). Data resulting from these efforts provided insight into the types of social support and coping strategies commonly used by African American cancer survivors (Hamilton & Sandelowski; Henderson & Fogel; Henderson et al.), the influence of the social support on adherence with recommended breast cancer screening guidelines in African American and Hispanic women (Katapodi et al.), the spiritual needs of African American cancer survivors and cosurvivors (Kinney et al.; Taylor; Underwood & Powell), relationships between acculturation and access to cancer care (Chen & Bakken), and the influence of cultural affiliation on the breast cancer screening practices of Asian immigrant women (Yu et al.) and Native American women (Canales & Rakowski). However, the data challenge current assumptions about the impact of acculturation on access and utilization of cancer care and the influence of religion and spirituality on cancer-related attitudes, beliefs, and behaviors (Underwood & Powell; Kinney et al.).

Conclusion

Despite the increased focus on health disparities, underserved populations, and access to cancer care over the past two decades, research that addresses these issues is still well behind studies that address cancer-related issues in non-Hispanic Caucasian populations. Although it may be argued that the attention to the types of cancers affecting racial and ethnic populations has narrowed and become more focused over time, the lack of research that aims to explore the cancer experiences of Native American/Alaskan Native populations; the lack of research on the cancers that disproportionately affect racial and ethnic minority populations, such as lung, bronchial, and stomach; the paucity of research that addresses the cancer care needs and concerns of ethnic and racial minority cancer survivors; and the paucity of research that addresses cancer in men remains of particular concern. Especially disconcerting is the absence of reports of nursing research outcomes that focus on lung and bronchial cancer detection and control in nursing journals dedicated to eliminating health-related disparities or emphasizing multicultural nursing, oncology nursing, and nursing research.

A substantive body of knowledge related to cancer among racial and ethnic minority population groups has developed as a result of nurse scientists' efforts. Although providing a beginning foundation, in order for the profession to fully contribute to the elimination of cancer-related disparities, a need exists to further expand this body of science. More focused reviews of the existing nursing literature that describes outcomes of nursing science focused on cancer prevention and control among racial and ethnic population groups are needed. Also needed is the development of theoretically based and methodologically rigorous programs of research that

- Examine issues and concerns associated with cancers having the greatest morbidity and mortality among African American, Native American and Alaskan Native, Asian/Pacific Islander, and Hispanic population groups
- Explore variations in cancer knowledge, beliefs, and perceptions between and among African Americans, Native Americans and Alaskan Natives, Asians/Pacific Islanders, and Hispanic population groups
- Explore cancer risk and risk management among African American, Native American and Alaskan Native, Asian/Pacific Islander, and Hispanic population groups
- Examine the manner and extent to which cancer care is delivered to African American, Native American and Alaskan Native, Asian/Pacific Islander, and Hispanic populations across the cancer care continuum (e.g., cancer prevention, screening, risk management, diagnosis, treatment, symptom management, palliative and end-of-life care)
- Examine the manner and extent to which cancer care is delivered to priority groups (e.g., male, female, older adult, urban, rural, economically disadvantaged, underinsured, immigrant, refugee, medically underserved, at-risk populations) within the African American, Native American and Alaskan Native, Asian/Pacific Islander, and Hispanic communities
- Evaluate (and/or validate) the mediating influence of culture and cultural phenomena on cancer prevention and control in African American, Native American and Alaskan Native, Asian/Pacific Islander, and Hispanic population groups

- Evaluate interventions that aim to reduce cancer morbidity and mortality among African American, Asian American, Hispanic, and Native American populations.

Research designed to enhance cancer prevention and cancer care among racial and ethnic minority groups must increase substantially if the goal of eliminating cancer-related health disparities is to become a reality. The need to expand the scope of nursing research designed to address the elimination of cancer-related disparities in U.S. racial and ethnic populations is pronounced. If the goal of eliminating cancer-related health disparities is to be achieved, oncology nurse scientists, both individually and collectively, must undertake concerted efforts to do so.

References

Adams, M.L., Becker, H., Stout, P.S., Coward, D., Robertson, T., Winchell, M., et al. (2004). The role of emotion in mammography screening of African-American women. *Journal of National Black Nurses Association, 15*(1), 17–23.

American Cancer Society. (2008). *Cancer facts and figures, 2008.* Atlanta, GA: Author.

Andrews, M.M., & Boyle, J.S. (2008). *Transcultural concepts in nursing care* (5th ed.). Philadelphia: Lippincott Williams & Wilkins.

Antle, A. (1987). Ethnic perspectives of cancer nursing: The American Indian. *Oncology Nursing Forum, 14*(3), 70–73.

Baldwin, D.M., & Williams-Brown, S. (2005). Uncovering homeless African-American women's knowledge of breast cancer and their use of breast cancer screening services. *Journal of National Black Nurses Association, 16*(1), 24–30.

Bradley, P.K. (2005). The delay and worry experience of African American women with breast cancer. *Oncology Nursing Forum, 32*(2), 243–249.

Bradley, P.K., Berry, A., Lang, C., & Myers, R.E. (2006). Getting ready: Developing an educational intervention to prepare African American women for breast biopsy. *Journal of the Association of Black Nursing Faculty, 17*(1), 15–19.

Brant, J.M., & Vanderhoof, D. (1994). Blending cultural beliefs with conventional treatments enhances patient care. *Oncology Nursing Forum, 21*(10), 1737.

Burchard, E.G., Ziv, E., Coyle, N., Gomez, S.L., Tang, H., Karter, A.J., et al. (2003). The importance of race and ethnic background in biomedical research and clinical practice. *New England Journal of Medicine, 348*(12), 1170–1175.

Burnett, C.B., Steakley, C.S., & Tefft, M.C. (1995). Barriers to breast and cervical cancer screening in underserved women of the District of Columbia. *Oncology Nursing Forum, 22*(10), 1551–1557.

Busch, S. (2003). Elderly African American women's knowledge and belief about colorectal cancer. *Journal of the Association of Black Nursing Faculty, 14*(5), 99–103.

Campinha-Bacote, J. (2002). The process of cultural competence in the delivery of healthcare services: A model of care. *Journal of Transcultural Nursing, 13*(3), 181–184.

Canales, M.K., & Rakowski, W. (2006). Development of a culturally specific instrument for mammography screening: An example with American Indian women in Vermont. *Journal of Nursing Measurement, 14*(2), 99–115.

Canto, M.T., & Chu, K.C. (2000). Annual cancer incidence rates for Hispanics in the United States: Surveillance, Epidemiology, and End Results, 1992–1996. *Cancer, 88*(11), 2642–2652.

Chen, W.T., & Bakken, S. (2004). Breast cancer knowledge assessment in female Chinese immigrants in New York. *Cancer Nursing, 27*(5), 407–412.

Clarke-Tasker, V. (2003). Socioeconomic status and African Americans' perceptions of cancer. *Journal of National Black Nurses Association, 14*(1), 13–19.

Clarke-Tasker, V.A., & Dutta, A.P. (2005). African-American men and their reflections and thoughts on prostate cancer. *Journal of National Black Nurses Association, 16*(1), 1–7.

Clarke-Tasker, V.A., & Wade, R. (2002). What we thought we knew: African American males' perceptions of prostate cancer and screening methods. *Journal of the Association of Black Nursing Faculty, 13*(3), 56–60.

Clegg, L.X., Li, F.P., Hankey, B.F., Chu, K., & Edwards, B.K. (2002). Cancer survival among U.S. whites and minorities: A SEER (Surveillance, Epidemiology and End Results) Program population-based study. *Archives of Internal Medicine, 162*(17), 1985–1993.

Coleman, E.A., Lord, J., Heard, J., Coon, S., Cantrell, M., Mohrmann, C., et al. (2003). The Delta project: Increasing breast cancer screening among rural minority and older women by targeting rural healthcare providers. *Oncology Nursing Forum, 30*(4), 669–677.

Collins, F.S. (2004). What we do and don't know about "race," "ethnicity," genetics and health at the dawn of the genome era. *Nature Genetics, 36*(Suppl. 11), S13–S15.

Cooper, H.M. (1982). Scientific guidelines for conducting integrative research reviews. *Review of Educational Research, 52*(2), 291–302.

Dirksen, S.R., & Erickson, J.R. (2002). Well-being in Hispanic and non-Hispanic white survivors of breast cancer. *Oncology Nursing Forum, 29*(5), 820–826.

Douglass, M., Bartolucci, A., Waterbor, J., & Sirles, A. (1995). Breast cancer early detection: Differences between African American and white women's health beliefs and detection practices. *Oncology Nursing Forum, 22*(5), 835–837.

Eversley, R., Estrin, D., Dibble, S., Wardlaw, L., Pedrosa, M., & Favila-Penney, W. (2005). Post-treatment symptoms among ethnic minority breast cancer survivors. *Oncology Nursing Forum, 32*(2), 250–256.

Ford, M.E., Hill, D.D., Blount, A., Morrison, J., Worsham, M., Havstad, S.L., et al. (2002). Modifying a breast cancer risk factor survey for African American women. *Oncology Nursing Forum, 29*(5), 827–834.

Fowler, B.A. (2006). Claiming health: Mammography screening decision making of African American women. *Oncology Nursing Forum, 33*(5), 969–975.

Fowler, B.A., Rodney, M., Roberts, S., & Broadus, L. (2005). Collaborative breast health intervention for African American women of lower socioeconomic status. *Oncology Nursing Forum, 32*(6), 1207–1216.

Frank, D., Swedmark, J., & Grubbs, L. (2004). Colon cancer screening in African American women. *Journal of the Association of Black Nursing Faculty, 15*(4), 67–70.

Frank-Stromborg, M., & Olsen, S.J. (Eds.). (2001). *Cancer prevention in diverse populations: Cultural implications for the multidisciplinary team* (2nd ed.). Pittsburgh, PA: Oncology Nursing Society.

Freeman, H.P. (1998). The meaning of race in science—considerations for cancer research: Concerns of special populations in the National Cancer Program. *Cancer, 82*(1), 219–225.

Gelfand, D.E., Parzuchowski, J., Cort, M., & Powell, I. (1995). Digital rectal examinations and prostate cancer screening: Attitudes of African American men. *Oncology Nursing Forum, 22*(8), 1253–1255.

Giger, J.N., & Davidhizar, R.E. (Eds.). (2008). *Transcultural nursing: Assessment and intervention* (5th ed.). St. Louis, MO: Mosby.

Gill, K.M., Mishel, M., Belyea, M., Germino, B., Germino, L.S., Porter, L., et al. (2004). Triggers of uncertainty about recurrence and long-term treatment side effects in older African American and Caucasian breast cancer survivors. *Oncology Nursing Forum, 31*(3), 633–639.

Graham, M.E., Liggons, Y., & Hypolite, M. (2002). Health beliefs and self breast examination in black women. *Journal of Cultural Diversity, 9*(2), 49–54.

Green, P.M., & Kelly, B.A. (2004). Colorectal cancer knowledge, perceptions, and behaviors in African Americans. *Cancer Nursing, 27*(3), 206–215.

Grindel, C.G., Brown, L., Caplan, L., & Blumenthal, D. (2004). The effect of breast cancer screening messages on knowledge, attitudes, perceived risk, and mammography screening of African American women in the rural South. *Oncology Nursing Forum, 31*(4), 801–808.

Guillory, J. (1987). Ethnic perspective of cancer nursing: The Black American. *Oncology Nursing Forum, 14*(3), 66–69.

Gutoski, M. (1995). Study verifies lack of ethnic diversity in bone marrow donors. *Oncology Nursing Forum, 22*(4), 717.

Hall, C.P., Wimberley, P.D., Hall, J.D., Pfrieme, J.T., Hubbard, E., Stacy, A.S., et al. (2005). Teaching breast cancer screening to African American women in the Arkansas Mississippi River Delta. *Oncology Nursing Forum, 32*(4), 857–863.

Hamilton, J.B., & Sandelowski, M. (2004). Types of social support in African Americans with cancer. *Oncology Nursing Forum, 31*(4), 792–800.

Henderson, P.D., & Fogel, J. (2003). Support networks used by African American breast cancer support group participants. *Journal of the Association of Black Nursing Faculty, 14*(5), 95–98.

Henderson, P.D., Gore, S.V., Davis, B.L., & Condon, E.H. (2003). African American women coping with breast cancer: A qualitative analysis. *Oncology Nursing Forum, 30*(4), 641–647.

Ho, V., Yamal, J.M., Atkinson, E.N., Basen-Engquist, K., Tortolero-Luna, G., & Follen, M. (2005). Predictors of breast and cervical screening in Vietnamese women in Harris County, Houston, Texas. *Cancer Nursing, 28*(2), 119–129.

Itano, J.K., & Taoka, K.N. (Eds.). (2005). *Core curriculum for oncology nursing* (4th ed.). St. Louis, MO: Elsevier Saunders.

Kagawa-Singer, M. (1987). Ethnic perspectives of cancer nursing: Hispanics and Japanese-Americans. *Oncology Nursing Forum, 14*(3), 59–65.

Katapodi, M.C., Facione, N.C., Miaskowski, C., Dodd, M.J., & Waters, C. (2002). The influence of social support on breast cancer screening in a multicultural community sample. *Oncology Nursing Forum, 29*(5), 845–852.

Kim, J., Ashing-Giwa, K.T., Kagawa-Singer, M., & Tejero, J.S. (2006). Breast cancer among Asian Americans: Is acculturation related to health-related quality of life? [Online exclusive]. *Oncology Nursing Forum, 33*(6), E90–E99. Retrieved January 1, 2008, from http://ons.metapress.com/content/77632w7745620554/fulltext.pdf

Kim, Y.H., & Sarna, L. (2004). An intervention to increase mammography use by Korean American women. *Oncology Nursing Forum, 31*(1), 105–110.

Kinney, A.Y., Emery, G., Dudley, W.N., & Croyle, R.T. (2002). Screening behaviors among African American women at high risk for breast cancer: Do beliefs about God matter? *Oncology Nursing Forum, 29*(5), 835–843.

Kleier, J.A. (2004). Using the Health Belief Model to reveal the perceptions of Jamaican and Haitian men regarding prostate cancer. *Journal of Multicultural Nursing and Health, 10*(3), 41–48.

Lacey, L.P., Phillips, C.W., Ansell, D., Whitman, S., Ebie, N., & Chen, E. (1989). An urban community-based cancer prevention screening and health education intervention in Chicago. *Public Health Reports, 104*(6), 536–541.

Lambert, S., Fearing, A., Bell, D., & Newton, M. (2002). A comparative study of prostate screening health beliefs and practices between African American and Caucasian men. *Journal of the Association of Black Nursing Faculty, 13*(3), 61–63.

Leininger, M. (1985). Transcultural care, diversity, and universality: A theory of nursing. *Nursing and Health Care, 6*(4), 209–212.

Leininger, M., & McFarland, R. (2002). *Transcultural nursing: Concepts, theories, research, and practice* (3rd ed.). New York: McGraw-Hill.

Lovejoy, N.C., Jenkins, C., Wu, T., Shankland, S., & Wilson, C. (1989). Developing a breast cancer screening program for Chinese-American women. *Oncology Nursing Forum, 16*(2), 181–187.

Lu, Z.J. (1995). Variables associated with breast self-examination among Chinese women. *Cancer Nursing, 18*(1), 29–34.

Manfredi, C., Lacey, L., & Warnecke, R. (1990). Results of an intervention to improve compliance with referrals for evaluation of suspected malignancies at neighborhood public health centers. *American Journal of Public Health, 80*(1), 85–87.

Mickley, J., & Soeken, K. (1993). Religiousness and hope in Hispanic- and Anglo-American women with breast cancer. *Oncology Nursing Forum, 20*(8), 1171–1177.

Miller, B.A., Kolonel, L.N., Bernstein, L., Young, J.L., Jr., Swanson, G.M., West, D., et al. (Eds.). (1996). *Racial/ethnic patterns of cancer in the United States 1988–1992* [NIH Publication No. 96-4104]. Bethesda, MD: National Cancer Institute.

Millon-Underwood, S., & Sanders, E. (1990). Factors contributing to health promotion behaviors among African-American men. *Oncology Nursing Forum, 17*(5), 707–712.

Millon-Underwood, S., & Sanders, E. (1991). Testicular self-examination among African-American men. *Journal of National Black Nurses Association, 5*(1), 18–28.

Millon-Underwood, S., Sanders, E., & Davis, M. (1993). Determinants of participation in state-of-the-art cancer prevention, early detection/screening, and treatment trials among African-Americans. *Cancer Nursing, 16*(1), 25–33.

Morgan, P.D., Barnett, K., Perdue, B., Fogel, J., Underwood, S.M., Gaskins, M., et al. (2006). African American women with breast cancer and their spouses' perception of care received from physicians. *Journal of the Association of Black Nursing Faculty, 17*(1), 32–37.

Morgan, P.D., Fogel, J., Rose, L., Barnett, K., Mock, V., Davis, B.L., et al. (2005). African American couples merging strengths to successfully cope with breast cancer. *Oncology Nursing Forum, 32*(5), 979–987.

National Center for Health Statistics. (2008). *Health, United States, 2007.* Hyattsville, MD: U.S. Department of Health and Human Services, Centers for Disease Control and Prevention, National Center for Health Statistics.

Nemcek, M.A. (1989). Factors influencing black women's breast self-examination practice. *Cancer Nursing, 12*(6), 339–343.

Nielsen, B.B. (1989). The nurse's role in mammography screening. *Cancer Nursing, 12*(5), 271–275.

O'Hare, P.A., Malone, D., Lusk, E., & McCorkle, R. (1993). Unmet needs of Black patients with cancer posthospitalization: A descriptive study. *Oncology Nursing Forum, 20*(4), 659–664.

Oncology Nursing Society. (1999). *Multicultural outcomes: Guidelines for cultural competence.* Pittsburgh, PA: Author.

Oncology Nursing Society. (2001). *Multicultural toolkit: Moving toward cultural competence.* Pittsburgh, PA: Author.

Orque, M.S., Bloch, B., & Monrroy, L.S.A. (1983). *Ethnic nursing care: A multicultural approach.* St. Louis, MO: Mosby.

Otto, S.E. (Ed.). (2001). *Oncology nursing.* St. Louis, MO: Mosby.

Phillips, J.M., & Wilbur, J. (1995). Adherence to breast cancer screening guidelines among African-American women of differing employment status. *Cancer Nursing, 18*(4), 258–269.

Powe, B.D. (1994). Perceptions of cancer fatalism among African Americans: The influence of education, income, and cancer knowledge. *Journal of National Black Nurses Association, 7*(2), 41–48.

Powe, B.D. (1995a). Cancer fatalism among elderly Caucasians and African Americans. *Oncology Nursing Forum, 22*(9), 1355–1359.

Powe, B.D. (1995b). Fatalism among elderly African Americans. Effects on colorectal cancer screening. *Cancer Nursing, 18*(5), 385–392.

Powe, B.D., & Finnie, R. (2004). Knowledge of oral cancer risk factors among African Americans: Do nurses have a role? *Oncology Nursing Forum, 31*(4), 785–791.

Purnell, L.D., & Paulanka, B.J. (2003). *Transcultual healthcare: A culturally competent approach* (2nd ed.). Philadelphia: F.A. Davis.

Ries, L.A.G., Harkins, D., Krapcho, M., Mariotto, A., Miller, B.A., Feuer, E.J., et al. (Eds.). (2006). *SEER cancer statistics review, 1975–2003*. Bethesda, MD: National Cancer Institute. Retrieved January 1, 2008, from http://seer.cancer.gov/csr/1975_2003

Robertson, E.M., Franklin, A.W., Flores, A., Wherry, S., & Buford, J. (2006). African American community breast health education: A pilot project. *Journal of the Association of Black Nursing Faculty, 17*(1), 48–51.

Russell, K.M., Champion, V.L., & Perkins, S.M. (2003). Development of cultural belief scales for mammography screening. *Oncology Nursing Forum, 30*(4), 633–640.

Russell, K.M., Champion, V.L., & Skinner, C.S. (2006). Psychosocial factors related to repeat mammography screening over 5 years in African American women. *Cancer Nursing, 29*(3), 236–243.

Russell, K.M., Perkins, S.M., Zollinger, T.W., & Champion, V.L. (2006). Sociocultural context of mammography screening use. *Oncology Nursing Forum, 33*(1), 105–112.

Sanders, L.D., Wilmoth, M.C., & Lowry, B. (2004). Overcoming: Breast cancer and its effect on intimacy in middle aged African-American women. *Journal of National Black Nurses Association, 15*(2), 32–39.

Spector, R. (2004). *Cultural diversity in health and illness* (6th ed.). Upper Saddle River, NJ: Prentice Hall.

Spurlock, W.R., & Cullins, L.S. (2006). Cancer fatalism and breast cancer screening in African American women. *Journal of the Association of Black Nursing Faculty, 17*(1), 38–43.

Sugarek, N.J., Deyo, R.A., & Holmes, B.C. (1988). Locus of control and beliefs about cancer in a multi-ethnic clinic population. *Oncology Nursing Forum, 15*(4), 481–486.

Swinney, J.E. (2002). African Americans with cancer: The relationships among self-esteem, locus of control, and health perception. *Research in Nursing and Health, 25*(5), 371–382.

Taylor, E.J. (2003). Spiritual needs of patients with cancer and family caregivers. *Cancer Nursing, 26*(4), 260–266.

Thomas, E.C. (2004). African American women's breast memories, cancer beliefs, and screening behaviors. *Cancer Nursing, 27*(4), 295–302.

Thompson, H.S., Littles, M., Jacob, S., & Coker, C. (2006). Post-treatment breast cancer surveillance and follow-up care experiences of breast cancer survivors of African descent: An exploratory qualitative study. *Cancer Nursing, 29*(6), 478–487.

Underwood, S. (1992). Cancer risk reduction and early detection behaviors among Black men: Focus on learned helplessness. *Journal of Community Health Nursing, 9*(1), 21–31.

Underwood, S.M. (1991). African-American men. Perceptual determinants of early cancer detection and cancer risk reduction. *Cancer Nursing, 14*(6), 281–288.

Underwood, S.M. (2004). Promoting breast health among African American women in community-based settings: Identifying good, better and best practices. *Journal of Chi Eta Phi Sorority, 50*(1), 1–8.

Underwood, S.M., Powe, B., Canales, M., Meade, C.D., & Im, E.O. (2004). Cancer in U.S. ethnic and racial minority populations. *Annual Review of Nursing Research, 22,* 217–263.

Underwood, S.M., & Powell, R.L. (2006). Religion and spirituality: Influence on health/risk behavior and cancer screening behavior of African Americans. *Journal of the Association of Black Nursing Faculty, 17*(1), 20–31.

U.S. Department of Commerce. (1978). Directive No. 15. Race and ethnic standards for federal statistics and administrative reporting. In *Statistical Policy Handbook*. Washington, DC: U.S. Department of Commerce, Office of Federal Statistical Policy and Standards.

U. S. Department of Health and Human Services. (2000). *Healthy people 2010: Understanding and improving health.* Washington, DC: U.S. Government Printing Office.

U.S. Office of Management and Budget. (1994). *Statistical policy directive No. 15: Race and ethnic standards for federal statistics and administrative reporting: Standards for the classification of federal data on race and ethnicity.* Office of Management and Budget, Federal Register, 60FR44674-44693, August 28, 1995.

Varricchio, C.G. (Ed.). (2004). *A cancer source book for nurses* (8th ed.). Sudbury, MA: Jones and Bartlett.

Weinrich, S., Royal, C., Pettaway, C.A., Dunston, G., Faison-Smith, L., Priest, J.H., et al. (2002). Interest in genetic prostate cancer susceptibility testing among African American men. *Cancer Nursing, 25*(1), 28–34.

Weinrich, S.P., Faison-Smith, L., Hudson-Priest, J., Royal, C., & Powell, I. (2002). Stability of self-reported family history of prostate cancer among African American men. *Journal of Nursing Measurement, 10*(1), 39–46.

Weinrich, S.P., Seger, R., Miller, B.L., Davis, C., Kim, S., Wheeler, C., et al. (2004). Knowledge of the limitations associated with prostate cancer screening among low-income men. *Cancer Nursing, 27*(6), 442–453.

Weinrich, S.P., Weinrich, M.C., Priest, J., & Fodi, C. (2003). Self-reported reasons men decide not to participate in free prostate cancer screening [Online exclusive]. *Oncology Nursing Forum, 30*(1), E12–E16. Retrieved January 1, 2008, from http://ons.metapress.com/content/b743120318h46670/fulltext.pdf

Williams, D.R., Lavizzo-Mourey, R., & Warren, R.C. (1994). The concept of race and health status in America. *Public Health Reports, 109*(1), 26–41.

Willis, M.A., Davis, M., Cairns, N.U., & Janiszewski, R. (1989). Inter-agency collaboration: Teaching breast self-examination to black women. *Oncology Nursing Forum, 16*(2), 171–177.

Wood, R.Y., Duffy, M.E., Morris, S.J., & Carnes, J.E. (2002). The effect of an educational intervention on promoting breast self-examination in older African American and Caucasian women. *Oncology Nursing Forum, 29*(7), 1081–1090.

Wu, T.-Y., & Bancroft, J. (2006). Filipino American women's perceptions and experiences with breast cancer screening [Online exclusive]. *Oncology Nursing Forum, 33*(4), E71–E78. Retrieved January 1, 2008, from http://ons.metapress.com/content/e81vt241817p2p50/fulltext.pdf

Wu, T.Y., & Yu, M.Y. (2003). Reliability and validity of the mammography screening beliefs questionnaire among Chinese American women. *Cancer Nursing, 26*(2), 131–142.

Yu, M.Y., Wu, T.Y., & Mood, D.W. (2005). Cultural affiliation and mammography screening of Chinese women in an urban county of Michigan. *Journal of Transcultural Nursing, 16*(2), 107–116.

CHAPTER 11

Development and Maintenance of Interdisciplinary Research Teams

Christine A. Miaskowski, RN, PhD, FAAN

Introduction

Many successful nurse scientists have developed strong, sustained, and collaborative multidisciplinary research teams. However, as science has become more complex, a shift has occurred in the development of research teams. Through the Roadmap Initiative for Medical Research at the National Institutes of Health, members of the scientific community are engaged in the development of interdisciplinary research teams (Check, 2003; Goodman, 2004; Huerta et al., 2005; Wang, 2003; Zerhouni, 2003). The purposes of this chapter are to define interdisciplinary research, to describe the current trends in science that require the development of interdisciplinary research teams, to discuss the principles involved in the development of this type of team, and to explore ways to sustain interdisciplinary research teams.

Interdisciplinary Research: What It Is and Why It Is Needed

The concept of interdisciplinary research is evolving within the U.S. academic community (Conley & Tinkle, 2007; Hall, Long, Bermbach, Jordan,

& Patterson, 2005; Herndon, 2007; McGuire, 1999). In 2004, the National Academy of Sciences Committee on Facilitating Interdisciplinary Research (2004) defined *interdisciplinary research* as

> A mode of research by teams or individuals that integrates information, data, techniques, tools, perspectives, concepts, and/or theories from two or more disciplines or bodies of specialized knowledge to advance fundamental understanding or to solve problems whose solutions are beyond the scope of a single discipline or field of research practice. (p. 26)

Figure 11-1 illustrates the composition of an interdisciplinary research team.

According to Domino, Smith, and Johnson (2007), this comprehensive definition extends the concept of multidisciplinary research teams. *Multidisciplinary teams* are teams that work on the same problem with different approaches and tools. For example, two multidisciplinary research teams could be working on chemotherapy-induced peripheral neuropathy (CIPN). The first team is composed of a neurophysiologist, a neurologist, and a medical oncologist. They propose to evaluate the sensory changes that occur in patients with CIPN using electromyography and detailed somatosensory testing. The

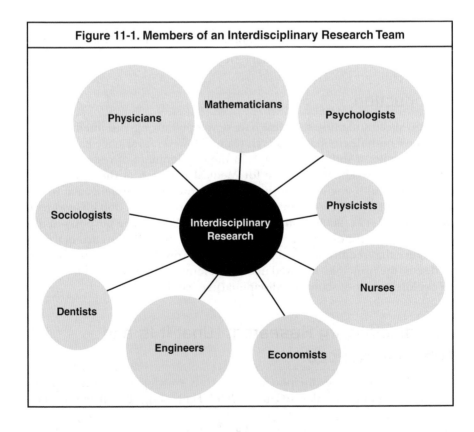

Figure 11-1. Members of an Interdisciplinary Research Team

second team is composed of a medical oncologist, a nurse, a physical therapist, and a neurologist. They propose to evaluate the sensory changes that occur in patients with CIPN using a neurologic examination, an assessment of pain qualities and pain intensity, and an evaluation of balance, gait, and coordination. Domino et al. posited that an interdisciplinary team would extend and broaden these two teams by encouraging the scientists to use each other's disparate skills to reframe research questions, to build new areas of research, and to quicken the pace of clinically useful discoveries.

One can ask the question Why are interdisciplinary research teams needed at the present time? In a commentary on the value of "big science," Esparza and Yamada (2007) outlined the evolution of biomedical research. In its earliest years, most scientists published alone. Many of the advances in science occurred through informal communications among a network of scholars. In the 20th century, science became more collaborative, but usually the collaborations occurred in small groups. For example, Watson and Crick, who won the Nobel Prize for the characterization of the double helix structure of DNA, worked as a research team. However, many other advances in science were slowed because communications only took place among a limited number of individuals who often received similar training and shared similar points of view.

The 21st century is characterized as the era of *big science*. The term was coined more than 40 years ago by nuclear physicist Alvin Weinberg to describe the large-scale approaches that were needed to develop modern nuclear technologies. Currently, the term refers to large-scale, complex scientific projects that require interdisciplinary collaboration. The exemplar of big science in the 21st century is the Human Genome Project. Prior to its initiation, a significant amount of debate occurred within the scientific community. A number of scientists were concerned that the costs of the project would monopolize research funds. In addition, several scientists argued that the project was of limited value because it was not hypothesis driven. Despite numerous objections, the Human Genome Project was funded and completed in 2001 through the efforts of an interdisciplinary team of scientists from around the world (Esparza & Yamada, 2007). This major scientific achievement, which required an enormous amount of collaboration among individuals from a large number of disciplines, will change the face of health care for years to come.

The second major reason why interdisciplinary research teams are a current necessity is because of the need to translate research findings into practice. Recent estimates suggest that it takes 17 years for a new discovery to reach clinical practice. In addition, estimates suggest that only 14% of new scientific discoveries result in advances in clinical care (Westfall, Mold, & Fagnan, 2007). These data suggest that changes need to occur in how scientists ask research questions, how they design research studies, how they execute those studies, and how they interpret the study findings. Many scientists hope that the creation of interdisciplinary research teams will facilitate the conduct of science and enable the movement of scientific discoveries from the "bench to the bedside" in a more expeditious manner.

Development and Maintenance of Interdisciplinary Research Teams

The development and maintenance of a strong, collaborative research team requires time, effort, and careful planning. The next section of this chapter reviews some of the general principles to consider during the development and maintenance of a research team (see Figure 11-2).

Figure 11-2. General Principles to Consider in the Development and Maintenance of a Research Team

- Start with small research teams.
- Select team members based on the scope of the research project.
- Establish clear expectations.
- Negotiate rewards and responsibilities.
- Maintain ongoing communication.

Initiation of a Research Team

The initiation and maintenance of a research team is a developmental process. Early in one's career, initial research studies are more exploratory or pilot in nature. Often, these studies are conducted with small budgets; therefore, the research team is smaller because of the size of the project and the limited resources that are available to support team members.

However, just as these preliminary or pilot studies can serve as the foundation for a program of research, the creation of an initial research team can lay the foundation for the development of a larger team. As the size and scope of research projects grow, research teams will enlarge by necessity. However, no matter how small or large the research team is, the researcher needs to follow some general principles to guide the development and maintenance of a successful research team.

Table 11-1 provides three examples from my program of research that illustrate the growth and development of my research teams as my research studies increased in size and complexity. The first descriptive, longitudinal study was designed to evaluate the prevalence of cancer pain in the outpatient setting and to evaluate the impact of the pain on patients and their family caregivers (Burrows, Dibble, & Miaskowski, 1998; Glover, Dibble, Dodd, & Miaskowski, 1995; Miaskowski, Kragness, Dibble, & Wallhagen, 1997; Stevens, Dibble, & Miaskowski, 1995; Yeager, Miaskowski, Dibble, & Wallhagen, 1995). Because I was a novice researcher, my research team required an experienced nurse scientist. In addition, to facilitate the recruitment of patients and their family caregivers, clinical nurse specialists at each of the study sites were an integral part of the research team. The team also included a part-time project director, a statistician, and graduate research assistants.

Table 11-1. Examples of Research Projects and Research Teams

Project	Description	Team Members
Project 1—small pilot study	Descriptive, correlational study • Evaluate the prevalence of cancer pain in an outpatient population. • Evaluate the impact of cancer pain on patients and their family caregivers.	• Senior nurse scientist • Clinical nurse specialists in outpatient settings • Statistician • Project director • Graduate student research assistants
Project 2—first large, federally funded research grant	Randomized clinical trial of a psychoeducational intervention to improve cancer pain management • 10 outpatient settings • 300 patients enrolled in a six-week nursing intervention	• Senior nurse scientist • Medical oncologist • Pharmacist • Nurse scientist with expertise in qualitative research • Clinical nurse specialists in outpatient settings • Statistician • Project director • Graduate student research assistants
Project 3—second large, federally funded research grant	Changes in symptom trajectories in patients undergoing radiation therapy for breast, lung, prostate, and brain cancers • Fatigue • Pain • Sleep disturbance • Anxiety • Depression	• Two radiation oncologists • Expert in fatigue • Expert in sleep • Oncology nurses in the research settings • Two statisticians • Psychiatrist • Project director • Nurse scientists • Graduate student research assistants

This study provided the preliminary data for my first federally funded grant that was a randomized clinical trial of a psychoeducational intervention to improve cancer pain management (Kim et al., 2004; Miaskowski et al., 2004; Paul, Zelman, Smith, & Miaskowski, 2005; Schumacher et al., 2002; Villars et al., 2007; West et al., 2003). This study enrolled more than 300 patients for a six-week intervention. As shown in Table 11-1, the size of the team grew substantially, and the expertise needed to complete this project expanded. In addition, the team became more interdisciplinary in its nature.

The third research project listed in Table 11-1 was a large, federally funded study that focused on the evaluation of symptom trajectories in patients who underwent radiation therapy for prostate, breast, lung, or brain cancer. The same symptoms were evaluated in family caregivers. Both patients and family caregivers were followed for a total of six months. In addition to the subjective assessment of symptoms, actigraphy was done to evaluate sleep patterns, and blood samples were obtained for serum cytokine and genetic analyses. Completing this complex study required a large interdisciplinary research team. The research team evolved in its scope as the data were analyzed, and different types of expertise were required to interpret the study findings. For example, when some of the longitudinal data on anxiety and depression in men with prostate cancer were analyzed, explanations for the findings were not readily apparent. The original research team did not include a member with expertise in depression and anxiety. However, we then recruited a psychiatrist who had an interest in psychological symptoms in patients with cancer to be part of the research team.

The composition of a research team can evolve during the course of a project. The types of expertise required to complete the study and analyze the findings are important to consider, not only at the initiation of the study but also as the study unfolds.

Select Research Team Members

The initial step in the development of a research team is to draft specific aims for the grant and a general outline of the methods for the research project. This approach allows for the identification of the scope and magnitude of the project. In addition, it allows for the determination of the type of expertise needed to carry out the study. Particularly for clinical studies, the researcher should consider the types of research expertise (e.g., specific analytic methods, specific physiologic measures) as well as the clinical expertise (e.g., expertise in a particular disease associated with a symptom under investigation, expertise in accessing the study population or clinical setting) that are required to complete the project successfully.

Important considerations in the selection of research team members are the personalities of the team members and the recognition that some individuals will need to be included on the research team because they are key stakeholders. Team organizers need to consider who has to be included on the research team to ensure the success of the project. This may involve considerations such as who controls access to certain patient populations or who, because of their international reputation, would be expected by the grant reviewers to be included on the research team. An important consideration in choosing team members is whether potential team members are dependable team players. An additional consideration is the academic rank of the individual. Depending on where the researcher is in his or her own scientific career, the researcher may need to include one or more senior scientists on the research team. In contrast, if the researcher is more senior, he or she may be able to invite more junior scientists and/or clinicians onto the team and mentor them in research. The actual composition of the research team is extremely important. A critical part of the grant review process is determining that the appropriate number of coinvestigators with the requisite expertise among the members is part of the research team to ensure success of the project.

An initial step in the selection of team members is to inquire with colleagues about the potential team member's particular attributes to determine if he or she is appropriate. The second step is to interview the potential team members to learn about their interest and availability to participate in the research project. At a minimum, the researcher should bring the specific aims and an outline of the methods for the grant application to the meeting. In addition, he or she should have clear expectations for what the potential team member would do on the grant. If the potential team member declines to participate, an alternate person with the requisite expertise is important to have. In some cases, the individual who declined to participate can recommend a colleague.

Establish Clear Expectations

Once a person has agreed to become a member of the research team, an important aspect of the team member's development is the establishment of clear expectations. Specific areas to address include expectations regarding the preparation and submission of the grant application, the individual's specific roles and responsibilities once the grant is funded, and the establishment of clear and specific timelines. One of the most difficult challenges is the establishment and maintenance of specific timelines. If timelines are not established, it can lead to significant delays in grant submission.

Negotiate Rewards and Responsibilities

The researcher needs to discuss with each team member his or her responsibilities prior to submission of the grant application, as well as when the grant is funded. In addition, a discussion should occur about the rewards of participating as a member of this particular research team.

In terms of expectations regarding the preparation and submission of the grant application, the major area that needs to be discussed in advance is the level of involvement that the researcher expects from an individual team member, as well as from the team as a whole. Expectations can include participating in refinement of the specific aims of the grant application, writing specific sections of the grant application, providing preliminary data, providing data on the clinical site and the potential for participant recruitment, or critiquing the grant application prior to submission. The researcher needs to consider the specific areas of expertise of each of the team members. For example, if a team member is included because of his or her expertise with a particular procedure or methodology, asking this individual to write that specific section of the grant application is reasonable. The researcher needs to be clear about timelines and deadlines. In addition, remembering that team members who participate in the development of the research grant are doing the work gratis in the hopes that the grant application will be funded is important.

In the initial meetings with team members, the lead researcher must discuss each member's responsibilities once the grant is funded. Figure 11-3 provides a list of potential responsibilities. The researcher must be specific with each team member about what his or her roles and responsibilities will be once the grant is funded prior to the grant submission. Once the grant is funded, team members should be reminded of these ongoing responsibilities.

Figure 11-3. Potential Responsibilities for Research Team Members

- Assist with the finalization of the study protocol.
- Assist with the recruitment of patients.
- Assist with data analysis.
- Assist with the interpretation of the study findings.
- Assist with the development and review of abstracts and publications.

An important part of the initial and ongoing discussions with research team members is the topic of rewards for participation in the grant and on the team. Prior to grant submission, team members will be able to participate in intellectually stimulating conversations. In addition, they are acknowledged for their specific level of expertise. Finally, being part of a research team allows for scholarly interaction with colleagues.

A number of rewards occur once the grant is funded. For most academic team members, publication is the most obvious and most important reward. The researcher needs to discuss with each team member individually, as well as when the team meets as a whole, his or her philosophy toward publications. Areas that need to be addressed regarding publications include the specific level of contribution of each team member to a particular paper, each team member's specific areas of interest, the order of authorship, who will be first author on which publications, timelines for publications, and order of publications. The research team also needs to determine the role of students on publications. In many cases, research teams develop a list of guidelines for publications, which are reviewed at every team meeting. In addition, the team develops a publication plan and reviews it at every team meeting.

Additional rewards that occur for individual team members after the grant is funded include intellectual stimulation and scholarly interaction with colleagues from other disciplines. Furthermore, the recognition of an individual's expertise is enhanced within the research team. Finally, a potential reward for some individuals is the opportunity for research training for graduate students and clinicians.

Maintain Ongoing Communication

The initial development of a research team and its sustainability depends on ongoing communication. One of the biggest struggles as a researcher is deciding how much communication is enough. During the grant development phase, the researcher may meet with individual team members about specific aspects of the application. Prior to the actual submission, a team meeting is useful. At this meeting, the team members have an opportunity to meet each other and to begin to interact with each other. Time should be spent with detailed introductions so that the team members become acquainted with each other's areas of expertise. In addition, the researcher should spend some time sharing with the team members the reason that each individual was selected to participate in this research team. Finally, this meeting can serve as an opportunity to review, critique, and make any final revisions to the grant application.

Once the grant is funded, the team should be notified and should celebrate their success. The researcher can use e-mail as a major communication tool to keep team members updated on a variety of grant-related activities. Sometimes, a monthly e-mail update serves as a great communication tool.

Meetings should be scheduled with the "smaller team" on a regular basis depending on the requirements of the specific research project. The *smaller team* consists of the principal investigator, the project director, and the research staff directly involved in recruitment, data collection, and data entry and analysis. These individuals need to meet on a regular basis to maintain the ongoing activities of the grant. Sometimes these meetings occur weekly, bimonthly, or monthly. The nature of the grant and the work that needs to be accomplished dictates the frequency of the meetings.

In a similar fashion, regular meetings need to be scheduled with the "larger team," usually about twice per year. These meetings include all of the coinvestigators and often the consultants on the grant application. The focus of these meetings may vary depending on the phase of the grant (e.g., the start or the end of the grant) but often include a reorientation to the grant, the presentation of preliminary findings, a discussion of the ongoing challenges and opportunities with the grant, plans for a new grant application, and a review of the publication plan. These meetings need to be well planned in order to be as productive as possible.

Nurse Scientists as Team Leaders and Team Members

Nurse scientists have all of the requisite skills to be successful leaders as well as members of a research team. Based on their clinical experience, they often may lead meetings of interdisciplinary colleagues to achieve a specific goal or objective. In some cases, a meeting will center on the coordination of care for a particular patient. In other situations, meetings will focus on the establishment of policies or procedures. However, for the nurse scientist, this level of involvement facilitates the development of leadership skills.

A successful research team consists of individuals who want to work together for a common goal. In most cases, this goal centers on answering an important scientific question. The nurse scientist needs to keep the team focused on that goal. If the team members feel individually and collectively that they are working toward the same goal, the team will be successful. The development and maintenance of a research team requires a time commitment from all members of the team. The scientist who builds a successful research team will spend a substantial amount of time nurturing the team, as well as mentoring individual team members and the team as a whole.

Conclusion

In order to advance nursing science, nurse scientists will need to build interdisciplinary research teams. Through the collective expertise of the members of these teams, more comprehensive research questions will be asked and answered to improve the care of patients with chronic medical conditions.

References

Burrows, M., Dibble, S.L., & Miaskowski, C. (1998). Differences in outcomes among patients experiencing different types of cancer-related pain. *Oncology Nursing Forum, 25*(4), 735–741.

Check, E. (2003). NIH "roadmap" charts course to tackle big research issues. *Nature, 425*(6957), 438.

Committee on Facilitating Interdisciplinary Research. (2004). *Facilitating interdisciplinary research.* Washington, DC: National Academies Press.

Conley, Y.P., & Tinkle, M.B. (2007). The future of genomic nursing research. *Journal of Nursing Scholarship, 39*(1), 17–24.

Domino, S.E., Smith, Y.R., & Johnson, T.R. (2007). Opportunities and challenges of interdisciplinary research career development: Implementation of a women's health research training program. *Journal of Women's Health, 16*(2), 256–261.

Esparza, J., & Yamada, T. (2007). The discovery value of "big science." *Journal of Experimental Medicine, 204*(4), 701–704.

Glover, J., Dibble, S.L., Dodd, M.J., & Miaskowski, C. (1995). Mood states of oncology outpatients: Does pain make a difference? *Journal of Pain and Symptom Management, 10*(2), 120–128.

Goodman, L. (2004). Clearing a roadmap. *Journal of Clinical Investigation, 113*(11), 1512–1513.

Hall, W.A., Long, B., Bermbach, N., Jordan, S., & Patterson, K. (2005). Qualitative teamwork issues and strategies: Coordination through mutual adjustment. *Qualitative Health Research, 15*(3), 394–410.

Herndon, D.N. (2007). Building the research teams of the future: Changing the paradigm. *Journal of Burn Care and Research, 28*(4), 631–633.

Huerta, M.F., Farber, G.K., Wilder, E.L., Kleinman, D.V., Grady, P.A., Schwartz, D.A., et al. (2005). NIH roadmap interdisciplinary research initiatives. *PLoS Computational Biology, 1*(6), e59.

Kim, J.E., Dodd, M., West, C., Paul, S., Facione, N., Schumacher, K., et al. (2004). The PRO-SELF pain control program improves patients' knowledge of cancer pain management. *Oncology Nursing Forum, 31*(6), 1137–1143.

McGuire, D.B. (1999). Building and maintaining an interdisciplinary research team. *Alzheimer Disease and Associated Disorders, 13*(Suppl. 1), S17–S21.

Miaskowski, C., Dodd, M., West, C., Schumacher, K., Paul, S.M., Tripathy, D., et al. (2004). Randomized clinical trial of the effectiveness of a self-care intervention to improve cancer pain management. *Journal of Clinical Oncology, 22*(9), 1713–1720.

Miaskowski, C., Kragness, L., Dibble, S., & Wallhagen, M. (1997). Differences in mood states, health status, and caregiver strain between family caregivers of oncology outpatients with and without cancer-related pain. *Journal of Pain and Symptom Management, 13*(3), 138–147.

Paul, S.M., Zelman, D.C., Smith, M., & Miaskowski, C. (2005). Categorizing the severity of cancer pain: Further exploration of the establishment of cutpoints. *Pain, 113*(1–2), 37–44.

Schumacher, K.L., Koresawa, S., West, C., Dodd, M., Paul, S.M., Tripathy, D., et al. (2002). The usefulness of a daily pain management diary for outpatients with cancer-related pain. *Oncology Nursing Forum, 29*(9), 1304–1313.

Stevens, P.E., Dibble, S.L., & Miaskowski, C. (1995). Prevalence, characteristics, and impact of postmastectomy pain syndrome: An investigation of women's experiences. *Pain, 61*(1), 61–68.

Villars, P., Dodd, M., West, C., Koetters, T., Paul, S.M., Schumacher, K., et al. (2007). Differences in the prevalence and severity of side effects based on type of analgesic prescription in patients with chronic cancer pain. *Journal of Pain and Symptom Management, 33*(1), 67–77.

Wang, L. (2003). "Roadmap" gives new direction to trans-NIH research. *Journal of the National Cancer Institute, 95*(23), 1741.

West, C.M., Dodd, M.J., Paul, S.M., Schumacher, K., Tripathy, D., Koo, P., et al. (2003). The PRO-SELF pain control program—an effective approach for cancer pain management. *Oncology Nursing Forum, 30*(1), 65–73.

Westfall, J.M., Mold, J., & Fagnan, L. (2007). Practice-based research—"blue highways" on the NIH roadmap. *JAMA, 297*(4), 403–406.

Yeager, K.A., Miaskowski, C., Dibble, S.L., & Wallhagen, M. (1995). Differences in pain knowledge and perception of the pain experience between outpatients with cancer and their family caregivers. *Oncology Nursing Forum, 22*(8), 1235–1241.

Zerhouni, E. (2003). Medicine. The NIH roadmap. *Science, 302*(5642), 63–72.

CHAPTER 12

Conducting Oncology Evidence-Based Intervention Research

Merle H. Mishel, RN, PhD, FAAN, and Barbara B. Germino, PhD, RN

Introduction

The intervention studies presented in this chapter are theory-based in that a specific theory was used to identify the problem, and the same theory was used to design the intervention. The theory for both the problem and the intervention is the Uncertainty in Illness Theory, a middle range theory (Mishel & Clayton, 2008) that was first published in 1988 (Mishel, 1988), with a second, reconceptualized theory of Uncertainty in Illness published in 1990 (Mishel, 1990). The original Uncertainty in Illness Theory was used in four of the six studies to be discussed in this chapter. Those four studies focused on newly diagnosed patients with breast or prostate cancer or patients with breast or prostate cancer who were already in treatment. The remaining two studies focused on breast cancer survivors and involved a combination of both uncertainty theories.

Uncertainty is defined as the inability to determine the meaning of illness-related events. It indicates the absence of a cognitive structure. A cognitive structure is the meaning placed on events and is formed over time and experience with an illness. According to the original uncertainty theory, uncertainty has three categories of antecedents. The major category of antecedents is titled the *stimuli frame* and refers to the structure of the information in areas of symptom pattern, event familiarity, and event congruence. A second category of antecedents is *structure providers*, which are the resources available to the patient to help to provide meaning to events, thereby reducing uncertainty. The resources include the social network, healthcare providers, education, and faith. A third category is *cognitive capacity* and refers to the information-processing ability of the person. Information-processing ability can be compromised in illness by a number of factors including disease stage, medications, and symptoms such as fatigue and pain. Based on the impact of the antecedents on uncertainty, the person enters an appraisal situation where uncertainty is evaluated as either a threat or an opportunity. In most new illness situations, uncertainty is evaluated as a threat. However, if the patient's situation is one of negative certainty (a predicted downward course to the illness), then uncertainty is preferable because it offers hope and would be evaluated as an opportunity. Uncertainty as a threat elicits mainly emotion-oriented coping strategies, and uncertainty as an opportunity elicits strategies to maintain the sense of opportunity.

The second theory focuses on how uncertainty leads to a change in value systems and orientation toward life. It applies to people who have been cancer survivors for at least two or more years since treatment. It is a process that one enters when uncertainty continues over time and begins to invade multiple areas of the patient's life. The process gradually moves the person toward accepting uncertainty and no longer desiring certainty. It is demonstrated by behaviors such as exploring new areas and activities and opening multiple new areas in life. Concepts of this theory are variables measured in both survivor studies, but it is applied as a skill only in the second breast cancer survivor study.

Because uncertainty is a moving target, the focus in most of the intervention studies is not on eliminating uncertainty but on managing uncertainty. Uncertainty is managed by problem solving, cognitive reframing (the ability to reframe a concern into something that is manageable), cancer knowledge, and patient-provider communication.

This chapter will include descriptions of the use of the Uncertainty in Illness Theories in each of six intervention studies (over the period 1994–2007), funded by either the National Institute of Nursing Research (NINR) or the National Cancer Institute (NCI), or cofunded by both institutes. Of the six intervention studies, four were conducted with patients with cancer who were entering or were in treatment. Two studies focused on cancer survivors. Two cancer populations were targeted in the interventions: either prostate cancer or breast cancer. This review of the studies will be organized by interventions delivered during diagnosis or treatment and interventions delivered during the survivorship period.

Intervention Studies on Patients With Cancer Who Are Newly Diagnosed or in Treatment

Three studies focused on patients with cancer during their treatment: one was a study of older women with breast cancer, one of men being treated for localized prostate cancer, and one of men with recurrent or advanced prostate cancer. Another study, which was completed in 2007, involved patients with prostate cancer immediately following diagnosis and before starting treatment. This study focused on decision making under conditions of uncertainty. See Figure 12-1 for the key points of each study. All studies included both Caucasian Americans and African Americans in sufficient numbers to analyze results by race. The inclusion of minority men and women improved the ability to generalize the findings to the broader community (Hughes, Sellers, Fraser, Teague, & Knight, 2007) and identified issues in minority patients with cancer.

Figure 12-1. Uncertainty Management Intervention: Examples of Problems From Problem List

Problem Categories
- Cancer diagnosis
- Treatment concerns
- Responses to treatment
- Living with cancer
- Self-care
- Broader life issues

Responses to Treatment: Examples of Problems
(B = breast cancer; P = prostate cancer)
- Arm numbness (B)
- Fatigue (B)
- Future potency (P)
- Getting an erection (P)
- Nausea (B)
- Skin changes (B)

Living With Cancer: Examples of Problems
- Caregiving responsibilities
- Family concerns
- Managing intimate relationships
- Sexuality

Self-Care: Examples of Problems
- Functioning in expected/desired roles
- Communicating concerns to healthcare provider
- Implementing self-care behaviors

Living With Broader Life Issues: Examples of Problems
- Ability to continue life
- Change from previous lifestyle
- Employment issues
- Financial issues

Interventions to Manage Uncertainty During Cancer Treatment

In the three studies conducted during treatment, the problems that were targeted for intervention were the uncertainty surrounding treatment, treatment-related side effects, and issues of living with cancer. The specific issues in each of these areas were further defined by focus groups of patients similar to those in the study samples. The intervention was designed to help the patient to reduce uncertainty in these areas. These three intervention studies shared the same intervention framework.

Study #1: Men Under Treatment for Localized Prostate Cancer

The study on managing uncertainty in stage B prostate cancer was co-funded by NINR and NCI and targeted a sample of African American and Caucasian men who were diagnosed with localized prostate cancer and who were within two weeks after catheter removal following prostatectomy, and within three weeks of beginning radiation treatment. Because the studied problems were uncertainty about treatment, managing treatment side effects, and living with cancer, the time frame for recruitment of men for this study was designed to capture men likely to be experiencing these problems. The final sample consisted of 239 men (134 Caucasians and 105 African Americans).

Study #2: Men Under Treatment for Recurrent or Advanced Prostate Cancer

The NINR-funded study enrolled 155 Caucasian and 116 African American men. Of the participants, 79 Caucasian men and 76 African American men had advanced disease, and 76 Caucasian and 40 African American men had recurrent disease. These men were beyond the stages of localized prostate cancer, so they were treated mainly with hormone therapy to suppress androgen production or with experimental chemotherapies. None of these treatments are curative, and all have myriad side effects, thus promoting uncertainty about what to expect and how to manage these side effects along with disease progression.

Study #3: Older Women Who Were Being Treated for Breast Cancer

The NCI-funded study of older women receiving treatment for breast cancer targeted women from two ethnic groups after their initial breast cancer surgery and while they were receiving adjuvant treatment for breast cancer. The sample consisted of women older than age 50 and included 106

Caucasians and 104 African Americans. As noted previously, the uncertainty management intervention focused on management of treatment side effects and the uncertainty associated with their management. The post-surgery and adjuvant treatment period is the time when the women would begin to experience these problems.

Admission Criteria for Studies of Managing Uncertainty During Treatment

Because uncertainty naturally decreases when the person has had prior experience with a similar problem, admission criteria for these three studies included no prior or concurrent treatment for another form of malignancy (Mishel, 1988). Because these were all studies testing telephone-delivered interventions, access to a telephone was a criterion for participation. The research team documented that among individuals at poverty level in North Carolina, 97% of Caucasians and 98% of African Americans older than age 60 had telephones. (Note: These studies were conducted prior to the widespread use of cell phones by people of all socioeconomic levels.) All potential subjects had to pass an abbreviated form of the Mini-Mental State Examination to ensure their basic cognitive ability.

Study Designs for Studies of Patients in Treatment

The design for both studies of men being treated for prostate cancer was a three-by-two randomized block, repeated-measures design with three levels of intervention (uncertainty management direct, uncertainty management supplemented, and control) crossed with two levels of ethnicity (Caucasian American and African American). The level of intervention (uncertainty supplemented) was used in the prostate studies because of literature supporting the spouse's role in the family's health care (Bowie, Sydnor, Granot, & Pargament, 2004). All men who entered the prostate studies were required to include a spouse or another involved family member. In the uncertainty supplemented group, both the man and his family member separately received the intervention (Germino et al., 1998).

In the study of women during breast cancer treatment, the design was a two-by-two randomized block, repeated-measures design with two levels of intervention (uncertainty management and control) crossed with two levels of ethnicity (Caucasian American and African American) (Mishel, 1997). In all studies of patients during treatment, subjects were blocked on ethnicity and randomly assigned to a treatment or control group. The nurse intervener called treatment subjects every week for 8–10 weeks. He or she reviewed the most common problems with the participant and then proceeded through the assessment and intervention phases.

Because the intervention for the three studies of patients during treatment followed the same protocol, these three studies will be discussed as a group, to the extent possible. Focus groups were conducted with each subject population to identify the areas of concern that were consistent with the Uncertainty in Illness Theory. Using the information from the focus groups and also from the existing cancer literature, a problem list was constructed for each study. The problem lists contained the same major categories in each study but differed in the specific concerns. The major categories included cancer diagnosis, treatment concerns, responses to treatment, living with cancer, caring for oneself, and broader life issues. Figure 12-1 includes samples of specific concerns within these categories. The problem list corresponds to the stimuli frame, a concept in the Theory of Uncertainty in Illness (Mishel, 1988). The problem list was not read to the patient, but the most common problems were discussed while leaving opportunity for the patient to raise other problems. Major problems for these patients with cancer can be found in Figure 12-2. Once a problem was identified, the next phase was to classify it as to the type of uncertainty it engendered (see Figure 12-3).

In each of the three studies of patients under treatment, for each problem the participant identified, the intervener worked with the participant to determine where the uncertainty was most prominent. The five areas that were explored were

- Why the problem exists
- What the problem means
- How to manage the problem
- How long the problem will last
- What to expect as the outcome from the problem.

The next step was to consider the appraisal of the uncertainty as a danger (levels of danger were low, moderate, and high) or as an opportunity. This step corresponds with the appraisal process in the Uncertainty in Illness Theory (Mishel, 1988). Based upon the intervener's discussion with the participant and using the four criteria for each of the three degrees of danger or for opportunity, the intervener assigned a level to the appraisal categories (see Figure 12-4). The intervention was selected considering the area of uncertainty and the appraisal.

When the appraisal of the uncertainty was judged to be as an opportunity (i.e., expectation of a positive outcome for the uncertain situation), or when the appraisal of the uncertainty was judged to be a danger (i.e., only low level of danger), the uncertainty did not require further intervention. Instead, the nurse intervener helped the patient to identify the strategies that he or she currently was using by asking how he or she was managing the situation. In this type of appraisal, the patient usually had implemented strategies that could work to manage the uncertainty (see Figure 12-4). Therefore, in this situation, the nurse intervener only strengthened the patient's current view of the situation and reinforced an opportunity appraisal. This was done by using specific strategies, such as reinforcing the patient's ability to make choices, reinforcing their coping strategies, reinforcing their problem solving, and validating their view of the situation.

Figure 12-2. Problems Specific to Each Study Conducted During Treatment

Major Problems of Men With Localized Prostate Cancer
Caucasian men
- Leaking urine
- Erection problems
- Communication with healthcare providers
- General side effects
- Fatigue
- Pain

African American men
- Leaking urine
- Communication with healthcare providers
- General side effects
- Erection problems
- Fatigue
- Pain

Major Problems of Men With Recurrent and Advanced Prostate Cancer
- Lack of information about possible treatments
- Nontraditional treatments
- Expectations about treatment
- Side effects from hormone therapy
  - Hot flashes, sexual functioning, bone pain
  - Fluctuating prostate-specific antigen levels

Major Problems of Women With Breast Cancer
Caucasian women
- Fatigue
- Medical uncertainty
- Ability to cope
- Implementing self-care behaviors
- Treatment plan
- Finances
- Outcomes from treatment
- Comorbidity

African American women
- Finances
- Fatigue
- Implementing self-care behaviors
- Nausea
- Expectations
- Pain
- Recurrence
- Skin changes

Figure 12-3. Flowchart of Uncertainty Management Interventions

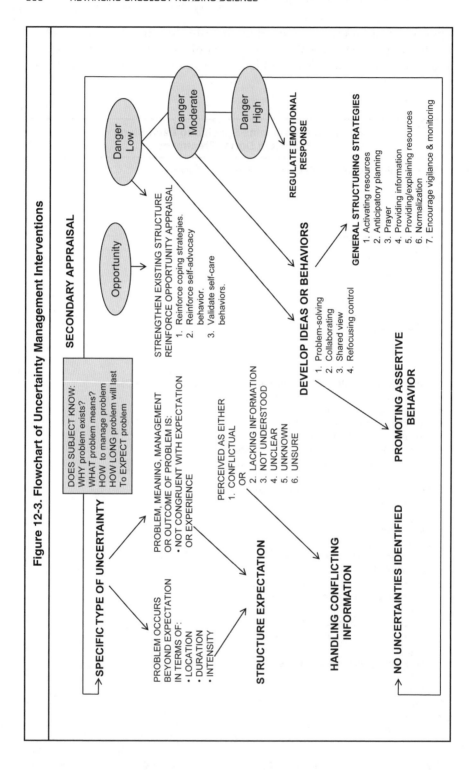

Figure 12-4. Appraisal of Threat: Secondary Appraisal

Appraisal Categories
- Opportunity
- Low danger
- Moderate danger
- High danger

Opportunity
- Positive emotion
- Sees positive outcomes
- Uses self-care behavior
- Prefers to maintain the uncertainty

Low Danger
- Emotional arousal low
- Seeking support for own ideas
- Good understanding of situation
- Mobilizing resources
- Well-structured rationale for uncertainty

Moderate Danger
- Heightened emotional arousal
- Seeking information for how to proceed
- Inadequate understanding of situation
- Limited mobilization of resources

High Danger
- High emotional arousal
- Difficulty problem solving
- Lack of rationale for problem/situation
- Absence of mobilization of resources

If the appraisal of the uncertainty was judged to be of moderate danger, then the problem was further categorized into one of the following areas.

1. The problem occurs beyond expectation in terms of either intensity frequency or duration.
2. The problem, meaning, management, or outcome is not congruent with experience or expectation.
3. The problem, meaning, management, or outcome is perceived as conflicting.
4. The problem, meaning, management, or outcome is perceived as either lacking information, not understood, unclear, unknown, or unsure.

If the problem was assigned to "1" or "2," the intervention was selected from the list of those under "structure expectation." If the problem was assigned to "3," then interventions from "handling conflicting information" were selected. If the problem was assigned to "4," then interventions were selected from the category "developing ideas or behaviors." From this category, the intervener could move either to promoting assertive behavior or general structuring strategies. If the appraisal of the uncertainty was judged to be high danger, then strategies to regulate the emotional response were offered to the subject. (See the following Specific Interventions section for further details.)

Specific Interventions

Structuring Expectations

Strategies to structure expectations were used when the uncertainty centered on a problem that occurred beyond expectations or was not congruent with experience in terms of duration, frequency, or intensity. The specific intervention strategies used in this type of situation involved attempts to provide a framework for expectations and to modify expectations. The most frequent approach was to provide information about the usual trajectory of the problem (e.g., telling the patient what to expect about when a problem might occur, how it might unfold, and how long it might last). Another approach was to provide the subjects with markers or timelines that they could use to gauge whether they were making progress or whether the problem was resolving. For example, the nurse might say to a patient with prostate cancer, "In about six months, your incontinence should have decreased." For a situation where the problem is not congruent with experience, the intervener usually pointed out why the expectation or experience did not fit in the current situation. For example, if a patient with breast cancer expected to feel less tired once treatment ended but feels more tired instead, the intervener would explain to her that the effects of radiation treatment are cumulative over time and last for several weeks or more after treatment ends. In other words, the patient's experience is actually consistent with what would be expected, although it is different from the patient's expectations.

Strategies for Handling Conflicting Information

Conflicting information was most often because of discrepancies between information resources. The strategies used to address this issue included supporting either the perspective of the doctor, patients, or others, depending on the patient's relationship with the information resources and the nature of the discrepancy. The focus was to change the patient's perspective from one of uncertainty because of conflicting information to that of less uncertainty by embracing one perspective. Another strategy was to promote the patient's awareness of options and the likely benefit of these being acceptable. The most common strategy used here was promoting assertive communication. The intervener worked with the participants in role-playing situations to strengthen their assertive behavior with health-care providers.

Strategies for Developing Ideas or Behaviors

Intervention strategies in this category were used when the problem, management, or outcomes were lacking information, were not understood, or were unclear, unknown, or unsure and when the danger level was moderate. The nurse intervener worked with the patient collaboratively to generate options and ideas. Problem solving is the modality used, and the intervener does not tell the patient what to do but joins him or her in investigating multiple alternatives.

Two other approaches are used in this category of interventions. One is to communicate a shared view of the situation. In this intervention, the intervener is able to say, "Yes, I understand what you are experiencing here. I have seen other people who have had a very similar experience, and this is the kind of thing they have done." It is important not to minimize the value of the patient's experience; however, it often helps the patient to realize that their experience is similar to the experiences of others. The second approach used in this category of interventions is refocusing control to controllable areas of life. In this intervention, the intervener is attempting to "wall off" the feeling that events are out of control. To do this, the intervener explores and emphasizes other areas of life where the person has control, is able to manage, and has solutions, so that the specific problem area becomes smaller in comparison to these other areas.

General Structuring Strategies

General structuring strategies include a variety of intervention activities that were selected according to the nature of the uncertainty. Some of the most frequently used strategies are

- Activating resources that can help the participant to clarify the situation: This includes exploring the patient's usual resources, such as church, fraternal, or social organizations; cancer-related support groups, such as Man to Man; and helper networks of spouses, children, siblings, and friends.
- Encouraging vigilance and monitoring to enlarge the subject's pool of information: In this intervention, the intervener encourages patients to observe themselves, to be aware of their environment, to pay attention to what is occurring around them in order to use this information to have a clearer view of the situation.
- Providing information and linking the participant's previous experience and current situation: Information is provided in a way that is compatible with the patient's beliefs and educational level. It is provided in small doses and not in a lecture format but rather in a conversational manner. Information is targeted so after it is provided, the intervener clarifies that the topic of discussion was fact and *not* simply the intervener's opinion. The information is then sent to the patient in written, CD, video, or another form so that it functions as a lasting resource.

- Providing and explaining resources: For these studies, the scientists developed lists of resources for each community in the state. These were shared with the patient, and those of interest were mailed to him.
- Normalizing: Normalizing was also included under general structuring strategies because the focus was on putting the problem or situation into a perspective where it fit into the participant's life and overlapped with strategies the subject used for other purposes. For example, in the prostate cancer studies, approaches for men dealing with erectile dysfunction as a result of treatment included suggesting alternative methods for lovemaking and intimacy and providing information about potency-enhancement methods. For men experiencing urinary incontinence during treatment, strategies included teaching them methods to control leakage/incontinence and providing information about how to manage treatment side effects in the context of their ongoing life. In the study of women in breast cancer treatment, normalizing was implemented by helping the participant find resources for breast prostheses and wigs, which, in turn, reduced uncertainty about managing certain aspects of her daily life such as maintaining her appearance.

Other general structuring strategy interventions that helped to manage uncertainty included compartmentalizing the uncertainty by imagining it becoming small and placing it into a small box; anticipatory planning; and encouraging the use of prayer if that was part of the patient's belief system. These were the major specific strategies included in the area of general structuring strategies.

Regulating the Emotional Response

When the danger level of the uncertainty was seen as high, the subject was not ready to learn a new management strategy and usually exhibited anxiety. The focus in this situation was on regulating the emotional response before moving on to other strategies. The strategies used included communicating a shared view of the situation, encouraging positive self-talk, and encouraging the ventilation of feelings. The intervener acknowledged to the subject how hard it was to be positive and emphasized his or her availability. These methods usually helped to reduce the emotional response. The most common interventions used in these three studies appear in Figure 12-5.

All the intervention activities were recorded in a client intervention log, which enabled the intervener to record the week, the call, the problem, who made the call, and the date. The intervener then completed a notation on the problem list, including the category and specific problem. All possibilities had been keyed into the program. This was followed by a notation regarding the nature of the uncertainty followed by the appraisal information. After this, the intervener selected interventions used from the list of interventions and was free to record any relevant comments in the log. From the second

---

**Figure 12-5. Interventions Most Frequently Used by Patients
With Breast or Prostate Cancer During the Study**

Interventions Used Most Frequently Among Older Women With Breast Cancer
Caucasian
• Provide information and resources.
• Validate self-care behaviors.
• Communicate and validate views.
• Clarify expectations.
African American
• Provide information.
• Validate self-care behaviors.
• Encourage vigilance.
• Put symptoms in treatment context.
• Reinforce self-advocacy behaviors.

Interventions Used Most Frequently Among Men With Localized Prostate Cancer
Caucasian
• Provide information on usual trajectory.
• Promote assertive communication.
• Provide information to manage incontinence.
• Share experience with others.
• Validate self-care.
African American
• Provide information on usual trajectory.
• Promote assertive communication.
• Provide information to manage incontinence.
• Encourage a positive view of situation.

**Interventions Used Most Frequently Among Men With Recurrent and Advanced
Prostate Cancer**
• Provide information to address specific concerns.
• Provide and explain resources.
• Provide information on treatment options.
• Support self-care behaviors.
• Teach assertive behavior.
• Activate resources.

---

call to the end of calls, the problems from the prior calls were reviewed and then coded in the current log by code number. Finally, the intervener noted whether suggested interventions were used or not used or whether the problem was resolved.

Outcomes

The outcomes for these three studies were similar. The focus was not on eliminating uncertainty but on managing uncertainty through problem solving, cognitive reframing, cancer knowledge, and patient-provider communication. The other major outcome was symptom management. In the study of older women during breast cancer treatment, cognitive reframing ($F_{2,272}$ = 3.76, p = .03) cancer knowledge ($F_{2,265}$ = 6.35, p = .002), and patient-provider communication ($F_{2,270}$ = 3.03, p = .05) were significantly higher over time for all women who received the intervention as compared to control subjects. Significant improvement in symptom management was found for African American women who received the intervention. They reported better symptom management and had fewer treatment side effects over time ($F_{2,278}$ = 7.58, p = .001) than control subjects, including significant reduction in symptom intensity ($F_{2,278}$ = 4.20, p = .02), fatigue ($F_{2,276}$ = 9.18, p = .001), and nausea ($F_{2,277}$ = 3.42, p = .04) (Mishel, 1997; Mishel, Germino, Belyea, & Harris, 1996).

For the study of men in treatment for localized prostate cancer, the majority of benefits from the intervention occurred at four months after baseline, when treatment side effects were most intense. All men receiving the intervention improved on two uncertainty management methods, cognitive reframing ($F_{4,456}$ = 3.81, p = .005) and problem solving ($F_{4,456}$ = 2.40, p = .05). African American men in the intervention groups, as compared to controls, also improved in control of urinary incontinence ($F_{2,212}$ = 3.71, p = .03) and in sexual satisfaction ($F_{1,186}$ = 6.57, p = .01) (Mishel et al., 2002). In the treatment-supplemented group, improvements in doctor-patient communication were found with the moderator of lower extrinsic religiosity scores in cancer knowledge ($F_{24,396}$ = 1.90, p = .007); similar improvements were found with the moderator of less education ($F_{24,386}$ = 1.76, p = .02) (Mishel et al., 2003).

For the study of men in treatment for recurrent and advanced prostate cancer, uncertainty management was measured by cognitive reframing, cancer knowledge, and doctor-patient communication. Symptom control was measured by the Southwest Oncology Group's Symptom Scale. Findings differed by specific outcome variable in interaction with disease status (e.g., recurrent versus advanced) for both uncertainty management and symptom management. Findings were significant for two of the four uncertainty management scales: cognitive reframing ($F_{4,496}$ = 3.16, p = .01) and cancer knowledge ($F_{4,496}$ = 5.18, p = .0004). Both ethnic groups that received the intervention and both categories of disease status benefited more than control subjects from the intervention. For symptom management, in both ethnic groups and disease categories, a significant difference occurred over time, with treatment groups benefiting more than controls ($F_{32,468}$ = 1.45, p = .05). Those in the intervention reported a decrease in symptom intensity in back pain, constipation, erection difficulty, breast enlargement, body fat, hot flashes, hair loss, and weight gain.

The interventions done during treatment demonstrated effectiveness both in managing uncertainty and managing symptoms. These interventions can be integrated into advanced practice and would provide oncology nurses with a tested protocol that can be delivered via telephone to patients during treatment.

Intervention Studies: Decision Making for Prostate Cancer

The need for a decision-making study was communicated to the investigators by the men who participated in the earlier study on managing uncertainty during treatment for recurrent and advanced prostate cancer. Men with recurrent disease frequently complained that they regretted the treatment they had selected. They said that they felt pushed into a specific treatment, depending on the specialty of the doctor they saw to discuss treatment. These men also complained that they felt they had to make a treatment decision with very limited information. This led the research team to design a study focused on reducing decisional regret. In order to deliver the intervention prior to the patient meeting with the doctor to discuss treatment choices, men were enrolled in the study as soon as they could be contacted after a biopsy report that was positive for early-stage prostate cancer. The intervention focused on producing a competent patient who knew how to communicate concerns and issues to the physician and who would therefore be an informed and active participant in the treatment decision. The design of the intervention followed the design of the prior interventions with patients with prostate cancer in treatment. All patients entering the study had to bring in a primary support person, but only the primary support people of subjects in the treatment-supplemented group received the intervention. The blocking of subjects by ethnicity and random assignment to one of the two treatment arms (treatment supplemented and treatment direct [patient only]) was the same as in studies of patients with prostate cancer in treatment.

The intervention developed for the study was specific to the aims of producing a well-informed patient who was able to communicate effectively with the physician. It had three key components: (a) an investigator-developed book titled *Patients' Questions—Doctors' Answers*, which was a patient-focused, evidence-based guide to treatment issues for early-stage prostate cancer, (b) a professionally produced videotape, scripted by the investigators, designed to teach subjects skills for effective communication with their physician and showing both Caucasian and African American men as patients with prostate cancer, and (c) four telephone calls to the participant by nurse interventionists. The purposes of the calls were to help subjects learn to use the booklet, to provide subjects with practice using the booklet to find information and to generate questions for their physicians, and to allow them to practice targeting communication skills for interacting with their physicians.

The booklet developed by the research team was organized by a patient question-and-answer format and was designed to provide information on prostate cancer and possible treatment options, so that men were well informed and able to formulate specific questions before meeting with their physicians. The concerns about prostate cancer that were addressed in the book, including specific information about treatment options, were identified through three studies conducted by members of the Radiation Oncology Research Unit in Canada from discussion groups and surveys of patients, family members, and treatment providers (Feldman-Stewart, Brundage, Van Manen, Skarsgard, & Siemens, 2003). For this intervention, the book was designed to be user-friendly, featuring its organization by potential subject questions, about such topics as the prostate-specific antigen (PSA) test, prostate cancer staging and diagnosis, and treatment options. A personal information form was included where subjects wrote in their specific diagnostic information, including their Gleason score and PSA results. Using this form and information provided in the book, participants could formulate questions to ask their physician about the probability of specific treatment- and disease-related events happening to them and to record answers to their questions. The booklet also included a tear-out sheet that subjects could use to write down other questions they wanted to ask as they worked with the nurse intervener on using the intervention materials. The booklet included a tabbed format, table of contents, background information including male urogenital anatomy, a list of other places to find information and support, and a glossary of terms they were likely to encounter in the staging and treatment discussions. An index was included to make the book user-friendly and to allow subjects to easily access information on their most pressing issues or concerns. The 10 tabbed sections in the booklet were (a) Understanding My Prostate Cancer, (b) About to Make a Decision, (c) Issues Around Treatments, (d) People Involved in My Case, (e) A Closer Look at Treatments, (f) Looking Into the Future, (g) My Usual Activities, (h) Summing Up the Side Effects, (i) Monitoring My Situation, and (j) If My Cancer Gets Worse. Each section was further divided into specific questions in that topic area.

Along with the booklet, a professional CD-ROM was developed in which actors playing the roles of patients and physicians provided examples of four types of communication strategies. In the CD-ROM, patients are talking with their doctors about treatment options. The specific scenarios were designed to exemplify common communication issues in physician-patient interactions and to demonstrate four essential communication skills. The skills demonstrated in the CD-ROM were giving information to the doctor, asking questions in a clear and specific manner, obtaining the information that is needed by verifying and persisting until the patient receives an answer, and clarifying information, including medical terms that are not understood. The CD-ROM was supplemented by handouts designed to assist subjects to become "competent" patients who were able to give and receive the information they needed, and to participate effectively in the treatment decision discussion.

The nurse intervention calls began as soon as the subject had received the intervention materials and continued for four calls over 7–10 days, depending on the window of time available until the treatment consultation and on the subject's convenience. All calls were audiotaped and reviewed by the investigators for quality control and maintaining the fidelity of the intervention. For subjects in the treatment-supplemented arm of the intervention, both the patient and the primary support person received the four phone calls separately from the same nurse intervener. The calls were scripted in the sense that they had specific objectives, identified components of the call, and both questions and directions for the nurse intervener. The objectives of the first call were for the nurses to introduce themselves; to perform a crisis assessment because many men were within a few days of having been told they had a positive biopsy, to review a handout titled *The Competent Patient*, which discussed the importance of being an informed patient and being ready for the treatment decision-making meeting by identifying questions and other strategies; and to help the participants learn how to use the book and to practice using it. The second call's objectives included helping the participants to identify questions that they wanted to ask, helping them to formulate questions that were specific and direct, and helping them to practice reformulating questions in that way. In preparation for the third call, the participants were asked to watch the CD-ROM. The objectives of this call included reviewing the first three communication skills and strategies for each skill and practicing these. The final call included reviewing the fourth skill—clarifying information—and the strategies for using it, as well as practicing this skill with the nurse. This last call ended with the nurse reminding the subject to take a copy of their questions to the meeting with their doctor and to review the handout and the CD-ROM the day before the meeting.

The components of the Uncertainty in Illness Theory that guided this intervention were the uncertainty of the stimuli frame variables (symptom pattern and event familiarity) and enhancing the use of the structure provider variable (the healthcare provider) (Mishel, 1988). Outcomes included improving patient communication with the physician, measured by coded doctor-patient interviews and other outcome measures. This study was completed in June 2007, and data analyses are ongoing. Early findings indicate that the men in the treatment-supplemented group had more interaction with their physician compared to men in the other intervention group or in the control group. The improvement in communication occurred because 92% of spouses in the treatment-supplemented group attended and participated in the doctor-patient interview compared with 70% in the treatment-direct group and 72% in the control group. Similarly, spouses in the treatment-supplemented group had a significantly higher percentage of participation over all content areas compared with spouses in the other two groups. This was particularly evident in content related to treatments and procedures. In question asking, both patients and spouses in the treatment-supplemented group had a significantly higher level of direct questions concerning prognosis. On outcome measures, the treatment groups were significantly higher than controls on doctor-patient communication ($F_{4,341} = 3.19$, $p = .01$), cancer knowledge ($F_{4,341} = 7.08$, $p = .0001$), and communication competence ($F_{4,339} = 3.271$, $p = .01$), and were lower than control groups on decisional regret ($F_{2,223} = 4.73$, $p = .01$). Early findings indicate that the intervention was successful.

The next study was on older, long-term survivors of breast cancer, and the sixth study (ongoing at the time of this publication) focuses on younger survivors of breast cancer. The survivor studies target the uncertainty of recurrence, long-term treatment side effects, and other issues specific to the age of the survivors.

After Treatment: Managing Uncertainty in Younger and Older Breast Cancer Survivors

The final two studies to be discussed focused on the period of time after treatment was completed and, specifically, on breast cancer survivors. The completed survivor study funded by NCI focused on older women with breast cancer who were five to seven years post-treatment. The sample consisted of 509 recurrence-free women, with 360 Caucasians and 149 African Americans who had a mean age of 64. Women were assigned randomly to either the intervention or usual care control condition. These women were post-treatment, so the focus of the study was on managing the uncertainties of survivorship, which do not occur at any particular time but may be triggered by a variety of events. The research team needed to design a portable intervention that could be sent to survivors for use at home when uncertainties arose. The intervention consisted of CD-ROMs on cognitive strategies to use whenever they encountered a trigger that generated thoughts about the uncertainty of recurrence and a self-help manual designed to help women to understand and manage the uncertainties related to long-term treatment side effects and other symptoms. The intervention is described in depth in the publication by Gil et al. (2005). This intervention was built on components of the original Uncertainty in Illness Theory and the reconceptualized Uncertainty in Illness Theory (Mishel, 1988, 1990).

A new measure of growth through uncertainty was one of the outcome measures. The expectation was that women would gradually move their view of uncertainty from a threat to an opportunity for new avenues in life. This change would be reflected in the Growth Through Uncertainty Scale (GTUS).

After intervention, subjects received the book and CD-ROM and a nurse phoned them once a week for four weeks to help them to personalize the uncertainty management strategies and to locate symptom concerns in the manual for times when uncertainties arose in those areas. Following the four weeks of nurse support, women in the treatment group received a call biweekly for four months to determine their use of the intervention materials and the frequency of their treatment-related concerns. Women in this study reported approximately two triggers of uncertainty per month, and 75% of the women receiving the intervention reported symptoms of fatigue, joint stiffness, and pain during the 10 months of the study (Gil et al., 2004). Study outcomes were measured at baseline and at 10 months and 20 months after baseline. From 10–20 months after the intervention, women in the treatment and control groups were contacted monthly by letters to retain them in the study.

At the 10-month follow-up, training in uncertainty management resulted in improvements in cognitive reframing ($F_{1,505}$ = 6.66, p = 0.01), cancer knowledge ($F_{1,505}$ = 22.41, p = .001), and patient-provider communication (specifically in how much the patient told the nurse among African American women in the intervention group) ($F_{1,504}$ = 10.83, p = .001). Caucasian women in the intervention group showed improvements in the specific coping strategies of coping self-statements ($F_{1,505}$ = 4.11, p = .04), behavioral activities ($F_{1,505}$ = 14.95, p = .001), and diverting attention ($F_{1,505}$ = 21.82, p = .001). Among African American women in the intervention group, as compared to controls, there was a decrease in catastrophizing ($F_{1,505}$ = 5.18, p = .02). The treatment group improved significantly in accessing symptom-related resources ($F_{1,505}$ = 98.87, p = .001), particularly in accessing lymphedema resources (Mishel et al., 2005).

Women in the study were not contacted for another 10 months and then were measured again on the outcome variables. Twenty-month outcomes included maintenance or improvement for intervention subjects in cognitive reframing ($F_{1,479}$ = 3.94, p = .05), cancer knowledge ($F_{1,479}$ = 17.85, p = .0001), accessing resources (particularly in accessing lymphedema and symptom resources) ($F_{1,479}$ = 77.56, p = .0001), and diverting attention ($F_{1,479}$ = 4.71, p = .03), as well as declines in illness uncertainty ($F_{1,479}$ = 4.85, p = .03). African American women in the treatment group reported greater positive expectations for the future (a subscale of the GTUS) ($F_{1,479}$ = 5.65, p = .02). Significant results shortly after an intervention are common. However, in this study, the research team waited 10 months from the last measurement time to see if the effects of the intervention would hold. The results strongly supported that women learned from the intervention and were able to maintain many of the gains made at the first follow-up time (Gil et al., 2006). The intervention and the results from this intervention are now available on NCI's Web site (NCI, 2005).

Based on the strong results from the first survivor study, the scientists decided to modify the intervention for the concerns of younger women. The research team was funded in 2006 by NINR to test a revised intervention with breast cancer survivors who are younger than 50 years old and have been survivors for two to four years. The concerns and issues of these women are vastly different from those of older breast cancer survivors. The researchers plan on recruiting 120 Caucasian American and 120 African American younger breast cancer survivors. The format of the intervention remains as a CD-ROM and manual; however, the contents of both have been changed markedly. The CD-ROM contains three of the strategies to help women in managing uncertainty about recurrence, but two new strategies to facilitate communication with significant others and to find positive experiences in life are included. The manual has been updated and extended to include areas of concern to younger survivors of breast cancer, such as premature menopause, sexuality, and fertility. Recruitment for this study is under way.

Conclusion

The six studies described all shared the same theory base but were modified to address the concerns of the specific population under study and the timing of the study along the cancer trajectory. They demonstrate how a program of research can proceed and extend the evidence for both the theory and its application. The interventions can be transferred to practice and can be tested during ongoing treatment and also in centers focused on survivorship. The studies conducted with patients with cancer during treatment can be useful for promoting an evidence-based patient navigation system. The studies on survivorship can be used with cancer survivors for management of post-treatment concerns.

References

Bowie, J.V., Sydnor, K.D., Granot, M., & Pargament, K.I. (2004). Spirituality and coping among survivors of prostate cancer. *Journal of Psychosocial Oncology, 22*(2), 41–56.

Feldman-Stewart, D., Brundage, M.D., Van Manen, L., Skarsgard, D., & Siemens R. (2003). Evaluation of a question and answer booklet on early stage prostate cancer. *Patient Education and Counseling, 49*(2), 115–124.

Germino, B., Mishel, M.H., Belyea, M., Harris, L., Ware, A., & Mohler, J. (1998). Uncertainty in prostate cancer: Ethnic and family patterns. *Cancer Practice, 6*(2), 107–113.

Gil, K.M., Mishel, M.H., Belyea, M., Germino, B., Germino, L.S., Porter, L., et al. (2004). Triggers of uncertainty about recurrence and long-term treatment side effects in long-term older breast cancer survivors. *Oncology Nursing Forum, 31*(3), 633–639.

Gil, K.M., Mishel, M.H., Belyea, M., Germino, B., Porter, L.S., & Clayton, M. (2006). Benefits of the uncertainty management intervention for African American and Caucasian older breast cancer survivors: 20-month outcomes. *International Journal of Behavioral Medicine, 13*(4), 285–294.

Gil, K.M., Mishel, M.H., Germino, B., Porter, L.S., Carlton-LaNey, I., & Belyea, M. (2005). Uncertainty management intervention for older African American and Caucasian long-term breast cancer survivors. *Journal of Psychosocial Oncology, 23*(2–3), 3–21.

Hughes, G.D., Sellers, D.B., Fraser, L., Teague, R., & Knight, B. (2007). Prostate cancer community collaboration and partnership: Education, awareness, recruitment and outreach to southern, African American males. *Journal of Cultural Diversity, 14* (2), 68–73.

Mishel, M.H. (1988). The theory of uncertainty in illness. *Image: The Journal of Nursing Scholarship, 20*(4), 225–232.

Mishel, M.H. (1990). Reconceptualization of the uncertainty in illness theory. *Image: The Journal of Nursing Scholarship, 22*(4), 256–262.

Mishel, M.H. (1997). The efficacy of the uncertainty management intervention for older white and African-American women with breast cancer. *Proceedings of the 11th Annual Conference of the Southern Nursing Research Society, 7,* 11.

Mishel, M.H., Belyea, M., Germino, B.B., Stewart, J.L., Bailey, D.E., Robertson, C., et al. (2002). Helping patients with localized prostate cancer manage uncertainty and treatment side effects: Nurse-delivered psycho-educational intervention via telephone. *Cancer, 94*(6), 1854–1866.

Mishel, M.H., & Clayton, M.F. (2008). Theories of uncertainty in illness. In M.J. Smith & P.R. Liehr (Eds.), *Middle range theory for nursing* (pp. 55–88). New York: Springer.

Mishel, M.H., Germino, B., Belyea, M., & Harris, L. (1996). A self-help intervention for older white and minority women with breast cancer. *Proceedings of the American Psychological Association Conference, 9,* 13.

Mishel, M.H., Germino, B.B., Belyea, M., Stewart, J.L., Bailey, D.E., Mohler, J., et al. (2003). Moderators of an uncertainty management intervention for men with localized prostate cancer. *Nursing Research, 52*(2), 89–97.

Mishel, M.H., Germino, B.B., Gil, K.M., Belyea, M., LaNey, I.C., Stewart, J., et al. (2005). Benefits from an uncertainty management intervention for African-American and Caucasian older long-term breast cancer survivors. *Psycho-Oncology, 14*(11), 962–978.

National Cancer Institute. (2005). *Research-tested intervention programs.* Retrieved September 1, 2008, from http://rtips.cancer.gov/rtips/rtips_search.do?topicid=12&choice =default&cg=

CHAPTER 13

The Role of National Cancer Institute–Funded Cooperative Groups

Ellen M. Lavoie Smith, PhD, APRN-BC, AOCN®,
and Carol Estwing Ferrans, PhD, RN, FAAN

The Clinical Trials Cooperative Group Program

Introduction

Historically, clinical intervention studies in nursing science have been hindered by relatively small samples collected from a limited number of institutions. Because of the logistical issues involved in intervention studies, using a large number of institutions scattered over a wide geographic area generally has not been feasible. These studies require trained research staff and clinical collaborators within each participating institution to recruit participants, administer the intervention, and measure the outcomes. All sites need to be monitored closely to ensure the fidelity of the intervention and the quality of the research. Traditionally, these factors have limited the number of institutions that could participate in any one study because of the effort required and the expense.

The Clinical Trials Cooperative Group Program of the National Cancer Institute (NCI) is a resource that has great potential as a vehicle for conducting nursing intervention studies. Although oncology nurses have always played a

The authors are grateful to Ann O'Mara, PhD, RN, FAAN, of the National Cancer Institute for her thoughtful critique of this chapter.

major role in the execution of studies within the cooperative groups (CGs), relatively few nurse scientists have been principal investigators (PIs). However, this situation is now changing, and for the first time, oncology nurses hold primary leadership roles within almost all of the CGs.

The CGs provide a number of advantages. First, if a study is opened within a CG, all the member institutions throughout the country potentially are available as study sites. Because they receive various types of rewards for participation, institutions are more willing to participate than if approached by a PI working alone. In addition, payments to participating sites are handled by the CG's Central Office, which frees the PI from the burden of negotiating subcontracts and handling billing for each one. Second, each institution already has CG-specific research staff in place who will be assigned to the study. Since the implementation of the privacy rules of the Health Insurance Portability and Accountability Act (HIPAA), this has become critically important because the research staff has access to protected health information within their institution. In addition, because the research staff is shared among studies, the expense for any one study is reduced. Third, the research staff at each participating institution is responsible for obtaining institutional review board (IRB) approvals and HIPAA authorization, both initially and annually for renewals. Fourth, the CGs provide an additional source of National Institutes of Health (NIH) funding for research, which is outside the R-series (R01, R03, and R21) grants that are awarded by NIH to support various types of research projects and are traditionally utilized by oncology nurse scientists. Funding for both pilot and large studies is available through the CGs, and oncology nurse scientists have competed successfully for both types. Therefore, many benefits are inherent within the CG system. A comprehensive description of this system follows.

The Clinical Trials Cooperative Group Program is a complex system of interlinked universities, community hospitals, and small clinical practices and is sponsored by NCI. This program can be credited with significant successes over the past 50 years because through this mechanism, major advances have been made in cancer treatment (Comis, 1998). Most specifically, this program is designed to promote and support clinical trials investigating new cancer treatments as well as approaches to early detection and cancer prevention. Research focused on improving quality-of-life (QOL) and supportive care outcomes is also a priority. The program involves more than 1,700 institutions. Institutional groupings comprise unique CGs, and participating investigators employed at these institutions accrue more than 22,000 patients to CG-conducted clinical trials each year (NCI, n.d.-b).

Who Are the Cooperative Groups?

The CG network was established in 1955 and is composed of 12 multisite research groups—10 based in the United States, 1 Canadian group, and 1

European group (NCI, n.d.-b). Each CG is a system of linked research sites, some of which are organized by their distinct scientific focus, whereas others are defined by geography. For example, the Radiation Therapy Oncology Group (RTOG) designs and implements studies to advance the science of radiation oncology (RTOG, n.d.). A second example, the Gynecologic Oncology Group, focuses its efforts on the study of a group of related cancers. This is in contrast to the Southwest Oncology Group (SWOG), whose name is descriptive of its original geographic domain. Its member institutions are located primarily on the West Coast, and its scientific mission is to conduct clinical research related to the prevention and cure of cancer in adults (SWOG, n.d.). Although each CG varies slightly with respect to its main focus, in general, the missions of all 12 CGs are similar: to develop and conduct large-scale trials in multi-institutional settings (Comis, 1998). All the groups focus on adults with cancer with the exception of the Children's Oncology Group (COG). The names of the CGs, their acronyms, and their research missions are summarized in Table 13-1.

Community Cancer Oncology Program

The Community Cancer Oncology Program (CCOP) is another NCI-funded network within which multisite research is conducted. Established in 1983, the main goal of this program is to provide clinical trial access to minority populations, as well as to patients in community settings (NCI Division of Cancer Prevention [DCP], n.d.-a). In addition to treatment trials, CCOP trials focus on cancer prevention and cancer control outcomes (e.g., symptom management, palliative care) (O'Mara, Bauer-Wu, Berry, & Lillington, 2007). For example, a cancer control trial might focus on evaluating the efficacy of interventions to improve chemotherapy-induced nausea and vomiting. Another type of cancer control study might investigate

Table 13-1. The Cooperative Groups	
Group	**Research Mission**
American College of Surgeons Oncology Group (ACOSOG, n.d.)	To evaluate the surgical management of patients with malignant solid tumors
American College of Radiology Imaging Network (ACRIN, n.d.)	To screen high-risk populations for cancer To diagnose and stage disease to guide therapy To investigate biomarkers of treatment response
	(Continued on next page)

Table 13-1. The Cooperative Groups *(Continued)*

Group	Research Mission
Cancer and Leukemia Group B (CALGB, n.d.-a)	To answer important therapeutic questions through large clinical trials To develop a strong multidisciplinary approach to cancer treatment and prevention To integrate information obtained from basic science and from economic and psychosocial investigations with information from clinical trials To explore the relationship between dose density and therapeutic outcome To systematically explore methods for optimizing treatment for individual patients To introduce novel therapies and treatment approaches for patients with poor prognoses To study quality of life and financial impact on patients with cancer To encourage fresh and innovative ideas of new investigators To involve community hospitals in CALGB cancer research To maintain a high degree of quality control in all CALGB science To increase participation of minority populations, older adults, and women in clinical trials To collect, analyze, and publish the results of CALGB studies
Children's Oncology Group (COG, n.d.)	To cure and prevent childhood and adolescent cancer through scientific discovery and compassionate care
Eastern Cooperative Oncology Group (ECOG, n.d.)	To control, effectively treat, and ultimately cure cancer
European Organisation for Research and Treatment of Cancer (EORTC, 2002)	To develop, conduct, coordinate, and stimulate translational and clinical research in Europe to improve the management of cancer and related problems by increasing survival but also patients' quality of life
Gynecologic Oncology Group (GOG, 2006)	To promote excellence in the quality and integrity of clinical and basic scientific research in the field of gynecologic malignancies

(Continued on next page)

Table 13-1. The Cooperative Groups *(Continued)*	
Group	**Research Mission**
National Cancer Institute of Canada, Clinical Trials Group (NCIC, n.d.)	To develop and conduct clinical trials aimed at improving the treatment and prevention of cancer with the ultimate goal of reducing morbidity and mortality from this disease
National Surgical Adjuvant Breast and Bowel Project (NSABP, n.d.)	To improve the treatment and prevention of breast and bowel cancers
North Central Cancer Treatment Group (NCCTG, n.d.)	To improve the survival of and quality of life for patients with cancer
Radiation Therapy Oncology Group (RTOG, n.d.)	To increase the survival of patients with malignant diseases in which control of the local-regional tumor is a major determinant of outcome To improve quality of life by preserving structure and function while maintaining or increasing survival To provide palliation and to preserve patient dignity To prevent second and subsequent malignant tumors To seek greater understanding of the biology of several cancer types
Southwest Oncology Group (SWOG, n.d.)	To conduct clinical research in the prevention and cure of cancer in adults

QOL outcomes related to specific cancer types, treatments, or symptoms. The CCOP network comprises academic centers, referred to as research bases, and community oncology practices located throughout the United States and Puerto Rico (NCI DCP, n.d.-a). A *research base* might be an NCI-designated cancer center or an entire CG. The research base receives NCI funding to design and conduct minimally complex cancer prevention and cancer control trials that are feasible for conduct at nonacademic centers. *Community oncology practices* receive NCI funding to accrue patients to treatment, prevention, and control trials. Additionally, some community-based sites are designated as Minority-Based CCOPs. Forty percent of newly diagnosed patients with cancer at these sites must be a member of a minority population (NCI DCP, n.d.-a).

The funding received by a CCOP site is targeted specifically to support data management and is paid by NCI on a case-by-case basis. Therefore, the more patients accrued, the greater the funding stream. Because of this unique funding structure and the less complex nature of studies that are feasible for conduct at CCOP institutions, CCOP sites often are eager to accrue patients to the types of studies that are typically designed by nurse scientists.

Cooperative Group Program Funding

Two distinct NCI-based funding mechanisms support the Clinical Trials Cooperative Group Program. The first of these programs is the Division of Cancer Treatment and Diagnosis, Cancer Therapy Evaluation Program (NCI CTEP, 2006). CTEP sponsors clinical trials evaluating new anticancer interventions (e.g., chemotherapeutic agents, radiation therapy, surgery), with a particular emphasis on translational and basic science research (CTEP). The second mechanism for funding CG studies is via the Community Oncology and Prevention Trials Research Group of the DCP. Studies typically funded by the DCP investigate cancer control, genetics, and screening outcomes, in addition to prevention (NCI DCP, n.d.-b).

Although government funds have been the main source of support for the CG program, budgetary cuts to NCI threaten future CG research. In light of shrinking resources, many CGs are working to improve organizational efficiency and are forming new alliances with the pharmaceutical industry and other funding organizations.

Cooperative Group Internal Structure

Numerous smaller committees exist within each CG, each with a distinct research agenda that is determined by the purpose for the committee. These committees may be organized by cancer type (e.g., breast, lung, leukemia) or by a modality focus. Examples of modality-focused committees are those which concentrate on designing and implementing patient QOL, symptom management, or healthcare economic trials. Other modality committees are discipline-specific. For instance, many CGs have nursing, pharmacy, and/or clinical research associate (CRA) committees.

With the exception of discipline-specific committees, committee membership typically is quite diverse and includes physicians, basic and behavioral scientists, statisticians, CRAs, pharmacists, patient advocates, research nurses, and oncology nurse scientists. The fact that these members volunteer their time is important to note. Other members include CG-funded staff. These staff members are employed at a central office, which historically has been located at the CG chair's base institution. These staff members are responsible for editorial, budgetary, legal, regulatory, and other administrative issues. All volunteer and CG-funded committee members work collaboratively to design and implement studies for the purpose of preventing and curing cancers, as well as to decrease treatment- and disease-related morbidity.

Accrual to Cooperative Group Trials

Once a CG trial has been developed and approved by NCI, patients may be accrued from institutions within the sponsoring CG network. For example, any participating RTOG institution may accrue patients to RTOG trials. Normally, member institutions enter patients on trials opened within their own CG, although main members of the CGs actually are permitted to accrue patients to other CG trials using the Cancer Trials Support Unit (CTSU). In addition, non-CG individual physicians, as well as nonmember institutions, may accrue patients to select high-priority phase III trials if the trial has been registered with the CTSU. NCI established the CTSU as a pilot project for the purpose of meeting the following objectives (NCI CTSU, n.d.).

- To increase physician and patient access to NCI-sponsored clinical trials
- To streamline and standardize trial data collection and reporting
- To reduce regulatory/administrative burden on investigators participating in NCI-sponsored CG clinical trials

Since its inception in 2000, the CTSU has been effective in achieving these goals, with an unprecedented increase of 18% in accrual to NCI-sponsored cancer treatment trials in the first year alone (NCI, n.d.-a).

Nursing Roles Within Cooperative Groups

Main Membership

A CG's main nursing membership consists of the hundreds of oncology nurses throughout the world who are employed at CG member institutions. CG nurses fulfill a variety of roles. These roles include facilitating patient recruitment, screening for eligibility, facilitating informed consent, providing patient and family education, coordinating and/or administering clinical trial–specific tests and treatments, monitoring and managing treatment-related side effects, educating staff regarding relevant nursing care issues, performing specimen and data collection, and carrying out administrative functions (Aikin, 2000; Ruccione, Hinds, Wallace, & Kelly, 2005; Smith et al., 2006).

Core Committee Membership

In addition to performing many important functions as CG main members, smaller subsets of oncology nurses may become even more involved as core members of CG committees. Core committee members offer consultative support by reviewing clinical trials for the inclusion and accuracy of drug administration, research implementation feasibility, and patient educational components. In many CGs, core members function as liaisons to other disease and modality committees, ensuring that oncology nursing care is woven into all newly developed trials. Core committee members also are responsible for patient, family, and professional education via publication mechanisms. Additionally, CG nurses and CRA committee members are responsible for the planning and execution of educational sessions targeting the larger CG nurse and CRA membership. Critical for keeping abreast of emerging new therapies, these educational sessions are offered to any CG member, irrespective of discipline at the CG's annual to semiannual group meetings (Aikin, 2000; Hinds et al., 2003; Ruccione & Kelly, 2000; Smith et al., 2006).

Nurses who are interested in becoming core committee members should contact the committee chair. Typically, candidates are asked to submit a résumé or curriculum vitae, as well as a cover letter stating interest in a core committee position. Core committee nurses typically are chosen based on educational background, clinical or research focus, and prior demonstrated involvement within the CG arena. In addition, core nurse members must negotiate with their employers for time to work on CG activities. Funding to attend meetings is available to core members. However, additional funds may be required from the candidate's employer and should be negotiated prior to acceptance of a core committee position. For example, in Cancer and Leukemia Group B (CALGB), funding for travel is provided to core members to attend core meetings only. For CALGB group meetings, the employer is expected to provide for travel expenses.

Cooperative Group Nursing Research

Historical milestones: Prior to offering further discussion of how CG nursing research can be implemented, the history of CG nurses' progress is important to understand. To date, very few studies have been conducted within the CG network where nurses have been PIs (referred to as the study chair within the CGs). The first nurse-led study was conducted in 1994 by a group of SWOG nursing investigators (O'Mara et al., 2007) and compared three breast self-examination educational interventions (Strickland et al., 1997). However, of all the CGs, the COG has made the most significant progress in developing nurse-initiated studies. It was one of the first groups to take systematic steps to interject nursing research priorities into the CG's overall research portfolio. Following decades of slow and steady progress, the COG Nursing Discipline Committee successfully created an environment that values and supports pediatric oncology CG nursing research. In February 2000, this group held the first CG-specific State of the Science Nursing Research Summit. The purpose of this summit was to provide a collaborative opportunity where nursing leaders could outline a nursing-specific scientific agenda and plan for how pediatric oncology staff nurses, advanced practice nurses, and nurse scientists could work together to weave this agenda into the COG's overall mission (Hinds & DeSwarte-Wallace, 2000). Summit participants defined nursing research priorities for future focus (see Figure 13-1) and acknowledged the importance of fostering transdisciplinary collaboration as a key strategy for moving nursing science forward.

Figure 13-1. Priority Areas for Cooperative Group Nursing Research

- Disease prevention
- End of life
- Health promotion in diverse populations
- Immune responses and oncology
- Minority health issues
- Neurologic function and sensory conditions
- Symptom management

A second CG-led summit held in Washington, DC, in 2002 was another important milestone in CG nursing history (Smith et al., 2006). The CALGB Nursing Committee led and sponsored this national initiative. The objectives of the meeting were to

1. Understand the nursing research structure and culture of all CGs
2. Investigate funding opportunities for CG nursing research
3. Establish a collaborative network of nurses interested in fostering CG nursing research
4. Increase national awareness of nursing research opportunities within CG settings
5. Develop strategies to integrate nursing research into CG research agendas.

Nine CGs were represented at the meeting (Smith et al., 2006). Additional participants included nursing leaders from NCI, the National Institute of Nursing Research (NINR), Susan G. Komen for the Cure, the American Cancer Society, and the Oncology Nursing Society (ONS) (Smith et al.). Both the COG- and CALGB-sponsored summits were instrumental as initial steps toward equipping nurses to change the culture and the environment within CGs, thereby opening the door to new opportunities.

Since these initial summits, CG leaders, oncology nurse scientists, NCI, and ONS have continued to collaborate on initiatives addressing knowledge-deficit barriers to conducting CG research and have worked toward the development of a strategic plan for the purpose of fostering nurse-led CG trials (O'Mara et al., 2007). As a component of this strategic plan, ONS conducted a needs assessment survey in March 2005 to determine (a) whether its members were aware of CG function and infrastructure, (b) the current level of ONS member participation in CG activities, and (c) perceptions regarding the advantages and disadvantages of conducting a CG study (O'Mara et al.). More than

3,000 ONS members were surveyed using Web-based technology. Of the 682 (19.3%) who responded, approximately 50% reported being involved and familiar with CGs, but only 5% reported CG involvement as a CG trial PI or coinvestigator (O'Mara et al.).

Nurse scientists: The CG network historically has been underutilized by nurse scientists for the purpose of designing and implementing studies that address nurse-generated research questions or hypotheses. More recently, oncology nurse scientists have become valuable members and leaders of CG committees. Nurse scientists' main functions are to design and to implement studies aimed at discovering new ways to improve QOL and supportive care outcomes for patients with cancer. Nurse scientists also collaborate in the development of CG studies emerging from disease and other modality committees, frequently serving as coinvestigators. Another newer role of CG nurse scientists includes serving as a member of their respective CG's executive-level scientific review committee. These prestigious positions traditionally have been reserved for physicians. However, with the increase in QOL, behavioral, and symptom management research in the CGs, nurse scientists are being recognized for providing a unique perspective and are well-prepared to provide expert peer review for these studies.

Writing a Cooperative Group Study

Challenges

Inefficient processes: Many challenges arise when embarking on a CG research path. One main challenge is that the CG system is known for its inefficient and bureaucratic processes (Dilts et al., 2006; O'Mara et al., 2007). For example, the time from the initial idea generation to study implementation is estimated to take as long as three to five years. In contrast, a study performed by a single institution most likely would be completed within the same time frame, but with a significantly smaller sample size and limited generalizability. Historically, this has posed a significant disincentive for faculty members whose academic promotion is based on prolific research and publication productivity. Therefore, these delays have led to significant frustration, particularly for nurse scientists in tenured academic positions. This painfully slow study development time frame is the main reason why many nurse scientists previously abandoned the prospect of using CG networks (Ruccione & Kelly, 2000). However, the situation is changing, as the small number of nurse scientists who have successfully conducted studies within the CGs is growing. As nurses have gained credibility and experience navigating the network within the CGs, they have learned how to obtain approval for their studies more quickly.

Dealing with constituents: Dealing with constituents can pose another difficult challenge when collaborating with coinvestigators and other CG members to develop a CG research study. Collaboration is essential within the CG culture, and "study design by consensus" is a real yet unstated expectation. The benefit of the consensual approach is that the strength of a CG study improves greatly when a variety of experts provide feedback throughout the design process. Members of the sponsoring committee, such as the Nursing or Symptom Management committees, typically provide this feedback. Then, the study usually is presented to other cosponsoring committees, such as the Quality of Life Committee, and/or disease-specific committees, based upon the patient population of interest. The study concept is presented multiple times to the associated committees at semiannual CG meetings over the course of a year or more. With each presentation, the investigators seek advice regarding problematic design and methodologic issues, as well as work to convince the committee members that the study is worth supporting. At any one of these committee gatherings, anywhere from 10–40 CG members may be offering opinions regarding how to improve the study. During this phase, the PI and coinvestigators must synthesize and incorporate the best suggestions. At the same time, they must ensure that the cosponsoring committees support the study concept and that the committees will encourage and facilitate study accrual at their respective institutions. At some point along this feedback trajectory, the PI and coinvestigators need to decide when the study is ready to be presented for approval to the Executive Committee or Scientific Review Committee. Making further presentations to cosponsoring committees at this point produces continued "tinkering" that can compromise and slow study development.

Incongruent values and language: Another challenge impeding the advancement of nursing research within the CGs is related to differences in training and focus, resulting in incongruent values and language within nursing versus medical domains (Hinds et al., 2003). Hinds et al. described and made visible this incongruence. Nurse scientists may place a greater value on research targeted to improve overall *health*, symptom distress, and QOL. In contrast, CG clinical trials have historically been designed within a medical framework for the purpose of treating *disease* (cancer) and increasing survival. However, this incongruence in research values is now becoming less relevant. Today, studies designed to influence symptom management, QOL, and economic outcomes have become critical to achieving the CG mission.

In addition, the gold standard for research designs in the CGs is the experimental design to test an intervention, such as a new drug or combination of drugs, radiation dose or novel sequencing, or surgical technique. However, in addition to experimental designs, oncology nurse scientists have interest in addressing research questions that require historical, qualitative, descriptive, or correlational designs. These research designs, and their associated methodologies, are unfamiliar to many medical scientists and may be perceived as less compelling. Moreover, research using these designs may not be feasible to conduct within multiple CG institutions across the country because of the need for specialized training of data collectors or complex and time-consuming data collection methods.

Knowledge deficits: Many oncology nurse scientists do not receive formal training via their graduate programs regarding CG structure and function and are unaware that CGs even exist (Hinds et al., 2003; O'Mara et al., 2007). In addition, even upon becoming involved in a CG, few senior nurse mentors are available to provide guidance to new PIs. One strategy for combating this problem has been to pair nurse scientists new to CGs with advanced practice nurses possessing clinical and CG systems expertise. Through this coupling, the oncology nurse scientist gains access to a complex network of resources. This relationship also assists the scientist in assimilating CG language (Given, 2001). The CG advanced practice nurse offers perspective to the nurse scientist regarding clinical problems worthy and feasible for additional investigation within the CG setting. In turn, the advanced practice nurse receives mentorship regarding research design, methodology, and utilization. Another strategy for educating new CG nurse scientists regarding the CG process has been via newly emerging CG training programs. One such program, funded by the pharmaceutical industry and the ONS Foundation, was offered to several CGs in 2006. Key program topics included values and language of clinical trials; nursing in CGs; examples of research conducted by nurse scientists in CGs; CG values, mission, aims, and group infrastructure; cancer control/CCOP studies; writing in clinical trials and CG protocol language; concept development; minority recruitment in clinical trials; and monitoring strategies.

Drug acquisition: Drug acquisition can pose another significant barrier for nurse scientists with interest in testing pharmacologic agents, such as in studies designed to alleviate symptoms or treatment-related side effects. More specifically, drug acquisition becomes a concern when designing trials investigating the effectiveness of a commercially available drug, herbal supplement, or nutritional product for the treatment or prevention of a new clinical problem. For example, if conducting a phase III trial to test the effect of a dietary supplement or drug, the scientist normally must provide the study drug to study participants without cost. If a placebo is to be used, this also needs to be obtained. The drug manufacturer may be willing to provide the drug and placebo free of charge, but only if the research promises to provide an economic advantage to the manufacturer in the future. Instances have occurred in which the development of CG trials designed to test the efficacy of currently available drugs for the treatment of a new problem were unsuccessful because of the inability to obtain the study drug. To address this problem, the PI should consult the drug manufacturer in the *initial* stages of study development to determine whether collaboration is feasible.

Securing Funding

As for any study, securing funding for research conducted in the CGs can be a significant challenge. The following section discusses various funding sources and highlights the unique aspects of each within the context of CG research. As described in this chapter, a significant amount of time is invested in developing a study and presenting it to the relevant committees at CG meetings. Unless the PI is the chair of one of the core committees, normally no monetary compensation is available from the CG for this investment of time. This and the limited funding for travel have been identified as disincentives for conducting CG research (O'Mara et al., 2007). The CG reimburses for expenses for travel to CG meetings only if the PI is a member of a core committee. However, in some cases, the nurse scientist's home institution may provide funding for travel through its cancer center or CCOP grant.

Funding from NCI: The most common source of funding for CG studies is NCI, either through CTEP or DCP's Community Oncology and Prevention Trials Research Group. These provide two separate sources of funding, and the nature of the study determines which one is appropriate. In general, CTEP funds clinical trials that evaluate new anticancer interventions (e.g., chemotherapy, radiation therapy, surgery), and DCP sponsors clinical trials focusing on cancer prevention and control, which includes symptom management and QOL. Studies need to be reviewed and approved at three levels: (a) CG core committee, (b) CG Executive Committee or Scientific Review Committee, and (c) CTEP or DCP Review Committee at NCI. Approvals are based on the strength of the study design, as well as the importance of the topic addressed and feasibility, all of which determine the priority rankings at each level. The entire review process at NCI, from concept to final approval of the full study, often takes more than a year to complete.

Although the mission of DCP clearly falls within the purview of many oncology nurse scientists, only a few have obtained approval for implementation of their studies through this mechanism. Part of the reason is that the CG mechanism provides no salary support for PIs or coinvestigators. This mechanism also does not pay for any intervention, including drugs or placebos. If they are needed, approval for funding will hinge on the pharmaceutical company's promise to provide these free of charge. Funding from NCI is limited to data collection at the participating sites and data management and analysis at the CG statistical center, which is important because no indirect cost recovery exists for the PI's home department and institution. Based on these considerations, nurse scientists may choose to pursue funding through the R01 mechanism for studies carried out in the CGs. The R01 research project grant is one of several NIH R-series awards. R01s typically are awarded to the most experienced and successful scientists. This is a relatively new approach within the CGs, but a few nurse scientists already have done this successfully.

Pharmaceutical industry sponsorship: Pharmaceutical industry sponsorship can range from supplementing studies funded by NCI to funding entire research projects. Given the limited funding from CTEP and DCP, the pharmaceutical industry plays a critically important role in determining which studies are conducted. In addition to donating drugs and placebos, they also can pay for data collection and statistical analysis, salary for investigators, and per-case payments for the number of patients accrued to the study.

NIH-funded R01 research grant: An NIH-funded R01 research grant is ideal for oncology nurse scientists working with the CGs because it is large enough to fund multisite data collection activities, as well as provide salary support for investigators and indirect cost recovery for the PI's home institution. If the study entails a behavioral intervention, it also will provide salary support for the interveners. Before submitting the grant proposal for review through the standard R01 review process, the study needs to be reviewed and approved by the CG core committee and the Executive Committee or Scientific Review Committee. The chair of the CG then provides a letter of support to accompany the grant application, and the CG Central Office and Statistical Center provide subcontract budgets that are worked into the overall budget for the grant application. The grant application then is submitted for review to NIH using the standard process for R01s. If the study is selected for funding by NCI or another institute, such as NINR, it will undergo an expedited DCP review because it has already undergone scientific review.

Pilot study funding sources: Funding for pilot studies can come from a variety of sources. Some of the CGs have special funds that can support small studies conducted at a limited number of institutions. For example, the CALGB Foundation was formed to provide additional support for research within CALGB, including that of junior investigators. It has provided support for cancer control research as well as therapeutic clinical trials. An example of one of the recent initiatives supported by the foundation was a study to improve the QOL of patients with cancer and their caregivers (CALGB, n.d.-b).

In addition to the CGs, oncology nurse scientists can submit their studies through one of the CCOP Research Bases. The mission of the CCOP Research Bases is to design and implement cancer prevention and control clinical trials (NCI DCP, n.d.-a). In a process similar to that of the CGs, studies are submitted through the CCOP Research Base for final approval through CTEP or DCP.

Smaller grants funded by NIH also can be used to obtain pilot data, such as the R03 (small research grant for new investigators) or R21 (exploratory/ developmental grant) mechanisms. Generally, grants funded by either of these mechanisms are limited to two years. Because of this time limit and smaller budgets, these mechanisms are better suited for studies involving a small number of institutions rather than the entire CG network.

Benefits

Enhanced generalizability: Although the challenges to conducting CG nursing research may seem daunting, many advantages of the CG system also exist. Most nursing research to date has been performed at single institutional sites using small and minimally diverse patient populations, limiting generalizability. However, the main advantage of the CG network is that large numbers of diverse patients can be accrued to a trial, thus enhancing the external validity of the trial's findings (O'Mara et al., 2007). Also, the time required to accrue large numbers of diverse patients is significantly shortened; therefore, scientific discoveries can be disseminated more rapidly to patients and their families. Multisite CG accrual is particularly advantageous when studying rare diseases or conditions where too few patients would be available to participate at any single site.

For example, one CALGB study, activated in April 2008, is investigating the efficacy of duloxetine for patients with painful chemotherapy-induced peripheral neuropathy. Patients must have moderate to severe neuropathy-related pain in order to participate. Although neuropathy in the cancer population is common, finding an adequate number of patients with painful neuropathy at a single institution to satisfy statistical power requirements would be difficult. Also, study findings could be generalized to only the sample population accrued at that one site. When considering the major benefits, multisite nursing research clearly must be a priority for the future.

An existing collaborative network: A second advantage is that semiannual CG meetings provide an opportunity for nurse scientists to meet with coinvestigators with similar interests, thus minimizing feelings of isolation. Group meetings also may be utilized to provide specialized training to nurses and CRAs regarding study-specific interventional or data collection techniques.

Access to resources: A third advantage of CG participation is that the oncology nurse scientist has access to many resources (O'Mara et al., 2007). Highly trained protocol editors, statisticians, individuals who design data collection forms, pharmacists, CRAs, and many others work collaboratively with the nurse scientist throughout study design, implementation, data collection, and analysis phases. For example, individuals with expertise in peer-review processes and drug acquisition mechanisms are available to support the nurse scientist from the start. In addition, a statistician is assigned to the study to work closely with the nurse investigator to design the statistical analysis for the study. Skilled CRAs located at each accruing institution identify patients who meet the study criteria, perform recruitment, and obtain informed consent. Simple data collection, such as handing a questionnaire to a patient, sometimes can be performed by CRAs, but the time they have to spend on any one study is very limited. The data are then entered into the CG database, which is managed by the CG's statistical center. In addition, systems are in place for monitoring data integrity and patient safety.

Opportunities for collaboration: A fourth advantage of the CG system is that it allows the nurse scientist the opportunity to collaborate with nationally recognized CG members who are experts in their fields and have experience with leading CG trials. This transdisciplinary collaboration and mentorship is an invaluable benefit of the CG system (O'Mara et al., 2007).

Increased visibility: A final yet under-realized advantage of nurse scientist utilization of CG mechanisms for advancing oncology nursing science is that through this process, healthcare professionals, patients and their families, the pharmaceutical industry, and advocacy groups can have a greater understanding of the nature and importance of nurse-led research. Through implementation of large, multisite studies, nursing research priorities will become more visible and perceptions of its importance will improve.

Cooperative Group Study Types

The three types of CG studies are (a) freestanding primary or main studies, (b) companion studies, and (c) imbedded studies. A *freestanding study* is one that accrues independently of other studies, meaning that its research objectives are not linked to another CG study. Extramural funding outside of the CG is easier to obtain for such a study when compared to studies where the research objective has been imbedded within a complex treatment trial (Hinds et al., 2003). Also, these studies typically are less complicated to move through the CG peer-review process when compared to companion or embedded studies.

A *companion study* is one that is linked to a freestanding primary or main study. A companion study is offered to the patient concurrently with the main study. Participation in a companion study may be optional or mandatory. If mandatory, the patient is offered both the main and companion studies as an interdependent duo, and the patient has the choice of participating in both or neither. If the companion study is optional, the patient may choose to participate in the main study but decline participation in the companion. For example, the main study may involve randomization of patients to one of several breast cancer chemotherapy programs. When patients are entered on the breast cancer treatment trial, they also may be offered participation in a linked companion study investigating the differences in QOL of patients undergoing the various treatments being investigated in the primary study. Several advantages to this approach exist. Using the breast cancer and QOL example, data regarding QOL outcomes can be collected simultaneously without requiring patients to return for additional data collection. Also, findings from the QOL study can be useful when interpreting the findings of the main treatment trial. However, disadvantages to the companion trial approach also exist. Patients are sometimes too overwhelmed to agree to participate in more than one study, so they may agree to the primary treatment trial because this is perceived to have "life or death" implications. However, in this circumstance, an optional companion may be considered as less vital to survival, and when given the option, the patient may decline participation in the companion trial because simultaneous consideration of a second protocol may be too overwhelming.

Ideally, companion studies should be developed concurrently with the main study. With this approach, the studies are optimally interwoven. Moreover, CG and NCI reviews will occur simultaneously and more efficiently. Also, both studies will be simultaneously activated. However, if the companion study is developed at a later date *following* activation of the main study, accrual to the companion study will decrease. Another disadvantage of the companion study approach is that if the main study suffers from suboptimal accrual, so will the companion study.

The third option is for the oncology nurse scientist to imbed research objectives within a main treatment trial. This option is very similar to the mandatory companion study approach, except that the patient is accrued to one study and the imbedded research objectives are listed as secondary hypotheses. Therefore, when compared to companion studies, embedded studies have fewer accrual barriers. For example, only one consent form and one IRB approval need to be obtained at each participating institution for the entire study, rather than two with a companion study.

Secondary data analysis opportunities also exist within the CG system. In this regard, the nurse scientist would develop a formal research study, which would undergo peer review at the committee and CG executive level in the same way as other studies. In developing this proposal, the nurse scientist would establish relationships with the PIs who are responsible for the initial data collection, as well as with CG administrative and statistical staff. Following approval, the nurse scientist would be allowed access to the relevant database housed at the CG's statistical center. Authorship negotiations are determined prospectively. The main advantages of this approach include rapid access to data and minimal cost; however, the PI would need to obtain funding for the analysis through the CG or extramural funding outside of the CG.

An additional consideration for the nurse scientist is whether the study will be open to all CG institutions versus being available to only select institutions, termed a *limited access study*. Limiting patient accrual to select institutions may be important if the intervention or data collection process is costly and/or complex, requiring specialized training of nursing and other research staff. This allows the nurse scientist to provide focused, more extensive training and supervision at only a few sites. Access also may be limited when the main purpose of the study is to pilot an intervention or methodologic approach prior to developing a larger scale study.

Study Development Details

Although many details regarding the CG study development process have been described previously, more specific details will now be explained. However, this process description is still rather general and not CG-specific. Nurse scientists must work within their respective CGs to learn of CG-specific varia-tions in process. Figure 13-2 summarizes suggestions for optimizing success when working within a CG.

Figure 13-2. Suggestions for Success With Cooperative Group Studies

- Gain early support for the research idea from well-respected members of cosponsoring committees. Include them as coinvestigators.
- Collaborate early with the cooperative group (CG) statistician as a coinvestigator on the study.
- Establish a relationship with a *mentor*, someone who is knowledgeable regarding the CG study development process.
- Seek funding sources as early as possible.
- If designing an intervention study utilizing a pharmacologic agent, secure funding for drug (and placebo, if relevant) early.
- Design a study that is consistent with national research priorities, as well as the priori-ties of the sponsoring CG committee.
- Design a study that is likely to still address an important issue three to five years from its inception.
- Present the study concept to a variety of constituents at CG meetings, to obtain valu-able feedback and buy-in. Incorporate this feedback as appropriate.
- Organize and lead conference calls with coinvestigators between group meetings to address issues in a timely manner.
- Design the study so that it is as simple as possible, to increase the likelihood of expedi-tious accrual.
- Ensure that the study is feasible for conduct within a CG setting.
- After obtaining consensus regarding the research design and methodology, write the remaining concept sheet using the CG's template.
- Establish respectful relationships with CG staff. These individuals will be instrumental in moving the study through the system.
- Following peer review, take suggestions seriously, because incorporation of the peer reviewers' ideas usually will strengthen the study. If not incorporating the suggestions, provide well-justified reasons for not doing so.

The initial concept: The CG study development process begins with an idea. Initially, this idea is presented informally at a CG committee meeting, such as at a Nursing, Quality of Life, Prevention, or Symptom Intervention Core Committee meeting. If the study falls within the committee's research priorities, then the nurse scientist is encouraged to develop the idea into an initial concept. The term *concept* is used by many CGs to mean a preliminary draft of the research study.

Formalizing a team: At this time, the nurse scientist establishes a team of coinvestigators who have expertise and are willing to participate in writing and reviewing the study concept. Members might include a physician, behavioral scientist, and research nurse, as well as an administrative representative from the CG's central office. In addition, including a statistician as a team member is critical. However, because of the many competing requests for a CG statistician's time, the statistician will not develop the concept's statistical section until the study design has been determined more definitively.

Writing the concept: The PI takes the lead in writing the concept. The key components of the concept are similar to the key components of any research study proposal (i.e., background, specific aims, design, eligibility, data collection, statistical methods). Including a graphic representation of randomization and treatment phases (schema) also is important. If applying for extramural funding, the concept should mirror grant application requirements. The work of writing the concept occurs between group meetings. Therefore, conference calls and e-mail communications must be used to collaborate with coinvestigators when finalizing design and methodologic details. Throughout this process, key questions will arise that require input from other CG experts. These issues will be raised when presenting the concept at the next group meeting, and at this time, further advice is solicited from group participants.

Study design by consensus: Preliminary concepts are first presented to nursing colleagues, possibly at the CG's Nursing Committee meeting. This provides an opportunity for the investigator to receive feedback in a safe and mentoring environment. During these initial committee meetings, the nurse investigator receives feedback regarding design, methodology, and statistical issues. Also during this early phase of concept development, the nurse investigator begins to modify nursing research language into CG language. As described previously, the concept also is presented at other key CG committee meetings. At this phase, keeping an open mind and structuring the group presentation in a way that solicits input from others are important. Asking a colleague to take notes during the presentation ensures that important points are not forgotten. Suggestions from CG members are incorporated as appropriate, followed by presentation of the modified concept at subsequent group meetings.

Peer review: Once the concept is developed adequately, it undergoes peer review by the CG's Scientific Review Committee. If the concept receives an adequate priority score, it progresses to the first NCI review. All prevention and cancer control studies are submitted to the DCP regardless of study phase or sample size. In cases where the nurse scientist is seeking drug and/or placebo from an industry sponsor, the concept must undergo an additional pharmaceutical company review process. At any point along the review process trajectory, the concept usually will not be approved the first time. In this circumstance, the study team works together to make revisions based upon peer reviewer feedback. In most cases, the concept may then be resubmitted for review again, depending on CG policy.

Once NCI approves the concept, the central office staff works with the PI to transform the concept into a full protocol based on a CG-specific protocol template. The full protocol undergoes review by a variety of CG members, and further revisions are made. Also at this time, protocol-specific regulatory and drug acquisition details are determined, and data collection forms are developed. Following final revisions, the full protocol undergoes NCI review.

NCI provides a written review within approximately 30 days. Further revisions may be required before the study is approved. This entire process may transpire over the course of several years. However, once it becomes an approved NCI protocol, study activation finally can take place. For example, development of the previously mentioned CALGB intervention study of duloxetine for painful chemotherapy-induced peripheral neuropathy began in March 2005. The study was activated in November 2007, two years and eight months from conception. Thus, perseverance in this process is critically important.

Conclusion

When weighing the challenges against the benefits of CG involvement, the overall gains must be determined while maintaining a patient-centered perspective. Continued reliance on small, single-site studies results in limited contributions to science and health care because the findings generated from these investigations frequently lack adequate statistical power and cannot be generalized to the larger population. For years, nurses have been well-situated within the core of CG organizations, with access to vast resources. Oncology nurses need to take full advantage of the resources available through the CGs to advance the science of oncology nursing.

References

Aikin, J.L. (2000). Nursing roles in clinical trials. In A.D. Klimaszewski, J.L. Aikin, M.A. Bacon, S.A. DiStasio, H.E. Ehrenberger, & B.A. Ford (Eds.), *Manual for clinical trials nursing* (pp. 273–285). Pittsburgh, PA: Oncology Nursing Society.

American College of Radiology Imaging Network. (n.d.). *Major research objectives.* Retrieved June 23, 2008, from http://www.acrin.org/RESEARCHERS/CONDUCTING RESEARCH/SCIENTIFICPLAN20082012/tabid/67/Default.aspx

American College of Surgeons Oncology Group. (n.d.). *ACSOG history.* Retrieved January 15, 2007, from https://www.acosog.org/about/history.jsp

Cancer and Leukemia Group B. (n.d.-a). *About the Cancer and Leukemia Group B.* Retrieved January 15, 2007, from http://www.calgb.org/Public/about/about.php

Cancer and Leukemia Group B. (n.d.-b). *CALGB Foundation.* Retrieved March 18, 2007, from http://www.calgb.org/Public/foundation/foundation.php

Children's Oncology Group. (n.d.). Retrieved January 15, 2007, from http://www.childrensoncologygroup.org

Comis, R.L. (1998). The cooperative groups: Past and future. *Cancer Chemotherapy and Pharmacology, 42*(Suppl.), S85–S87.

Dilts, D.M., Sandler, A.B., Baker, M., Cheng, S.K., George, S.L., Karas, K.S., et al. (2006). Processes to activate phase III clinical trials in a cooperative oncology group: The case of Cancer and Leukemia Group B. *Journal of Clinical Oncology, 24*(28), 4553–4557.

Eastern Cooperative Oncology Group. (n.d.). *Introduction to ECOG.* Retrieved June 23, 2008, from http://www.ecog.org/general/intro.html

European Organisation for Research and Treatment of Cancer. (2002). *EORTC: Aims and mission.* Retrieved January 15, 2007, from http://www.eortc.be/about/Directory2008-2009/01%20Background.htm

Given, B. (2001). Into the millennium: Open the door and let the future in for cancer nursing research. *Oncology Nursing Forum, 28*(4), 647–654.

Gynecologic Oncology Group. (2006). Retrieved January 15, 2007, from http://www.gog.org

Hinds, P.S., Baggott, C., DeSwarte-Wallace, J., Dodd, M., Haase, J., Hockenberry, M., et al. (2003). Functional integration of nursing research into a pediatric oncology cooperative group: Finding common ground [Online exclusive]. *Oncology Nursing Forum, 30*(6), E121–E126. Retrieved December 2, 2006, from http://ons.metapress.com/content/v73v86m24mlm8271/fulltext.pdf

Hinds, P.S., & DeSwarte-Wallace, J. (2000). Positioning nursing research to contribute to the scientific mission of the pediatric oncology cooperative group. *Seminars in Oncology Nursing, 16*(4), 251–252.

National Cancer Institute. (n.d.-a). *Building the nation's cancer research capacity: National Clinical Trials Program in treatment and prevention.* Retrieved September 28, 2007, from http://plan2004.cancer.gov/capacity/trials.htm

National Cancer Institute. (n.d.-b). *NCI's Clinical Trials Cooperative Group Program.* Retrieved December 20, 2006, from http://www.cancer.gov/cancertopics/factsheet/NCI/clinical-trials-cooperative-group

National Cancer Institute Cancer Therapy Evaluation Program. (2006). *The mission of the Cancer Therapy Evaluation Program (CTEP).* Retrieved January 15, 2007, from http://ctep.info.nih.gov/about/mission.html

National Cancer Institute Cancer Trials Support Unit. (n.d.). *About the CTSU.* Retrieved December 20, 2006, from http://www.ctsu.org

National Cancer Institute Division of Cancer Prevention. (n.d.-a). *About the Community Clinical Oncology Program: Facts about the CCOP network.* Retrieved May 28, 2008, from http://prevention.cancer.gov/programs-resources/programs/ccop/about/facts

National Cancer Institute Division of Cancer Prevention. (n.d.-b). *Community oncology and prevention trials: About the research group.* Retrieved May 28, 2008, from http://prevention.cancer.gov/programs-resources/groups/copt/about

National Cancer Institute of Canada, Clinical Trials Group. (n.d.). *About us: Mission.* Retrieved January 15, 2007, from http://www.ctg.queensu.ca

National Surgical Adjuvant Breast and Bowel Project. (n.d.). *Fifty years of NSABP history: Accomplishments in breast and colorectal cancers.* Retrieved January 15, 2007, from http://foundation.nsabp.org/about_nsabp.asp

North Central Cancer Treatment Group. (n.d.). *About NCCTG.* Retrieved January 15, 2007, from http://ncctg.mayo.edu/about.html

O'Mara, A., Bauer-Wu, S., Berry, D., & Lillington, L. (2007). A needs assessment of oncology nurses' perceptions of National Cancer Institute (NCI)-supported clinical trials networks [Online exclusive]. *Oncology Nursing Forum, 34*(2), E23–E27. Retrieved December 20, 2007, from http://ons.metapress.com/content/kn0385xvx518j658/fulltext.pdf

Radiation Therapy Oncology Group. (n.d.). *Mission statement.* Retrieved January 15, 2007, from http://www.rtog.org/history.html

Ruccione, K., & Kelly, K.P. (2000). Pediatric oncology nursing in cooperative group clinical trials comes of age. *Seminars in Oncology Nursing, 16*(4), 253–260.

Ruccione, K.S., Hinds, P.S., Wallace, J.S., & Kelly, K.P. (2005). Creating a novel structure for nursing research in a cooperative clinical trials group: The Children's Oncology Group experience. *Seminars in Oncology Nursing, 21*(2), 79–88.

Smith, E.L., Skosey, C., Armer, J., Berg, D., Cirrincione, C., & Henggeler, M. (2006). The Cancer and Leukemia Group B Oncology Nursing Committee (1983–2006): A history of passion, commitment, challenge, and accomplishment. *Clinical Cancer Research, 12*(11, Pt. 2), 3638s–3641s.

Southwest Oncology Group. (n.d.). *Visitors.* Retrieved January 15, 2007, from http://www.swog.org/Visitors/Index.asp

Strickland, C.J., Feigl, P., Upchurch, C., King, D.K., Pierce, H.I., Grevstad, P.K., et al. (1997). Improving breast self-examination compliance: A Southwest Oncology Group randomized trial of three interventions. *Preventive Medicine, 26*(3), 320–332.

SECTION V

RESEARCH TRAINING AND EDUCATION

Role of Professional Organizations and Nonprofit Organizations in Advancing Oncology Nursing Research

Gail A. Mallory, PhD, RN, NEA-BC

Introduction

Professional and nonprofit organizations have contributed significantly to the advancement of oncology nursing research. The Oncology Nursing Society (ONS) and the ONS Foundation, in particular, have provided pivotal leadership facilitating nurse scientist communication, thus enabling the growth and development of oncology nursing science. Several other professional and nonprofit organizations, notably the American Cancer Society (ACS), have contributed significantly over the years to the advancement of oncology nursing research.

As oncology nursing science develops, oncology nurse scientists increasingly are contributing to the interdisciplinary development of new knowledge and the translation of that knowledge to patient-centered approaches for people experiencing cancer and their caregivers (from prevention to survival and/or palliative care). This chapter will use the ONS Research Agenda as a framework to address the role of organizations in advancing oncology nursing research and to discuss examples of the increasing interaction among oncology nurse scientists and cancer research funding and policy agencies, all with the goal of providing quality cancer care.

Oncology Nursing Society and ONS Foundation Background

ONS's mission is to promote excellence in oncology nursing and quality cancer care. ONS traces its origin to the first National Cancer Nursing Conference, supported by the American Nurses Association and ACS in 1973. Following this conference, a small group of oncology nurses met to discuss the need for a national organization to support their profession. ONS was founded in 1975 and has facilitated education, research, and collaboration among oncology nurses and oncology nurse scientists since its inception (ONS, n.d.-a). The ONS Foundation has provided funding for oncology nursing research, scholarships, awards, and educational programs since its inception in 1981. The ONS logo, which was redesigned in 2006, states "ONS—Where Oncology Nurses Connect." The synergy created through connections among oncology nurses and nurse scientists at ONS Congresses and National Cancer Nursing Research Conferences (the first four research conferences were supported by ACS), early research committee work, mentoring, project teams, educational programs, advisory panels, and collaborative projects, along with the ONS Foundation's financial support of research initiatives, has led to the recognition of ONS as a leader nationally and internationally in nursing research. As of June 26, 2008, of the 36,827 ONS members, 765 were doctorally prepared (133 reported "nurse scientist" as their primary role) and 463 reported being enrolled either part-time or full-time in doctoral programs. The ONS Advanced Nursing Research (ANR) Special Interest Group (SIG) had 520 members, and the ONS Clinical Trial Nurses (CTN) SIG had 936 members (J. Brown, personal communication, June 26, 2008). The growing number of ONS members with research experience and training provides an incredible opportunity for ONS to continue to facilitate the growth and development of oncology nursing research.

The ONS Foundation had funded 443 research grants for a total of $8,618,687 as of early 2007 (ONS Foundation, 2008). In 1999, the ONS Foundation Board of Trustees launched a capital campaign, "Leading the Transformation," to support the virtual ONS Foundation Center for Leadership, Information, and Research (CLIR) (ONS Foundation, 1999). The research component of CLIR was designed to "shape the future of oncology nursing by conducting nursing intervention studies, training new nurse scientists, and informing cancer professionals and the public about advances in cancer care" (ONS Foundation, 1999). The capital campaign raised more than $16 million, of which nearly $4 million was allocated for research. In 2006, the ONS Foundation launched a major endowment campaign, the Silver Anniversary Campaign, to increase total endowment to $10 million. The campaign focused on creating three endowment pillars for research, education, and leadership development in order to benefit the future of cancer nursing care (C. Byrum, personal communication, June 24, 2008).

The success of the 1999 ONS Foundation capital campaign and the history of ONS research priorities surveys (see Chapter 1) led the 1999 ONS Research Advisory Panel to recommend to the ONS Steering Council and Board of Directors that the 2000 ONS Research Priorities Survey be utilized, along with the research priorities of other cancer and nursing nonprofit organizations and government agencies, to create an ONS Research Agenda (ONS, 2000b). A project team convened in February 2001 at the 5th National Conference on Cancer Nursing Research to develop an ONS Research Agenda (see Chapter 1). The three major goals of the ONS Research Agenda are (www.ons.org/research/information/agenda.shtml)

1. To increase the knowledge base for oncology nursing practice through identifying cutting-edge/critical priority areas of oncology nursing research and recommend mechanisms of support
2. To prepare future oncology nursing researchers who will be well trained and prepared to implement ongoing programs of research and to seek support from major sponsors such as the National Institutes of Health (NIH) and ACS
3. To prepare clinical nurses as critical consumers of research findings that can be applied to practice.

Increasing the Knowledge Base for Oncology Nursing Practice

Many of the strategies utilized by ONS, the ONS Foundation, professional nursing organizations, and nonprofit cancer research funding organizations that have affected oncology nursing research will be described in this section (some have been detailed in other chapters).

Oncology Nursing Society

McGuire and Ropka (2000) provided a summary of ONS's contributions to oncology nursing research from the 1970s to the 1990s. The major ONS strategies to increase the knowledge base for oncology nursing practice in the 1970s included the formation of the ONS Research Committee and the presentation of research sessions at the annual ONS Congress. The ONS Research Committee provided the infrastructure that enabled oncology nurse scientists within ONS to collaborate, leading to the increased research activity and knowledge generation of the 1980s and beyond. The presentation of research sessions at the annual ONS Congress and research publications in the *Oncology Nursing Forum* fostered the dissemination of new knowledge and increased the ability of other oncology nurse scientists to build on that knowledge.

In the 1980s, ONS began conducting oncology nursing research priorities surveys (see Chapter 1). Research sessions continued to be presented at the annual ONS Congress, and the ONS/Schering Excellence in Research Award was initiated. The *Oncology Nursing Forum* incorporated a column authored by ONS Research Committee members on measuring clinical phenomena (McGuire & Ropka, 2000).

The ONS ANR SIG was formed in 1989. The 2008 ANR SIG membership of more than 500 demonstrates the important role that the ANR SIG continues to play in facilitating communication among oncology nurse scientists toward the development of new knowledge for practice. The ONS Excellence in Cancer Nursing Research Award is still in existence "to recognize and support excellence in cancer nursing research likely to make a significant contribution to the body of nursing knowledge" (ONS, n.d.-e).

In the 1990s, the groundwork that had been built in the 1970s and 1980s within ONS to support knowledge generation came to fruition in a variety of ways. A special advanced research session at the annual ONS Congress, the ONS Distinguished Researcher Award, was initiated in 1992 (see Chapter 2); ONS state-of-the knowledge conferences were held on fatigue, outcomes, pain, and quality of life ("Conference Addresses Nurse Sensitive Outcomes," 1999; King et al., 1997; "State-of-the-Knowledge Conference," 1994; Winningham et al., 1994); and an ONS research director was hired. ONS restructured from committees to an innovative model utilizing a Steering Council, including the ONS research director as a standing member, specific project teams, and advisory panels (research, education, and membership). The ONS research director and the Research Advisory Panel work closely to advance the generation of new knowledge for practice. The ONS Board of Directors also supported a nursing researcher liaison role to three National Cancer Institute (NCI) cooperative groups (Southwest Oncology Group, Eastern Cooperative Oncology Group, and Children's Oncology Group) in the late 1990s, thus increasing the opportunities for interdisciplinary knowledge generation (McGuire & Ropka, 2000). These liaisons from ONS to the NCI cooperative groups laid some of the groundwork for interdisciplinary cancer research knowledge development.

In 1999, ONS took over the management of the National Conference on Cancer Nursing Research, which had been managed by ACS from 1989 to 1997. The 5th National Conference on Cancer Nursing Research was held February 10–13, 1999, in Newport Beach, CA. The purpose of the conference was "to provide a forum for scholarly exchange related to the foundation and advancement of cancer nursing science and practice" (ONS, 1999). Ada M. Lindsey, PhD, RN, FAAN, provided the keynote address, "Cancer Nursing Research: The Next Generation." The conference included 2 plenary sessions, 3 symposia, and 15 abstract sessions (3–4 research presentations each). Lillian Nail, PhD, RN, FAAN, presented the closing session, "Oncology Nursing Research: Inspiration and Challenges of the Future." The attendance was 187 (ONS, 2005b).

The ONS infrastructure to support the generation of new knowledge for practice continued to develop into the 21st century with the addition of ONS Expert Panels, which review the state of the science and knowledge and make research recommendations for specific topics such as nursing-sensitive patient outcomes (NSPOs) (Given & Sherwood, 2005), biotherapy, neutropenia (Nirenberg et al., 2006a, 2006b), and sleep-wake disturbances (Berger, Parker, et al., 2005). The ONS Research Priorities Surveys were conducted in 2000 (Ropka et al., 2002) and 2004 (Berger, Berry, et al., 2005) and were utilized to develop and update the ONS Research Agenda (see Chapter 1) (ONS, 2007b).

In 2005, the ONS Board of Directors requested multiyear strategic plans for NSPOs and for multisite research. Special project teams of ONS members were established to develop these plans. The Outcomes Strategic Plan Project Team included scientists and advanced practice nurses. The ONS Board of Directors approved a five-year outcomes strategic plan in July 2005. *NSPOs* are defined as "patient outcomes that are amenable to nursing interventions" (Given & Sherwood, 2005, p. 773). Examples of symptom management NSPOs include anorexia, constipation, dyspnea, fatigue, nausea and vomiting, pain, and peripheral neuropathy. Economic, functional, and health status NSPOs also are identified (Given & Sherwood). Figure 14-1 summarizes the major goals of the Outcomes Strategic Plan. Outcomes research knowledge has been disseminated through ONS national conferences, regional conferences, and ONS chapters and at non-ONS meetings.

The Multisite Research Project Team included researchers and clinical trial nurses. The ONS Board of Directors approved a three-year multisite research strategic plan (see Table 14-1) in August 2005 (ONS, 2005c). The ONS Multisite Research Strategic Plan led to the organization of two project teams, Data Sharing in 2006 and Core Data Set in 2007, with the charge of developing

---

Figure 14-1. Oncology Nursing Society Nursing-Sensitive Patient Outcomes Strategic Goals, 2006–2010

- To increase ONS member awareness and ability to identify nursing-sensitive patient outcomes
- To obtain and distribute funding for nursing-sensitive patient outcomes research guided by the ONS Research Agenda
- To increase consumer awareness of the value of oncology nurses to nursing-sensitive patient outcomes
- To increase awareness of oncology nurses' contributions to patient outcomes through policy activities
- To identify core clinical and research instruments and database structure to collect and analyze nursing-sensitive patient outcomes
- To develop and maintain up-to-date recommendations for appropriate outcomes measurement tools and levels of evidence for interventions for outcomes

Note. Based on information from "ONS Outcomes Strategic Plan 2006–2010," Oncology Nursing Society Internal Report, July 2005.

Table 14-1. Oncology Nursing Society (ONS) Multisite Research Strategic Plan, 2006–2008

Group	Goals
Top Priority	
Education	Educate target audiences about multisite research and role-related opportunities. Target audiences include nurse scientists, project managers, clinical trial nurses, clinical research associates, and data collectors.
Mentorship	Develop a mentorship program for ONS nurse scientists and advanced practice nurses to facilitate their participation in multisite research groups and networks, including leadership roles.
National Research Advocacy	Create one or more proactive mechanisms to monitor and influence the national research agendas.
Marketing	Initiate a national marketing campaign for the public about nursing multisite research.
Second Priority	
Data Cooperative	Explore the possibility of creating a nursing network data cooperative and/or adding oncology nursing variables to existing research networks where participants agree to use common data elements and to share their data.
Multisite Research Language	Insert language regarding multisite research in existing and future ONS documents.
Partnership	Explore potential opportunities for ONS partnerships with existing multisite research groups and networks.
Third Priority	
Expanded Marketing	Motivate deans, nursing administrators, funding agencies, and consumers to become involved in nursing multisite research.
ONS Membership Involvement	Facilitate ONS membership involvement in multisite research.

Note. Based on information from Oncology Nursing Society, 2005c.

recommendations for ONS's role in facilitating data sharing across research projects and clinical settings. The 2006 Data Sharing Project Team identified issues and made recommendations, including suggesting that the Core Data Set Project Team be formed to identify and implement a process to reach consensus on core research and clinical measures for specific patient outcomes (ONS, 2006c). The use of these measures in research and clinical practice will facilitate consistent measurement of key oncology nursing variables so that knowledge can be measured and synthesized across settings and studies to generate new knowledge.

ONS continued to manage the biennial National Conference on Cancer Nursing Research in 2001 (211 participants), 2003 (349 participants), 2005 (377 participants), and 2007 (497 participants) (ONS, 2005b). The 9th National Conference on Cancer Nursing Research was held February 8–10, 2007, in Hollywood, CA. The target audience was expanded to include advanced practice nurses and clinical trial nurses. More than 105 doctoral students attended the conference, demonstrating a strong interest in the development of new knowledge for oncology nursing practice within ONS membership (ONS, 2007a).

ONS Foundation

The mission of the ONS Foundation is "to improve cancer care and the lives of people with cancer by funding oncology nursing research, scholarships, awards, and educational programs" (ONS Foundation, n.d.). The ONS Foundation has provided major financial support for the generation of new knowledge for oncology nursing practice. The ONS Foundation Small Research Grants Program started in the 1980s and expanded to include major research grants ($25,000–$500,000) in the 1990s and 2000s through the 1999 capital campaign and subsequent funding.

In 1995, the ONS Foundation funded an innovative five-year project through a professional education, public education, and research initiative known as FIRE® (the Fatigue Initiative through Research and Education). The purpose of FIRE® was to improve the basic understanding of the biophysical mechanisms and social/personal consequences of cancer-related fatigue. The research components of the FIRE® initiative included (ONS, 2003)

- Three $50,000 Development Grants to promote the design of pilot projects that would lead to the application for a FIRE® Fatigue Multi-Institutional Research Grant (awarded in December 1995)
- One Fatigue Clinical Research Scholar, funded 1996–1998
- Three $50,000 Cancer-Related Fatigue Instrumentation Grants, funded 1997–1998 (Hockenberry et al., 2003; Piper et al., 1999; Schwartz et al., 2002)
- The $500,000 FIRE® Fatigue Multi-Institutional Research Grant, funded 1997–2000 (Mock et al., 2005).

The ONS Foundation FIRE® initiative was a unique opportunity to influence the generation of knowledge related to cancer treatment–related fatigue. Several recipients of these grants were invited to present at a 2002 NIH State-of-the-Science Conference on Symptom Management in Cancer: Pain, Depression, and Fatigue, demonstrating the impact of the FIRE® initiative on the generation of knowledge related to cancer treatment–related fatigue (Beck, 2004; Mock, 2004; Mock, Nail, & Grant, 1998; Nail, 2004).

Several other ONS Foundation major grants have been funded since 1998 and are summarized in Table 14-2. In 2007, three calls for proposals for Major

Research Grants for a total of more than $500,000 were distributed (ONS, n.d.-b):
* Adherence to oral chemotherapeutic agents—Two $200,000 grants
* Certification and outcomes (Oncology Nursing Certification Corporation)—$60,000
* Breast cancer—$100,000

Table 14-2. ONS Foundation Major Grant Funding, 1998–2007			
Type of Grant	Grant Year	Number Funded	Amount Awarded
Acute Care Outcomes Study	1998	1	$418,395
Adherence to Oral Chemotherapeutic Agents	2007	2	$399,938
Biotherapy Grant Phase I	2000	3	$199,972
Biotherapy Grant Phase II	2001	1	$169,236
Biotherapy Grant Phase III	2002	0	$0
Breast Cancer Research Grant	2006	1	$100,000
Breast Cancer Research Grant	2007	1	$100,000
Lung Cancer Study	1999	1	$400,000
Nausea and Vomiting Study	1999	1	$200,025
Neutropenia Grant Phase I	2001	3	$207,533
Neutropenia Grant Phase II	2002	0	$0
Neutropenia Grant Phase III	2003	1	$277,947
Outcomes Grant Phase I	2001	3	$74,056
Outcomes Grant Phase II	2001	3	$216,217
Outcomes Grant Phase III	2002	1	$100,000
Outcomes Grant Phase IV	2004	4	$178,556
Practice Change Grant Phase I	2003	1	$49,006
Practice Change Grant Phase II	2004	2	$100,000
Symptom Cluster Grant	2004	2	$360,000
Symptom Management Grant Phase I	2001	4	$199,937
Symptom Management Grant Phase II	2002	2	$400,000
Symptom Management Grant Phase III	2004	2	$149,967
Note. Based on information from ONS Foundation, 2008.			

Clearly, ONS Foundation research grant funding has significantly supported the ONS Research Agenda's objective of generating new knowledge.

Other Cancer Research Nonprofit Organizations

As mentioned earlier, ACS initiated several of the strategies that laid the groundwork for the generation of new knowledge related to oncology nursing research and its impact on practice and patient care. Barckley (1964) noted that ACS has supported cancer nursing since the 1940s, and the ONS Web site noted that an ACS conference in 1973 provided the impetus for the creation of ONS (ONS, n.d.-a). The ACS research grant program funded more than $20 million in psychosocial and behavioral research in fiscal year 2005–2006. Oncology nurse scientists have received funding from ACS and serve on the Peer Review Committee for Cancer Control and Prevention: Psychosocial and Behavioral Aspects of Cancer Research (ACS, n.d.).

The ACS Professorship in Oncology Nursing was awarded from 1981 to 1994 to outstanding oncology nursing faculty through a very competitive review process. The goal of the program was "to enhance the care of cancer patients and their families and those at risk for cancer" (V. Krawiec, personal communication, April 10, 2007).

ACS's initiation and management of the first four National Conferences on Cancer Nursing Research were a significant contribution to the dissemination of new knowledge. The first conference was held November 30–December 1, 1989, in Atlanta, GA. The purpose of the conference was to "bridge the gap between nursing research and practice and to create a milieu for scholarly exchange" (ACS, 1989, p. 5). The conference chair was Jean Johnson, PhD, RN, FAAN, and the program committee consisted of ACS professors of oncology nursing from around the country. Karin Kirchhoff, PhD, RN, FAAN, presented the keynote address, "Bridging the Gap Between Research and Practice." Jeanne Quint Benoliel, DNSc, RN, FAAN, presented the conference summary, "From Research to Scholarship: Personal and Collective Transitions" (ACS, 1989). The ACS Nursing Committee noted in 1990 that the first conference was evaluated positively and that the participants requested that the conference continue to be held on a regular basis (V. Krawiec, personal communication, April 10, 2007). The 4th National Conference on Cancer Nursing Research was managed by ACS in cooperation with the Association of Pediatric Oncology Nurses and ONS and was held January 23–25, 1997, in Panama City, FL (ACS, 1996). The ONS/ACS State-of-the-Science Lectureship Award was first awarded in 2001 at the 6th National Conference on Cancer Nursing Research and was supported by an ACS donation (ONS, 2001), and ACS also sponsored the conference in 2003, 2005, and 2007. ACS also has provided scholarships for master's-prepared nurses and graduate and doctoral students to attend the research conference. ACS clearly has been a leader in supporting the generation of new knowledge for oncology nursing practice through its research grants and the initiation of the conference.

Other cancer research funding organizations, such as Susan G. Komen for the Cure (www.komen.org) and the Lance Armstrong Foundation (www.livestrong.org), and several government agencies, such as NCI (www.cancer.gov), the National Institute of Nursing Research (NINR) (2006), and the U.S. Congressionally Directed Medical Research Programs (http://cdmrp.army.mil), have funded cancer nurse scientists and significantly affected new knowledge growth related to oncology nursing practice (see Chapter 22). The American Brain Tumor Association provides support for an annual $10,000 ONS Foundation Small Grant for neuro-oncology nursing research (ONS, n.d.-f).

Nursing Professional Organizations

Several nursing professional organizations fund research grants that contribute to the generation of new nursing knowledge. The American Nurses Foundation (ANF) has awarded more than 950 nursing research grants since 1955 totaling more than $3.5 million (ANF, 2007). Several of the ANF grants were awarded for oncology nursing research. Sigma Theta Tau International Honor Society of Nursing and its chapters have been funding nursing research since 1936 and provided the first nursing research grant in the United States. Sigma Theta Tau International (2007a) funds more than $650,000 annually through its chapters and grant partners. Sigma Theta Tau International and the ONS Foundation jointly fund a $10,000 small grant annually, and other Sigma Theta Tau research grants fund research related to the care of people with cancer. In addition, other 2005 and 2006 Sigma Theta Tau International research grants were awarded for studies related to cancer (Sigma Theta Tau, 2007b). The four regional organizations, the Eastern Nursing Research Society (www.enrs-go.org), the Midwest Nursing Research Society (www.mnrs.org), the Southern Nursing Research Society (www.snrs.org), and the Western Institute of Nursing (www.ohsu.edu/son/win), also accept applications for small research grants related to the care of people with cancer. Clearly, numerous nursing professional organizations fund research grants that increase the knowledge base related to the care of people with cancer.

In addition to research grants, many nursing professional organizations and regional nursing research societies provide awards for outstanding contributions to research. The Association of Pediatric Hematology/Oncology Nurses (APHON) awards the APHON Distinguished Researcher Award (APHON, n.d.-a) and the APHON Novice Researcher Award annually (APHON, n.d.-b). Oncology nurse scientists frequently have received prestigious research awards from national and regional nursing professional organizations.

Preparing Future Oncology Nurse Scientists

Oncology Nursing Society

Many of the ONS strategies to increase the knowledge base for nursing practice also provide a mechanism to prepare future scientists. The ANR SIG and the CTN SIG both provide communication opportunities through the SIG Virtual Communities and newsletters. Articles in the newsletters from members and from the ONS Research Team staff frequently describe opportunities for mentoring. The ONS Research Team manages a Research Consultation Program (ONS, n.d.-b) in which members who have questions related to research are paired with doctorally prepared ONS nurse scientists with expertise in the consultee's area of interest. The nurse scientist consults with, mentors, and provides assistance to the consultee. ONS members can access the e-mail addresses of other members through the online membership directory, facilitating communication for mentoring and collaboration.

As mentioned previously, the biennial National Conference on Cancer Nursing Research provides excellent opportunities for networking and learning about issues and methods related to conducting research. Sessions at the annual ONS Congress, the Institutes of Learning, the Advanced Practice Nursing Conference, and regional conferences frequently include sessions related to conducting research. All of these educational programs offered by ONS also contribute to the preparation of new oncology nurse scientists. The research sessions at general ONS conferences have kindled the enthusiasm of nonresearchers to consider a research career.

From 1983 to 2004, the ONS/NCI Cancer Nursing Research Short Course was offered through funding from an NCI R25 grant. The objectives of the course were to

> (a) Conduct a national forum for exchange between distinguished oncology nursing faculty and competitively selected pre- and postdoctoral nurses from different institutions and (b) use the critique process as an innovative approach to strengthen the scientific nature of the competitively selected research proposals. (Grant, Mooney, Rutledge, Gerard, & Eaton, 2004, p. E33)

The ONS/NCI Research Short Course provided new investigators with critique and guidance from experienced oncology nurse scientists. Many of the new investigators came from institutions where minimal to no resources were available for mentorship in the conduct of oncology nursing research. In a follow-up evaluation of the participants from 1984 to 1998, many reported "the course was a turning point in their research development" (Grant et al., 2004, p. E36). The experienced research members of ONS worked within the ONS infrastructure and the funding provided by NCI to create a strong and long-lasting mechanism to prepare future oncology nurse scientists.

An additional contribution toward education and training of nurse scientists developed from the ONS Multisite Research Strategic Plan. A framework and set of core competencies for investigators for the conduct of multisite research were developed and have been validated in 2007. Instructional sessions related to conducting multisite research have been presented at ONS national meetings (ONS, n.d.-d).

ONS Foundation

The ONS Foundation has implemented several strategies to support the development of new scientists. One to four ONS Foundation fellowships have been awarded annually since 1993. The purpose of the fellowship is to support short-term oncology research training and mentorship. The amount of the fellowship was $13,700 from 1993 until it was raised to $18,700 in 2005 and then to $20,000 in 2006 (ONS, n.d.-i). The ONS Foundation initiated a New Investigator Award in 2001 to be awarded biennially at the National Conference on Cancer Nursing Research. This award recognizes the contributions of new investigators in building a scientific foundation for oncology nursing practice (ONS, n.d.-j). In 2007, this award was renamed the Victoria Mock New Investigator Award. The ONS Foundation provides three scholarships for doctoral study (two $3,000 scholarships and one $5,000 scholarship) annually to provide support for nurses pursuing doctoral education. The recognition and support of the ONS Foundation through the fellowships, awards, and doctoral and research conference scholarships provide strong resources for the preparation of new scientists and their ongoing development.

The ONS Foundation also has supported creative strategies to complement the researcher development strategies offered by ONS through conferences and the ONS/NCI Research Short Course (1984–2004). In 2004 and 2006, ONS Foundation Research Grant-Writing Education Mentorship Programs were held to assist master's-prepared nurses to develop grant-writing skills. In 2004, four master's-prepared nurses whose ONS Foundation Small Research Grant applications were not funded were selected to work closely with a recently retired oncology nursing researcher to resubmit their grant applications. In 2006, four master's-prepared nurses were selected through a competitive application process to work with a recently retired oncology nurse scientist to prepare and submit an ONS Foundation Small Research Grant proposal based on a clinical problem identified in their practice. This intensive research coaching program for master's-prepared nurses helped them to develop a research team and prepare a research proposal for submission or resubmission, a very innovative strategy to prepare future oncology nurse scientists (ONS, 2006a).

In 2006, the ONS Foundation Research Institute took place. The institute provided training and mentorship to doctorally prepared nurse scientists who had received previous research funding and submitted a plan to build their program of research by obtaining funding at the next level. Twelve applicants were selected to work with four experienced research mentors over a three-day intensive weekend program (ONS, 2006b).

The ONS Foundation Small Grants Program has provided Novice Investigator Research Awards and in 2006 developed a grant funding mechanism to enable new investigators to work with a mentor to prepare an application for the ONS Foundation Small Grants Program (ONS, n.d.-g).

In 2006, the ONS Foundation supported an innovative ONS Foundation Interdisciplinary Multisite Research Training Program. Five interdisciplinary research teams within the NCI cooperative groups led by oncology nurse scientists new to research worked with NCI cooperative group leaders, NCI staff, and other nurse scientists with research funded through the cooperative group to develop a proposal to submit through the cooperative group research review infrastructure. The goals of the program were to

1. Describe the mechanism for developing a research concept that contributes to the science of NCI cooperative groups
2. Explain issues related to clinical trial research
3. Identify strategies for implementing interdisciplinary research within an NCI cooperative group.

Several sessions from the program are on the ONS Web site as webcasts (ONS Foundation, 2006). The support of this program by the ONS Foundation demonstrated a significant step toward the development of nurse scientists as leaders within interdisciplinary research teams.

Cancer Research Nonprofit Organizations

ACS created several innovative strategies in the 1980s to assist in the development of oncology nurse scientists. ACS developed its Scholarship and Professorships in Oncology Nursing Program to enhance the care of people with and at risk for cancer and their families by strengthening nursing practice. It accomplishes this goal by providing assistance for advanced preparation in research, education, administration, and clinical practice in cancer nursing (ACS Scholarships in Cancer Nursing and Professorships in Oncology Nursing Report, 1995, V. Krawiec, personal communication, April 13, 2007). In 1986, the ACS Nursing Advisory Group recommended that ACS support three $8,000 doctoral scholarships in response to the need to prepare expert clinicians, educators, and scientists in cancer nursing. Although the national ACS office no longer supports the ACS Professorship in Oncology Nursing, ACS has supported more than 20 professorships beginning in 1981. The ACS funding of ACS Professors in Oncology Nursing enabled several oncology nursing faculty scientists to mentor and educate new oncology nurse scientists throughout the years that the program was in existence (V. Krawiec, personal communication, April 10, 2007).

Nursing Professional Organizations

Several professional nursing organizations have enhanced the preparation of oncology nurse scientists. Regional nursing research societies, Sigma Theta

Tau International, the International Society of Nurses in Cancer Care, ANF, and the Council for the Advancement of Nursing Science (2007) all provide education, collaboration, and mentorship opportunities that facilitate the development of nurse scientists.

Preparing Clinical Nurses as Critical Consumers of Research Findings

Oncology Nursing Society and ONS Foundation

Since 1996, when the investigators of the ONS/NCI Research Short Course proposed offering a Research Utilization (RU) Short Course, ONS has initiated several strategies to prepare its clinical members (staff nurses and advanced practice nurses) to be critical consumers of research. The one-day ONS/NCI RU Short Course (funded by an NCI R25 grant) was modeled after the ONS/ NCI Research Short Course described previously. The course joined faculty experts in RU methodology with nurses proposing research-based practice changes involving patients with cancer (Rutledge, Mooney, Grant, & Eaton, 2004). The course involved didactic content and a participant presentation of a proposed RU practice change with discussion of the strengths and weaknesses of the proposed project by faculty. An evaluation of the long-term impact of the program on the participants' practices confirmed the difficulty of implementing evidence-based practice (EBP) changes in the practice setting. Despite the barriers in the practice setting, several of the participants were able to successfully carry out their proposed practice changes, and some of the participants went on to implement other EBP changes in their settings (Rutledge et al.).

The ONS Steering Council identified the need to educate ONS members about EBP (ONS, 2000a). At the 2000 Advanced Practice Nursing (APN) Retreat (funded by the ONS Foundation), EBP content was presented as one of the sessions. In 2001, a project team convened to develop an online EBP Resource Area on the ONS Web site (ONS, n.d.-c). The ONS EBP Resource Area was launched at the 2001 Institutes of Learning conference and provided the basis for the next step in ONS's journey toward educating its members to become consumers of research. At the December 2001 APN Retreat, a project team met to determine the available evidence base for specific patient-related oncology topics. The project team members reviewed and critiqued systematic reviews and summarized them for the ONS EBP Resource Area and for publication (Clark, Cunningham, McMillan, Vena, & Parker, 2004; Joyce, McSweeney, Carrieri-Hohlman, & Hawkins, 2004). The 2002/2003 APN Retreat (funded by the ONS Foundation) also focused on EBP by educating all of the participants about the process of finding and critiquing systematic reviews for selected patient-related oncology topics. The process and the examples of the critiques were added to the ONS EBP Resource Area. Also in 2003, an ONS Outcomes Project Team was established and continued to develop the concept of EBP as it applied to oncology NSPOs (see Chapter 17). A five-year ONS Outcomes Strategic Plan was developed in 2005 (ONS, 2005d). The ONS EBP Resource Area and the ONS Outcomes Resource Area continue to develop and expand through the work and advice of the Evidence-Based Practice/Outcomes Subgroup of the Research Advisory Panel and the Outcomes Project Teams (ONS, n.d.-h).

In March 2007, the ONS Board of Directors approved the formation of the Evidence-Based Practice Change Focus Group (www.ons.org/membership/ focusgroups.shtml), indicating that enough interest exists within the membership to begin networking about EBP. Many ONS focus groups become SIGs. The Evidence-Based Practice Change Focus Group may develop into an ONS SIG devoted to preparing clinical nurses as critical consumers of research.

As advanced practice nurses became more involved with EBP, more topic and discussion group submissions have been received and accepted by ONS Congress, Institutes of Learning, and APN Conference planning teams over the past few years, so more education is occurring throughout ONS in a variety of educational venues. A CD-ROM of the 2005 Institute on Nursing-Sensitive Patient Outcomes (funded by the ONS Foundation) was distributed to all ONS members (ONS, 2005a).

Clearly, ONS and the ONS Foundation have made significant progress toward the ONS Research Agenda's aim of preparing clinical nurses as critical consumers of research findings to affect practice.

Nursing Professional Organizations

Other nursing organizations, such as the American Nurses Credentialing Center (ANCC), which approves facilities as Nurse Magnet™ hospitals, and Sigma Theta Tau International, also have made significant contributions to the preparation of clinical nurses to be critical consumers of research. ANCC developed the Magnet Recognition Program® to recognize healthcare organizations that meet its nursing excellence criteria. The program is also an avenue for the dissemination of successful nursing practices and strategies (ANCC, 2008a).

The research/EBP requirement for achieving Magnet status states

> The nursing organization must be able to demonstrate the presence of well established and operationalized structures and processes for research and evidence-based practice. The sources of evidence must demonstrate several examples of the integration and acculturation of evidence-based practice and nursing research by direct care nurses. The Nursing Research Council/Committee or a similar type of structure must be well established. The outcomes from the council or committee must demonstrate how nursing research and evidence-based practice is supported and implemented throughout the organization. (ANCC, 2008b)

This research/EBP component of the ANCC Magnet Recognition Program has contributed significantly to the preparation of clinical nurses in hospitals to utilize research findings in their practices.

The Sigma Theta Tau International journal, *Worldviews on Evidence-Based Nursing*, has provided additional resources for EBP. *Worldviews* is a quarterly, peer-reviewed journal that provides knowledge synthesis and research articles on best evidence to support best practices globally for nurses in a wide range of roles, from clinical practice and education to administration and public healthcare policy (Sigma Theta Tau International Honor Society of Nursing, 2007c).

As research generates more knowledge for nursing practice, more print, online, and educational resources from nursing organizations will be available to prepare clinical nurses as critical consumers of research findings.

Oncology Nursing Science Contributions to Cancer Research Funding Organizations and Selected Government Agencies

This summary of some of the contributions of professional organizations and nonprofit organizations to the advancement of nursing science has demonstrated how nursing science has grown significantly through these relationships. As nursing science has developed, the opportunity for nurse scientists, clinical trial nurses, and cancer scientists of other professions to interact has increased. Cancer clinical trial nurses have been key members of interdisciplinary research teams within the NCI cooperative group structure (see Chapter 13). As ONS multisite research initiatives develop, increased collaboration between nurse scientists and clinical trial nurses is influencing the design and patient focus of cancer clinical trials.

Several other national and international cancer research funding organizations have gained increased awareness of the types of research conducted by oncology nurse scientists through the ONS Foundation's membership in the International Cancer Research Portfolio (ICRP). The ICRP partners are international cancer funding organizations and government agencies that agreed in September 2000 to code their research portfolios with a Common Scientific Outline, to use the information in the ICRP database to analyze research trends, and to use these trends to develop international cancer research priorities (ICRP, n.d.) The research grants funded by the ONS Foundation since 2004 are on the ICRP Web site along with the research grants funded by the ICRP partner organizations.

Another significant contribution of oncology nursing science to interdisciplinary cancer research was several oncology nurse scientists' participation in the NIH State-of-the-Science Conference on Symptom Management in Cancer: Pain, Depression, and Fatigue held in Bethesda, MD, July 15–17, 2002. An expert panel listened to the presentations and prepared a consensus statement

(NIH State-of-the-Science Panel, 2004). Oncology nurse scientists presented papers on fatigue (Mock, 2004; Nail, 2004), pain (McGuire, 2004), and symptom clusters (Beck, 2004; Dodd, Miaskowski, & Lee, 2004; Miaskowski, 2004; Paice, 2004). The strong involvement of nurse scientists as leaders in cancer symptom management and quality-of-life research continues within NCI and NINR as new initiatives within the field of cancer research develop.

One of the top priority initiatives from the ONS Multisite Research Strategic Plan included increased advocacy and partnerships to influence the national cancer research agenda. The 2006 Multisite Research Advocacy and Partnership Project Team participated in the ONS Board recommendation of oncology nurse scientists to key NCI cancer panels and committees and set up a process for monitoring and responding to opportunities for involvement in cancer research leadership panels.

Conclusion

This chapter has summarized many of the extensive contributions of professional and nonprofit organizations to the advancement of oncology nursing science. The continued involvement of oncology nurse scientists, clinical trial nurses, advanced practice nurses, and staff nurses in nursing and interdisciplinary organizations will ensure that the infrastructure and the opportunity for connections provided by the organizations will continue to contribute significantly to the delivery of high-quality cancer care.

References

American Cancer Society. (1989). *1st National Conference on Cancer Nursing Research program.* Atlanta, GA: Author.

American Cancer Society. (1996). *4th National Conference on Cancer Nursing Research call for abstracts.* Atlanta, GA: Author.

American Cancer Society. (n.d.). *Peer review committee on scholarships and professorships in oncology nursing.* Retrieved April 7, 2007, from http://www.cancer.org/docroot/RES/content/RES_4_1x_Peer_Review_Committee_on_Scholarships_and_Professorships_in_Oncology_Nursing

American Nurses Credentialing Center. (2008a). *Magnet manual updates.* Retrieved June 4, 2008, from http://www.nursecredentialing.org/magnet/apply/updates.html

American Nurses Credentialing Center. (2008b). *What is the magnet recognition program?* Retrieved June 4, 2008, from http://www.nursecredentialing.org/magnet/index.html

American Nurses Foundation. (2007). *History of the American Nurses Foundation.* Retrieved June 4, 2008, from http://anfonline.org/anf/history.htm

Association of Pediatric Hematology/Oncology Nurses. (n.d.-a). *APHON Distinguished Researcher Award.* Retrieved June 4, 2008, from http://www.apon.org/i4a/pages/Index.cfm?pageID=3636

Association of Pediatric Hematology/Oncology Nurses. (n.d.-b). *APHON Novice Researcher Award.* Retrieved June 4, 2008, from http://www.apon.org/i4a/pages/Index.cfm?pageID=3638

Barckley, V. (1964). Enough time for good nursing. *Nursing Outlook, 12*(4), 44–48.

Beck, S.L. (2004). Symptom clusters: Impediments and suggestions for solutions [Abstract]. *Journal of the National Cancer Institute Monographs, 2004*(32), 137–138.

Berger, A.M., Berry, D.L., Christopher, K.A., Greene, A.L., Maliski, S., Swenson, K.K., et al. (2005). Oncology Nursing Society year 2004 research priorities survey. *Oncology Nursing Forum, 32*(2), 281–290.

Berger, A., Parker, K., Young-McCaughan, S., Mallory, G., Barsevick, A., Beck, S., et al. (2005). Sleep/wake disturbances in people with cancer and their caregivers [Online exclusive]. *Oncology Nursing Forum, 32*(6), E98–E126. Retrieved April 7, 2007, from http://ons .metapress.com/content/7244v4525u2j6408/fulltext.pdf

Clark, J., Cunningham, M., McMillan, S., Vena, C., & Parker, K. (2004). Sleep-wake disturbances in people with cancer part II: Evaluating the evidence for clinical decision making. *Oncology Nursing Forum, 31*(4), 747–771.

Conference addresses nurse sensitive outcomes. (1999). *ONS News, 14*(2), 5.

Council for the Advancement of Nursing Science. (2007). *Goals.* Retrieved April 7, 2007, from http://www.nursingscience.org

Dodd, M.J., Miaskowski, C., & Lee, K.A. (2004). Occurrence of symptom clusters. *Journal of the National Cancer Institute Monographs, 2004*(32), 76–78.

Given, B.A., & Sherwood, P.R. (2005). Nursing-sensitive patient outcomes: A white paper. *Oncology Nursing Forum, 32*(4), 773–784.

Grant, M., Mooney, K., Rutledge, D., Gerard, S., & Eaton, L. (2004). Cancer nursing research short course: Long-term follow-up of participants, 1984–1998 [Online exclusive]. *Oncology Nursing Forum, 31*(2), E32–E38. Retrieved April 7, 2007, from http://ons.metapress .com/content/p828320638455455/fulltext.pdf

Hockenberry, M.J., Hinds, P.S., Barrera, P., Bryant, R., Adams-McNeil, J., Hooke, C., et al. (2003). Three instruments to assess fatigue in children with cancer: The child, parent and staff perspectives. *Journal of Pain and Symptom Management, 25*(4), 319–328.

International Cancer Research Portfolio. (n.d.). *Frequently asked questions.* Retrieved April 14, 2007, from http://www.cancerportfolio.org

Joyce, M., McSweeney, M., Carrieri-Hohlman, V.L., & Hawkins, J. (2004). The use of nebulized opioids in the management of dyspnea: Evidence synthesis. *Oncology Nursing Forum, 31*(3), 551–561.

King, C.R., Haberman, M., Berry, D.L., Bush, N., Butler, L., Dow, K.H., et al. (1997). Quality of life and the cancer experience: The state-of-the-knowledge. *Oncology Nursing Forum, 24*(1), 27–41.

McGuire, D.B. (2004). Occurrence of cancer pain. *Journal of the National Cancer Institute Monographs, 2004*(32), 51–56.

McGuire, D.B., & Ropka, M.E. (2000). Research and oncology nursing practice. *Seminars in Oncology Nursing, 16*(1), 35–46.

Miaskowski, C. (2004). Gender differences in pain, fatigue, and depression in patients with cancer. *Journal of the National Cancer Institute Monographs, 2004*(32), 139–143.

Mock, V. (2004). Evidence-based treatment for cancer-related fatigue. *Journal of the National Cancer Institute Monographs, 2004*(32), 112–118.

Mock, V., Frangakis, C., Davidson, N.E., Ropka, M.E., Pickett, M., Poniatowski, B., et al. (2005). Exercise manages fatigue during breast cancer treatment: A randomized controlled trial. *Psycho-Oncology, 14*(6), 464–477.

Mock, V., Nail, L.M., & Grant, M. (1998). Implementing the FIRE® planning grant. *Oncology Nursing Forum, 25*(8), 1389–1412.

Nail, L.M. (2004). My get up and go got up and went: Fatigue in people with cancer. *Journal of the National Cancer Institute Monographs, 2004*(32), 72–75.

National Institute of Nursing Research. (2006). *Research funding.* Retrieved April 20, 2007, from http://www.ninr.nih.gov/ResearchAndFunding

National Institutes of Health State-of-the-Science Panel. (2004). National Institutes of Health state-of-the-science conference statement: Symptom management in cancer:

Pain, depression, and fatigue, July 15–17, 2002. *Journal of the National Cancer Institute Monographs, 2004*(32), 9–16.

Nirenberg, A., Bush, A.P., Davis, A., Friese, C.R., Gillespie, T.W., & Rice, R.D. (2006a). Neutropenia: State of the knowledge part I. *Oncology Nursing Forum, 33*(6), 1193–1201.

Nirenberg, A., Bush, A.P., Davis, A., Friese, C.R., Gillespie, T.W., & Rice, R.D. (2006b). Neutropenia: State of the knowledge part II. *Oncology Nursing Forum, 33*(6), 1202–1208.

Oncology Nursing Society. (1999). *5th National Conference on Cancer Nursing Research syllabus and conference guide.* Pittsburgh, PA: Author.

Oncology Nursing Society. (2000a). Online evidence-based practice toolkit. In *ONS Steering Council business plan.* (Available from Oncology Nursing Society, 125 Enterprise Drive, Pittsburgh, PA 15275-1214)

Oncology Nursing Society. (2000b). ONS Research Agenda. In *ONS Steering Council business plan.* (Available from Oncology Nursing Society, 125 Enterprise Drive, Pittsburgh, PA 15275-1214)

Oncology Nursing Society. (2001). *6th National Conference on Cancer Nursing Research syllabus and conference guide.* Pittsburgh, PA: Author.

Oncology Nursing Society. (2003). *FIRE® final report.* (Available from the Oncology Nursing Society, 125 Enterprise Drive, Pittsburgh, PA 15275-1214)

Oncology Nursing Society. (2005a). *Institutes of Learning syllabus.* (Available from the Oncology Nursing Society, 125 Enterprise Drive, Pittsburgh, PA 15275-1214)

Oncology Nursing Society. (2005b). *National Cancer Nursing Research Conference report.* (Available from the Oncology Nursing Society, 125 Enterprise Drive, Pittsburgh, PA 15275-1214)

Oncology Nursing Society. (2005c). *ONS Multisite Research Strategic Plan, 2006–2008.* (Available from the Oncology Nursing Society, 125 Enterprise Drive, Pittsburgh, PA 15275-1214)

Oncology Nursing Society. (2005d). *ONS Outcomes Strategic Plan, 2006–2010.* (Available from Oncology Nursing Society, 125 Enterprise Drive, Pittsburgh, PA 15275-1214)

Oncology Nursing Society. (2006a). *ONS Foundation research grant writing mentorship education program.* (Available from Oncology Nursing Society, 125 Enterprise Drive, Pittsburgh, PA 15275-1214)

Oncology Nursing Society. (2006b). *ONS Foundation research institute report.* (Available from Oncology Nursing Society, 125 Enterprise Drive, Pittsburgh, PA 15275-1214)

Oncology Nursing Society. (2006c). *ONS multisite research data sharing report.* (Available from Oncology Nursing Society, 125 Enterprise Drive, Pittsburgh, PA 15275-1214)

Oncology Nursing Society. (2007a). *9th National Conference on Cancer Nursing Research: Highlights from the conference.* Retrieved April 19, 2007, from http://www.ons.org/research/documents/pdfs/Research_Conf_Highlights.pdf

Oncology Nursing Society. (2007b). *Oncology Nursing Society 2005–2009 Research Agenda.* Retrieved June 4, 2008, from http://www.ons.org/research/information/documents/pdfs/ONSResAgendaFinal10-24-07.pdf

Oncology Nursing Society. (n.d.-a). *About ONS.* Retrieved April 19, 2007, from http://www.ons.org/about/index.shtml

Oncology Nursing Society. (n.d.-b). *Consult an expert.* Retrieved April 19, 2007, from http://www.ons.org/research/projects/index.shtml

Oncology Nursing Society. (n.d.-c). *Evidence-based practice resource area.* Retrieved April 19, 2007, from http://www.ons.org/evidence

Oncology Nursing Society. (n.d.-d). *Multisite research initiatives: Core competencies in multisite research.* Retrieved June 25, 2008, from http://www.ons.org/research/multisite/core

Oncology Nursing Society. (n.d.-e). *ONS excellence awards.* Retrieved April 19, 2007, from http://www.ons.org/awards/onsawards/cancerNursing.shtml

Oncology Nursing Society. (n.d.-f). *ONS Foundation small research grants.* Retrieved April 19, 2007, from http://www.ons.org/awards/foundawards/neurooncology.shtml

Oncology Nursing Society. (n.d.-g). *ONS Foundation small research grants: 2009 mentored planning grant funding (RE 01A).* Retrieved June 4, 2008, from http://www.ons.org/awards/foundawards/mentoring.shtml

Oncology Nursing Society. (n.d.-h). *Outcomes resource area.* Retrieved April 19, 2007, from http://www.ons.org/outcomes

Oncology Nursing Society. (n.d.-i). *Research fellowship award.* Retrieved April 20, 2007, from http://www.ons.org/awards/foundawards/fellowships.shtml

Oncology Nursing Society. (n.d.-j). *10th National Conference on Cancer Nursing Research Award: Victoria Mock New Investigator Award.* Retrieved June 4, 2008, from http://www.ons.org/awards/onsawards/investigator.shtml

ONS Foundation. (1999). *Leading the transformation* [Brochure]. Pittsburgh, PA: Author.

ONS Foundation. (2006). *Interdisciplinary multi-site research training program.* Retrieved April 14, 2007, from http://onsopcontent.ons.org/education/webcasts/msr/index.shtml

ONS Foundation. (2008). *Summary of research awards, 1984–2007.* (Available from ONS Foundation, 125 Enterprise Drive, Pittsburgh, PA 15275-1214)

ONS Foundation. (n.d.). *Home.* Retrieved April 19, 2007, from http://www.onsfoundation .org

Paice, J.A. (2004). Assessment of symptom clusters in people with cancer. *Journal of the National Cancer Institute Monographs, 2004*(32), 98–102.

Piper, B.F., Dodd, M.J., Ream, E., et al. (1999). Improving the clinical measurement of cancer treatment-related fatigue [Abstract]. In *Better health through nursing research: International state of the science* (p. 99). Washington, DC: American Nurses Association.

Ropka, M.E., Guterbock, T.M., Krebs, L.U., Murphy-Ende, K., Stetz, K.M., Summers, B., et al. (2002). Year 2000 Oncology Nursing Society research priorities survey. *Oncology Nursing Forum, 29*(3), 481–491.

Rutledge, D.N., Mooney, K., Grant, M., & Eaton, L. (2004). Implementation and refinement of a research utilization course for oncology nurses. *Oncology Nursing Forum, 31*(1), 121–126.

Schwartz, A.L., Meek, P.M., Nail, L.M., Fargo, J., Lundquist, M., Donofrio, M., et al. (2002). Measurement of fatigue: Determining minimally important clinical differences. *Journal of Clinical Epidemiology, 55*(3), 239–244.

Sigma Theta Tau International Honor Society of Nursing. (2007a). *About the foundation, board of directors, mission, and annual report.* Retrieved June 4, 2008, from http://www .nursingsociety.org/Foundation/About/Pages?AbouttheFoundation.aspx

Sigma Theta Tau International Honor Society of Nursing. (2007b). *2007–2008 Sigma Theta Tau International Grant Recipients.* Retrieved June 25, 2008, from http://www.nursingsociety .org/Research/SmallGrants/Pages/2007GrantRecipients.aspx

Sigma Theta Tau International Honor Society of Nursing. (2007c). *Worldviews on evidence based nursing.* Retrieved April 18, 2007, from http://www.nursingsociety.org/Publications/ Journals/Pages/worldviews.aspx

State-of-the-knowledge conference on cancer pain identifies nursing's challenges in managing pain. (1994). *ONS News, 9*(6), 5.

Winningham, M.L., Nail, L.M., Burke, M.B., Brophy, L., Cimprich, B., Jones, L.S., et al. (1994). Fatigue and the cancer experience: The state of the knowledge. *Oncology Nursing Forum, 21*(1), 23–36.

CHAPTER 15

Accelerating the Research Translation Continuum to Improve Oncology Patient Outcomes

Ann M. Berger, PhD, RN, AOCN®, FAAN,
and Sandra A. Mitchell, PhD, CRNP, AOCN®

Introduction

The National Cancer Act of 1971 was the primary stimulus that encouraged biomedical research focused on the etiology, treatment, and supportive care related to cancer. During the past 35 years, major advances in basic science have led to the discovery of molecular and epidemiologic factors involved in the etiology of cancer cells. The development of pharmacologic and non-pharmacologic interventions to prevent and treat cancer has accompanied these advances. Early and late translation activities (see Table 15-1) have resulted in regulatory approval of numerous drugs and devices. Supportive care interventions to manage many symptoms have been tested and synthesized into evidence-based guidelines. Yet, widespread dissemination and adoption of these advances have not occurred in practice or in policy and are needed to provide access for all Americans to these scientific breakthroughs (U.S. Department of Health and Human Services [USDHHS], National Institutes of Health [NIH], & National Cancer Institute [NCI], 2006).

Special thanks to Ilisa Halpern Paul, MPP, and Clare Hastings, RN, PhD, FAAN, for their assistance with this chapter.

Table 15-1. Definitions Related to Translation and Dissemination of Research	
Term	**Definition**
Research translation	Encompasses all of the processes involved in developing promising basic laboratory and epidemiologic discoveries into cancer-related drugs and biologics, medical devices, behavioral interventions, methodologies, and instruments, and making these readily available to all segments of the public with cancer and those at risk for cancer
Basic science discovery	Refers to identification of a promising molecule or gene target, a candidate protein biomarker, or a basic epidemiologic finding related to cancer
Early translation	Generally refers to development activities that begin following a promising discovery in the laboratory or in basic epidemiology and continues to the point at which an intervention undergoes initial (phase I/II) testing in the clinic or the community
Late translation	Begins when an intervention demonstrates efficacy in a larger population, receives regulatory approval, if required, and is commercialized or produced so that it can be made available to the public
Dissemination of the intervention	Occurs when information, training, and resources pertaining to the intervention are shared with the providers and/or the public
Adoption of the intervention	Refers to the uptake of new interventions into standard practice by providers or the acceptance of behavioral interventions by patients and the public. This phase also includes postmarketing data collection to support intervention refinement; outcomes, health services, and other research; and provider practice pattern analysis.

Note. Based on information from U.S. Department of Health and Human Services, National Institutes of Health, & National Cancer Institute, 2005.

This chapter focuses on the opportunities that exist for oncology nurse scientists, advanced practice nurses, clinical research nurses, and clinicians to improve oncology nursing-sensitive patient outcomes (NSPOs). Collaboration along the discovery, development, and delivery continuum will lead to improved NSPOs. This chapter addresses individual, cooperative, and interdisciplinary approaches to close the gap between practice and research. The initiatives integrate discovery activities, promote the translation of research into improvements in service delivery, and harness the knowledge gained from clinical application to inform further discovery. The chapter also addresses five major content areas. First, the chapter reviews the process by which discoveries are developed and disseminated into supportive care interventions. Next, contemporary forces are examined that have influenced a focus on evidence-based practice (EBP) and outcomes. Using cancer-related fatigue (CRF) as an exemplar, its evolution is traced from research into practice and policy. The interface between the discovery of new knowledge and the development of that knowledge for application in practice is emphasized. The next segment of the chapter proposes knowledge transfer strategies that may enhance uptake of innovations and promote sustained adoption. The chapter concludes by identifying future directions to accelerate the translation of research into practice and policy.

The Translational Research Continuum

Translational research activities are designed to transform ideas, insights, and discoveries generated through basic scientific inquiry and from clinical or population studies into effective and widely available clinical applications. These applications reduce the incidence and associated morbidity and mortality of cancer. A variety of models of the translational research process have been proposed. Although these models employ various descriptive terms and include a varying number of phases, all describe activities along a continuum from basic science discoveries through adoption in clinical practice (Sussman, Valente, Rohrbach, Skara, & Pentz, 2006). After reviewing the literature, the Translation Continuum Model (USDHHS, NIH, & NCI, 2005) of several processes involved in the discovery, development, dissemination, and adoption of advances in cancer-related care was adapted to guide this chapter (see Figure 15-1). Definitions of key terms related to translating and disseminating knowledge are included in Table 15-1. In Figure 15-1, the process is initiated with basic science discoveries. In the early translation phase, discoveries are developed and tested using phase I/II clinical trials. If the phase I/II trials are not successful, early translation activities are continued. If promising results are obtained, these developments next proceed to later translation through phase III clinical trials and replication studies. The process may once again need to return to the early translation phase or may be ready to move to dissemination, depending on the results of phase III trials. As an innovation enters the adoption phase of the continuum, clinical outcomes data are collected to establish the effectiveness of the intervention. These data may lead to refinement of the intervention and further translational testing (phase IV trials) in this iterative and bidirectional model (Ginexi & Hilton, 2006).

National Efforts to Promote Evidence-Based Practice and Translational Research

The 2004–2005 President's Cancer Panel (USDHHS et al., 2005) identified complex barriers that are related to the current culture of research, including dissemination efforts and regulatory issues that limit access to state-of-the-art cancer information and care. The panel concluded that the academic research

Figure 15-1. Translating Research to Reduce the Burden of Cancer

The Translation Continuum

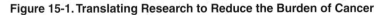

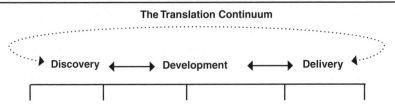

Discovery ⟷ Development ⟷ Delivery

Basic Science Discovery	Early Translation	Late Translation	Dissemination	Adoption
• Descriptive, correlational, qualitative studies • Explanatory mechanisms • Measurement • Analytic techniques developed through simulation studies and secondary data analyses	• Phase I/II trials • Theory building • Intervention development: tailoring, dose finding • Outcomes measure refinement (adaptation for language, educational level) • Comparative studies of analytic techniques • Partnerships and collaboration	• Phase III trials • Replication studies • Partnerships • Production/commercialization • Standardizing methods, materials and messages for intervention delivery • Payment mechanisms • Regulatory approval	• Communication to patients, public, clinicians, administrators, advocates, community leaders • Refinement of intervention to permit widespread use • Partnership to ensure sustained adoption • Outcomes evaluation to examine the external effectiveness of an intervention as it receives widespread use. Patient, clinician, organizational, and societal outcomes should be measured, including effectiveness, feasibility, intervention tailoring, acceptability, and cost.	• Incorporated into training/education curricula • Continued data collection to support intervention effectiveness and to inform provider practices • Payment mechanisms in place to ensure sustained adoption • Innovation reflected in policies of regulatory agencies, accreditation standards, and certification examinations

Note. From *President's Cancer Panel 2004–2005 Annual Report—Translating Research Into Cancer Care: Delivering on the Promise* (p. ii), by U.S. Department of Health and Human Services, National Institutes of Health, and National Cancer Institute, 2005, Bethesda, MD: Author. Copyright 2005 by U.S. Department of Health and Human Services. Adapted with permission.

culture and its structures, practices, and reward systems must be redesigned. This change is needed to remove the significant barriers to collaborative multi- and transdisciplinary research to enhance the widespread adoption of currently available therapies. Factors that slow or impede the transfer of research into practice may be historical, political, economic, scientific, cultural, or organizational (Glasgow & Emmons, 2007). Traditional methods of knowledge dissemination have had a low impact on implementation of new approaches in practice or policy (Grunfeld et al., 2004). Newer dissemination methods need to capture the impact of the adoption of evidence-based interventions on outcomes, cost, and quality (Donaldson, Rutledge, & Ashley, 2004). A number of national agencies have identified translational research among their funding priorities (Laurence, 2006). The NIH Roadmap Initiative (2007) is designed to accelerate fundamental discovery and translation of that knowledge into effective prevention strategies and new treatments. The National Institute of Nursing Research's (NINR's) mission statement includes an imperative to translate scientific advances into cost-effective, high-quality health care. The NINR areas of research priority collectively address projects at all phases in the translation continuum (Grady, 2006, 2007). The recently initiated NIH Institutional Clinical and Translational Science Awards program has been designed to energize the discipline of clinical and translational science in academic health centers (Zerhouni, 2005; Zerhouni & Alving, 2006).

Rogers (2003) has suggested that the properties of the change agent, in addition to the properties of the innovation, are critical to the speed and extent of innovation adoption and diffusion. Rogers developed the stages in the innovation-decision process based on prior work on the hierarchy-of-effects and stages-of-change models. Stages in the innovation-decision process include knowledge, persuasion, decision, implementation, and confirmation. Understanding these stages can help to guide efforts to enhance adoption of research. The limited workforce of translational and clinical scientists in comparison to basic scientists has weakened the national efforts to promote the translation of cancer-related research into practice. Appropriate mentors have been scarce, and grant funding has been limited to disseminate EBP guidelines. The translational research infrastructure currently is inadequate for the required work and is in dire need of additional resources (USDHHS et al., 2005). A variety of approaches to promote the adoption of scientific advances need to be pilot tested to identify models for wider dissemination.

The federal and state regulatory structure affecting translation of cancer-related research is complex and was designed to protect the public's safety. Many current regulations instead impede the pace of new discoveries, developments, and delivery to the public. Managing the maze of regulations from the U.S. Food and Drug Administration, institutional review boards, scientific review committees, and the Health Insurance Portability and Accountability Act is daunting and limits public access to advances in cancer care (USDHHS et al., 2005).

In 1989, the U.S. Congress created the Agency for Health Care Policy and Research (AHCPR) to foster research in healthcare outcomes and to support the development of clinical practice guidelines (Hadorn, Baker, Hodges, & Hicks, 1996). An outcome of AHCPR, which was reauthorized in 1999 as the Agency for Healthcare Research and Quality (AHRQ), was the creation of a mechanism for rating the quality of evidence for clinical practice guidelines. This attempt to ensure the reliability and validity of research study results was an essential step in the process of promoting EBP. The *evidence-based medicine movement*, by definition, combines the integration of clinical expertise with the best available evidence from systematic research and patient/family preferences. This movement has been a major impetus to transferring research results to the bedside (Sackett, Rosenberg, Gray, Haynes, & Richardson, 1996).

Efforts to Promote Evidence-Based Oncology Nursing Practice

The Oncology Nursing Society (ONS) initiated efforts to promote EBP through sponsorship of the Priority Symptom Management (PRISM) project (Ropka & Spencer-Cisek, 2001). Prior to this project, nurses had used the term *research utilization* to denote the process of incorporating research findings into practice (McGuire & Ropka, 2000; Rutledge, Ropka, Greene, Nail, & Mooney, 1998). The PRISM project was a multiphase, multiyear initiative to identify symptom management as a priority for oncology nurses in education, research, healthcare services, and health policy. From these efforts, the PRISM Levels of Evidence were developed based on Hadorn et al.'s (1996) work. Fatigue was one of the first symptoms identified for further discovery, development, and dissemination.

With the focus on symptom management, ONS members proceeded to identify NSPOs that are defined as those patient outcomes that are amenable to nursing intervention. Discovering the independent nursing interventions that reduce symptom burden (e.g., for fatigue) is critical to achieving optimal patient outcomes. By improving NSPOs, oncology nurses are in a position to "drive quality oncology care through clinical practice, research, education, and policy" (Given & Sherwood, 2005, p. 773).

Oncology scientists need to evaluate NSPOs and to frame clinical research in the context of outcomes. One major barrier to outcomes research is the measurement of relevant indicators of the NSPOs. To fill this gap, expert ONS members developed summaries for measuring NSPOs of four outcomes, initially focusing on fatigue, nausea and vomiting, return to usual function, and prevention of infection (Friese & Beck, 2004; Gobel, Beck, & O'Leary, 2006). In the second phase of the project, teams were assembled to synthesize the evidence base for interventions designed to improve each of these outcomes. The teams were responsible for following a rigorous process of critically appraising the research and assigning a weight-of-evidence classification level to each intervention. The ONS Putting Evidence Into Practice® (PEP) Weight of Evidence Classification System (see Table 15-2) was developed by Mitchell and Friese (n.d.) based on the work of Hadorn et al. (1996), Ciliska, Cullum, and

Table 15-2. Oncology Nursing Society Putting Evidence Into Practice® (PEP) Weight of Evidence Classification System

Category	Description	Nature of Available Evidence
Recommended for Practice	Interventions for which effectiveness has been demonstrated by strong evidence from rigorously conducted studies, meta-analyses, or systematic reviews and for which expectation of harms is small compared with the benefits	Interventions with strong evidence from • At least two well-conducted randomized controlled trials each with a sample size of at least 100 participants, and each performed at more than one institutional site. In studies with fewer than 100 participants and a large effect size, observed power of greater than or equal to 80% should be reported or evident. • A meta-analysis of research studies that included a total of 100 participants or more in its estimate of effect size and confidence intervals for the size of the effect. • Systematic review or practice guidelines from a panel of experts that derive from an explicit literature search strategy and include thorough analysis, quality rating, and synthesis of the evidence.
Likely to Be Effective	Interventions for which effectiveness has been demonstrated by supportive evidence from a single rigorously conducted controlled trial, consistent supportive evidence from well-designed controlled trials using small samples, or guidelines developed from evidence and supported by expert opinion	Interventions with consistent supportive evidence from • A single well-conducted randomized controlled trial that included at least 100 participants. In a study with fewer than 100 participants and a large effect size, observed power of greater than or equal to 80% should be reported or evident. • Several rigorously conducted controlled trials using small samples (N < 100). • A meta-analysis that does not include a total of 100 participants or more in its estimate of effect size and confidence intervals for the size of the effect. • A systematic review that derives from an explicit literature search strategy and includes thorough analysis, quality rating, and synthesis of the evidence from rigorously conducted controlled trials using small samples (N < 100). • Guidelines or recommendations that include both expert opinion that an intervention is effective and positive findings from studies that were reviewed critically by a panel of experts.
Benefits Balanced With Harms	Interventions for which clinicians and patients should weigh the beneficial and harmful effects according to individual circumstances and priorities	• Supportive evidence from one or more randomized trials, meta-analyses, or systematic reviews but where the intervention has been associated with adverse effects in certain patient populations. • Such adverse effects include those that contribute or potentially contribute to mortality, significant morbidity, or functional disability, hospitalization, or excess length of stay.

(Continued on next page)

**Table 15-2. Oncology Nursing Society Putting Evidence Into Practice®
(PEP) Weight of Evidence Classification System** *(Continued)*

Category	Description	Nature of Available Evidence
Effective-ness Not Estab-lished	Interventions for which data are insufficient or conflicting or data of inadequate quality, with no clear indication of harm	Interventions with supportive evidence that is insufficient, conflicting, or of poor quality, such as from • A single well-conducted randomized controlled trial with a sample size of less than 100 participants. • A well-conducted case control study. • Conflicting evidence concerning the efficacy of an intervention but with no clear indication of harm. • Supportive or conflicting evidence from a poorly controlled or uncontrolled study. • Evidence from randomized clinical trials with one or more major or three or more minor methodologic flaws that could invalidate the results. • Evidence from nonexperimental studies with high potential for bias (such as case series with comparison to historical controls). • Evidence from case series or case reports.
Effective-ness Un-likely	Interventions for which lack of effectiveness has been demonstrated by negative evidence from a single rigorously conducted controlled trial, consistent negative evidence from well-designed controlled trials using small samples, or guidelines developed from evidence and supported by expert opinion	Interventions where evidence of ineffectiveness is consistent from • A single well-conducted randomized controlled trial that included at least 100 participants and was conducted at more than one institution and showed no evidence of effectiveness. • Several rigorously conducted randomized controlled trials using small samples (N < 100). • A well-conducted case control study, a poorly controlled or uncontrolled study, a randomized trial with major methodologic flaws, or an observational study (e.g., case series with historical controls) that showed no evidence of effectiveness together with a prominent and unacceptable pattern of adverse events and serious toxicities (National Cancer Institute Common Terminology Criteria for Adverse Events [CTCAE] grade III/IV). • Guidelines or recommendations that are supported both by expert opinion that an intervention lacks effectiveness and by negative findings from studies that were reviewed critically by a panel of experts.

(Continued on next page)

**Table 15-2. Oncology Nursing Society Putting Evidence Into Practice®
(PEP) Weight of Evidence Classification System *(Continued)***

Category	Description	Nature of Available Evidence
Not Recommended for Practice	Interventions for which lack of effectiveness or harmfulness has been demonstrated by strong evidence from rigorously conducted studies, meta-analyses, or systematic reviews, or interventions where the costs, burdens, or harms associated with the intervention exceed anticipated benefit	Interventions where strong evidence of ineffectiveness or harmfulness is based on • Two or more well-conducted randomized controlled trials with at least 100 participants and conducted at more than one site and which showed no benefit for the intervention and that excessive costs, burdens, or harms may accrue from the intervention. • A single trial that attributed a prominent and unacceptable pattern of life-threatening adverse events and toxicities (CTCAE grade IV/V) to the intervention. • A meta-analysis of research studies that included a total of 100 participants or more in its estimate of effect size and which demonstrated lack of benefit or prominent and unacceptable toxicities. • Systematic review or practice guidelines from a panel of experts that discourage use of the intervention based on an explicit literature search strategy and include thorough analysis, quality rating, and synthesis of the evidence.

Note. From *ONS PEP® (Putting Evidence Into Practice) Weight of Evidence Classification Schema: Decision Rules for Summative Evaluation of a Body of Evidence,* by S.A. Mitchell and C.R. Friese, n.d. Retrieved September 9, 2007, from http://www.ons.org/outcomes/tables/documents/woevidence.pdf. Copyright by Oncology Nursing Society. Adapted with permission.

Marks (2001), and Ropka and Spencer-Cisek (2001). The new product line, called ONS PEP, provides online and pocket-size resources to assist clinical nurses in gaining knowledge and selecting evidence-based interventions to improve outcomes for patients with cancer (Gobel et al.).

Translational Research in Cancer Symptom Management: Fatigue as an Exemplar

Interest in CRF continues to expand. This growing interest is based both on the prevalence of CRF and on a growing recognition of its contribution to symptom distress. Fatigue frequently occurs as a component of symptom clusters and results in deleterious consequences for functioning and health-related quality of life (QOL). As a model of translational research, CRF offers an example of what can be achieved across the discovery, development, and delivery continuum. An examination of the state of the science of CRF management can offer insights that may promote translational research efforts relative to other important and prevalent clinical problems in oncology nursing. Tracing progress along the discovery, development, and delivery continuum also exemplifies the iterative nature of these phases on the continuum. Problems identified in service delivery play a critical role in shaping the formulation of new discoveries. The problems also illustrate how scientific discoveries need to be further developed through synthesis, dissemination, and innovation adoption before they can achieve widespread application in care delivery.

Early Discoveries: Frameworks and Instruments

The National Comprehensive Cancer Network (NCCN, 2008) defines *cancer-related fatigue* as "a distressing, persistent, subjective sense of tiredness or exhaustion related to cancer or cancer treatment that is not proportional to recent activity and interferes with usual functioning" (p. FT 1). Informed by observations in clinical practice, early research on the problem of CRF employed descriptive and qualitative studies to define the problem. The research studies also helped to gauge CRF's extent and correlates in patients receiving surgical, chemotherapy, radiotherapy, biotherapy, or transplant cancer treatments. The very early research in CRF was conducted using items or subscales of measures developed by other disciplines, such as the Profile of Mood States (Derogatis & Melisaratos, 1983), the Beck Depression Inventory (Beck, Ward, Mendelson, Mock, & Erbaugh, 1961), or the Fatigue Feeling Tone Checklist (Pearson & Byars, 1956). Self-report of fatigue severity was included as a single item embedded in an early symptom checklist developed by nurse scientists (McCorkle & Young, 1978). Nurse scientists also made efforts to understand the biologic mechanisms of CRF through research exploring muscle function and its association with cytokine activity (St. Pierre, Kasper, & Lindsey, 1992).

Through these early discoveries, scholars identified the need to develop theoretical frameworks and explanatory models that could be used to guide fatigue research (Ream & Richardson, 1999). The earliest models proposed by Rhoten (1982) and Aistars (1987) hypothesized that fatigue was a response to the physiologic and psychological stressors associated with the cancer experience. Prolonged or intense exposure to these stressors led to energy depletion, fatigue, and ultimately exhaustion. In contrast, other fatigue models posited that fatigue was a symptom indicating an energy deficit (Irvine, Vincent, Graydon, Bubela, & Thompson, 1994; Piper, Lindsey, & Dodd, 1987; Winningham et al., 1994). These models suggested that fatigue occurred when the human response to illness, symptoms, treatment, and the environment interfered with maintaining energy balance (including energy intake, production, metabolism, and expenditure). Piper et al.'s (1987) Integrated Fatigue Model has had wide influence in both practice and research, creating an understanding of fatigue as a multidimensional sensation with behavioral, affective, sensory, and cognitive components. Olson (2007) hypothesized a model in which tiredness, fatigue, and exhaustion represent distinct states along an adaptation continuum. Each of these states is characterized by unique features in terms of sleep quality, cognition, stamina, emotional reactivity, social interaction, and control over body processes. Olson's model is based both on previously proposed fatigue theories and on empiric data derived from a series of qualitative studies.

Theory building for the phenomenon of CRF represents an important developmental step along the discovery-to-delivery continuum because it directly informs the design of instruments to measure fatigue. Through the evolution of theoretical insights, the conventional clinical wisdom regarding rest for fatigued patients was first challenged. This challenge opened the field to evaluate supportive care interventions such as exercise in CRF management (Winningham, 1992). Building on the conceptualization of fatigue as a multidimensional phenomenon, nurse scientists recognized that discovery could proceed more rapidly if more specific and psychometrically rigorous approaches to the measurement of fatigue were developed. Early efforts included the development of the Piper Fatigue Scale (Piper et al., 1987, 1998). More recent developments include the Situational Fatigue Scale (Yang & Wu, 2005) and fatigue item banks that permit computerized adaptive testing (Lai et al., 2005). These fundamental discoveries have since undergone development to permit their application to patients who speak languages other than English and to test their psychometric properties in various populations of patients with cancer.

Descriptive and Intervention Research

Supported by these fundamental discoveries and theoretical developments, the number of studies that describe the prevalence and correlates of fatigue has been steadily increasing (Barton-Burke, 2006; Bower, 2006; Davis, Khoshknabi, & Yue, 2006; De Jong, Courtens, Abu-Saad, & Schouten, 2002; Iop, Manfredi, & Bonura, 2004; Lawrence, Kupelnick, Miller, Devine, & Lau, 2004; Mock & Olsen, 2003; Morrow, Shelke, Roscoe, Hickok, & Mustian, 2005; Prue, Rankin, Allen, Gracey, & Cramp, 2006; Servaes, Verhagen, & Bleijenberg, 2002; Sood & Moynihan, 2005; Tavio, Milan, & Tirelli, 2002; Wagner & Cella, 2004; White, 2001; Winningham et al., 1994). The ONS Fatigue Initiative through Research and Education (FIRE®) awards gave prominence to the problem of CRF and generated significant research activity. Most of the work was conducted in adults receiving chemotherapy and women with breast cancer. More descriptive and correlational work is needed in understudied populations, including the medically underserved, individuals living in rural settings, and those with diverse racial and ethnic backgrounds. The experience of fatigue in patients with recurrent or terminal disease also has been under-researched. Descriptive studies also are needed that compare the experiences of men and women and increase scientists' understanding of the similarities and differences across various developmental phases. Continued research is needed to enhance the understanding of the association between fatigue and outcomes such as functional status, QOL, and psychological distress.

Cancer care providers and scientists still have a limited understanding of the complex etiology of CRF, despite the increased knowledge of its prevalence and correlates. Emerging research is identifying the multiple causative factors that contribute to the experience of CRF (Bower, 2005; Bower, Ganz, & Aziz, 2005; Bower, Ganz, Aziz, & Fahey, 2002; Bower et al., 2006; Payne, 2004; Schubert, Hong, Natarajan, Mills, & Dimsdale, 2006; Winningham et al., 1994; Wood, Nail, Gilster, Winters, & Elsea, 2006). However, the relative contribution of a range of biobehavioral factors to the development of fatigue syndromes in different populations of patients with cancer is largely unknown. A more thorough understanding of the etiologic factors discovered through basic scientific investigation is needed to inform future development of supportive care interventions and for tailoring of CRF management in specific patient populations.

Although some examples of intervention research in the early 1980s are available (Johnson, Nail, Lauver, King, & Keys, 1988; MacVicar, Winningham, & Nickel, 1989), most of the work testing pharmacologic and nonpharmacologic interventions to manage fatigue has been conducted during the past decade. Exercise, psychotherapy, energy conservation, educational interventions, complementary therapies, and measures to optimize sleep quality are examples of nonpharmacologic interventions. Pharmacologic therapies have included methylphenidate, paroxetine, modafinil, and bupropion. These interventions have been studied in randomized trials, single-arm studies, or small case series (Mitchell, Beck, Hood, Moore, & Tanner, 2007; Mock, 2003; Morrow et al., 2005; Nail, 2002; White, 2001; Winningham, 2001). Many more supportive care interventions need to be tested in phase III clinical trials (Jean-Pierre et al., 2006). Oncology scientists and clinicians are challenged and responsible for disseminating results into practice and to test their effects on patient outcomes as they are published. Curt and Johnston (2003) observed that CRF remains under-researched, and evidence suggests that CRF is suboptimally assessed and treated in clinical practice (Gibson, Garnett, Richardson, Edwards, & Sepion, 2005; Knowles, Borthwick, McNamara, Miller, & Leggot, 2000; Stone et al., 2003).

Promoting the Adoption of Interventions in Clinical Practice

Recently, national efforts have been undertaken to increase awareness among clinicians and scientists and to persuade them to support continued progress in terms of discoveries. These efforts promote the adoption in clinical practice of interventions that have shown at least preliminary effectiveness in preventing or treating CRF. In 2000, NCCN issued the first set of guidelines for the assessment, prevention, and management of CRF. NCCN revises the guidelines at approximately annual intervals and offers a tool to facilitate translation of research and expert consensus into best practices for patients.

In 2002, NIH brought together experts in the field to address key questions regarding the assessment and treatment of CRF, to examine barriers to effective treatment, and to propose directions for future research (NIH, 2002). This effort to achieve consensus and identify the direction for continued work by both scientists and clinicians was an important decisional stage for the translational research process (Patrick et al., 2004).

ONS also has recognized that effective management of CRF and other symptoms is an important responsibility of oncology nurses, whose disciplinary background uniquely positions them to address supportive care practices. ONS's Nursing-Sensitive Patient Outcomes Project identified CRF as one of the first outcomes to be addressed. In the initial phase of this project, several definitions of fatigue were proposed (Cella, Peterman, Passik, Jacobsen, & Breitbart, 1998; Mock et al., 2000; Nail, 2002). The available measures to evaluate fatigue were identified, and their measurement properties and strengths and limitations were summarized on the ONS Web site (ONS, 2004). In addition, interventions to manage CRF were identified for which evidence was at the highest level (multiple randomized trials summarized through meta-analyses) and consensus guidelines were available. Feedback from clinicians indicated that sorting through the burgeoning fatigue intervention literature to select appropriate interventions to apply in practice, and in particular specific patient group(s), increasingly was difficult. ONS then launched an ONS PEP initiative to translate available evidence for fatigue management into practice (Gobel et al., 2006).

ONS PEP teams systematically identified and critically examined all available evidence for the management of CRF. After the evidence supporting each intervention had been examined critically, the collective evidence for each intervention was classified using three criteria: evidence quality, magnitude of the outcome (effect size), and concurrence of the evidence among studies. This resulted in a summary of recommendations for clinical practice that are supported by evidence and are available to clinicians and patients via the Internet. Any individual who wants to examine the evidence used to develop the recommendations can access the evidence tables, which provide a detailed analysis of each study (ONS, n.d.).

Ongoing research includes studies to understand the mechanisms that produce CRF, the prevalence and correlation of fatigue associated with various treatments, and the systematic evaluation of pharmacologic and nonpharmacologic interventions designed to ameliorate CRF. Although guidelines distributed by organizations such as ONS or NCCN are a necessary developmental step in bringing discoveries to the clinic, they alone do not ensure that implementation that leads to optimal care delivery will occur.

To date, limited efforts have been made to design, measure, and evaluate the outcomes achieved through adoption of evidence-based CRF management guidelines in clinical practice. Similarly, few efforts have been made to apply what is known about CRF to the development of health policy that supports evidence-based CRF management. One example of the translation of research findings into health policy related to fatigue is the designation of cancer fatigue as a syndrome, with specific defining features by the International Classification of Disease, 10th revision (ICD-10) (Cella, Davis, Breitbart, & Curt, 2001). By assigning a specific ICD-10 code, these criteria for an official diagnosis of CRF create a mechanism through which services to treat fatigue can be reimbursed. Attention to payment policy thereby removes a previously identified barrier to effective fatigue management (Passik, 2004). Reimbursement also helps to create a climate for sustained adoption of fatigue interventions in clinical practice. Building on descriptive and epidemiologic studies of fatigue in cancer, this definition of CRF as a syndrome with defining features also is a necessary developmental step toward improved screening in clinical practice. Efforts are ongoing to test the sensitivity and specificity of fatigue measures primarily used in research as clinical screening tools for CRF syndrome as defined by the ICD-10 criteria (Van Belle et al., 2005). Similarly, empirical evidence supporting the ICD-10 criteria for CRF is now emerging (Young & White, 2006). This evidence represents an example of how gaps in the knowledge base are necessary to optimize service delivery and provide the momentum for new discoveries. Programs of research on CRF are needed in order to make substantial and sustained contributions to scientific knowledge.

Selected Knowledge Transfer Strategies

Strategies are needed that will promote the dissemination and adoption of research findings and innovations in clinical practice. Without use of effective strategies, new knowledge generated through discovery and development will not close the gap between research and practice, nor will it have a measurable effect on patient outcomes. Rogers (2003) differentiated the *diffusion* of information through communication, and its *adoption*, as demonstrated by the full use in practice of an innovation as the best course of action available. Other authors (Lomas & Haynes, 1988) described *dissemination* as the spread of knowledge from its source to practitioners, whereas *application* is the way those practitioners use knowledge in the delivery of service, including adaptations of knowledge to fit a particular setting. The rates of adoption and implementation of an innovation are influenced by the characteristics of the innovation (e.g., its relative advantage, complexity) and the characteristics of the social system (e.g., the presence of opinion leaders and the effect of change agents), as well as the tendencies of the individual members of that social system to be innovators or early adopters (Rogers).

A number of different strategies to transfer research into practice and to promote the adoption of innovation in the delivery of services can be identified in the literature, but the application of these strategies in cancer care has been limited, and few have undergone systematic evaluation for effectiveness (see Figure 15-2). Many unanswered questions still exist regarding the most effective strategies for dissemination of information (Thompson, Estabrooks,

---

Figure 15-2. Strategies to Promote Dissemination and Adoption of Research Findings and Innovations in Clinical Practice

- Organizational culture that is supportive of innovation and collective action
- Systematic reviews, standards of care, and practice guidelines
- Education
- Audit and feedback
- Dissemination research
- Policy development
- Community education to promote patient-mediated implementation
- Networks that bring together resources for dissemination research

---

Scott-Findlay, Moore, & Wallin, 2007). For instance, which approaches are most effective in promoting the adoption of new research findings or innovations? How should the outcomes of these initiatives be measured? Strategies range from the diffusion of information in which no special efforts are made to promote the spread or application of knowledge, to active efforts to study the effectiveness of an intervention in a population. At the same time, cancer care providers need to optimize organizational culture and build capacity to achieve sustained and widespread delivery of interventions. Rogers (2003) termed this the *confirmation stage.*

Organizational Culture Supportive of Innovation and Collective Action

The translation of discoveries into interventions that improve patient outcomes is optimized in a climate and culture characterized by effective communication and collaboration among scientists and clinicians (Chorpita & Nakamura, 2004). Rogers (2003) has suggested that the characteristics of the change agent are critical moderators of the speed and extent of innovation diffusion. Clinicians and scientists need to understand each other's language and evolve a shared understanding of patients' needs and the challenges of contemporary clinical practice in order to begin to form powerful partnerships for change. Sustaining effective partnerships requires respect for each interdisciplinary team member's unique contributions, talents, and skill set. Partners need to develop an appreciation for the special role each person brings to the relationship, as well as the competing demands and priorities, and perhaps differential organizational imperatives, reward structures, and incentives for collaboration (Fraser, 2004; Loeb et al., 2008; Stokols, Harvey, Gress, Fuqua, & Phillips, 2005). Trust develops among collaborators when the goal of improving clinical outcomes is shared and when all parties derive professional benefit from the collaboration (Krumm & Mock, 2005; Solberg, 2006).

Sussman et al. (2006) described a consensual model of inquiry, wherein people from different backgrounds form a partnership, pooling their complementary expertise as they progress through the phases of intervention program design and evaluation. Baumbusch et al. (2008) detailed a collaborative model for knowledge translation in clinical settings that emphasizes this interactive and reciprocal process. Within these models, technology and expertise flow bidirectionally between clinicians and scientists, and evidence-based practices supplement or are codeveloped with existing practices (Fox, 2003; Pearson, Wiechula, Court, & Lockwood, 2007).

A barrier to achieving this is the top-down lexicon surrounding research utilization, dissemination of research findings, and adoption of innovations. To speak of new interventions or technology being developed, tested, and subsequently dropped into the practice arena may inadvertently imply that clinicians possess little or no knowledge of effective practice (Addis, 2002). An assumption that current practice likely contains strategies that are acceptably evidence-based would result in dissemination efforts that begin with a baseline assessment of the current practices in a system so that attention can be focused on supplementing or adding in the missing features (Chorpita & Nakamura, 2004).

Emerging evidence also suggests that the social context, climate, and culture of an organization and team influence the adoption of innovation and the incorporation of new evidence into practice (Chaffin, 2006; Dopson, 2007; Squires, Moralejo, & Lefort, 2007). Organizational cultures that are more flexible, risk tolerant, innovative, and collaborative tend to be more open to change (Hemmelgarn, Glisson, & James, 2006). Supportive conditions for innovation and knowledge translation exist in organizational cultures that value scientifically sound evidence, focus on measurable outcomes and results, and are committed to continual improvement (Estabrooks, Kenny, Adewale, Cummings, & Mallidou, 2007; Glisson, 2002). Similarly, organizational climates conducive to the uptake of new knowledge tend to be those where providers feel a sense of personal accomplishment, experience lower levels of emotional exhaustion, and believe they are provided with the leadership, support, autonomy, and resources necessary to perform their job effectively (Cummings, Estabrooks, Midodzi, Wallin, & Hayduk, 2007; Estabrooks, Midodzi, Cummings, & Wallin, 2007).

Systematic Reviews, Standards of Care, and Practice Guidelines

Development and dissemination of standards of care and clinical practice guidelines are strategies that often are deployed to promote the translation of research findings into practice. Few of these guidelines or standards emphasize the achievement of specific outcomes, and most are problem focused. Guidelines or practice standards may be developed based predominantly on (a) consensus of expert opinion, (b) evidence from rigorously conducted trials or through a synthesis of expert consensus, and (c) best available evidence. Systematic reviews increasingly form the basis for EBP and for the development of guidelines and, consequently, for making individual and policy-level healthcare decisions. Systematic reviews or evidence-based technology assessments represent a rigorous method of compiling scientific evidence to answer questions regarding healthcare issues. They differ from opinion-based narrative reviews in that they attempt to minimize bias by the comprehensiveness and reproducibility of the search for and selection of articles for review (Whittemore, 2005). Systematic reviews assess the methodologic quality of the studies, together with an evaluation of the overall strength of that body of evidence. Systematic reviews, guidelines, and practice standards may offer an efficient way to critically appraise and summarize evidence related to a specific problem area (Mitchell et al., 2007; Page, Berger, & Johnson, 2006; Zitella et al., 2006) and may serve as a foundation for the introduction of practice changes (Hinds et al., 2003).

The extent to which oncology practitioners adhere to guidelines and the impact of adherence on patient outcomes are just beginning to be studied. Cunningham (2006) examined oncology advanced practice nurses' use of clinical practice guidelines and found that documentation was consistent with a high level of adherence to guidelines from AHRQ for the management of acute pain, depression, and urinary incontinence. Practitioners' adherence to guidelines was lowest for the detection and management of depression. Cunningham also studied the relationship between guideline adherence and outcomes but did not find a relationship between improved outcomes and adherence to guidelines in practice. Whether this was caused by the high level of guideline adherence and, thus, not enough variability was in the sample to permit an association, is unknown. Further research is needed to study the relationship in oncology between adherence to practice guidelines and patient outcomes and to examine the effectiveness of various approaches to guideline dissemination and implementation (Grimshaw et al., 2004, 2006).

Clinician Education

Training approaches such as train-the-trainer activities, involvement of opinion leaders, role modeling, educational workshops, and educational facilitators are applied widely and assumed to be effective in closing the gap between research and practice (Stetler et al., 2006). However, studies in primary care and those related to interventions, such as smoking cessation, suggest that training approaches may achieve only limited outcomes. Much of the research to date has focused on evaluating the efficacy of interventions to promote behavior change among healthcare providers through active interventions such as educational outreach and healthcare provider reminders (McAlister et al., 2005; Sterman, Gauker, & Krieger, 2003). Among the training approaches, a train-the-trainer approach and workshops to prepare role models and local facilitators for dissemination of an intervention have shown modest effectiveness as a strategy (Johnson et al., 2006; MacDermid, Solomon,

Law, Russell, & Stratford, 2006). Less active interventions, such as attending conferences, reading journals, or mailing clinical practice guidelines, were not effective overall in changing provider behavior.

Audit and Feedback

A quality improvement process known as *audit and feedback* seeks to improve patient care through systematic review of the processes and outcomes of care against explicit criteria, the provision of clinician feedback, and where indicated, the implementation of change (National Institute for Clinical Excellence, 2002). As a strategy for improving clinical practice guidelines adherence, this technique has been found to be variably effective (Foy et al., 2005; Jamtvedt, Young, Kristoffersen, O'Brien, & Oxman, 2006). Idell, Grant, and Kirk (2007) evaluated the effects of a combined intervention that included education, advanced practice nurse facilitation, and audit and feedback on pain reassessment practices. This multicomponent intervention was effective in strengthening knowledge and attitudes regarding pain, and pain reassessment practices were improved and brought into alignment with national guidelines. However, few studies have examined whether patient outcomes improve as a result of changes in clinician behavior to comply with guidelines. Further research is needed to determine the characteristics of effective feedback in terms of actionability, nonpunitiveness, and timeliness, as well as to examine the effectiveness of audit and feedback when applied with active educational approaches (Feifer et al., 2006; Hysong, Best, & Pugh, 2006).

Dissemination Research

The terms *dissemination research* and *implementation science* encompass a range of research activities. The diversity of terms used for this type of research (e.g., diffusion, dissemination, knowledge transfer, uptake, utilization, adoption and implementation), as well as inconsistent definition and application of these terms, has hampered progress in these areas (Kerner, Rimer, & Emmons, 2005). According to Titler, Everett, and Adams (2007), *implementation science* is "the investigation of methods, interventions (strategies), and variables to influence adoption of evidence-based healthcare practices by individuals and organizations to improve clinical and operational decision making" (p. S57). The term *dissemination research* may be somewhat broader and typically refers to studies designed to evaluate the *effectiveness* of an intervention in a population and/or to evaluate a process of transferring to a target audience the knowledge, skill, and systems support needed to deliver an intervention (Kerner, 2006; Robinson et al., 2005; Rohrbach, Grana, Sussman, & Valente, 2006; Rubenstein & Pugh, 2006). With the exception of tobacco cessation (Morgan et al., 2003; Stokols et al., 2005), cancer control (AHRQ, 2003; Harris et al., 2005), and behavioral health (Ellis et al., 2005; Kerner, Rimer, et al.), few examples of dissemination research in cancer care exist (Kerner, Guirguis-Blake, et al., 2005).

The example of fatigue will be used to illustrate where implementation science or dissemination research fits along the discovery, development, and delivery continuum. Basic nursing science involves describing relationships among variables and illuminating the etiology or causative factors for a given problem and the mechanisms by which interventions have an effect (Lobo, 2005). Clinical trials, whether a phase I, II, or III study design, help to capitalize on basic science discoveries of etiologies and mechanisms. They also help to develop and to test interventions that will ameliorate the problem of interest. These clinical trials typically examine an intervention in a very controlled setting, with a homogeneous patient population for greater control over covariates and confounding factors, and with strictly defined inclusion and exclusion criteria. The focus is on maximizing internal validity. In the example of fatigue, the scientist might ask, "What are the effects of aerobic exercise and muscle strengthening on fatigue, performance-based measures of physical function, and self-reported functional status in patients with localized prostate cancer who are undergoing a six-week course of radiotherapy?"

As research shifts to dissemination or implementation research, the concern is with both internal and external validity and with the intervention's effectiveness in a large and diverse population (Glasgow & Emmons, 2007). The emphasis also is on treatment fidelity, feasibility, cost, adherence, patient acceptability and satisfaction, participation rates, the characteristics of those who participate and those who do not, any complications that patients experience, and any necessary adjustments or tailoring of the intervention regimen (Bruckenthal & Broderick, 2007; Glasgow & Emmons; Glasgow, Vogt, & Boles, 1999; Perrin et al., 2006).

A key issue related to adoption of innovations is the extent to which an intervention should be adapted for clinical settings. Rogers (2003) suggested that some reengineering of an intervention is a component of the implementation stage of innovation adoption. A balance must be struck between intervention fidelity and feasibility of adoption into practice. As interventions are incorporated into practice, they likely will need to be modified to accommodate several challenges. Some of these challenges include lower motivation of participants than is typical of those who enroll in clinical trials, managed care limitations on the number of billable treatment sessions, and patients' varied reading or education levels. Such adaptations are best accomplished when scientists and clinicians blend their areas of expertise. Rigorously designed dissemination research has an essential role in evaluating the effectiveness of widespread intervention implementation on clinical outcomes, cost, and patient satisfaction.

In the example of fatigue, the dissemination research question might be, "What is the feasibility and effectiveness of delivering a group exercise program in conjunction with the daily appointment for radiotherapy?" This project might have several phases to it. These could include one for tailoring the

334 ····· ADVANCING ONCOLOGY NURSING SCIENCE

intervention for widespread application, for developing the systems and staff for delivery of the intervention (including reimbursement mechanisms), and for training the team to ensure the intervention's long-term sustainability—an important feature to evaluate in dissemination research.

Studies evaluating the application of evidence in practice to improve outcomes will require scientists to address a number of theoretical and methodologic challenges (Green & Glasgow, 2006; Titler, 2004). To date, theoretical development of individual and organizational behavior models related to practice change has been limited, and explicit theoretical models only rarely are applied in the planning and conduct of dissemination research (Rycroft-Malone, 2007). Sales, Smith, Curran, and Kochevar (2006) argued that without explicit attention to theory in dissemination research, study findings are difficult to interpret, and essential elements of strategy needed to promote practice change may be overlooked. Theoretical models such as the Promoting Action on Research Implementation in Health Services model (Doran & Sidani, 2007; Rycroft-Malone et al., 2002), the Pettigrew and Whipp Model of Strategic Change (Stetler, Ritchie, Rycroft-Malone, Schultz, & Charns, 2007), the Iowa Model of Evidence-Based Practice (Titler et al., 2001; Vratny & Shriver, 2007), and decision theory (Bucknall, 2007) are examples of theoretical models that may provide helpful guidance in the design, analysis, or interpretation of dissemination research.

Projects that measure the outcomes of adopting research evidence in clinical practice also may require somewhat different designs, sampling plans, and attention to whether the individual, the unit, or the organization will be the analysis subject. The randomized controlled trial is the gold standard for studies of the efficacy of an intervention. However, studies concerned with evaluating the outcomes of widespread adoption of effective interventions may use the group randomized trial or a quasi-experimental design (Rabin, Brownson, Kerner, & Glasgow, 2006). Dissemination research designs also are concerned with generating knowledge that has strong external validity to permit generalizability to a wider population while simultaneously striking a balance between intervention fidelity and adaptation to local settings (Fraser, 2004; Glasgow & Emmons, 2007; Persaud & Mamdani, 2006). Outcomes measurement in dissemination research must encompass effectiveness together with data about generalization, cost, and provider behavior change (Glasgow et al., 1999). Qualitative techniques may have a role in providing information about the context, culture, and characteristics of the settings in which a program is implemented (Glasgow, Magid, Beck, Ritzwoller, & Estabrooks, 2005).

One current challenge is that the pool of nurse scientists with expertise in the design, conduct, and analysis of dissemination research is limited. Funding of these studies is resource intensive, and staff members are needed for coordination and integration, particularly because much dissemination research is concerned not only with studying the effects of the intervention on individual-level end points but also with examining indicators of practitioner, organizational, and policy change. Resources also must be applied to promote the adoption of the intervention by practitioners and integration into the care delivery system, thereby ensuring sustainability of the intervention after the study has concluded (Manderson & Hoban, 2006; Spoth & Greenberg, 2005).

Policy Development

Health policy development can be a powerful strategy to promote the adoption of research innovations in clinical practice. Efforts to translate cancer research into practice through policy development have been described in the areas of supportive care (Butler et al., 2002), family caregiving (McCorkle, 2006; McCorkle & Pasacreta, 2001), and tobacco control (Malone, 2006; Sarna & Bialous, 2006). Other scientists promote innovation uptake through the creation of position papers (Mooney, 2004) or through the analysis of their results within a health policy framework (Poirier, 2005, 2006). Health policy development in conjunction with payers and regulatory agencies is another important interface in which scientists and clinicians can contribute to the implementation of research findings in clinical practice (American Society of Clinical Oncology, 2006; Gajewski et al., 2005). Scientists and clinicians must recognize that reimbursement substantially influences care delivery. Therefore, scientists, clinicians, and payers must work together so that the reimbursement policy reflects research evidence and that the research addresses important questions in developing reimbursement policies. A further area of health policy that could enhance the translation of research into practice is the establishment of research policies similar to those in the United Kingdom that mandate the involvement of clinicians and patients in the development of publicly funded health services research (Smith et al., 2008).

Community Education to Promote Patient-Mediated Implementation

Community education to promote implementation of research findings is an important strategy and one that scientists may not fully capitalize upon. Studies show that media awareness campaigns are an effective strategy to disseminate information about research innovations (Broadwater, Heins, Hoelscher, Mangone, & Rozanas, 2004; Papas, Logan, & Tomar, 2004). The results of research also can be disseminated directly to patients and caregivers through a poster placed in the office waiting room or through development of a pamphlet, video, or computer/Internet-based resource (Balmer, 2005; Trevena, Barratt, Butow, & Caldwell, 2006). In designing, conducting, and communicating the results of translational research initiatives, patient advocacy organizations also can be key allies. Scientists can utilize the strengths and capacity of the advocacy organizations to help to make information available to both patients and their practitioners (Hubbard, Kidd, Donaghy, McDonald, & Kearney, 2007; Kim, 2007).

Networks That Bring Together Resources for Dissemination Research

One of the other requirements to accelerating the discovery, development, and delivery continuum is a mechanism for sharing details about interventions that have been tested and found to be effective (Given & Given, 2004; Leeman, Jackson, & Sandelowski, 2006). Research-Tested Intervention Programs (http://rtips.cancer.gov/rtips/index.do) is a newly designed Web site within the Cancer Control P.L.A.N.E.T. (Plan, Link, Act, Network with Evidence-Based Tools) Web site (http://cancercontrolplanet.cancer.gov) to provide clinicians and scientists with access to more detailed information about the intervention approaches that have been studied and have achieved positive outcomes. Sharing details of specific program components, messages, and materials that have been shown to produce positive outcomes is critical for the dissemination and adoption of innovations. The site provides a list of programs that have been tested in one or more peer-reviewed studies and were found to be effective in the populations and settings in which they were studied. These materials are rated for their dissemination readiness and cultural, age, and gender appropriateness, as well as the research integrity and the intervention impact. Materials at the site can be downloaded for implementation. The site also provides further guidance in terms of adapting a program to a local community context. Another resource for both clinicians and scientists who wish to contribute to research translation is the Workgroup to Evaluate and Enhance the Reach and Dissemination of Health Promotion Interventions. The work group has developed the RE-AIM model to address five dimensions to be considered in disseminating interventions to change health behavior. These five dimensions are

- *Reach* the target population.
- Select interventions with known *efficacy* or *effectiveness.*
- Facilitate *adoption* by the target setting or institution.
- Promote consistency in *implementation* of the intervention.
- Ensure *maintenance* of intervention effects in individuals and populations over time.

Funded by the Robert Wood Johnson Foundation, the work group maintains a Web site with tools and other resources (www.re-aim.org) for planning, implementing, and evaluating behavioral interventions. Another important resource is the Veterans Administration (VA) Quality Enhancement Research Initiative (QUERI) (Demakis, McQueen, Kizer, & Feussner, 2000; Hagedorn et al., 2006; McQueen, Mittman, & Demakis, 2004). The mission of QUERI is to enhance the quality and outcomes of VA health care by systematically implementing clinical research findings and evidence-based recommendations in routine clinical practice. QUERI offers a Web-based implementation guide (www.hsrd.research.va.gov/queri/implementation/default.cfm) that features a number of tools and resources that investigators may find helpful in the design, execution, and report of dissemination research projects. These include a primer on theory and methods for integrating research into practice; tool kits created by QUERI project groups as part of their efforts to conduct dissemination research; information to guide formative, process, and summative evaluations; and a dissemination research project proposal template.

Accelerating Progress Across the Research Translation Continuum: Future Directions

If the discovery, development, delivery, and research translation process is to progress at a brisk pace, then strategic involvement of nurses at the local and national levels will be essential. The responsibilities of oncology nurses to accelerate knowledge translation are summarized in Figure 15-3. To overcome barriers at the national level, expanding the capacity of translational research training programs will be essential. Institutional Clinical and Translational Science Awards programs will play a significant role for building translational research in the future but will need to extend to more academic health centers to realize their full potential. Scientists and clinicians will need to create team research partnerships that are based on mutual respect and value for each member's areas of expertise (Sussman et al., 2006). Translational research training with skilled mentors also will be a key component to support successful grant funding and long-term partnerships (Williams, 2004) and to prepare advanced practice nurses for their critical role in adoption of innovation (Magyary, Whitney, & Brown, 2006; Peirce, Cook, & Larson, 2004). Collaboration with informatics professionals will contribute to necessary reengineering of information systems so that they evolve to support EBP and outcomes evaluation (Doebbeling, Chou, & Tierney, 2006). Inclusion of technology experts also is essential because information and communication technologies, such as computers, the Internet, PDAs, and videoconferencing,

---

Figure 15-3. Oncology Nurses' Responsibilities to Accelerate Knowledge Translation

- Demonstrate clinical curiosity and a spirit of inquiry.
- Cultivate innovation, flexibility, and openness to change.
- Focus on outcomes, not tasks.
- Commit to continuous improvement through the application of knowledge.
- Adopt a systematic approach to problem solving and care delivery.
- Contribute to a culture that embraces critical thinking, application of evidence, and collective decision making.
- Create partnerships among clinicians, scientists, and administrators.
- Participate actively in professional organizations that shape public policy.

can play a pivotal role in the synthesis of knowledge and can build capacity for knowledge exchange and just-in-time information retrieval (Doran et al., 2007; Ho, Chockalingam, Best, & Walsh, 2003).

A white paper on NSPOs prepared by Given and Sherwood (2005) clearly articulated how a focus on NSPOs in research and policy development will stimulate oncology nurses to drive quality oncology care in the future. The white paper provides a strong foundation for future directions, and the following section outlines additional strategies for translating research findings at both the national level and within the scope of ONS.

A major responsibility of oncology scientists will be to evaluate NSPOs and to frame clinical research in the context of clinical outcomes. Identifying the clinical tools to consistently measure NSPOs and gathering resources to implement wide adoption of the clinical tools will be a major activity. Standardizing key patient and organizational indicators for databases also will be an important step to take in the near future. Research in NSPOs will need to evaluate not only efficacy but also effectiveness in clinical care. Large, multisite intervention studies using heterogeneous samples, multiple outcome measures (including cost), and comparison conditions such as current standard of care or alternative programs will be needed. These will be essential to determine how the effectiveness of nursing interventions on NSPOs varies by disease or ethnic, racial, or cultural characteristics. These dissemination research studies also will provide empirical validation of intervention adaptation procedures (Solomon, Card, & Malow, 2006) and will develop the evidence supporting widespread applicability and generalizability of research findings (Glasgow & Emmons, 2007; Green & Glasgow, 2006; Sussman, 2006).

Within the scope of ONS members' practice, most have a strong history of providing quality care; others contribute to the profession by assuming researcher and educator roles. However, few have recognized that their work-related activities can contribute to public policy. Establishing NSPOs helps to quantify the valuable contribution that all clinical nurses make to quality healthcare outcomes. Oncology nurses are challenged to provide evidence of the extent and quality of their contributions to patient outcomes. Information regarding the impact of NSPOs will be of great interest to legislators, healthcare agencies, regulators, insurers, and consumers as decisions are being made regarding policies that outline access to and reimbursement for healthcare services. To prepare oncology nurses to actively participate in EBP activities, including NSPOs in all levels of nursing education is essential. Many implications for practice settings exist in regard to creating the infrastructure to initiate and sustain EBP. Clinical leaders will need to understand the characteristics of practice change in order to overcome clinical care inertia. Leaders will be called upon to develop a practice culture that promotes daily application of evidence in nursing care delivery and that clinical nurses embrace (Glasgow, Lichtenstein, & Marcus, 2003; Stetler et al., 2007). A culture that lists EBP functions for each committee and council and uses expectations for EBP in all performance appraisals has a greater likelihood of success than one that only speaks to the importance of EBP. Opportunities for staff orientation and education to learn essential knowledge and skills about EBP will need to be available to sustain an EBP culture (Milner, Estabrooks, & Humphrey, 2005; Milner, Estabrooks, & Myrick, 2006). ONS will be challenged to provide short courses and conferences to promote an EBP culture in a variety of settings.

In addition to the recommendations for NSPOs presented in Given and Sherwood's 2005 paper, the following points are proposed.

- Develop and build the capacity of the nursing workforce needed for knowledge translation and dissemination research.
- Clarify the roles of nurses with varying levels of preparation and role emphasis in translational research.
- Identify the knowledge and skills needed by nurses who are leading the translation of research into practice.
- Develop policy to improve access to and reimbursement for oncology advanced practice nurses who play a critical role in translating research into practice.
- Strengthen the link between translational research and patient outcomes for healthcare workers, the public, and patients.
- Explore methodologic issues, such as selection of outcome measures, external validity of study design, and consistency across sites.
- Overcome challenges of structuring research-practice partnerships.

In order to coordinate these efforts, now is the time to consider the creation of an ONS Outcomes Center of Excellence. The center will need to have the personnel and financial resources to support an infrastructure to guide research and to develop practice guidelines, educational programs, and policy initiatives on NSPOs. Improving scientists' understanding of the business side of research translation will be of great benefit and can lead to the inclusion of a translation plan for each research project.

Simply stated, cancer outcomes research should inform policy, which in turn should influence clinical care. ONS has taken a leading role in communicating with other agencies to set priorities for research in linking nursing interventions to NSPOs. ONS also has worked closely with leading funders in healthcare research. Members of ONS have taken an active role in developing patient guidelines for cancer care, including fatigue, with organizations such as NCCN. ONS will need to continue to expand its audiences and partnerships in order for NSPOs to be widely valued and incorporated into practice, research, and education. Oncology nurse leaders will need to step up and assume leadership positions when guidelines will have a direct impact on daily clinical practice, such as fatigue guidelines. ONS and its members must continue to provide leadership in communicating research results to agencies and funders in order to build science in a systematic fashion. Commissioning an annual review and update on the state of the science in cancer NSPOs by expert ONS members will ensure that the organization remains in the forefront of the national outcomes agenda. ONS can increase efforts to engage with patient advocacy groups to help them to place value on NSPOs and to discuss the relevance of outcomes to quality patient care. Government relations representatives at the national level will need to continue to represent ONS's interests that are affected by legislative actions.

Conclusion

This chapter has provided key information regarding the translation continuum by which cancer care research can be incorporated into practice and policy. The symptom of CRF has been an exemplar of this process. Currently, great interest in the continuum's delivery phase is present, but scientific knowledge is lacking regarding the best methods for dissemination and adoption of advances in cancer-related care. This chapter provides foundational knowledge and information for teams involved in developing new knowledge and translating research findings into practice and policy.

References

Addis, M.E. (2002). Methods for disseminating research products and increasing evidence-based practice: Promises, obstacles, and future directions. *Clinical Psychology: Science and Practice, 9*(4), 367–378.

Agency for Healthcare Research and Quality. (2003). *Diffusion and dissemination of evidence-based cancer control interventions* [Evidence report/technology assessment: Number 79]. Retrieved February 11, 2007, from http://www.ahrq.gov/clinic/epcsums/canconsum.htm

Aistars, J. (1987). Fatigue in the cancer patient: A conceptual approach to a clinical problem. *Oncology Nursing Forum, 14*(6), 25–30.

American Society of Clinical Oncology. (2006). Reimbursement for cancer treatment: Coverage of off-label drug indications. *Journal of Clinical Oncology, 24*(19), 3206–3208.

Balmer, C. (2005). The information requirements of people with cancer: Where to go after the "patient information leaflet"? *Cancer Nursing, 28*(1), 36–44.

Barton-Burke, M. (2006). Cancer-related fatigue and sleep disturbances: Further research on the prevalence of these two symptoms in long-term cancer survivors can inform education, policy, and clinical practice. *Cancer Nursing, 29*(Suppl. 2), 72–77.

Baumbusch, J.L., Kirkham, S.R., Khan K.B., McDonald, H., Semeniuk, P., Tan, E., et al. (2008). Pursing common agendas: A collaborative model for knowledge translation between research and practice in clinical settings. *Research in Nursing and Health, 31*(2), 130–140.

Beck, A.T., Ward, C.H., Mendelson, M., Mock, J., & Erbaugh, J. (1961). An inventory for measuring depression. *Archives of General Psychiatry, 4,* 561–571.

Bower, J.E. (2005). Prevalence and causes of fatigue after cancer treatment: The next generation of research. *Journal of Clinical Oncology, 23*(33), 8280–8282.

Bower, J.E. (2006). Management of cancer-related fatigue. *Clinical Advances in Hematology and Oncology, 4*(11), 828–829.

Bower, J.E., Ganz, P.A., & Aziz, N. (2005). Altered cortisol response to psychologic stress in breast cancer survivors with persistent fatigue. *Psychosomatic Medicine, 67*(2), 277–280.

Bower, J.E., Ganz, P.A., Aziz, N., & Fahey, J.L. (2002). Fatigue and proinflammatory cytokine activity in breast cancer survivors. *Psychosomatic Medicine, 64*(4), 604–611.

Bower, J.E., Ganz, P.A., Aziz, N., Olmstead, R., Irwin, M.R., & Cole, S.W. (2006). Inflammatory responses to psychological stress in fatigued breast cancer survivors: Relationship to glucocorticoids. *Brain, Behavior, and Immunity, 21*(3), 251–258.

Broadwater, C., Heins, J., Hoelscher, C., Mangone, A., & Rozanas, C. (2004, October). Skin and colon cancer media campaigns in Utah. *Preventing Chronic Disease, 1*(4), Article A18. Retrieved June 26, 2008, from http://www.cdc.gov/pcd/issues/2004/oct/pdf/04_0023.pdf

Bruckenthal, P., & Broderick, J.E. (2007). Assessing treatment fidelity in pilot studies assist in designing clinical trials: An illustration from a nurse practitioner community-based intervention for pain [Online exclusive]. *Advances in Nursing Science, 30*(1), E72–E84. Retrieved June 26, 2008, from http://www.advancesinnursingscience.com/pt/re/ans/abstract.00012272-200701000-00015.htm;jsessionid=LGRGjWrl5R96j8pgVHQnyXfkx1XDPmH5JTWsKcyw2f33NhmGflVV!536197444!181195628!8091!-1

Bucknall, T. (2007). A gaze through the lens of decision theory toward knowledge translation science. *Nursing Research, 56*(Suppl. 4), S60–S66.

Butler, L., Love, B., Reimer, M., Browne, G., Downe-Wamboldt, B., West, R., et al. (2002). Nurses begin a national plan for the integration of supportive care in health research, practice, and policy. *Canadian Journal of Nursing Research, 33*(4), 155–169.

Cella, D., Davis, K., Breitbart, W., & Curt, G. (2001). Cancer-related fatigue: Prevalence of proposed diagnostic criteria in a United States sample of cancer survivors. *Journal of Clinical Oncology, 19*(14), 3385–3391.

Cella, D., Peterman, A., Passik, S., Jacobsen, P., & Breitbart, W. (1998). Progress toward guidelines for the management of fatigue. *Oncology, 12*(11A), 369–377.

Chaffin, M. (2006). Organizational culture and practice epistemologies. *Clinical Psychology: Science and Practice, 13*(1), 90–92.

Chorpita, B.F., & Nakamura, B.J. (2004). Four considerations for dissemination of intervention innovations. *Clinical Psychology: Science and Practice, 11*(4), 364–367.

Ciliska, D., Cullum, N., & Marks, S. (2001). Evaluation of systematic reviews of treatment or prevention interventions. *Evidence-Based Nursing, 4*(4), 100–104.

Cummings, G.G., Estabrooks, C.A., Midodzi, W.K., Wallin, L., & Hayduk, L. (2007). Influence of organizational characteristics and context on research utilization. *Nursing Research, 56*(Suppl. 4), S24–S39.

Cunningham, R.S. (2006). Clinical practice guideline use by oncology advanced practice nurses. *Applied Nursing Research, 19*(3), 126–133.

Curt, G., & Johnston, P.G. (2003). Cancer fatigue: The way forward. *Oncologist, 8*(Suppl. 1), 27–30.

Davis, M.P., Khoshknabi, D., & Yue, G.H. (2006). Management of fatigue in cancer patients. *Current Pain and Headache Reports, 10*(4), 260–269.

De Jong, N., Courtens, A.M., Abu-Saad, H.H., & Schouten, H.C. (2002). Fatigue in patients with breast cancer receiving adjuvant chemotherapy: A review of the literature. *Cancer Nursing, 25*(4), 283–297.

Demakis, J.G., McQueen, L., Kizer, K.W., & Feussner, J.R. (2000). Quality Enhancement Research Initiative (QUERI): A collaboration between research and clinical practice. *Medical Care, 38*(6, Suppl. 1), I17–I25.

Derogatis, L.R., & Melisaratos, N. (1983). The Brief Symptom Inventory: An introductory report. *Psychological Medicine, 13*(3), 595–605.

Doebbeling, B.N., Chou, A.F., & Tierney, W.M. (2006). Priorities and strategies for the implementation of integrated informatics and communications technology to improve evidence-based practice. *Journal of General Internal Medicine, 21*(Suppl. 2), S50–S57.

Donaldson, N., Rutledge, D., & Ashley, J. (2004). Outcomes of adoption: Measuring evidence uptake by individuals and organizations. *Worldviews on Evidence-Based Nursing, 1*(Suppl. 1), S41–S52.

Dopson, S. (2007). A view from organizational studies. *Nursing Research, 56*(Suppl. 4), S2–S77.

Doran, D.M., Mylopoulos, J., Kushniruk, A., Nagle, L., Laurie-Shaw, B., Sidani, S., et al. (2007). Evidence in the palm of your hand: Development of an outcomes-focused knowledge translation intervention. *Worldviews on Evidence-Based Nursing, 4*(2), 69–77.

Doran, D.M., & Sidani, S. (2007). Outcomes-focused knowledge translation: A framework for knowledge translation and patient outcomes improvement. *Worldviews on Evidence-Based Nursing, 4*(1), 3–13.

Ellis, P., Ciliska, D.K., Sussman, J., Robinson, P., Armour, T., Brouwers, M., et al. (2005). A systematic review of studies evaluating diffusion and dissemination of selected cancer control interventions. *Health Psychology, 24*(5), 488–500.

Estabrooks, C.A., Kenny, D.J., Adewale, A.J., Cummings, G.G., & Mallidou, A.A. (2007). A comparison of research utilization among nurses working in Canadian civilian and United States Army healthcare settings. *Research in Nursing and Health, 30*(3), 282–296.

Estabrooks, C.A., Midodzi, W.K., Cummings, G.G., & Wallin, L. (2007). Predicting research use in nursing organizations: A multilevel analysis. *Nursing Research, 56*(Suppl. 4), S7–S23.

Feifer, C., Ornstein, S.M., Jenkins, R.G., Wessell, A., Corley, S.T., Nemeth, L.S., et al. (2006). The logic behind a multimethod intervention to improve adherence to clinical practice guidelines in a nationwide network of primary care practices. *Evaluation and the Health Professions, 29*(1), 65–88.

Fox, N.J. (2003). Practice-based evidence: Towards collaborative and transgressive research. *Sociology, 37*(1), 81–102.

Foy, R., Eccles, M.P., Jamtvedt, G., Young, J., Grimshaw, J.M., & Baker, R. (2005). What do we know about how to do audit and feedback? Pitfalls in applying evidence from a systematic review. *BMC Health Services Research, 5,* 50.

Fraser, I. (2004). Organizational research with impact: Working backwards. *Worldviews on Evidence-Based Nursing, 1*(Suppl. 1), S52–S59.

Friese, C.R., & Beck, S.L. (2004). Advancing practice and research: Creating evidence-based summaries on measuring nursing-sensitive patient outcomes. *Clinical Journal of Oncology Nursing, 8*(6), 675–677.

Gajewski, J.L., Simmons, A., Weinstein, R., Snyder, E., McMannis, J., Patashnik, B., et al. (2005). The new apheresis and blood and marrow transplantation-related current procedural terminology codes for payment of apheresis and blood and marrow transplantation services. *Biology of Blood and Marrow Transplantation, 11*(11), 871–880.

Gibson, F., Garnett, M., Richardson, A., Edwards, J., & Sepion, B. (2005). Heavy to carry: A survey of parents' and healthcare professionals' perceptions of cancer-related fatigue in children and young people. *Cancer Nursing, 28*(1), 27–35.

Ginexi, E.M., & Hilton, T.F. (2006). What's next for translation research? *Evaluation and the Health Professions, 29*(3), 334–347.

Given, B., & Given, C.W. (2004). Research for nursing practice: What do we tell practitioners about nursing interventions? *Research in Nursing and Health, 27*(5), 293–295.

Given, B.A., & Sherwood, P.R. (2005). Nursing-sensitive patient outcomes—A white paper. *Oncology Nursing Forum, 32*(4), 773–784.

Glasgow, R.E., & Emmons, K.M. (2007). How can we increase translation of research into practice? Types of evidence needed. *Annual Review of Public Health, 28,* 413–433.

Glasgow, R.E., Lichtenstein, E., & Marcus, A.C. (2003). Why don't we see more translation of health promotion research to practice? Rethinking the efficacy-to-effectiveness transition. *American Journal of Public Health, 93*(8), 1261–1267.

Glasgow, R.E., Magid, D.J., Beck, A., Ritzwoller, D., & Estabrooks, P.A. (2005). Practical clinical trials for translating research to practice: Design and measurement recommendations. *Medical Care, 43*(6), 551–557.

Glasgow, R.E., Vogt, T.M., & Boles, S.M. (1999). Evaluating the public health impact of health promotion interventions: The RE-AIM framework. *American Journal of Public Health, 89*(9), 1322–1327.

Glisson, C. (2002). The organizational context of children's mental health services. *Clinical Child and Family Psychology Review, 5*(4), 233–253.

Gobel, B., Beck, S., & O'Leary, C. (2006). Nursing-sensitive patient outcomes: The development of the Putting Evidence Into Practice resources for nursing practice. *Clinical Journal of Oncology Nursing, 10*(5), 621–624.

Grady, P.A. (2006). A discussion with Patricia A. Grady on the 20th anniversary of the National Institute of Nursing Research. Interview by Peter I. Buerhaus. *Journal of Nursing Scholarship, 38*(3), 208–212.

Grady, P.A. (2007). A blueprint for the future. *Nursing Outlook, 55*(1), 55–57.

Green, L.W., & Glasgow, R.E. (2006). Evaluating the relevance, generalization, and applicability of research: Issues in external validation and translation methodology. *Evaluations and the Health Professions, 29*(1), 126–153.

Grimshaw, J.M., Eccles, M.P., Greener, J., Maclennan, G., Ibbotson, T., Kahan, J.P., et al. (2006). Is the involvement of opinion leaders in the implementation of research findings a feasible strategy? *Implementation Science, 1*(3), 1–12.

Grimshaw, J.M., Thomas, R.E., MacLennan, G., Fraser, C., Ramsay, C.R., Vale, L., et al. (2004). Effectiveness and efficiency of guideline dissemination and implementation strategies. *Health Technology Assessment, 8*(6), 1–72.

Grunfeld, E., Zitzelsberger, L., Evans, W.K., Cameron, R., Hayter, C., Berman, N., et al. (2004). Better knowledge translation for effective cancer control: A priority for action. *Cancer Causes and Control, 15*(5), 503–510.

Hadorn, D.C., Baker, D., Hodges, J.S., & Hicks, N. (1996). Rating the quality of evidence for clinical practice guidelines. *Journal of Clinical Epidemiology, 49*(7), 749–754.

Hagedorn, H., Hogan, M., Smith, J.L., Bowman, C., Curran, G.M., Espadas, D., et al. (2006). Lessons learned about implementing research evidence into clinical practice. Experiences from VA QUERI. *Journal of General Internal Medicine, 21*(Suppl. 2), S21–S24.

Harris, J.R., Brown, P.K., Coughlin, S., Fernandez, M.E., Hebert, J.R., Kerner, J.F., et al. (2005, January). The cancer prevention and control research network. *Preventing Chronic Disease, 2*(1), Article A21. Retrieved June 26, 2008, from http://www.cdc.gov/pcd/issues/2005/jan/pdf/04_0059.pdf

Hemmelgarn, A., Glisson, C., & James, L. (2006). Organizational culture and climate: Implications for services and interventions research. *Clinical Psychology: Science and Practice, 13*(1), 73–89.

Hinds, P.S., Gattuso, J.S., Barnwell, E., Cofer, M., Kellum, L.K., Mattox, S., et al. (2003). Translating psychological research findings into practice guidelines. *Journal of Nursing Administration, 33*(7–8), 397–403.

Ho, K., Chockalingam, A., Best, A., & Walsh, G. (2003). Technology-enabled knowledge translation: Building a framework for collaboration. *Canadian Medical Association Journal, 168*(6), 710–711.

Hubbard, G., Kidd, L., Donaghy, E., McDonald, C., & Kearney, N. (2007). A review of literature about involving people affected by cancer in research, policy and planning and practice. *Patient Education and Counseling, 65*(1), 21–33.

Hysong, S.J., Best, R.G., & Pugh, J.A. (2006). Audit and feedback and clinical practice guideline adherence: Making feedback actionable. *Implementation Science, 1*(9), 1–10.

Idell, C.S., Grant, M., & Kirk, C. (2007). Alignment of pain reassessment practices and National Comprehensive Cancer Network guidelines. *Oncology Nursing Forum, 34*(3), 661–671.

Iop, A., Manfredi, A.M., & Bonura, S. (2004). Fatigue in cancer patients receiving chemotherapy: An analysis of published studies. *Annals of Oncology, 15*(5), 712–720.

Irvine, D., Vincent, L., Graydon, J.E., Bubela, N., & Thompson, L. (1994). The prevalence and correlates of fatigue in patients receiving treatment with chemotherapy and radiotherapy. A comparison with the fatigue experienced by healthy individuals. *Cancer Nursing, 17*(5), 367–378.

Jamtvedt, G., Young, J.M., Kristoffersen, D.T., O'Brien, M.A., & Oxman, A.D. (2006, April 19). Audit and feedback: Effects on professional practice and health care outcomes. *Cochrane Database of Systematic Reviews 1998*, Issue 1. Art. No.: CD000259. DOI: 10.1002/14651858 .CD000259.pub2.

Jean-Pierre, P., Mustian, K., Kohli, S., Roscoe, J.A., Hickok, J.T., & Morrow, G.R. (2006). Community-based clinical oncology research trials for cancer-related fatigue. *Journal of Supportive Oncology, 4*(10), 511–516.

Johnson, D.W., Craig, W., Brant, R., Mitton, C., Svenson, L., & Klassen, T.P. (2006). A cluster randomized controlled trial comparing three methods of disseminating practice guidelines for children with croup [ISRCTN73394937]. *Implementation Science, 28*(1), 10.

Johnson, J.E., Nail, L.M., Lauver, D., King, K.B., & Keys, H. (1988). Reducing the negative impact of radiation therapy on functional status. *Cancer, 61*(1), 46–51.

Kerner, J., Rimer, B., & Emmons, K. (2005). Introduction to the special section on dissemination—Dissemination research and research dissemination: How can we close the gap? *Health Psychology, 24*(5), 443–446.

Kerner, J.F. (2006). Knowledge translation versus knowledge integration: A "funder's" perspective. *Journal of Continuing Education in the Health Professions, 26*(1), 72–80.

Kerner, J.F., Guirguis-Blake, J., Hennessy, K.D., Brounstein, P.J., Vinson, C., Schwartz, R.H., et al. (2005). Translating research into improved outcomes in comprehensive cancer control. *Cancer Causes and Control, 16*(Suppl. 1), 27–40.

Kim, P. (2007). Cost of cancer care: The patient perspective. *Journal of Clinical Oncology, 25*(2), 228–232.

Knowles, G., Borthwick, D., McNamara, S., Miller, M., & Leggot, L. (2000). Survey of nurses' assessment of cancer-related fatigue. *European Journal of Cancer Care, 9*(2), 105–113.

Krumm, S., & Mock, V. (2005). Maximizing clinical-academic partnerships in studies of symptom management: Examples of success. *Advanced Studies in Nursing, 3*(5), 164–169.

Lai, J.S., Cella, D., Dineen, K., Bode, R., Von Roenn, J., Gershon, R.C., et al. (2005). An item bank was created to improve the measurement of cancer-related fatigue. *Journal of Clinical Epidemiology, 58*(2), 190–197.

Laurence, J. (2006). Translating translational research. *Translational Research, 148*(1), 1–3.

Lawrence, D.P., Kupelnick, B., Miller, K., Devine, D., & Lau, J. (2004). Evidence report on the occurrence, assessment, and treatment of fatigue in cancer patients. *Journal of the National Cancer Institute Monographs, 2004*(32), 40–50.

Leeman, J., Jackson, B., & Sandelowski, M. (2006). An evaluation of how well research reports facilitate the use of finding in practice. *Journal of Nursing Scholarship, 38*(2), 171–177.

Lobo, M.L. (2005). Descriptive research is the bench science of nursing. *Western Journal of Nursing Research, 27*(1), 5–6.

Loeb, S.J., Penrod, J., Kolanowski, A., Hupcey, J.E., Haidet, K.K., & Fick, D.M. (2008). Creating cross-disciplinary research alliances to advance nursing science. *Journal of Nursing Scholarship, 40*(2), 195–201.

Lomas, J., & Haynes, R.B. (1988). A taxonomy and critical review of tested strategies for the application of clinical practice recommendations: From "official" to "individual" clinical policy. *American Journal of Preventive Medicine, 4*(Suppl. 4), 77–94.

MacDermid, J., Solomon, P., Law, M., Russell, D., & Stratford, P. (2006). Defining the effect and mediators of two knowledge translation strategies designed to alter knowledge, intent and clinical utilization of rehabilitation outcome measures: A study protocol [NCT00298727]. *Implementation Science, 1*(1), 14.

MacVicar, M.G., Winningham, M.L., & Nickel, J.L. (1989). Effects of aerobic interval training on cancer patients' functional capacity. *Nursing Research, 38*(6), 348–351.

Magyary, D., Whitney, J.D., & Brown, M.A. (2006). Advancing practice inquiry: Research foundations of the practice doctorate in nursing. *Nursing Outlook, 54*(3), 139–151.

Malone, R.E. (2006). Nursing's involvement in tobacco control: Historical perspective and vision for the future. *Nursing Research, 55*(Suppl. 4), S51–S57.

Manderson, L., & Hoban, E. (2006). Cervical cancer services for indigenous women: Advocacy, community-based research and policy change in Australia. *Women and Health, 43*(4), 69–88.

McAlister, F.A., Man-Son-Hing, M., Straus, S.E., Ghali, W.A., Anderson, D., Majumdar, S.R., et al. (2005). Impact of a patient decision aid on care among patients with nonvalvular atrial fibrillation: A cluster randomized trial. *Canadian Medical Association Journal,* *173*(5), 496–501.

McCorkle, R. (2006). A program of research on patient and family caregiver outcomes: Three phases of evolution. *Oncology Nursing Forum, 33*(1), 25–31.

McCorkle, R., & Pasacreta, J.V. (2001). Enhancing caregiver outcomes in palliative care. *Cancer Control, 8*(1), 36–45.

McCorkle, R., & Young, K. (1978). Development of a symptom distress scale. *Cancer Nursing, 1*(5), 373–378.

McGuire, D.B., & Ropka, M.E. (2000). Research and oncology nursing practice. *Seminars in Oncology Nursing, 16*(1), 35–46.

McQueen, L., Mittman, B.S., & Demakis, J.G. (2004). Overview of the Veterans Health Administration (VHA) Quality Enhancement Research Initiative (QUERI). *Journal of the American Medical Informatics Association, 11*(5), 339–343.

Milner, M., Estabrooks, C.A., & Humphrey, C. (2005). Clinical nurse educators as agents for change: Increasing research utilization. *International Journal of Nursing Studies, 42*(8), 899–914.

Milner, M., Estabrooks, C.A., & Myrick, F. (2006). Research utilization and clinical nurse educators: A systematic review. *Journal of Evaluation in Clinical Practice, 12*(6), 639–655.

Mitchell, S., Beck, S., Hood, L., Moore, K., & Tanner, E. (2007). Putting Evidence Into Practice (PEP): Evidence-based interventions for fatigue during and following cancer and its treatment. *Clinical Journal of Oncology Nursing, 11*(1), 99–113.

Mitchell, S., & Friese, C. (n.d.). *ONS PEP® (Putting Evidence Into Practice) weight of evidence classification schema: Decision rules for summative evaluation of a body of evidence.* Retrieved September 9, 2007, from http://www.ons.org/outcomes/tables/documents/woevidence .pdf

Mock, V. (2003). Clinical excellence through evidence-based practice: Fatigue management as a model. *Oncology Nursing Forum, 30*(5), 787–796.

Mock, V., Atkinson, A., Barsevick, A., Cella, D., Cimprich, B., Cleeland, C., et al. (2000). NCCN practice guidelines for cancer-related fatigue. *Oncology, 14*(11A), 151–161.

Mock, V., & Olsen, M. (2003). Current management of fatigue and anemia in patients with cancer. *Seminars in Oncology Nursing, 19*(Suppl. 2), 36–41.

Mooney, K.H. (2004). Promoting professional oncology nursing practice through position papers. *Seminars in Oncology Nursing, 20*(2), 74–88.

Morgan, G.D., Kobus, K., Gerlach, K.K., Neighbors, C., Lerman, C., Abrams, D.B., et al. (2003). Facilitating transdisciplinary research: The experience of the transdisciplinary tobacco use research centers. *Nicotine and Tobacco Research, 5*(Suppl. 1), S11–S19.

Morrow, G.R., Shelke, A.R., Roscoe, J.A., Hickok, J.T., & Mustian, K. (2005). Management of cancer-related fatigue. *Cancer Investigation, 23*(3), 229–239.

Nail, L.M. (2002). Fatigue in patients with cancer. *Oncology Nursing Forum, 29*(3), 537.

National Comprehensive Cancer Network. (2008). *NCCN Clinical Practice Guidelines in Oncology™: Cancer-related fatigue* [v.1.2008]. Retrieved June 26, 2008, from http://www.nccn .org/professionals/physician_gls/PDF/fatigue.pdf

National Institute for Clinical Excellence. (2002). *Principles for best practice in clinical audit.* Abingdon, UK: Radcliffe Medical Press.

National Institutes of Health. (2002). State-of-the-science statement on symptom management in cancer: Pain, depression, and fatigue. *NIH Consensus Statement, 19*(4), 1–29.

National Institutes of Health. (2007). *NIH roadmap for medical research.* Retrieved February 11, 2007, from http://nihroadmap.nih.gov

Olson, K. (2007). A new way of thinking about fatigue: A reconceptualization. *Oncology Nursing Forum, 34*(1), 93–99.

Oncology Nursing Society. (2004). *Measuring oncology nursing-sensitive patient outcomes: Evidence-based summary.* Retrieved February 11, 2007, from http://onsopcontent.ons .org/toolkits/evidence/Clinical/pdf/Fatigue2.pdf

Oncology Nursing Society. (n.d.). *Fatigue: Evidence tables.* Retrieved February 11, 2007, from http://www.ons.org/outcomes/volume1/fatigue/fatigue_evidence.shtml

Page, M.S., Berger, A.M., & Johnson, L.B. (2006). Putting Evidence Into Practice: Evidence-based interventions for sleep-wake disturbances. *Clinical Journal of Oncology Nursing, 10*(6), 753–767.

Papas, R.K., Logan, H.L., & Tomar, S.L. (2004). Effectiveness of a community-based oral cancer awareness campaign. *Cancer Causes and Control, 15*(2), 121–131.

Passik, S.D. (2004). Impediments and solutions to improving the management of cancer-related fatigue. *Journal of the National Cancer Institute Monographs, 2004*(32), 136.

Patrick, D.L., Ferketich, S.L., Frame, P.S., Harris, J.J., Hendricks, C.B., Levin, B., et al. (2004). National Institutes of Health state-of-the-science conference statement: Symptom management in cancer: Pain, depression, and fatigue. *Journal of the National Cancer Institute Monographs, 2004*(32), 9–16.

Payne, J.K. (2004). A neuroendocrine-based regulatory fatigue model. *Biological Research for Nursing, 6*(2), 141–150.

Pearson, A., Wiechula, R., Court, A., & Lockwood, C. (2007). A re-consideration of what constitutes "evidence" in the healthcare professions. *Nursing Science Quarterly, 20*(1), 85–88.

Pearson, R.G., & Byars, G.E. (1956). *The development and validation of a checklist for measuring subjective fatigue* [Report No. 56-115]. Randolph Air Force Base, TX: School of Aviation Medicine, U.S. Air Force.

Peirce, A., Cook, S., & Larson, E. (2004). Focusing research priorities in schools of nursing. *Journal of Professional Nursing, 20*(3), 156–159.

Perrin, K., Burke, S., O'Connor, D., Walby, G., Shippey, C., Pitt, S., et al. (2006). Factors contributing to intervention fidelity in a multi-site chronic disease self-management program. *Implementation Science, 1*(1), 26.

Persaud, N., & Mamdani, M.M. (2006). External validity: The neglected dimension in evidence ranking. *Journal of Evaluation in Clinical Practice, 12*(4), 450–453.

Piper, B.F., Dibble, S.L., Dodd, M.J., Weiss, M.C., Slaughter, R.E., & Paul, S.M. (1998). The revised Piper Fatigue Scale: Psychometric evaluation in women with breast cancer. *Oncology Nursing Forum, 25*(4), 677–684.

Piper, B.F., Lindsey, A.M., & Dodd, M.J. (1987). Fatigue mechanisms in cancer patients: Developing nursing theory. *Oncology Nursing Forum, 14*(6), 17–23.

Poirier, P. (2005). Policy implications of the relationship of sick leave benefits, individual characteristics, and fatigue to employment during radiation therapy for cancer. *Policy, Politics and Nursing Practice, 6*(4), 305–318.

Poirier, P. (2006). The relationship of sick leave benefits, employment patterns, and individual characteristics to radiation therapy-related fatigue. *Oncology Nursing Forum, 33*(3), 593–601.

Prue, G., Rankin, J., Allen, J., Gracey, J., & Cramp, F. (2006). Cancer-related fatigue: A critical appraisal. *European Journal of Cancer, 42*(7), 846–863.

Rabin, B.A., Brownson, R.C., Kerner, J.F., & Glasgow, R.E. (2006). Methodologic challenges in disseminating evidence-based interventions to promote physical activity. *American Journal of Preventive Medicine, 31*(4, Suppl. 1), 24–34.

Ream, E., & Richardson, A. (1999). From theory to practice: Designing interventions to reduce fatigue in patients with cancer. *Oncology Nursing Forum, 26*(8), 1295–1303.

Rhoten, D. (1982). Fatigue and the postsurgical patient. In C.M. Norris (Ed.), *Concept clarification in nursing* (pp. 277–300). Rockville, MD: Aspen.

Robinson, K., Elliott, S.J., Driedger, S.M., Eyles, J., O'Loughlin, J., Riley, B., et al. (2005). Using linking systems to build capacity and enhance dissemination in heart health promotion: A Canadian multiple-case study. *Health Education Research, 20*(5), 499–513.

Rogers, E. (2003). *Diffusion of innovations* (5th ed.). New York: Free Press.

Rohrbach, L.A., Grana, R., Sussman, S., & Valente, T.W. (2006). Type II translation: Transporting prevention interventions from research to real-world settings. *Evaluation and the Health Professions, 29*(3), 302–333.

Ropka, M.E., & Spencer-Cisek, P. (2001). PRISM: Priority symptom management project phase I: Assessment. *Oncology Nursing Forum, 28*(10), 1585–1594.

Rubenstein, L.V., & Pugh, J. (2006). Strategies for promoting organizational and practice change by advancing implementation research. *Journal of General Internal Medicine, 21*(Suppl. 2), S58–S64.

Rutledge, D.N., Ropka, M., Greene, P.E., Nail, L., & Mooney, K.H. (1998). Barriers to research utilization for oncology staff nurses and nurse managers/clinical nurse specialists. *Oncology Nursing Forum, 25*(3), 497–506.

Rycroft-Malone, J. (2007). Theory and knowledge translation: Setting some coordinates. *Nursing Research, 56*(Suppl. 4), S78–S85.

Rycroft-Malone, J., Kitson, A., Harvey, G., McCormack, B., Seers, K., Titchen, A., et al. (2002). Ingredients for change: Revisiting a conceptual framework. *Quality and Safety in Health Care, 11*(2), 174–180.

Sackett, D.L., Rosenberg, W.M.C., Gray, J.A.M., Haynes, R.B., & Richardson, W.S. (1996). Evidence based medicine: What it is and what it isn't. It's about integrating individual clinical expertise and the best external evidence. *BMJ, 312*(7023), 71–72.

Sales, A., Smith, J., Curran, G., & Kochevar, L. (2006). Models, strategies, and tools. Theory in implementing evidence-based findings into health care practice. *Journal of General Internal Medicine, 21*(Suppl. 2), S43–S49.

Sarna, L., & Bialous, S.A. (2006). Strategic directions for nursing research in tobacco dependence. *Nursing Research, 55*(4, Suppl. 1), S1–S9.

Schubert, C., Hong, S., Natarajan, L., Mills, P.J., & Dimsdale, J.E. (2006). The association between fatigue and inflammatory marker levels in cancer patients: A quantitative review. *Brain, Behavior and Immunity, 21*(4), 413–427.

Servaes, P., Verhagen, C., & Bleijenberg, G. (2002). Fatigue in cancer patients during and after treatment: Prevalence, correlates and interventions. *European Journal of Cancer, 38*(1), 27–43.

Smith, E., Ross, F., Donovan, S., Manthorpe, J., Brearley, S., Sitzia, J., et al. (2008). Service user involvement in nursing, midwifery and health visiting research: A review of evidence and practice. *International Journal of Nursing Studies, 45*(2), 298–315.

Solberg, L. (2006). Recruiting medical groups for research: Relationships, reputation, requirements, rewards, reciprocity, resolution, and respect. *Implementation Science, 1*(1), 25.

Solomon, J., Card, J.J., & Malow, R.M. (2006). Adapting efficacious interventions: Advancing translational research in HIV prevention. *Evaluation and the Health Professions, 29*(2), 162–194.

Sood, A., & Moynihan, T.J. (2005). Cancer-related fatigue: An update. *Current Oncology Reports, 7*(4), 277–282.

Spoth, R.L., & Greenberg, M.T. (2005). Toward a comprehensive strategy for effective practitioner-scientist partnership and larger-scale community health and well-being. *American Journal of Community Psychology, 35*(3/4), 107–126.

Squires, J.E., Moralejo, D., & Lefort, S.M. (2007). Exploring the role of organizational policies and procedures in promoting research utilization in registered nurses. *Implementation Science, 2*, 17.

St. Pierre, B.A., Kasper, C.E., & Lindsey, A.M. (1992). Fatigue mechanisms in patients with cancer: Effects of tumor necrosis factor and exercise on skeletal muscle. *Oncology Nursing Forum, 19*(3), 419–425.

Sterman, E., Gauker, S., & Krieger, J. (2003). Continuing education: A comprehensive approach to improving cancer pain management and patient satisfaction. *Oncology Nursing Forum, 30*(5), 857–864.

Stetler, C., Legro, M., Rycroft-Malone, J., Bowman, C., Curran, G., Guihan, M., et al. (2006). Role of "external facilitation" in implementation of research findings: A qualitative evaluation of facilitation experiences in the Veterans Health Administration. *Implementation Science, 2*, 3.

Stetler, C.B., Ritchie, J., Rycroft-Malone, J., Schultz, A., & Charns, M. (2007). Improving quality of care through routine, successful implementation of evidence-based practice at the bedside: An organizational case study protocol using the Pettigrew and Whipp model of strategic change. *Implementation Science, 2,* 3.

Stokols, D., Harvey, R., Gress, J., Fuqua, J., & Phillips, K. (2005). In vivo studies of trans-disciplinary scientific collaboration: Lessons learned and implications for active living research. *American Journal of Preventive Medicine, 28*(2, Suppl. 2), 202–213.

Stone, P., Ream, E., Richardson, A., Thomas, H., Andrews, P., Campbell, P., et al. (2003). Cancer-related fatigue—a difference of opinion? Results of a multicentre survey of healthcare professionals, patients and caregivers. *European Journal of Cancer Care, 12*(1), 20–27.

Sussman, S. (2006). The transdisciplinary-translation revolution: Final thoughts. *Evaluation and the Health Professions, 29*(3), 348–352.

Sussman, S., Valente, T.W., Rohrbach, L.A., Skara, S., & Pentz, M.A. (2006). Translation in the health professions: Converting science into action. *Evaluation and the Health Professions, 29*(1), 7–32.

Tavio, M., Milan, I., & Tirelli, U. (2002). Cancer-related fatigue (review). *International Journal of Oncology, 21*(5), 1093–1099.

Thompson, D.S., Estabrooks, C.A., Scott-Findlay, S., Moore, K., & Wallin, L. (2007). Interventions aimed at increasing research use in nursing: A systematic review. *Implementation Science, 2,* 15.

Titler, M.G. (2004). Translation science: Quality, methods and issues. *Communicating Nursing Research, 37,* 15, 17–34.

Titler, M.G., Everett, L.Q., & Adams, S. (2007). Implications for implementation science. *Nursing Research, 56*(Suppl. 4), S53–S59.

Titler, M.G., Kleiber, C., Steelman, V.J., Rakel, B.A., Budreau, G., Everett, L.Q., et al. (2001). The Iowa model of evidence-based practice to promote quality care. *Critical Care Nursing Clinics of North America, 13*(4), 497–509.

Trevena, L.J., Barratt, A., Butow, P., & Caldwell, P. (2006). A systematic review on communicating with patients about evidence. *Journal of Evaluation in Clinical Practice, 12*(1), 13–23.

U.S. Department of Health and Human Services, National Institutes of Health, & National Cancer Institute. (2005, June). *President's cancer panel 2004–2005 annual report: Translating research into cancer care: Delivering on the promise.* Bethesda, MD: Author.

U.S. Department of Health and Human Services, National Institutes of Health, & National Cancer Institute. (2006, June). *President's cancer panel 2005–2006 annual report: Assessing Progress, advancing change.* Bethesda, MD: Author.

Van Belle, S., Paridaens, R., Evers, G., Kerger, J., Bron, D., Foubert, J., et al. (2005). Comparison of proposed diagnostic criteria with FACT-F and VAS for cancer-related fatigue: Proposal for use as a screening tool. *Supportive Care in Cancer, 13*(4), 246–254.

Vratny, A., & Shriver, D. (2007). A conceptual model for growing evidence-based practice. *Nursing Administration Quarterly, 31*(2), 162–170.

Wagner, L.I., & Cella, D. (2004). Fatigue and cancer: Causes, prevalence and treatment approaches. *British Journal of Cancer, 91*(5), 822–828.

White, A.M. (2001). Clinical applications of research on fatigue in children with cancer. *Journal of Pediatric Oncology Nursing, 18*(2, Suppl. 1), 17–20.

Whittemore, R. (2005). Combining evidence in nursing research: Methods and implications. *Nursing Research, 54*(1), 56–62.

Williams, C.A. (2004). Preparing the next generation of scientists in translation research. *Worldviews on Evidence-Based Nursing, 1*(Suppl. 1), S73–S77.

Winningham, M.L. (1992). The role of exercise in cancer therapy. In M. Eisinger & R.W. Watson (Eds.), *Exercise and disease* (pp. 63–70). Boca Raton, FL: CRC Press.

Winningham, M.L. (2001). Strategies for managing cancer-related fatigue syndrome: A rehabilitation approach. *Cancer, 92*(Suppl. 4), 988–997.

Winningham, M.L., Nail, L.M., Burke, M.B., Brophy, L., Cimprich, B., Jones, L.S., et al. (1994). Fatigue and the cancer experience: The state of the knowledge. *Oncology Nursing Forum, 21*(1), 23–36.

Wood, L.J., Nail, L.M., Gilster, A., Winters, K.A., & Elsea, C.R. (2006). Cancer chemotherapy-related symptoms: Evidence to suggest a role for proinflammatory cytokines. *Oncology Nursing Forum, 33*(3), 535–542.

Yang, C.M., & Wu, C.H. (2005). The situational fatigue scale: A different approach to measuring fatigue. *Quality of Life Research, 14*(5), 1357–1362.

Young, K.E., & White, C.A. (2006). The prevalence and moderators of fatigue in people who have been successfully treated for cancer. *Journal of Psychosomatic Research, 60*(1), 29–38.

Zerhouni, E.A. (2005). Translational and clinical science—time for a new vision. *New England Journal of Medicine, 353*(15), 1621–1623.

Zerhouni, E.A., & Alving, B. (2006). Clinical and translational science awards: A framework for a national research agenda. *Translational Research, 148*(1), 4–5.

Zitella, L.J., Friese, C.R., Hauser, J., Gobel, B.H., Woolery, M., O'Leary, C., et al. (2006). Putting Evidence Into Practice: Prevention of infection. *Clinical Journal of Oncology Nursing, 10*(6), 739–750.

CHAPTER 16

New Approaches to Conducting Oncology Nursing Research Using Technology

Usha Menon, PhD, RN, and Diana J. Wilkie, PhD, RN, FAAN

Introduction

Technology today is so pervasive and accessible that it influences almost every aspect of a person's life. Advanced technology is integrated into everything from grocery stores with self-checkout lines, to laser brain surgery, to self-management of chronic diseases. In health care, technologic advances are behind lifesaving diagnoses, treatments, and continued care. In the United States, chronic diseases are the major cause of disability and account for almost 70% of healthcare spending. The Institute of Medicine (2001) report *Cross-*

Usha Menon, PhD, RN, is supported in part by awards from the National Institutes of Health, National Institute of Nursing Research (R01 NR08425) and National Cancer Institute (R21 CA100566, R03 CA93184), and Diana J. Wilkie, PhD, RN, FAAN, is supported in part by the National Institutes of Health, National Institute of Nursing Research (R01 NR009092 and P30 NR010680) and National Cancer Institute (2 R01 CA081918).

The contents of this chapter are solely the responsibility of the authors and do not necessarily represent the official views of the National Institutes of Health, National Institute of Nursing Research, or National Cancer Institute.

ing the Quality Chasm: A New Health System for the 21st Century identified health information technology as one of four critical forces that could significantly improve clinical decision making, patient safety, and overall quality of care. For more than three decades, researchers have shown that health information technology (e.g., handheld devices for gathering data, clinical information databases, clinical decision-making aids, Internet resources) has increased the quality of health care. Inevitably, such technology has greatly influenced nursing research. Among nurses (the largest healthcare profession), technology-based research slowly has gained popularity. For example, nurses now conduct research using computer-based decision aids and interactive technology-based pain and symptom management.

Nursing research focuses on diverse aspects of health care. This chapter spotlights the use of advanced technology for data collection, information databases, clinical decision making, and interventions. The use of progressive technology has many advantages, such as reaching larger numbers of patients in less time, allowing for real-time tailoring of interventions, eliminating errors in data collection and data entry, and gathering a continuous flow of multimodal data. Although advanced technology is an important component of both behavioral and biologic research, this chapter will focus on the use of such technology in behavioral nursing research. One premier benefit is that successful advanced technologic methods may translate easily to clinical practice, thus creating better work environments and assisting in delivering high-quality health care.

Tailoring Interventions Using Computer Technology

Tailored interventions have shown great promise in recent years in improving health promotion behavior. Tailoring has been used to study health issues such as dietary behavior change, smoking cessation, mammography use, and symptom management (Campbell et al., 1994; Champion, 1994; Rakowski et al., 1998; Wilkie et al., 2001, in press). *Tailored interventions* are defined as any combination of information or change strategies intended to reach one specific person, based on characteristics that are unique to that person, related to the outcome of interest, and derived from an individual assessment (Kreuter, Farrell, Olevitch, & Brennan, 2000). Overall, computer-based education is fast becoming a valuable and effective way to change health promotion behavior by tailoring the education or information delivered to the individual. Investigators have conducted several studies that have documented the effectiveness of computer-based education related to various diseases, including cancer (Green, Biesecker, McInerney, Mauger, & Fost, 2001; Gustafson et al., 2001; Jones, Nyhof-Young, Friedman, & Catton, 2001; Kim et al., 2001; Nicholas, Huntington, Williams, & Vickery, 2001; Sutherland, Campbell, Ornstein, Wildemuth, & Lobach, 2001; Wilkie et al., in press). Touch screen and interactive computer programs are supported as practical, private, and user-friendly methods of collecting health-related data, as well as delivering education (Baratiny, Campbell, Sanson-Fisher, Graham, & Cockburn, 2000; DePalma, 2000; Pearson et al., 1999; Wilkie et al., 2001; Wofford, Smith, & Miller, 2005). Additionally, this form of health education delivers information that can be tailored to individual risk factors, diagnoses, or symptoms; is self-paced; and is considered more relevant by patients (Green et al., 2001; Jones et al., 1999; Pearson et al.; Wilkie et al., in press).

The most practical way to tailor is to use computers. Although the actual delivery of the tailored intervention can occur by any media, such as print, phone, or in person, the process of tailoring usually is accomplished by computer. For example, to tailor education on breast cancer screening to individual women, baseline information is entered into a database. Then, using preprogrammed algorithms, the relevant set of messages is drawn together for an individual. Figure 16-1 illustrates what happens when a 65-year-old woman is queried about barriers to completing a fecal occult blood test. Based on her response of "no symptoms," she receives an educational message that addresses the fact that colorectal cancer can occur without symptoms. In addition, her age and gender are worked into the message, making it tailored to her.

Tailoring has many advantages because the technology can be used via stand-alone computers or over the Internet for multiple health issues. As such, tailoring has been tested in cancer screening (Champion et al., 2003; Menon et al., 2007; Skinner et al., 2007), clinical decision making for breast cancer treatment (Keating, Guadagnoli, Landrum, Borbas, & Weeks, 2002; Mooney, Beck, Friedman, & Farzanfar, 2002), smoking cessation (Strecher et al., 2005), psychological functioning of newly diagnosed patients with cancer (Rawl et al., 2002), cancer risk assessment (Emmons et al., 2004), decision making about genetic testing for breast cancer (Green et al., 2004), and symptom management (Wilkie et al., 2001, in press). Although some of these interventions are delivered by computer, tailored scripts also can be used to guide counseling that is phone-based, in person, or mailed print materials. Tailoring decreases the amount of time to deliver personalized messages. For example, a clinician may take an hour to complete a baseline assessment of beliefs about cervical cancer screening. A touch screen computer program in the waiting room could be used to gather this information in 5–10 minutes. Additionally, the information then given to the patient can be made relevant and culturally appropriate. Software for tailoring can integrate culturally sensitive graphics, colors, words, and even language preferences in an educational program. In Figure 16-1, the 65-year-old patient's language preference and cultural orientation also could be integrated into the message on reducing barriers to colorectal cancer screening. Done manually without a computer, such tailoring would involve using multiple resources, such as clinician time, interpreters, and culturally competent personnel.

Tailored interventions also can be utilized to reach people in a multitude of settings, such as primary care, specialty clinics, community settings (e.g., faith-based organizations, beauty salons), and in the home (via the Internet,

Figure 16-1. Sample of a Tailored Algorithm for Fecal Occult Blood Test (FOBT) Barriers

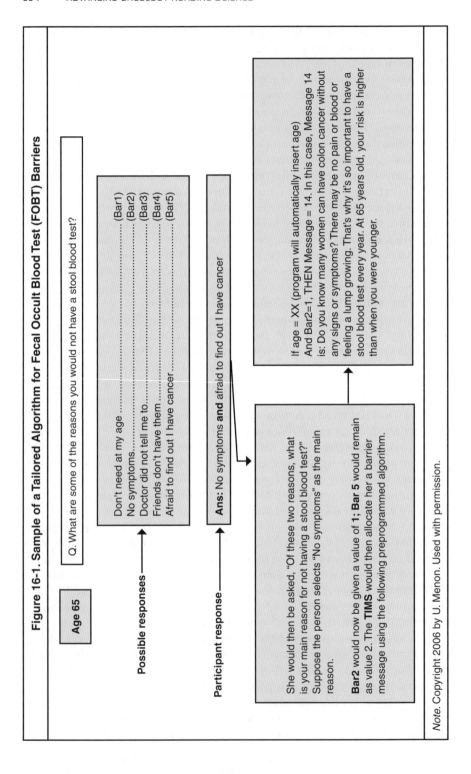

Age 65

Q. What are some of the reasons you would not have a stool blood test?

Possible responses

Don't need at my age .... (Bar1)
No symptoms .... (Bar2)
Doctor did not tell me to .... (Bar3)
Friends don't have them .... (Bar4)
Afraid to find out I have cancer ... (Bar5)

Participant response

Ans: No symptoms **and** afraid to find out I have cancer

She would then be asked, "Of these two reasons, what is your main reason for not having a stool blood test?" Suppose the person selects "No symptoms" as the main reason.

Bar2 would now be given a value of **1; Bar 5** would remain as value 2. The **TIMS** would then allocate her a barrier message using the following preprogrammed algorithm.

If age = XX (program will automatically insert age) And Bar2=1, THEN Message = 14. In this case, Message 14 is: Do you know how many women can have colon cancer without any signs or symptoms? There may be no pain or blood or feeling a lump growing. That's why it's so important to have a stool blood test every year. At 65 years old, your risk is higher than when you were younger.

DVDs, CD-ROMs, or other technology). Health education for health promotion or even support groups for patients with cancer can be delivered at home, thereby reducing the burden of travel on the patient.

However, tailoring has some disadvantages. The cost of initial setup of software and computers can be prohibitive. Some level of technology support is necessary to keep these systems—which often can be complex and large—functioning smoothly. Despite the access to technology in many aspects of people's lives, the digital divide still exists with older adults, those with low education and/or literacy, and underserved minorities. For such people, the use of the computer may be too impersonal or intimidating; for some cultures, computer-based education may indicate a lack of caring on the part of the health professional. Therefore, although tailoring has many advantages, such as being an effective way to reach an increasing number of patients with a health message and to deliver education that is relevant to each individual, its use must be judicious, based on the targeted population.

Computer-Assisted Telephone Interviews and Interactive Voice Recognition Calls

Computer-assisted telephone interviews (CATIs) have been used in research for several years. The most common forms of CATI allow the interviewer to read from a computer program and enter responses directly into it. Questions are programmed with automatic skip patterns and defined parameters for response values, minimizing data entry error and missing data. For the most part, researchers increasingly are using CATIs to collect data for various types of surveys (e.g., cross-sectional surveys, baseline interviews, follow-up interviews). CATIs are an effective data collection method as well, in that they can elicit adequate response rates (Albertsen, Andersen, Olsen, & Gronbaek, 2004; Allen, Bastani, Bazargan, & Leonard, 2002; Blyth, March, Shellard, & Cousins, 2002; Buckwalter, Crooks, & Petitti, 2002; Champion et al., 2002, 2003; Cherpitel, 2002, 2003; Rawl et al., 2005; Skinner, Champion, Menon, & Seshadri, 2002; Weinbaum et al., 2001). These studies encompass diverse health issues from domestic violence to mammography screening. More recently, CATIs also are being used to deliver interventions (Ketola & Klockars, 1999; Leon et al., 1999; Wilkins, Casswell, Barnes, & Pledger, 2003). A CATI-based intervention may take the form of simple reminders to either patients or providers about a screening examination or actual education or counseling calls (Crawford et al., 2005; Lee, Friedman, Cukor, & Ahern, 2003).

CATIs can be arranged through a variety of software programs. In the simplest version, the data collector reads questions from a computer screen and enters the responses as they are given. The responses are saved in a spreadsheet format for analysis. Programs such as Microsoft® Access™ or SPSS® Data or Builder are used for such CATIs. More complex CATIs include dialing functions and reminder prompts. For example, in an advanced CATI, the computer will dial phone numbers automatically and repeat dialing if a number is busy or if voice mail is reached.

Using CATIs for data collection has several advantages. They eliminate the potential for errors in data entry because data are entered into the database in real time, not double-entered on paper first and then into the computer. Automated dialing and tracking of busy numbers and answering machines allows for a participant to be called at various times during the day until he or she responds. Based on previous dialing outcomes, automation also permits easy follow-up with participants at times when they can be reached.

An intrinsic limitation of CATIs for data collection is that individuals without landline phone access are left out of the study, which can affect external validity. However, an Australian team successfully has conducted pilot tests using computer-assisted cell phone interviews to survey people living in households without landline phones (Wilkins et al., 2003). As with most computer-based programs, a certain degree of cost and labor is needed to develop, test, and implement CATIs. Other disadvantages are that CATI calls compete with numerous telemarketing calls. Answering machines, privacy management services, and caller ID allow potential study participants to "screen out" calls, leading to a passive form of refusal to enroll or continue in a research study.

The potential of interactive voice recognition (IVR) in research only recently has been addressed. IVR allows for the respondent to speak responses to questions rather than press number keys. This process can be less burdensome for the respondent. Many studies with IVR are pilot studies focused on developing and testing the feasibility of IVR use in research. In IVR technology, automated voice prompts over the phone guide the respondent to answer using the numbers on the touch phone. For example, the voice prompt may ask a patient with cancer if he or she has experienced any symptoms related to chemotherapy that day. The patient may be asked to press 1 for yes or 2 for no. In a review of 19 studies using voice-prompted phone calls, Krishna, Balas, Boren, and Maglaveras (2002) concluded that automated phone communication was acceptable to patients and improved the quality of care. Studies were focused on diverse areas, such as childhood immunizations, influenza vaccines, medication compliance, and chronic conditions such as diabetes, heart failure, and hypertension (Krishna et al.).

IVR has numerous advantages, including human labor cost reduction, autonomy, confidentiality, access to certain population groups, improved data quality, and standardized interviewing (Corkrey & Parkinson, 2002). Additionally, IVR can be adapted to language and accent by using appropriate voice recordings. Despite these advantages, applications of IVR have been limited in large clinical research studies. Literature searches produced only a couple of uses in cancer screening (White et al., 2006) and none in cancer treatment or symptom management.

IVR systems can be expensive to develop and require highly specialized personnel. Additionally, only a few easy-to-use software programs are available for IVR programming (Janda, Janda, & Tedford, 2001). IVR technology is touted as having substantial benefits, but many questions remain about its effectiveness in research. Studies that have systematically evaluated components of IVR, such as evaluation of voice, multilingual interfaces, touch-tone phone prevalence, survey response rates, and use by older adults, are lacking.

Handheld Devices

Investigators have used a variety of handheld devices to conduct research across the spectrum of cancer care, including prevention, early detection, supportive care during treatment, and palliative care. The devices include PDAs, pen tablet computers, and mini computers, such as those in accelerometers. A key commonality among these types of devices is their portability for use in the person's home, work, or clinical environment. The devices can be moved easily from one place to another, both indoors and outdoors. However, special screen settings may be needed for optimal outdoor viewing. Battery life also can limit use of these handheld devices when electricity or charging devices are not readily available. This limitation may be overcome by the efforts of people such as Nicholas Negroponte, originally from the Massachusetts Institute of Technology and now chair of One Laptop per Child, a nonprofit organization dedicated to developing inexpensive laptop computers for even the world's poorest children who live without electricity (see Figure 16-2). Such innovations could dramatically influence cancer research in the future.

Handheld devices differ dramatically in the types of operating systems that power their computing capabilities. Some devices, such as PDAs and smart phones, operate on propriety operating systems such as Palm OS®, for which research applications are not readily available or easily built. However, features that exist within the devices can be used to facilitate research. Turner, Mermelstein, and Flay (2004) led a team that adapted PDAs to collect ecologic momentary assessment data (real-time data) for smoking behavior and responses from adolescents in their everyday environments.

Other popular devices operate with Windows Embedded CE® or various versions of the Windows® operating system, for which software development is easily supported using Microsoft software application tools for developers or applications such as Microsoft Access. Windows-based point-of-care applications have been developed to support screening of patients for clinical trial eligibility (Breitfeld, Weisburd, Overhage, Sledge, & Tierney, 1999), for pain assessment in the community, cancer clinics, or inpatient settings (Wilkie et al., 2003), for patient education tailored to symptom level and beliefs (Wilkie et al., 2001, in press), to provide decision support for clinicians (Huang et al., 2003), for patients (Berry et al., 2006) in outpatient oncology clinics, and for cancer genetic risk assessment (Emery, 2005), to name a few examples. Figure 16-3 is an illustration of a section from a computerized fatigue intervention that was delivered on a pen tablet computer in oncology outpatient clinics.

Mini computer devices also use propriety systems, such as the Actiwatch®-Score actigraph, which has two sensors, one to detect acceleration (activity)

Figure 16-2. One Laptop per Child: An Inexpensive Laptop for Use in Developing Countries

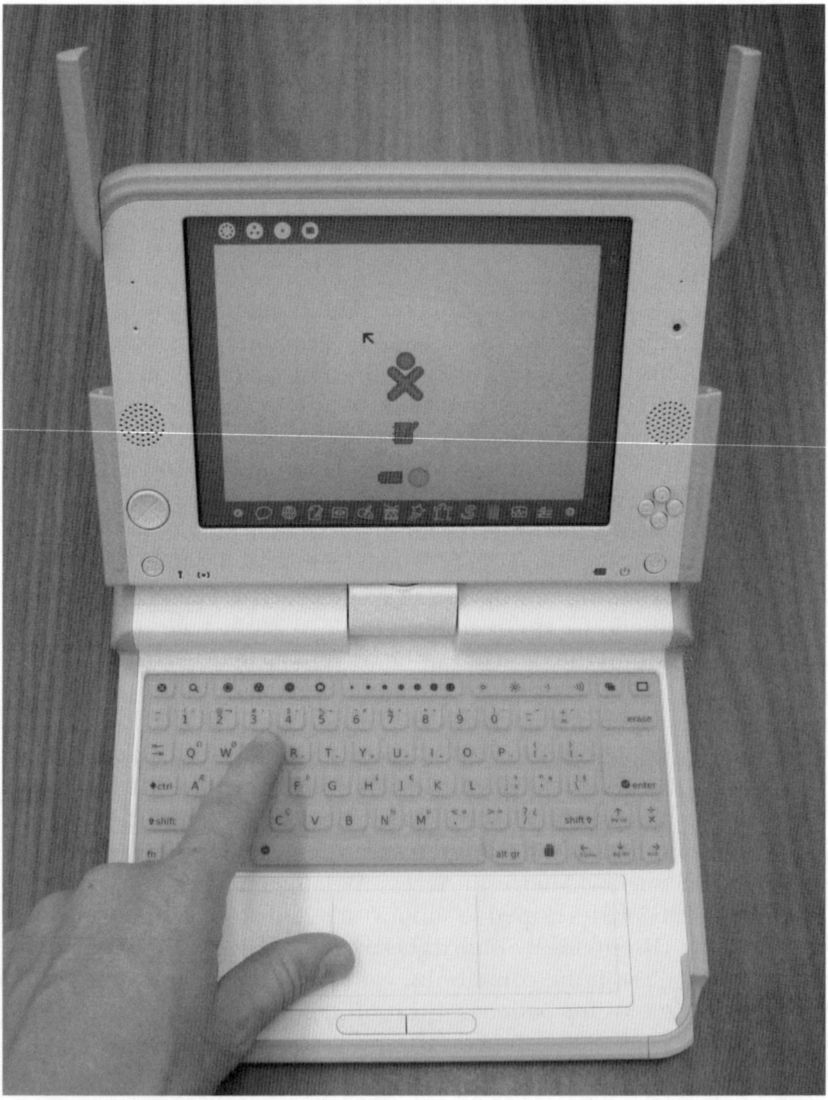

Note. Photo courtesy of D.J. Wilkie. Used with permission.

Figure 16-3. Examples of Screens From FatigueUCope—A Tailored Computerized Intervention Delivered on Pen Tablet Computers

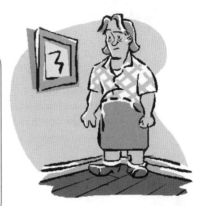

Managing Fatigue

Quit

Patients receiving treatment for cancer commonly experience fatigue. Exercise is one way you can reduce your feelings of fatigue.

Next

Screen 1 of 36

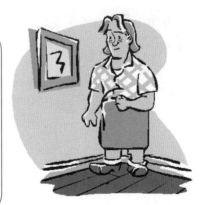

Managing Fatigue

Quit

Patients tell us that the most important time to exercise is often when their symptoms of fatigue and nausea are at their worst.

Back

Next

Screen 2 of 36

(Continued on next page)

Figure 16-3. Examples of Screens From FatigueUCope—A Tailored Computerized Intervention Delivered on Pen Tablet Computers *(Continued)*

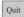

Managing Fatigue

We don't know how exercise works, but we do know that exercise makes you have more energy.

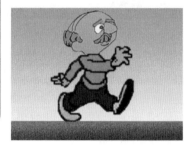

Screen 3 of 36

Managing Fatigue

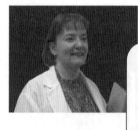

How often do I exercise aerobically?

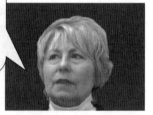

Screen 4 of 36

(Continued on next page)

Figure 16-3. Examples of Screens From FatigueUCope—A Tailored Computerized Intervention Delivered on Pen Tablet Computers *(Continued)*

Managing Fatigue

Quit

At least 4 days per week.

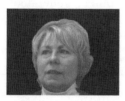

	November					
Sun	Mon	Tue	Wed	Thu	Fri	Sat
	1	2	3	4	5	6
⑦	8	⑨	10	⑪	12	⑬
14	15	16	17	18	19	20
21	22	23	24	25	26	27
28	29	30			1999	

Back

Next

Screen 5 of 36

Managing Fatigue

Quit

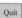

The Exercise Program

The exercise plan slowly increases the amount of exercise each week.

Week 1:	Day 1:	15 minutes
	Day 2:	18 minutes
	Day 3:	20 minutes
Week 2:	Day 1:	18 minutes
	Day 2:	22 minutes
	Day 3:	25 minutes
Week 3:	Day 1:	20 minutes
	Day 2:	24 minutes
	Day 3:	27 minutes
Week 4:	Day 1:	23 minutes
	Day 2:	26 minutes
	Day 3:	30 minutes

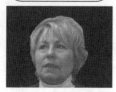

Back

Next

Screen 6 of 36

Note. Copyright 1999 by D.J. Wilkie. Used with permission.

and another to detect a selected score (e.g., pain, fatigue) (see Figure 16-4). Investigators download data stored in the Actiwatch-Score and then conduct analyses, such as relating activity to cancer symptoms or quality of life in transplant recipients (Hacker & Ferrans, 2007). The propriety operating systems provide less opportunity for researchers to tailor the devices to the research protocol. However, if the protocol fits the capabilities of the device, important cancer research can be facilitated by use of these innovations.

Scientists face important challenges when considering whether to use handheld devices. One challenge is to find a device that suits the research question and target population. The vast array of devices makes this challenge seem insurmountable to the novice technology user; a Google search on July 27, 2008, using "handheld computers" generated in 2,300,000 results.

Figure 16-4. Example of a Mini Computer Device: The Actiwatch®-Score Actigraph

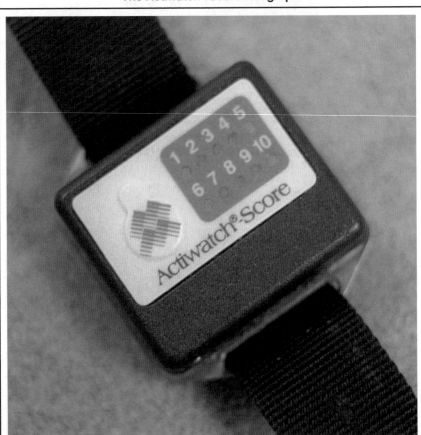

Note. Photo courtesy of D.J. Wilkie. Used with permission.

Discussions with researchers experienced in use of technology can reduce the burden of the search. Also, information technology specialists at most institutions are excellent resources for helping to find the latest and greatest devices; however, they may not fully understand the needs of the target population. Although some of the smaller, lighter-weight devices are very attractive, a major consideration is the screen size and brightness, especially for older adults and people with visual impairments or motor difficulties such as paralyses or tremors. The clinical wisdom of the scientist along with pilot testing of the various devices should guide selection of a device for a particular study.

The disadvantages of using handheld devices in research require careful consideration before using these tools in cancer nursing research. Collecting data with the technology is costly. Examples of costs include device purchase, extended warranty, maintenance, theft insurance, and software development for the research tools, as well as data downloading and conversion to statistical analysis software. The form in which the data are captured on the device can make the data conversion a time-consuming and, therefore, costly activity that requires special expertise. Loss of equipment is a concern that often is overlooked as a major limitation when the devices are used in clinics or home settings with adult subjects. Scientists should be prudent and plan for some loss of equipment, especially when the devices are carried by the research participant from place to place or when studies extend beyond the warranty period of the device, typically three years. Some costs of using the technology are offset by reduced personnel costs, particularly for data collection and double data entry. Availability of adequate programming and information technology expertise minimizes some of the cost burdens of using handheld devices in oncology nursing research.

Computer Adaptive Testing

The power of computing in the 21st century enables researchers to provide a tailored process of administering questions to subjects. *Computer adaptive testing* (CAT) is the term applied to such tailored testing. The original concept of CAT focused on item level of difficulty and has been used extensively in testing situations, such as professional competency examinations (e.g., NCLEX® examinations, Graduate Record Examinations®). In cancer research, the CAT concept has been applied to assessment of multidimensional phenomena, such as quality of life (Petersen et al., 2006). From a bank of items and based on the subject's response to a particular item, the CAT process selects the next logical item to present to the respondent that will provide maximal new information about the phenomenon as experienced by the respondent. This CAT measurement process is more efficient than standard questionnaires and reduces respondent burden because redundant items are not presented. As many as 30%–50% fewer questions may be required to obtain maximal information with CAT (Petersen et al.). This feature of CAT is attractive for research with people living with cancer.

Few scientists have used CAT in cancer research. Important disadvantages of CAT are the requirement of a large pool of calibrated items, the need for large samples in the development of the algorithms for the CAT process, and a solid theoretical understanding of the dimensional properties of the phenomenon. Scientists have used CAT to reduce the number of items required for a quality-of-life tool, but they found that the number of calibrated items was insufficient for optimal performance of the tool for people with scores in the tails of the distribution curve (Petersen et al., 2006). Although CAT theoretically holds promise for cancer research, lack of instruments with sufficient numbers of calibrated items may limit application of this innovation in oncology nursing research.

Web-Based Surveys and Interventions

The Internet has become a pervasive element of society, with information on almost anything available within the reach of a few computer keystrokes. Health care is no exception; information is available on the Web about myriad subjects, including medications, symptoms, diseases, and genetics. Research indicates that the Web is a primary source of information for cancer survivors (Mayer et al., 2007).

Scientists use the Web to collect data as well as to deliver education and information. Studies focus on everything from Internet-based support groups (Owen, Klapow, Roth, Nabell, & Tucker, 2004), to decision-making aids (Molenaar et al., 2007), to multimedia interactive risk communication (Strecher, Greenwood, Wang, & Dumont, 1999). Using the Web for research has many advantages. The Web provides access to a large and diverse sample that need not be geographically limited. Web-based education allows for interactive communication that is accessible in the convenience of the individual's home, is timely, and can be self-paced. Information can be made culturally appropriate, as evidenced in a recent innovative CD-ROM and Web-based program called *Breast Cancer Detective* (Roubidoux, 2005). *Breast Cancer Detective* is a computer game designed to teach medical students about early detection of breast cancer. It has been successfully adapted for Native American women.

Other examples include self-guided support groups on the Web for women with early-stage cancer that provide opportunities for psychological support and coping skills training (Owen et al., 2004). Even areas typically considered highly individualized and tied to faith-based centers are incorporated into the convenience of Web-based support groups. Religious expression and prayer expressed in computer-based support groups have improved psychosocial outcomes for breast cancer survivors (Shaw et al., 2007).

The use of the Web has several limitations. Research is limited on response rates and the underlying factors that influence the success of Web-based studies.

Security is an increasing problem, with the growing numbers of spammers, hackers, and messages that often not only clutter e-mail and sites but also may cause breakdown of systems. Research sites must use foolproof security to ensure that information is kept confidential and not vulnerable to outside hackers. People in rural areas where Internet connections still are not available may not benefit as yet from such information on the Web. Additionally, as people become more entranced with high-tech gadgetry, such as Adobe® Flash media, interactive graphics, music, and voice-over, high-speed Internet connections are necessary to be able to download such information. For those with low-speed or dial-up modem connections, these advanced media can be a deterrent to obtaining the information intended for them. Web-based surveys also can be accessed by people other than the intended audience, especially if incentives are involved for completing surveys. Security measures, such as using passwords, may alleviate some of the problem but can create an additional step for the respondent. Other measures include recording the Internet protocol numbers; if an individual logs in from the same computer to complete a survey a second time, the person will be blocked from taking the survey again. This security procedure, however, does not preclude someone from gaining access from a different computer.

Another limitation is the need to hire trained professionals to develop such Web-based research protocols. Maintenance must be built into any budget, as no system is foolproof. Additionally, development and testing of such programs can take several months to a year, which scientists also must account for in their timeline and budget.

Conclusion

Overall, some forms of technology have gained a solid foothold in oncology nursing research. These technologies include using CATIs for data collection and using computer-based tools for decision support, interactive support groups, and tailored patient education. The many advantages to using advanced technology include human labor cost reduction, convenient access for patients from home or while waiting for provider appointments, and access to diverse samples not limited by geographical boundaries. Using advanced technology in data collection may reduce errors. Another great advantage is the ability to personalize an intervention using interactive programs to make it most relevant to the targeted audience. Despite the many advantages, some forms of technology, such as IVR, CATI, and CAT, are less used, probably because of the need for skilled programmers, easy-to-use software programs, and calibrated items. More evaluation of these successful innovations is needed, especially for acceptability and use by low-literacy and marginalized populations as well as ethnic minority groups. The ability to personalize interventions to meet the unique needs of each individual can only increase the quality of care that nurses deliver, and as such, the integration of technology into nursing research is a necessary and valuable step.

The authors would like to thank Kelly Martin and Kevin Grandfield for their editorial assistance in preparing this chapter.

References

Albertsen, K., Andersen, A.M., Olsen, J., & Gronbaek, M. (2004). Alcohol consumption during pregnancy and the risk of preterm delivery. *American Journal of Epidemiology, 159*(2), 155–161.

Allen, B., Jr., Bastani, R., Bazargan, S., & Leonard, E. (2002). Assessing screening mammography utilization in an urban area. *Journal of the National Medical Association, 94*(1), 5–14.

Baratiny, G.Y., Campbell, E.M., Sanson-Fisher, R.W., Graham, J., & Cockburn, J. (2000). Collecting cancer risk factor data from hospital outpatients: Use of touch-screen computers. *Cancer Detection and Prevention, 24*(6), 501–507.

Berry, D.L., Wolpin, S.E., Lober, W.B., Ellis, W.J., Russell, K.J., & Davison, B.J. (2006). Actual use and perceived usefulness of a Web-based, decision support program for men with prostate cancer. In H.A. Parks, P. Murray, & C. Delaney (Eds.), *Consumer-centered computer-supported care for healthy people* (pp. 781–782). Amsterdam: IOS Press.

Blyth, F.M., March, L.M., Shellard, D., & Cousins, M.J. (2002). The experience of using random digit dialing methods in a population-based chronic pain study. *Australia and New Zealand Journal of Public Health, 26*(6), 511–514.

Breitfeld, P.P., Weisburd, M., Overhage, J.M., Sledge, G., Jr., & Tierney, W.M. (1999). Pilot study of a point-of-use decision support tool for cancer clinical trials eligibility. *Journal of the American Medical Informatics Association, 6*(6), 466–477.

Buckwalter, J.G., Crooks, V.C., & Petitti, D.B. (2002). A preliminary psychometric analysis of a computer-assisted administration of the Telephone Interview of Cognitive Status-modified. *Journal of Clinical and Experimental Neuropsychology, 24*(2), 168–175.

Campbell, M.K., DeVellis, B.M., Strecher, V.J., Ammerman, A.S., DeVellis, R.F., & Sandler, R.S. (1994). Improving dietary behavior: The effectiveness of tailored messages in primary care settings. *American Journal of Public Health, 84*(5), 783–787.

Champion, V.L. (1994). Beliefs about breast cancer and mammography by behavioral stage. *Oncology Nursing Forum, 21*(6), 1009–1014.

Champion, V.L., Maraj, M., Hui, S., Perkins, A.J., Tierney, W., Menon, U., et al. (2003). Comparison of tailored interventions to increase mammography screening in nonadherent older women. *Preventive Medicine, 36*(2), 150–158.

Champion, V.L., Skinner, C.S., Menon, U., Seshadri, R., Anzalone, D.C., & Rawl, S.M. (2002). Comparisons of tailored mammography interventions at two months postintervention. *Annals of Behavioral Medicine, 24*(3), 211–218.

Cherpitel, C.J. (2002). Screening for alcohol problems in the U.S. general population: Comparison of the CAGE, RAPS4, and RAPS4-QF by gender, ethnicity, and service utilization. Rapid Alcohol Problems Screen. *Alcoholism, Clinical and Experimental Research, 26*(11), 1686–1691.

Cherpitel, C.J. (2003). Changes in substance use associated with emergency room and primary care services utilization in the United States general population: 1995–2000. *American Journal of Drug and Alcohol Abuse, 29*(4), 789–802.

Corkrey, R., & Parkinson, L. (2002). Interactive voice response: Review of studies 1989–2000. *Behavior Research Methods, Instruments, and Computers, 34*(3), 342–353.

Crawford, A.G., Sikirica, V., Goldfarb, N., Popiel, R.G., Patel, M., Wang, C., et al. (2005). Interactive voice response reminder effects on preventive service utilization. *American Journal of Medical Quality, 20*(6), 329–336.

DePalma, A. (2000). Prostate cancer shared decision: A CD-ROM educational and decision-assisting tool for men with prostate cancer. *Seminars in Urologic Oncology, 18*(3), 178–181.

Emery, J. (2005). The GRAIDS trial: The development and evaluation of computer decision support for cancer genetic risk assessment in primary care. *Annals of Human Biology, 32*(2), 218–227.

Emmons, K.M., Wong, M., Puleo, E., Weinstein, N., Fletcher, R., & Colditz, G. (2004). Tailored computer-based cancer risk communication: Correcting colorectal cancer risk perception. *Journal of Health Communication, 9*(2), 127–141.

Green, M.J., Biesecker, B.B., McInerney, A.M., Mauger, D., & Fost, N. (2001). An interactive computer program can effectively educate patients about genetic testing for breast cancer susceptibility. *American Journal of Medical Genetics, 103*(1), 16–23.

Green, M.J., Peterson, S.K., Baker, M.W., Harper, G.R., Friedman, L.C., Rubinstein, W.S., et al. (2004). Effect of a computer-based decision aid on knowledge, perceptions, and intentions about genetic testing for breast cancer susceptibility: A randomized controlled trial. *JAMA, 292*(4), 442–452.

Gustafson, D.H., Hawkins, R., Pingree, S., McTavish, F., Arora, N.K., Mendenhall, J., et al. (2001). Effect of computer support on younger women with breast cancer. *Journal of General Internal Medicine, 16*(7), 435–445.

Hacker, E.D., & Ferrans, C.E. (2007). Ecological momentary assessment of fatigue in patients receiving intensive cancer therapy. *Journal of Pain and Symptom Management, 33*(3), 267–275.

Huang, H.Y., Wilkie, D.J., Zong, S.P., Berry, D., Hairabedian, D., Judge, M.K., et al. (2003). Developing a computerized data collection and decision support system for cancer pain management. *Computers, Informatics, Nursing, 21*(4), 206–217.

Institute of Medicine. (2001). *Crossing the quality chasm: A new health system for the 21st century.* Washington, DC: National Academies Press.

Janda, L.H., Janda, M., & Tedford, E. (2001). IVR test and survey: A computer program to collect data via computerized telephonic applications. *Behavior Research Methods, Instruments, and Computers, 33*(4), 513–516.

Jones, J.M., Nyhof-Young, J., Friedman, A., & Catton, P. (2001). More than just a pamphlet: Development of an innovative computer-based education program for cancer patients. *Patient Education and Counseling, 44*(3), 271–281.

Jones, R., Pearson, J., McGregor, S., Cawsey, A.J., Barrett, A., Craig, N., et al. (1999). Randomised trial of personalised computer based information for cancer patients. *BMJ: Clinical Research Edition, 319*(7219), 1241–1247.

Keating, N.L., Guadagnoli, E., Landrum, M.B., Borbas, C., & Weeks, J.C. (2002). Treatment decision making in early-stage breast cancer: Should surgeons match patients' desired level of involvement? *Journal of Clinical Oncology, 20*(6), 1473-1479

Ketola, E., & Klockars, M. (1999). Computer-assisted telephone interview (CATI) in primary care. *Family Practice, 16*(2), 179–183.

Kim, S.P., Knight, S.J., Tomori, C., Colella, K.M., Schoor, R.A., Shih, L., et al. (2001). Health literacy and shared decision making for prostate cancer patients with low socioeconomic status. *Cancer Investigation, 19*(7), 684–691.

Kreuter, M.W., Farrell, D.W., Olevitch, L.K., & Brennan, L.R. (2000). *Tailoring health messages: Customizing communication with computer technology.* Mahwah, NJ: Lawrence Erlbaum.

Krishna, S., Balas, E.A., Boren, S.A., & Maglaveras, N. (2002). Patient acceptance of educational voice messages: A review of controlled clinical studies. *Methods of Information in Medicine, 41*(5), 360–369.

Lee, H., Friedman, M.E., Cukor, P., & Ahern, D. (2003). Interactive voice response system (IVRS) in health care services. *Nursing Outlook, 51*(6), 277–283.

Leon, A.C., Kelsey, J.E., Pleil, A., Burgos, T.L., Portera, L., & Lowell, K.N. (1999). An evaluation of a computer assisted telephone interview for screening for mental disorders among primary care patients. *Journal of Nervous and Mental Disease, 187*(5), 308–311.

Mayer, D.K., Terrin, N.C., Kreps, G.L., Menon, U., McCance, K., Parsons, S.K., et al. (2007). Cancer survivors information seeking behaviors: A comparison of survivors who do and do not seek information about cancer. *Patient Education and Counseling, 65*(3), 342–350.

Menon, U., Champion, V.L., Monahan, P.O., Daggy, J., Hui, S., & Skinner, C.S. (2007). Health Belief Model variables as predictors of progression in stage of mammography adoption. *American Journal of Health Promotion, 21*(4), 255–261.

Molenaar, S., Sprangers, M., Oort, F., Rutgers, E., Luiten, E., Mulder, J., et al. (2007). Exploring the black box of a decision aid: What information do patients select from an interactive CD-ROM on treatment options in breast cancer? *Patient Education and Counseling, 65*(1), 122–130.

Mooney, K.H., Beck, S.L., Friedman, R.H., & Farzanfar, R. (2002). Telephone-linked care for cancer symptom monitoring: A pilot study. *Cancer Practice, 10*(3), 147–54.

Nicholas, D., Huntington, P., Williams, P., & Vickery, P. (2001). Health information: An evaluation of the use of touch screen kiosks in two hospitals. *Health Information Library Journal, 18*(4), 213–219.

Owen, J.E., Klapow, J.C., Roth, D.L., Nabell, L., & Tucker, D.C. (2004). Improving the effectiveness of adjuvant psychological treatment for women with breast cancer: The feasibility of providing online support. *Psycho-Oncology, 13*(4), 281–292.

Pearson, J., Jones, R., Cawsey, A., McGregor, S., Barrett, A., Gilmour, H., et al. (1999). The accessibility of information systems for patients: Use of touchscreen information systems by 345 patients with cancer in Scotland. *Proceedings of the American Medical Informatics Association Annual Symposium*, pp. 594–598.

Petersen, M.A., Groenvold, M., Aaronson, N., Fayers, P., Sprangers, M., & Bjorner, J.B. (2006). Multidimensional computerized adaptive testing of the EORTC QLQ-C30: Basic developments and evaluations. *Quality of Life Research, 15*(3), 315–329.

Rakowski, W., Ehrich, B., Goldstein, M.G., Rimer, B.K., Pearlman, D.N., Clark, M.A., et al. (1998). Increasing mammography among women aged 40–74 by use of a stage-matched, tailored intervention. *Preventive Medicine, 27*(5, Pt. 1), 748–756.

Rawl, S.M., Given, B.A., Given, C.W., Champion, V.L., Kozachik, S.L., Kozachik, S.L., et al. (2002). Intervention to improve psychological functioning for newly diagnosed patients with cancer. *Oncology Nursing Forum, 29*(6), 967–975.

Rawl, S.M., Menon, U., Champion, V.L., May, F.E., Loehrer, P., Sr., Hunter, C., et al. (2005). Do benefits and barriers differ by stage of adoption for colorectal cancer screening? *Health Education Research, 20*(2), 137–148.

Roubidoux, M.A. (2005). Breast cancer detective: A computer game to teach breast cancer screening to Native American patients. *Journal of Cancer Education, 20*(Suppl. 1), 87–91.

Shaw, B., Han, J.Y., Kim, E., Gustafson, D., Hawkins, R., Cleary, J., et al. (2007). Effects of prayer and religious expression within computer support groups on women with breast cancer. *Psycho-Oncology, 16*(7), 676–687.

Skinner, C.S., Champion, V., Menon, U., & Seshadri, R. (2002). Racial and educational differences in mammography-related perceptions among 1,366 nonadherent women. *Journal of Psychosocial Oncology, 20*(3), 1–17.

Skinner, C.S., Kobrin, S.C., Monahan, P.O., Daggy, J., Menon, U., Todora, H.S., et al. (2007). Tailored interventions for screening mammography among a sample of initially non-adherent women: When is a booster dose important? *Patient Education and Counseling, 65*(1), 87–94.

Strecher, V.J., Greenwood, T., Wang, C., & Dumont, D. (1999). Interactive multimedia and risk communication. *Journal of the National Cancer Institute Monographs, 1999*(25), 134–139.

Strecher, V.J., Marcus, A., Bishop, K., Fleisher, L., Stengle, W., Levinson, A., et al. (2005). A randomized controlled trial of multiple tailored messages for smoking cessation among callers to the cancer information service. *Journal of Health Communication, 10*(Suppl. 1), 105–118.

Sutherland, L.A., Campbell, M., Ornstein, K., Wildemuth, B., & Lobach, D. (2001). Development of an adaptive multimedia program to collect patient health data. *American Journal of Preventive Medicine, 21*(4), 320–324.

Turner, L., Mermelstein, R., & Flay, B. (2004). Individual and contextual influences on adolescent smoking. *Annals of the New York Academy of Sciences, 1021,* 175–197.

Weinbaum, Z., Stratton, T.L., Chavez, G., Motylewski-Link, C., Barrera, N., & Courtney, J.G. (2001). Female victims of intimate partner physical domestic violence (IPP-DV), California 1998. *American Journal of Preventive Medicine, 21*(4), 313–319.

White, M., Stark, J.R., Luckmann, R., Rosal, M.C., Clemow, L., & Costanza, M.E. (2006). Implementing a computer-assisted telephone interview (CATI) system to increase colorectal cancer screening: A process evaluation. *Patient Education and Counseling, 61*(3), 419–428.

Wilkie, D.J., Huang, H.Y., Berry, D.L., Schwartz, A., Lin, Y.C., Ko, N.Y., et al. (2001). Cancer symptom control: Feasibility of a tailored, interactive computerized program for patients. *Family and Community Health, 24*(3), 48–62.

Wilkie, D.J., Judge, M.K., Berry, D.L., Dell, J., Zong, S., & Gilespie, R. (2003). Usability of a computerized PAINReportIt in the general public with pain and people with cancer pain. *Journal of Pain and Symptom Management, 25*(3), 213–224.

Wilkie, D.J., Schwartz, A., Huang, H.Y., Ko, N.Y., Liao, W.C., Hairabedian, D., et al. (in press). Computerized exercise education for patients reduces cancer-related fatigue. *Cancer.*

Wilkins, C., Casswell, S., Barnes, H.M., & Pledger, M. (2003). A pilot study of a computer-assisted cell-phone interview (CACI) methodology to survey respondents in households without telephones about alcohol use. *Drug and Alcohol Review, 22*(2), 221–225.

Wofford, J.L., Smith, E.D., & Miller, D.P. (2005). The multimedia computer for office-based patient education: A systematic review. *Patient Education and Counseling, 59*(2), 148–157.

CHAPTER 17

Advancing Oncology Nursing Science: Focus on Nursing-Sensitive Patient Outcomes

Susan L. Beck, PhD, APRN, FAAN, AOCN®,
Danielle Pierotti May, RN, MSN, AOCN®,
and Darryl Somayaji, MSN, RN, CCRC

Introduction

The focus on quality in healthcare delivery has shifted from process to outcomes for individual patients, families, and populations. Healthcare organizations and providers now are accountable not only for performance or the quality of care delivered but also for the end results of their care—outcomes. Drivers of this new era of accountability include national leadership organizations, legislators, regulators, payers, and consumers. Each constituent group is interested in knowing to what extent practice actually brings about improvement in health—in other words, whether the patient achieves the desired outcome (Given et al., 2003).

This chapter provides a review of historical developments leading to a focus on outcomes, discusses issues related to measuring performance and outcomes, and makes recommendations for advancing oncology nursing science.

Historical Perspectives

Since 1990, the Institute of Medicine (IOM), an independent scientific advisory body, has released a series of landmark reports (see Figure 17-1) that

---

Figure 17-1. Landmark Reports From the Institute of Medicine of the National Academies That Have Shaped the Outcomes Imperative in Oncology

1990—*Medicare: A Strategy for Quality Assurance*
1998—*Statement on Quality of Care—National Roundtable on Health Care Quality: The Urgent Need to Improve Health Care Quality*
1999—*Measuring the Quality of Health Care*
1999—*Ensuring Quality Cancer Care*
1999—*To Err Is Human: Building a Safer Health System*
2001—*Crossing the Quality Chasm: A New Health System for the 21st Century*
2003—*Priority Areas for National Action: Transforming Health Care Quality*
2003—*Keeping Patients Safe: Transforming the Work Environment of Nurses*
2004—*Patient Safety: Achieving a New Standard of Care*
2005—*Quality Through Collaboration: The Future of Rural Health Care*
2006—*Rewarding Provider Performance: Aligning Incentives in Medicare*
2007—*Advancing Quality Improvement Research: Challenges and Opportunities, Workshop Summary*
2008—*Knowing What Works in Healthcare: A Roadmap for the Nation*

Note. Based on information from Institute of Medicine of the National Academies, 2008.

---

repeatedly call for dramatic changes to improve the quality of health care in the United States. In one such report, *quality of care* was defined as "the degree to which services for individuals and populations increase the likelihood of desired health *outcomes* and are consistent with current professional knowledge" (Lohr, 1990, p. 4). This definition provides an essential framework to posit that consistent practice, based on evidence including research, ultimately can improve the quality of care as measured by patient outcomes.

This outcomes imperative gained increased momentum with the 2003 Medicare Prescription Drug, Improvement, and Modernization Act, which set the stage for pay-for-performance. Since then, Medicare has launched a number of initiatives to encourage improved quality of care in all healthcare settings that serve Medicare beneficiaries. The settings include ambulatory care clinics and physicians' offices, hospitals, home healthcare agencies, and nursing homes (Centers for Medicare and Medicaid Services [CMS], 2007). These initiatives have been particularly wide reaching because of the involvement of numerous partner organizations, including the National Quality Forum (NQF), the Joint Commission on Accreditation of Healthcare Organizations, the National Committee for Quality Assurance, the Agency for Healthcare Research and Quality (AHRQ), the American Medical Association, and many others (CMS, 2005).

One example of the Medicare Hospital Quality Initiative calls for hospitals to report data related to specific quality indicators to CMS. Although not mandatory, hospitals that do not participate do not receive 100% of the allowable diagnosis-related group reimbursement. A critical component of such CMS quality initiatives is that data are available to consumers on a searchable Web site, such as www.hospitalcompare.hhs.gov. The Web site allows comparison of hospitals by specific indicators. Plans are now in place to extend this initiative to providers.

The focus to date has been on performance, which is documenting delivery of evidence-based care. The goals to align payment with performance were outlined in the 2006 IOM report titled *Rewarding Provider Performance: Aligning Incentives in Medicare* (IOM, 2006). The report recommended that CMS reward care based on three criteria: high clinical quality, patient-centeredness, and efficiency. A staged implementation is planned that includes all provider organizations as well as clinicians, including advanced practice nurses. New initiatives to measure and report patient outcomes and patient-centered care, such as those proposed by NQF and the Hospital Consumer Assessment of Healthcare Providers and Systems (HCAHPS®) survey, a unified patient satisfaction survey sponsored by CMS, will extend accountability beyond performance to outcomes (CMS & AHRQ, 2005). As other payers adopt such approaches, the monitoring, reporting, and improving of quality indicators, including both performance and outcomes, will become integral to the business of healthcare delivery.

In the Oncology Nursing Society (ONS) white paper on nursing-sensitive patient outcomes (NSPOs), Given and Sherwood (2005) reviewed the historical contexts and national trends that are driving organizations such as ONS to develop strategic initiatives to improve patient outcomes. Figure 17-2 summarizes and updates their review of the milestones that have occurred in oncology nursing.

The focus on hospital quality of care began in earnest in the 1990s as the American Nurses Association (ANA) responded to restructuring and downsizing initiatives of hospitals trying to reduce costs (Bolton, Donaldson, Rutledge, Bennett, & Brown, 2007). ANA led the development of a national nursing quality database, which has grown into an extensive resource on nurse and patient outcomes in hospitalized patients. The National Database of Nursing Quality Indicators (NDNQI®) is only one example of an important advance in health services research—the explosion of databases. Table 17-1 provides examples of multiple types of databases that may inform oncology nursing science and practice. These databases have extended beyond the hospital setting and include ambulatory care, home care, and long-term care (Alexander, 2007; Needleman, Kurtzman, & Kizer, 2007; Rantz & Connolly, 2004).

The *outcomes movement* notably has gained in strength as a result of the synergistic efforts of multiple partnering organizations. For example, as of 2006, the National Comprehensive Cancer Network (NCCN) and the American Society of Clinical Oncology began collaborating on the National Initiative on Cancer Care Quality. During the first phase, providers are collecting and reporting data on seven indicators for breast and colorectal cancer (NCCN, 2007). Oncology nursing is well positioned to actively be engaged in these partnership initiatives through participation of individual nurse scientists as leaders within these organizations and through organizational partnerships via ONS.

Figure 17-2. Historical Milestones in the Movement to Improve Oncology Nursing-Sensitive Patient Outcomes (NSPOs)

1995—American Nurses Association (ANA) Nursing Report for Acute Care Settings was released.

1998—Oncology Nursing Society (ONS) State-of-the-Science Conference on Nursing-Sensitive Patient Outcomes was held.

2000—ONS Outcomes Expert Panel identified gaps and goals for outcomes research.

2002—Nursing-sensitive quality indicators for community-based nonacute care settings were established.

2002—ANA launched its Safety and Quality Initiative.

2002—Focus groups from ONS Special Interest Groups convened at ONS Congress.

2003—ONS research agenda prioritized research on effectiveness of nursing care on outcomes.

2003—ONS Outcomes Project Team developed definition of NSPOs.

2004—APRN retreat identified the need for additional products for evidence-based practice.

2004—National Quality Forum established national voluntary consensus standards for nursing-sensitive care, and an annual performance measure was set.

2005—Given and Beck gave the keynote address on NSPOs at the 8th National Conference on Cancer Nursing Research.

2005—Given and Sherwood's commissioned white paper on NSPOs was published in the *Oncology Nursing Forum*.

2005—The first volume of evidence-based summaries on measuring symptoms was completed by multiple teams of researchers and clinicians.

2005—The ONS Outcomes Strategic Planning Team was commissioned to develop a detailed strategic plan to improve NSPOs.

2005—ONS evidence-based teams developed the first Putting Evidence Into Practice® (PEP) products.

2005—Representatives from each ONS PEP Team developed and presented an institute on evidence-based practice at the ONS Institutes of Learning (IOL) in Arizona.

2006—A CD-ROM of the IOL presentation was distributed to ONS members.

2006—The first wave of ONS PEP products was launched.

2006—ONS PEP reviews were published in the *Clinical Journal of Oncology Nursing*.

2006—Beck, Joyce, and Mitchell made a presentation at ONS Congress on the ONS journey to improve NSPOs.

2007—Volume 2 of ONS PEP products were published.

2008—Volumes 3 and 4 of ONS PEP products were published.

Note. Based on information from Given & Sherwood, 2005.

Nursing-Sensitive Patient Outcomes

NQF provided a broad definition of *nursing-sensitive performance measures* as processes and outcomes, and the structural proxies for these processes and outcomes (for example, skill mix and staffing hours), that are affected, provided, or influenced by nursing personnel but for which nursing is not exclusively responsible (NQF, 2006). Within this framework, outcomes that result from the impact of nursing interventions on patients and their healthcare problems have been called NSPOs (Given et al., 2003). NQF has recom-

Table 17-1. Examples of Outcomes Databases Valuable for Advancing Oncology Nursing Science

Name and Web Address	Description
CaPSURE™ database www.capsure.net	Created in 1995, the CaPSURE™ database has enrolled more than 11,000 patients and provides one of the most extensive sets of data available today on prostate cancer. Physicians provide comprehensive clinical assessment of their patients with prostate cancer over the course of their treatment, including method of diagnosis, pathologic staging, medications, and the results of all procedures and lab tests such as biopsies, imaging, and blood tests.
Home Care: Outcome and Assessment Information Set (OASIS) www.cms.hhs.gov/OASIS	OASIS is a group of data elements that represent core items of a comprehensive assessment for an adult homecare patient and form the basis for measuring patient outcomes for purposes of outcome-based quality improvement. OASIS was designed to provide the necessary data items to measure both outcomes and patient risk factors. OASIS data items address sociodemographic, environmental, support system, health status, functional status, and health service utilization characteristics of the patient.
IKnowMed www.iknowmed.com/home.html	IKnowMed is an oncology database that captures treatment outcomes including treatment response, toxicities, treatment regimen, relative dose intensity, chemotherapy dosing, tests, and lab results. The databse is now used by U.S. Oncology, a network of more than 900 physicians practicing in approximately 460 locations, including 85 outpatient cancer centers in 32 states for more than 350,000 patients with cancer per year—more than any other single medical organization in the world.
Minimum Data Set (MDS) www.cms.hhs.gov/Minimum DataSets20	The MDS is part of the federally mandated process for clinical assessment of all residents in Medicare- or Medicaid-certified nursing homes. This process provides a comprehensive assessment of each resident's functional capabilities and helps nursing home staff to identify health problems.
The National Cancer Institute (Surveillance, Epidemiology and End Results [SEER])-Medicare Datalink http://healthservices.cancer.gov/seermedicare/aboutdata	This linkage of two large population-based sources of data provides detailed information about older adults with cancer. The current SEER-Medicare linkage includes all Medicare-eligible people appearing in the SEER database through 2002 and their Medicare claims through 2005.

(Continued on next page)

Table 17-1. Examples of Outcomes Databases Valuable for Advancing Oncology Nursing Science *(Continued)*

Name and Web Address	Description
The National Health Interview Survey (NHIS) www.cdc.gov/nchs/nhis.htm	The main objective of the NHIS is to monitor the health of the U.S. population through the collection and analysis of data on a broad range of health topics. The annual nation-wide survey of about 36,000 households in the United States determines knowledge, attitudes, and practices concerning cancer-related health behaviors and cancer screening modalities.
Patient Care Monitor www.supportiveoncologyservices .com	Patient Care Monitor is a tablet computer–based self-assessment that yields a review of symptoms and family history. Data are collected at the time of a patient visit to more than 100 community-based oncology practices in the United States.

mended voluntary consensus standards for nursing performance that include patient-centered, nursing-centered, and system-centered outcome measures (NQF; Naylor, 2007).

An ONS project team defined *NSPOs* in a definition statement as follows.

> Outcomes, which focus on how patients and their health care problems are affected by nursing interventions, have been identified and are described as Nursing-Sensitive Outcomes. Nursing-sensitive outcomes are those outcomes arrived at, or significantly impacted, by nursing interventions. The interventions must be within the scope of nursing practice and integral to the processes of nursing care; an empirical link must exist. Nursing-Sensitive Outcomes represent the consequences or effects of nursing interventions and result in changes in patients' symptom experience, functional status, safety, psychological distress, and/or costs. . . . Nursing-Sensitive Outcomes are outcomes that are sensitive to nursing care or care rendered in collaboration with other healthcare providers. (Given et al., 2003)

Several classification schemas have been published within nursing journals to provide an organizing framework for NSPOs, which are compared in Table 17-2. The ONS definition includes five categories that are identified as being critical to oncology nursing: the symptom experience, functional status, safety (preventable adverse events), psychological distress, and economic outcomes. Examples are provided for each category in Figure 17-3.

Table 17-2. Comparison of Classification Schema for Nursing-Sensitive Patient Outcomes	
Source	**Classification Schema**
Hegyvary, 1991	Clinical (patient's responses to interventions) Functional (improvement or decline in functioning) Financial (cost and length of stay) Perceptual (patient satisfaction with care)
Mitchell et al., 1998	Appropriate self-care Demonstration of health-promoting behaviors Health-related quality of life Patient perception of receiving quality care Symptom management
Jennings et al., 1999	Patient-focused (e.g., diagnosis-focused and holistically focused) Care provider–focused (e.g., complication rates) Organization-focused (e.g., falls)
Given et al., 2003	Symptom experience Functional status Safety (preventable adverse events) Psychological distress Economic

The classification could be strengthened by the addition of a category related to healthy self-care or health-promoting behaviors as intermediate outcomes that affect cancer morbidity and mortality. Across the spectrum of care, from cancer prevention to long-term follow-up in the growing numbers of cancer survivors, outcomes such as smoking cessation, adopting and maintaining physical activity, and eating a healthy diet are behaviors that oncology nurses should target.

The Need for Good Measures of Patient Outcomes and Nursing Care

To understand the relationship between nursing care and patient outcomes, investigators must be able to reliably measure care quality and patient outcomes at the nurse-patient level in a time frame that is sensitive to change. Reliability and validity are two essential qualities of effective measurement tools. *Reliability* is an indicator of the consistency or stability of a measure and reflects the proportion of variance that is attributable to the true score of a latent variable versus random error (Carmines & Zeller, 1979). Key types of reliability that are important to consider are stability, internal consistency, and equivalence (American Educational Research Association, American Psychological Association, & National Council on Measurement in Education, 1999). The type of reliability that is relevant varies depending on the tool. *Validity* commonly is defined as whether a tool measures what it claims to measure and historically has included the three Cs: content, criterion-related, and construct validity.

Figure 17-3. Oncology Nursing-Sensitive Outcomes: A Classification With Exemplars

Symptom Experience
• Pain
• Fatigue
• Insomnia
• Nausea
• Constipation
• Anorexia
• Breathlessness
• Diarrhea
• Altered skin/mucous membranes
• Neutropenia

Functional Status
• ADL (activities of daily living)
• IADL (instrumental activities of daily living)
• Role functioning
• Activity tolerance
• Ability to carry out usual activities
• Nutritional status

Safety (preventable adverse events)
• Infections
• Falls
• Skin ulcers
• Extravasation incidents
• Hypersensitive reactions

Psychological Distress
• Anxiety
• Depression
• Spiritual distress

Economic (incorporate this category into all categories)
• Length of stay
• Unexpected readmissions
• Emergency visits
• Out-of-pocket costs (family)
• Cost per patient day
• Cost per episode of care

Note. From *Nursing-Sensitive Patient Outcomes,* by B. Given, S.L. Beck, C. Etland, B.H. Gobel, L. Lamkin, and V.D. Marsee, 2003. Retrieved May 20, 2007, from http://www.ons .org/outcomes/measures/outcomes.shtml. Copyright by the Oncology Nursing Society. Reprinted with permission.

More recent conceptualizations define validity as the degree to which evidence and theory support the interpretations of test scores entailed by the proposed use of tests (American Educational Research Association et al.). Five types of evidence are considered: (a) test content, (b) response processes, (c) internal structure, (d) relations to other variables, and (e) consequences of testing.

Three other factors are important to consider in measurement. If an instrument is to be useful in intervention studies, it must be *sensitive*—meaning it changes over time as hypothesized. Sensitivity is an essential quality to consider in a tool to measure outcomes of the quality of nursing care. Clinical utility is an extremely important factor if a tool is to be integrated into a practice setting for ongoing measurement and quality improvement. Finally, issues of literacy, readability, language, and cultural equivalency must be considered if surveys or questionnaires are used (Frank-Stromborg & Olsen, 2004).

Measuring Nursing-Sensitive Patient Outcomes

Numerous and varied approaches are available when measuring patient outcomes. These commonly include self-report measures such as surveys, questionnaires, and diaries. Such tools can be self-administered via paper and pencil or electronically administered using a telephone, a PDA, or a computer. Biophysiologic variables can be measured with equipment such as thermometers, sphygmomanometers, electrocardiographs, and actigraphs or via a laboratory. Measures may be directly obtained prospectively or indirectly abstracted from medical records using a retrospective approach.

In 2001, Spilsbury and Meyer indicated that the manner in which patient outcomes have been measured and documented varies widely. Therefore, inconsistent measurement has hampered efforts to build the evidence to better describe and test nursing interventions. Decisions about which tool to use must be made based on evidence related to the reliability, validity, and sensitivity of measures in the population that will be studied. Thus, one of the significant accomplishments in this area has been the work supported by ONS to develop a resource that summarizes the evidence related to measuring NSPOs in oncology populations (Friese & Beck, 2004). ONS commissioned specific project teams of scientists and clinicians to develop a summary of information related to outcomes in the following categories: definitions, integrated reviews and meta-analyses, guidelines and standards, tables of tools, references related to specific instruments to measure the outcome, summary of key evidence that nursing interventions influence this outcome, gaps in the current evidence base, recommendations, electronic links, and links to current research. Depending on the outcome, specific inclusion criteria for reviewing measures were specified. The authors provided summaries of each tool, including a description of the tool's constructs or domains, scaling, scoring, and language availability. Specific findings to support reliability, validity, sensitivity or responsiveness, and clinical usefulness, including language availability, were summarized (Friese & Beck). References related to each summary, including links to abstracts or electronically available manuscripts, are provided. Table 17-3 provides an example of a table of evidence related to measuring fatigue. The ONS Web site (www.ons.org/outcomes/measures/summaries.shtml) provides the most up-to-date resource for each outcome.

Outcomes must be evaluated across the continuum of care and will vary by setting (Given & Sherwood, 2005). Nurses need to include short-term, intermediate, and long-term outcome evaluations that incorporate preventive, interventional, supportive, and quality-of-life cancer care. Diverse types of measures need to be applied across nursing practice in a variety of clinical settings. Outcomes of choice will vary depending on the role and level of nursing practice. For example, a staff nurse in a homecare agency would be interested in different outcomes than an advanced practice nurse in an ambulatory treatment center.

Measuring Quality of Nursing Care

Nursing care can be measured in a variety of ways: nursing workforce and staffing, medical records, observations, and surveys. Measures related to nursing staff, also known as workforce measures, might include staffing variables (e.g., hours per patient day, caseload, total hours, staff mix), as well as characteristics of nurses hypothesized to be important (e.g., education, age, certification, experience). Several large nursing-quality databases, including the NDNQI, the California Nursing Outcomes Coalition, and the Veterans Administration Nursing Outcomes Database project, have included such workforce and nurse variables as quality indicators (Alexander, 2007; Brown, Donaldson, Aydin, & Carlson, 2001). These databases provide a resource to examine questions such as the relationship of variables (e.g., the number of nursing care hours per patient day) with specific patient outcomes (e.g., falls, skin breakdown). Data elements focus on the overall outcomes of care and are aggregated at the hospital and/or unit level. Both nurse and patient data are aggregated, and differences are examined from the collective perspective. Thus, individual patient outcomes cannot be linked to individual nursing interventions in these databases. For example, specific nursing interventions, such as adherence to a turning schedule for a bed-bound patient, cannot be examined specifically in relation to pressure ulcers. More research also is necessary to examine the relationship between specific oncology nursing characteristics, such as certification status, and NSPOs.

Medical records provide documentation of the interventions provided to a specific patient in chronologic order (Aaronson & Burman, 1994). They offer a single location to look for both intervention and outcome. Data can be extracted manually using a checklist or audit tool or can be integrated into an electronic medical record reporting system. Unfortunately, medical records vary from location to location. The language used is widely variable, and the documentation requirements differ—sometimes even from unit to unit within a facility. Additionally, much is assumed in medical records. The

Table 17-3. Examples From Tables of Evidence Related to Measuring Fatigue in Patients With Cancer

Sample Oncology Nursing Society Putting Evidence Into Practice® (PEP) Table of Evidence: Description of Tools

Name of Tool	Author/Year	Domains or Factors	# of Items	Scaling	Scoring	Language
Brief Fatigue Inventory (BFI)	Mendoza et al., 1999	Severity and impact of fatigue	9	0–10; 11-point Likert scale	A global fatigue score can be obtained by averaging all the items on the BFI. Severity of fatigue: sum of 3 items; Impact of fatigue: sum of 6 items	English, German, Japanese, Chinese-Taiwanese versions

Sample Oncology Nursing Society PEP Table of Evidence: Psychometric Properties of Tools

Name of Tool	Populations*	Reliability and Validity	Sensitivity	Clinical Utility	Comment
Brief Fatigue Inventory (BFI)	1. 305 adult inpatients and outpatients with a variety of cancer diagnoses and 290-member healthy group, 81% Caucasian (Mendoza et al., 1999)	Reliability 1. Internal consistency: Cronbach's alpha coefficient = 0.89–0.96 (Mendoza et al., 1999; Okuyama et al., 2003; Radbruch et al., 2003) 2. Test-retest: r = .79–.91 (Radbruch et al., 2003)	Patients with cancer reported higher levels of fatigue compared with control group (members of service groups) (Mendoza et al., 1999).	Rapid identification of those patients with clinically significant fatigue, and easy for intervention study to follow up on the impact of interventions on fatigue	The study found that the optimal cut point for "mild" and "moderate" fatigue severity should be investigated further (Mendoza et al., 1999).

(Continued on next page)

Table 17-3. Examples From Tables of Evidence Related to Measuring Fatigue in Patients With Cancer *(Continued)*

Sample Oncology Nursing Society PEP Table of Evidence: Psychometric Properties of Tools

Name of Tool	Populations	Reliability and Validity	Sensitivity	Clinical Utility	Comment
	2. 252 adults with a variety of cancer diagnoses in outpatient clinics in Japan (Okuyama et al., 2003) 3. 22 adults with chronic cancer-related and 95 non-cancer-related pain treated in a tertiary pain center in Germany (Radbruch et al., 2003)	Validity 1. Construct: factor analysis verified it is one factor (Mendoza et al., 1999; Okuyama et al., 2003; Radbruch et al., 2003) 2. Convergent: FACT (anemia subscales) (Mendoza et al., 1999); EORTC Global QOL (r = –.51), POMS depression subscale (r = .52) (Okuyama et al., 2003) 3. Convergent validity: correlations with Cancer Fatigue Scale (r = .64–76), POMS fatigue (r = .60–70), and vigor subscales (r = –.23—.28), and EORTC QLQC-C 30 fatigue subscale (r = .59–.72) (Okuyama et al., 2003); MIDOS (r = .46–.76), SF-36 (r = –.51—.67), ECOG-PSR (with decreased rating of the performance status both BFI mean scores also did increase) (Radbruch et al., 2003)			

Note. From *Measuring Oncology Nursing Sensitive Outcomes: Evidence-Based Summaries—Fatigue,* by S.L. Beck, S.S. Shun, and J. Erickson, 2004. Retrieved August 3, 2008, from http://www.ons.org/outcomes/measures/pdf/FatigueSummary.pdf. Copyright by the Oncology Nursing Society. Adapted with permission.

philosophy of charting by exception creates a hindrance to anyone trying to draw conclusions about the intervention/outcome connection. All the nursing interventions and all the patient's responses possibly were considered to be expected, thereby resulting in severely limited charting. In this case, institutional guidelines about both interventions and outcomes would have to be assumed. Deviations considered too minor to chart would be lost to the scientist.

Direct scientist observation of the nurse could reduce the assumptions found in the medical record by charging the observer with responsibility for documenting steps in care. Such observation could systematically note minor deviations in practice or response as well as behaviors that do not rise to the level of an "exception" for charting purposes. The observer could identify the many actions in nursing care that are left assumed in the medical record. This method could resolve many of the drawbacks of medical record audits for research purposes but certainly could become burdensome. A project built entirely on direct observation would require such resource intensity as to render it virtually impossible on a wide scale. Another limitation is the inability to observe important cognitive tasks that are essential to nursing care.

Surveys or questionnaires administered to nurses and/or patients and families can be informative tools for measuring nursing care. Surveys measure the respondent's perceptions and can be influenced by social desirability. In the case of nurses, they may be reluctant to report less than ideal adherence with care quality. In the case of patients and families, they may be concerned about criticizing their nurse caregivers. When the outcome of interest is comfort or trust, then patient perceptions are most appropriate measures. Moreover, a patient-centered care philosophy supports the critical nature of soliciting patient and family perceptions of the care delivered. The national HCAHPS survey specifically measures patient perceptions of care quality based on the dimensions of patient-centered care identified by the IOM (CMS & AHRQ, 2005). The survey includes 18 items across 7 topics. Topics relevant to nursing care include communication with nurses, pain management, communication about medicines, and discharge information. The tool has been tested in more than 3,000 hospitals and will be a required quality indicator nationwide (CMS, 2008).

Another tool that has been developed to measure the quality of nursing care in oncology is the Oncology Patients' Perception of Quality of Nursing Care Scale–Short Form (Radwin, Alster, & Rubin, 2003). The tool was used to measure the patients' perception of the care they received from nurse practitioners (NPs) during their hospitalization. This scale was developed based on concepts and data from a grounded theory study of patients' perspectives of the quality of their nursing care. The scale includes 40 items (alpha = 0.99) in four subscales: responsiveness (22 items, alpha = 0.99), individualization (10 items, alpha = 0.97), coordination (3 items, alpha = 0.87), and proficiency (5 items, alpha = 0.95) (Radwin et al.). A series of studies funded by the Robert Wood Johnson Foundation in 2006 are developing and testing tools to measure specific aspects of nursing care quality (Interdisciplinary Nursing Quality Research Initiative, 2007).

Does Nursing Care Improve Patient Outcomes?

Challenges in Establishing a Causal Link

Research about the impact of nursing care on NSPOs has been challenging. One major challenge is that correlating an individual nurse's manner of caregiving to a specific patient's outcome has not been possible in large-scale studies. Most studies to date have instead linked measures of nursing care at the institutional or unit level (aggregated across nurses) to individual patient outcomes. In this process, one first computes a mean score for all nurses on a given unit for measures of nursing care. Then, these aggregated scores are associated with the outcomes for individual patients treated on that unit. Thus, the patient outcomes on a given unit vary, but the measures of nursing care are fixed because they are aggregated at the unit level. These aggregated variables tend to show little variability across units; therefore, the power of the analyses is reduced because of this lack of variability in the measures of nursing care. Although mixed models can address some of these concerns, large samples are needed and the richness of the data across nurses is lost to aggregation. Thus, most research has been unsuccessful in capturing an association between the quality of nursing care and patient outcomes.

A second challenge relates to measurement of both patient outcomes and nursing care quality. First, patient outcome measures often are cross-sectional or aggregated across a hospital stay, care experience, or group of patients. Such an approach loses the variability that occurs during a hospital stay as the experience unfolds. Second, little research has been conducted to develop measures of nursing care quality. Thus, the nursing side of the outcomes equation has been fairly elusive and often measured by proxy indicators such as education, experience, and certification. These methodologic issues often have resulted in negative findings or weak and questionable causal links when findings are positive.

A third challenge that exists is studying NSPOs in the complex care environments of today's healthcare system. Most of the NSPOs that are relevant to individuals with cancer are not specific to a certain setting (Given & Sherwood, 2005). Unlike urinary tract infections, patient falls, or nosocomial infections, which are all outcomes measures that are important in the hospital, issues such as nausea, fatigue, and pain are not limited to the in-hospital experience. These patient outcomes are centered on the known issues that face the cancer population regardless of where they receive care or even the level of nurse that provides it. Both RNs and advanced practice nurses could potentially influence these types of NSPOs. In addition, most care is provided within the context of an interdisciplinary team. As patients with cancer move between care environments and multiple providers, directly linking an outcome to the interventions of any nurse in one location becomes difficult. This dynamic care system creates challenges and opportunities to examine the link between nursing intervention and outcome both within and across care settings and types of providers. Future oncology nurse scientists and health services scientists will need to create methods for addressing these complex structure and process questions in new ways.

Evidence That Nurses Influence Patient Outcomes

One area of research focus has linked nursing characteristics with outcomes. Aiken, Clarke, Cheung, Sloane, and Silber (2003) demonstrated a link between nursing educational background and surgical mortality. They reported that surgical patients had lower mortality rates in hospitals with higher proportions of baccalaureate-prepared nurses. Scott, Sochalski, and Aiken (1999) reviewed the research on Magnet hospitals and concluded that "research has demonstrated the beneficial relationships between magnet hospitals as an organizational form and patient outcomes" (p. 13). Magnet hospital is a designation bestowed by the American Nurses Credentialing Center on hospitals that have achieved success in a series of criteria designed to measure the strength, professionalism, and quality of nursing care. The same group went on to point out that Magnet hospitals demonstrated lower mortality and higher patient satisfaction when compared to non-Magnet hospitals. The impact that various other nurse resources may have on patient outcomes has yet to be included in outcomes research. Nurse educators, clinical specialists, mentoring programs, IV teams, and specialty certification are unexplored as structural variables in the patient outcomes equation. Even the effect of the nursing experience is explored only minimally. Questions about the effect of the continuity of care, care models, and assistive personnel have not been considered in this research.

Advanced practice nurses in the acute care setting are another aspect of hospital nursing that is only beginning to be explored. Hoffman, Tasota, Zullo, Scharfenberg, and Donahoe (2005) compared NP/attending physician teams to pulmonary fellow/attending physician teams on a subacute unit and found no differences in a number of medical outcomes, including mortality and readmission to acute care. All the patient outcomes measures were medical; therefore, NSPOs were not examined in this work. Dulko et al. (2008) found that improved adherence with NCCN cancer pain guidelines by acute care NPs improved acceptability of pain management to patients and decreased interference with function. Pain intensity did not improve significantly.

In a paper commissioned by the Robert Wood Johnson Foundation, Bolton et al. (2007) conducted a systematic review of the impact of nursing interventions on patient outcomes. They considered cross-cutting patient outcomes where sufficient research had led to systematic/integrative reviews and meta-analyses published in 1999–2004. They concluded that evidence was limited to support a relationship between nursing care processes and specific patient care outcomes. Most studies failed to utilize standardized, evidence-based tools that have been tested over time across care settings and across different populations. The strongest evidence published in the literature was risk assessment (Bolton et al.). However, the authors concluded that multiple interventions are ready to be translated into practice. These included specific strategies related to (Bolton et al.)

- Assessment using tested standardized tools
- Planning for care delivery and monitoring to reduce patient risk and incidence of adverse events
- Provision of patient education and self care
- Practices to promote reduction of risky behaviors and prevent progression of disease
- Decision support for management of anxiety, depression, asthma, and symptoms
- The promotion of health and disease prevention.

Evidence That Oncology Nurses Influence Patient Outcomes

Within oncology nursing, the ONS Patient Outcomes Survey (Mallory & Thomas, 2004) included descriptive information regarding beliefs about oncology NSPOs and assessed the value, use, and education needs of the oncology nurse related to NSPOs (www.ons.org/outcomes/measures/survey.shtml). The survey's primary focus was the five categories of symptoms in the ONS outcomes definition. Most of the 1,327 survey respondents, who were nurses from Pennsylvania, reported that nursing care does make a positive difference in the care of patients with cancer in the areas of symptoms, functional status, safety, psychological distress, and economic values. Overall, the respondents valued oncology nursing-sensitive patient issues and were interested in additional education in the areas of psychological distress, functional status, and safety outcomes, with additional support in symptom management outcomes and economic outcomes. The majority of respondents, despite differences found in the response mode, felt that information about NSPOs should be accessible on the ONS Web site. Overall, the survey provided important and necessary information regarding the nursing knowledge, nursing perceptions, values of oncology nurses, and NSPOs.

The ONS Putting Evidence Into Practice® (PEP) project, launched in 2005, has led to systematic reviews of whether specific interventions are efficacious in addressing targeted patient outcomes in oncology (Gobel, Beck, & O'Leary, 2006). Project teams focused on particular outcomes combined the expertise of scientists, advanced practice nurses, and staff nurses. Each team used a systematic process to ask relevant clinical questions, identify potential interventions, search and critique the evidence, and rate and classify the results (Gobel et al.). The process is remarkable in its inclusive and thorough review of multiple sources of evidence, including meta-analyses and integrated reviews, clinical practice guidelines, and primary research studies. As of May 2008, 16 reviews had been completed. The interventions that have been classified as "Recommended for Practice" for the two example outcomes of fatigue and prevention of infection are summarized in Table 17-4. The thoroughness of the reviews led to inclusion of interventions that may not be nursing-specific and yet may be utilized either directly or indirectly (via referral) by nurses depending on their role. Overall, the evidence for many interventions is limited. The project highlights the urgent need for research to link specific nursing interventions to patient outcomes of importance to individuals with cancer.

The ONS PEP products have been disseminated in multiple formats, including ONS PEP short cards for the practicing clinician; a Web site that includes definitions, detailed cards, and all tables of evidence; and review articles published in the *Clinical Journal of Oncology Nursing* (Gobel et al., 2006). The most current source of information is on the ONS Web site (www.ons .org/outcomes/index.shtml), from which materials can be printed easily. The project also resulted in a revision in the ONS Levels of Evidence that

**Table 17-4. Oncology Nursing Society Putting Evidence Into Practice®
(PEP) Recommendations for Two Examples of Specific Patient Outcomes**

Outcome	Recommendations From Evidence-Based Reviews
Fatigue	Recommended for practice • Exercise in patients with breast cancer, in patients with solid tumors, and in those undergoing hematopoietic stem cell transplantation
Prevention of Infection	Recommended for practice • Hand hygiene using soap and water or an antiseptic hand rub • Colony-stimulating factors for all patients undergoing chemotherapy with > 20% risk of febrile neutropenia • Influenza vaccine annually for all patients with cancer • 23-valent pneumococcal polysaccharide vaccine for all patients with cancer who are older than five years of age and 7-valent pneumococcal polysaccharide protein-conjugate vaccine for all patients with cancer who are younger than five years of age • Trimethoprim-sulfamethoxazole to prevent *Pneumocystis carinii* pneumonia for all patients at risk • Antifungal drugs absorbed or partially absorbed from the gastrointestinal tract to prevent oral candidiasis in patients with cancer undergoing chemotherapy • Antifungal prophylaxis for severely neutropenic afebrile patients (absolute neutrophil count < 1,000 for more than one week) • Antibacterial prophylaxis with quinolones for high-risk afebrile neutropenic patients with cancer undergoing chemotherapy • Herpes viral prophylaxis (acyclovir or valacyclovir) for selected seropositive patients with cancer • Protective gowns if soiling with respiratory secretions is anticipated • Prohibiting visitors with symptoms of respiratory infections • Environmental interventions

were adapted originally from Hadorn, Baker, Hodges, and Hicks (1996). In this model, evidence is ranked hierarchically into three categories from levels I (strongest) to III (weakest). In addition, Mitchell, Friese, Mallory, Eaton, and Beck (2007) developed a classification schema to categorize the weight of evidence across multiple sources. Categories include recommended for practice, likely to be effective, benefits balanced with harm, effectiveness not established, effectiveness unlikely, not recommended for practice, and expert opinion.

Clearly, evidence exists for interventions that improve patient outcomes that are ready for translation into practice. Yet, little evidence is available within nursing about what strategies are effective in achieving adoption of evidence-based practice. In its research priorities, ONS has identified the need for translational research. Specific priorities that have been identified include (Berry, 2005)

- Identifying barriers and facilitators in the clinical practice setting for translational research
- Creating and implementing methods to translate the research into the practice setting
- Comparing implementation methods in a variety of practice settings.

Future research also will be informed by the large and growing number of national databases. The nursing databases mentioned previously are only a select few of many available to connect nursing care and outcomes. Table 17-1 provides a brief description of other large databases that may inform outcomes research. National efforts are under way to provide an information network linking data from various sources through the Cancer Biomedical Information Grid, sponsored by the National Cancer Institute (2006). As the clinical data component of this network grows, enormous opportunities for research will arise that link multiple sources of data, including molecular and biomedical imaging data, with clinical outcomes.

Future Directions and Recommendations

A great many opportunities exist for future research in oncology NSPOs. The following recommendations are consistent with the research priorities from the review and analysis of research on nursing interventions and patient outcomes (Bolton et al., 2007) and with the ONS research agenda related to NSPOs (see Figure 17-4) (Berry, 2005).

1. Develop a core of clinical measures of NSPOs that are reliable, valid, and clinically useful in multiple oncology populations. Integrate these measures into electronic medical records and a national database.
2. Develop reliable and valid tools to measure the quality of nursing care and integrate these tools into clinical practice settings and databases.
3. Continue to conduct research on the efficacy and effectiveness of specific theoretically based nursing interventions and roles. Examination of nurs-

---

Figure 17-4. The Oncology Nursing Society 2005–2009 Research Agenda Related to Improving Nursing-Sensitive Patient Outcomes

Research in Nursing-Sensitive Patient Outcomes
Rationale: The demand for professional accountability regarding outcomes dictates that nurses are able to identify and document outcomes that are attributable to nursing care.

Priority Topics
1. The effectiveness and quality of nursing care on nursing-sensitive patient outcomes within the context of the healthcare system to prevent adverse events
   1.1 Infection
   1.2 Prevention of adverse events related to cancer treatment modalities
   1.3 Workforce issues that promote or threaten quality care
2. The effectiveness and quality of nursing care on nursing-sensitive patient outcomes within the context of health management for individuals
   2.1 Maintain or promote physical function, functional status, or functional ability of individuals who receive cancer treatment.
   2.2 Nursing interventions to prevent or decrease fatigue in individuals with cancer

---

Note. From *Oncology Nursing Society 2005–2009 Research Agenda*, by D.L. Berry, 2005. Retrieved June 23, 2007, from http://www.ons.org/research/information/documents/pdfs/executive05.pdf. Copyright 2005 by the Oncology Nursing Society. Reprinted with permission.

---

ing should include setting, role, and distinct aspects of nursing care. The focus of work to date on NSPOs as a hospital-based issue must expand to include multiple other locations of care: acute care, outpatient care, home care, and long-term care. The role of nursing varies by position. NSPO research should include and distinguish staff nurse, manager, advanced practice nurse, and other roles. Distinct aspects of direct care also will be important to specify (e.g., assessment, counseling, teaching, psychosocial support, promoting self-care, referrals) and to distinguish the role of the nurse from the interdisciplinary team. The dose of a nursing intervention that is needed also must be addressed. The ability to tailor interventions and measurement of certain outcomes using technology will provide important opportunities for advances in intervention research.

4. Expand and maintain the currency of tools, such as the products of the ONS PEP initiative, which provide a review of evidence with recommendations for practice.

5. Continue to evaluate the influence of workforce variables on NSPOs. The effect of nursing leaders (Boyle, 2004; Houser, 2003; Hughes et al., 2001; Manojlovich, 2005) has emerged as an important factor in the effectiveness of unit-level nursing teams. Concepts such as autonomy, collaboration, and control over practice distinguish Magnet hospitals but have not been directly linked to patient outcomes (Scott et al., 1999).

6. Maintain the currency of the outcomes of interest in oncology care. Add outcomes related to health-promoting behaviors as well as symptoms associated with monoclonal antibodies and other targeted therapies.

7. Conduct translational research that evaluates strategies to improve evidence-based practice and NSPOs.
8. Utilize national databases to answer important questions related to NSPOs and nursing care.

Conclusion

In summary, societal and professional mandates are increasing to show that nursing care results in optimal patient outcomes. Numerous national forces, driven by a variety of motives, are interested in understanding the impact that nursing care has on individuals. The body of evidence that specific nursing interventions result in improved outcomes is limited but growing. The challenge now is to translate this evidence into practice. The desire to establish a causal link between nursing care and patient outcomes has faced multiple challenges. The challenge of oncology nursing researchers is to define and measure these variables in unified, valid, and reliable ways that capture the diversity of both nursing practice and individual responses. Nurse scientists and clinicians must unite to establish reliable and valid core measures of outcomes and nursing care and integrate these measures into clinical databases. Advances in technology and information management will enable linkages of information with tremendous power to demonstrate the impact of nursing care on patient outcomes.

References

Aaronson, L.S., & Burman, M.E. (1994). Use of health records in research: Reliability and validity issues. *Research in Nursing and Health, 17*(1), 67–73.

Aiken, L.H., Clarke, S.P., Cheung, R.B., Sloane, D.M., & Silber, J.H. (2003). Educational levels of hospital nurses and surgical patient mortality. *JAMA, 290*(12), 1617–1623.

Alexander, G.R. (2007). Nursing sensitive databases: Their existence, challenges, and importance. *Medical Care Research and Review, 64*(Suppl. 2), 44S–63S.

American Educational Research Association, American Psychological Association, & National Council on Measurement in Education. (1999). *Standards for educational and psychological testing.* Washington, DC: American Educational Research Association.

Berry, D.L. (2005). *Oncology Nursing Society 2005–2009 research agenda.* Retrieved June 23, 2007, from http://www.ons.org/research/information/documents/pdfs/executive05.pdf

Bolton, L.B., Donaldson, N.E., Rutledge, D.N., Bennett, C., & Brown, D.S. (2007). The impact of nursing interventions: Overview of effective interventions, outcomes, measures, and priorities for future research. *Medical Care Research and Review, 64*(Suppl. 2), 123S–143S.

Boyle, S.M. (2004). Nursing unit characteristics and patient outcomes. *Nursing Economics, 22*(3), 111–119, 123, 127.

Brown, D.S., Donaldson, N., Aydin, C.E., & Carlson, N. (2001). Hospital nursing benchmarks: The California Nursing Outcomes Coalition project. *Journal for Healthcare Quality, 23*(4), 22–27.

Carmines, E.G., & Zeller, R.A. (1979). *Reliability and validity assessment.* Thousand Oaks, CA: Sage.

Centers for Medicare and Medicaid Services. (2005, January 31). *Medicare "pay for performance (p4p)" initiatives.* Retrieved June 14, 2007, from http://www.cms.hhs.gov/apps/media/press/release.asp?Counter=1343

Centers for Medicare and Medicaid Services. (2007). *Quality initiatives: General overview.* Retrieved June 14, 2007, from http://www.cms.hhs.gov/QualityInitiativesGenInfo

Centers for Medicare and Medicaid Services. (2008). *HCAHPS: Hospital care quality information from the consumer perspective/CAHPS hospital survey.* Retrieved August 3, 2008, from http://hcahpsonline.org

Centers for Medicare and Medicaid Services & Agency for Healthcare Research and Quality. (2005). *Hospital CAHPS® (HCAHPS®) fact sheet.* Retrieved June 14, 2007, from http://www.cms.hhs.gov/HospitalQualityInits/downloads/HospitalHCAHPSFactSheet200512.pdf

Dulko, D., Bacik, J., Hertz, E., Osoria, J., Beck, S.L., Coyle, N., et al. (2008). *Implementation of national cancer pain guidelines by acute care nurse practitioners using an audit and feedback strategy.* Manuscript submitted for publication.

Frank-Stromborg, M., & Olsen, S.J. (Eds.). (2004). *Instruments for clinical health-care research* (3rd ed.). Sudbury, MA: Jones and Bartlett.

Friese, C.R., & Beck, S.L. (2004). Advancing practice and research: Creating evidence-based summaries on measuring nursing-sensitive patient outcomes. *Clinical Journal of Oncology Nursing, 8*(6), 675–677.

Given, B., Beck, S.L., Etland, C., Gobel, B.H., Lamkin, L., & Marsee, V.D. (2003). *Nursing-sensitive patient outcomes.* Retrieved May 20, 2007, from http://www.ons.org/outcomes/measures/outcomes.shtml

Given, B.A., & Sherwood, P.R. (2005). Nursing sensitive patient outcomes—a white paper. *Oncology Nursing Forum, 32*(4), 773–784.

Gobel, B.H., Beck, S.L., & O'Leary, C. (2006). Nursing sensitive patient outcomes: The development of the Putting Evidence Into Practice resources for nursing practice. *Clinical Journal of Oncology Nursing, 10*(5), 621–624.

Hadorn, D.C., Baker, D., Hodges, J.S., & Hicks, N. (1996). Rating the quality of evidence for clinical practice guidelines. *Journal of Clinical Epidemiology, 49*(7), 749–754.

Hegyvary, S.T. (1991). Issues in outcomes research. *Journal of Nursing Quality Assurance, 5*(2), 1–6.

Hoffman, L.A., Tasota, F.J., Zullo, T.G., Scharfenberg, C., & Donahoe, M.P. (2005). Outcomes of care managed by an acute care nurse practitioner/attending physician team in a subacute medical intensive care unit. *American Journal of Critical Care, 14*(2), 121–130.

Houser, J. (2003). A model for evaluating the context of nursing care delivery. *Journal of Nursing Administration, 33*(1), 39–47.

Hughes, L.C., Ward, S., Grindel, C.G., Coleman, E.A., Berry, D.L., Hinds, P.S., et al. (2001). Relationships between certification and job perceptions of oncology nurses. *Oncology Nursing Forum, 28*(1), 99–107.

Institute of Medicine. (2006). *Rewarding provider performance: Aligning incentives in Medicare.* Washington, DC: National Academies Press.

Institute of Medicine. (2008). *The Institute of Medicine Report Index.* Retrieved June 16, 2008, from http://www.iom.edu/CMS/2955.aspx

Interdisciplinary Nursing Quality Research Initiative. (2007). *Interdisciplinary nursing quality research initiative.* Retrieved June 21, 2007, from http://www.inqri.org/ProgramOverview.html

Jennings, B.M., Staggers, N., & Brosch, L.R. (1999). A classification scheme for outcome indicators. *Image: The Journal of Nursing Scholarship, 31*(4), 381–388.

Lohr, K.N. (Ed.). (1990). *Medicare: A strategy for quality assurance* (Vol. 1, p. 4). Washington, DC: National Academies Press.

Mallory, G., & Thomas, R. (2004). *Oncology Nursing Society patient outcomes survey.* Retrieved December 1, 2007, from http://www.ons.org/outcomes/measures/survey.shtml

Manojlovich, M. (2005). Predictors of professional nursing practice behaviors in hospital settings. *Nursing Research, 54*(1), 41–47.

Mendoza, T.R., Wang, X.S., Cleeland, C.S., Morrissey, M., Johnson, B.A., Wendt, J.K., et al. (1999). The rapid assessment of fatigue severity in cancer patients: Use of the Brief Fatigue Inventory. *Cancer, 85*(5), 1186–1196.

Mitchell, P.H., Ferketich, S., & Jennings, B.M. (1998). Quality Health Outcomes Model. American Academy of Nursing Expert Panel on Quality Health Care. *Image: The Journal of Nursing Scholarship, 30*(1), 43–46.

Mitchell, S.A., Friese, C.R., Mallory, G., Eaton, L., & Beck, S.L. (2007). *Oncology Nursing Society Putting Evidence Into Practice (PEP)—development of a classification for determining the collective strength of evidence for an intervention.* Unpublished manuscript.

National Cancer Institute. (2006). *Welcome to caBIG™ community web site.* Retrieved August 3, 2008, from https://cabig.nci.nih.gov

National Comprehensive Cancer Network. (2007). *Oncology groups publish seven measures of quality care for breast and colorectal cancers.* Retrieved June 1, 2007, from http://www.nccn.org/about/news/newsinfo.asp?NewsID=79

National Quality Forum. (2006). *Nursing care quality at NQF.* Retrieved June 14, 2007, from http://216.122.138.39/nursing/#measures

Naylor, M.D. (2007). Advancing the science in the measurement of health care quality influenced by nurses. *Medical Care Research and Review, 64*(Suppl. 2), 144S–169S.

Needleman, J., Kurtzman, E.T., & Kizer, K.W. (2007). Performance measurement of nursing care: State of the science and the current consensus. *Medical Care Research and Review, 64*(Suppl. 2), 10S–43S.

Okuyama, T., Wang, X.S., Akechi, T., Mendoza, T.R., Hosaka, T., Cleeland, C.S., et al. (2003). Validation study of the Japanese version of the Brief Fatigue Inventory. *Journal of Pain and Symptom Management, 25*(2), 106–117.

Radbruch, L., Sabatowski, R., Elsner, F., Everts, J., Mendoza, T., & Cleeland, C. (2003). Validation of the German version of the Brief Fatigue Inventory. *Journal of Pain and Symptom Management, 25*(5), 449–458.

Radwin, L., Alster, K., & Rubin, K.M. (2003). Development and testing of the oncology patients' perceptions of the quality of nursing care scale. *Oncology Nursing Forum, 30*(2), 283–290.

Rantz, M.J., & Connolly, R.P. (2004). Measuring nursing care quality and using large data sets in nonacute care settings: State of the science. *Nursing Outlook, 52*(1), 23–37.

Scott, J.G., Sochalski, J., & Aiken, L. (1999). Review of magnet hospital research: Findings and implications for professional nursing practice. *Journal of Nursing Administration, 29*(1), 9–19.

Spilsbury, K., & Meyer, J. (2001). Defining the nursing contribution to patient outcome: Lessons from a review of the literature examining nursing outcomes, skill mix and changing roles. *Journal of Clinical Nursing, 10*(1), 3–14.

CHAPTER 18

Qualitative Oncology Nursing Science

Richard H. Steeves, RN, PhD, Barbara Parker, RN, PhD, FAAN,
and Kathryn Laughon, RN, PhD

Introduction

In this chapter, we will review the intellectual ideas that oncology nurse scientists use to form the basis and background for qualitative research. However, the best way to learn how to evaluate and use findings from qualitative studies is to learn how to conduct one; therefore, this chapter describes the practical steps that oncology nurse scientists use to conduct qualitative studies. Examples are provided throughout regarding an ongoing cutting-edge oncology nursing study, An Exploration of Breast Cancer and Intimate Partner Abuse (BC&IPA). This is a phenomenologic study that we, the authors of this chapter, designed to understand the experiences of women who were in an abusive intimate relationship when they were diagnosed with breast cancer.

Qualitative oncology nurse scientists often call what they do *naturalistic* or *interpretive* research, which probably are better descriptors of what they do than the word *qualitative*, which seems to suggest only that the data are not numbers. Also, scientists who do this kind of research often call it the *received view* or *majority* science. In this chapter, the terms *qualitative* and *quantitative* will be used because they are the terms in most common usage.

Qualitative science requires a slightly different way of looking at the world and a different way of thinking about what science should and can do. One difference the reader may have already noticed is that qualitative oncology nurse scientists often write in the first person and occasionally even the second person as we talk directly to the reader. Although this grammatical approach is frowned upon in writing associated with quantitative science, it is well accepted in qualitative reports and discussions. Now that the vocabulary and grammatical boundaries are set, we can begin the discussion.

The Intellectual Background of Qualitative Science

Thick Description

Qualitative research is scientific and empirical and should be rigorous. Thus, it shares a great deal with quantitative science. However, the two kinds of science do not share some characteristics, and these differences are important. First among these differences is the goal of qualitative research, which is to produce a thick description. The term *thick description* was made famous by Geertz (1973), an anthropologist who wanted to distinguish qualitative findings from thin or broad descriptions such as those that are produced by a questionnaire or other kind of instrument. For instance, in the BC&IPA study, we are using a brief questionnaire, Women's Experience of Battering (Smith, Smith, & Earp, 1999), to screen potential participants for abuse when they were diagnosed. The questionnaire has 10 items, and each item includes a 6-point Likert scale, for a total possible score of 60 points. Any score greater than 20 indicates an abusive relationship. The 10 items represent 6 domains: perceived threat, managing, yearning, altered identity, entrapment, and disempowerment. These domains are thought of as variables that offer some description of the experience of battered women, enough to determine if abuse is present or absent. Albeit very useful, this is a thin description of what is going on in the lives of the participants.

When we interview participants one-on-one in our study as oncology nurse scientists, we want a thick description of their lives. The thickness comes from the accumulated details of what their relationships were like with their intimate partners, as well as their experience of being diagnosed with and treated for breast cancer. For instance, instead of asking if a participant was hit, we ask for the entire story. We want to hear about the circumstances, the reasons for her reactions, the results, the emotions, and how she understood and gave meaning to the hit. A thick description can only come from one point of view at a time. That is, we ask questions to learn about the woman's experience while recognizing that the abuser has his or her own experience that could be the object of another study. The point is that qualitative studies seek understanding about a phenomenon from the participant's point of view and not from the view of an outside objective observer, even if such a creature could exist.

Instead of identifying variables, such as the presence or absence of disempowerment or entrapment, we gather descriptions. The important difference here is that we do not see the world as divisible into specific variables that can be turned into questions that can be answered "yes" or "no" or into statements that can be responded to with numbers like those on a Likert scale. The world view in qualitative research is too complicated, too multifaceted, and too thick for the identification of discrete variables.

The Social World

One cannot conduct qualitative research in physics, chemistry, or physiology. What happens between and among people is the object of study for qualitative oncology nurse scientists. In our BC&IPA study, we could not address what was happening at the cellular level in our participants' bodies. Although this is perhaps the most important aspect of the lives of these women from the point of view of some of the people who are treating them, our methods could not address this aspect. Our purpose was to investigate what the women thought was going on in their bodies and how they behaved in terms of the meaning they assigned to what was happening.

In a 1998 paper considering the effects of breast cancer, several oncology nurse scientists (Cohen, Kahn, & Steeves, 1998) catalogued what the breast might mean to a woman undergoing breast cancer treatment. First, a breast is a social object, in that it is part of the way a woman is perceived by others; that is, we see each other as bodies and behave differently toward people with different kinds of bodies. We do not treat older adults and babies the same even if their physical appearance is all we are given. Next, a breast or any other body part can be an object to oneself. Thus, a patient may say "My breast hurts me" or "I want my breast removed because it has cancer." The self and the breast are not the same thing. The breast is a separate object in the world, an object that can be looked at as the thing in the world that has malfunctioned. Lastly, a breast can be part of the self and not divisible from the self. This is the same as saying that our bodies are our access to existence—without them, we are not anything. When the breast is incised, the whole woman feels the pain; when the breast has a malignant tumor, the whole woman is sick.

Over the years, identifying the parts of human experience that are open to qualitative research has been controversial. Some qualitative scientists argue that all three aspects of how a breast is experienced are amenable to research, that private internal experiences are amenable to research just as social ones are (Merleau-Ponty, 1945/1962). Others confine the purview of qualitative research to only the first, the social aspects of experience, arguing that internal psychological and existential states are not open to interpretation and should not be the object of qualitative research (Kockelmans, 1970). This divergence of opinion is both philosophical and methodologic. For this discussion, we will concentrate on the social dimension.

Another way to talk about the social world is to talk about culture. Social scientists have defined *culture* a number of ways. In fact, defining this term often is the end result of many studies by anthropologists, in that anthropologists set out to study culture but only know exactly what they are studying after they have completed the study. We will not attempt a definition of the term here but will say that culture is a way of talking about social worlds. We all live in a social world—most of us live in many social worlds—and social worlds differ from each other in how the members define acceptable behaviors and shared meanings. Culture is a useful way of talking about the differences between social worlds. Thus, to some extent, all qualitative research is research about culture, and for qualitative nurse scientists, the culture is different than the culture for other qualitative scientists.

What Can Be Known

In the middle of the past century, behaviorism became an influential social-scientific approach, and to some extent, qualitative research was a response to behaviorism. In its most simple terms, *behaviorism* is the notion that all we can know is what people do. We cannot know what they were thinking when they did it. The mind is a black box that neither the researcher nor, in fact, the participants themselves have access to. The qualitative scientists, refusing to accept this unknowability, argued that people do understand what they are doing and why they are doing it. All one has to do is ask. For instance, a behaviorist might look at a woman with breast cancer in an abusive relationship and think of the situation as an invitation to change behavior. The behaviorist might think, "What is the level of incentive that needs to be offered to have women leave the abusive relationship?" The thinking is that we cannot know how the women understand their situation, nor do we need to. We merely need to apply force in the form of incentives or punishment until a behavior is changed. The qualitative oncology nurse scientist wants to know why a woman with breast cancer stays in or does not stay in an abusive relationship. The interest here is in meaning, not in changing behavior. The qualitative oncology nurse scientist believes that behavior is interpretable and is best interpreted by the one behaving. Women have complex relationships with their abusive partners, and they understand the meaning of those relationships and base their behavior on that meaning. The way to discover the meaning of a behavior is to ask the woman. Individuals generally know what it is they are thinking, and if asked, they can tell an interviewer.

Theory

Theory generally is a group of linked statements about the world that can be used to generate falsifiable statements. For instance, gravity is a theory from which we can derive the statement that because gravity is a constant force of attraction between two objects, the force should not vary with the masses of the objects. Therefore, objects of different weights dropped from the Leaning Tower of Pisa at the same time should hit the ground at the same time.

In qualitative research proposals and in the reports of qualitative research findings, the reader should not find a theory that guided the study. The point of theory is to produce a special kind of understanding of the world, an understanding of the world that usually can be expressed in numbers (e.g., according to the theory of gravity, objects on Earth fall at a rate of 32 ft/s^2), an understanding that is meant to lead to manipulation, an understanding of the world that usually only can be verified by manipulation of the world in some manner. In cancer research, the template for this kind of study is a drug study. This is quantitative research. The driving theory may be about how cells work. For instance, a scientist starts with a theory about how cancer cells divide and hypothesizes that if a certain chemical were introduced to the cell, then it would not divide. The hypothesis is a statement that is falsifiable, but only by introducing the chemical into the cell.

Qualitative oncology nursing research is aimed at a different kind of understanding of the world. The understanding is local and specific: How do women experience being diagnosed with breast cancer when they are living with an intimate partner who is abusive? No theory exists to guide this kind of work, only an observation that, indeed, some women must go through this experience. The result of the study is going to be complex and intricate because the lives of these women are complex and their understanding of their experience is going to be intricate. The findings will not be reducible to a string of statements that can be expressed in numbers.

In the special case of *grounded theory* research, the result of a qualitative study is a theory. The orthodoxy in grounded theory is to express the findings in the form of a theory with statements linked together in causal relationships. The differences between these grounded theories and those theories of quantitative research are many, but the most important one is that the grounded theory is a way of understanding a particular situation for a specific group of people. For instance, a grounded theory concerning women in abusive relationships who are diagnosed with breast cancer would apply only to that one study and that one sample of women. The grounded theory is not meant to apply to all women in abusive situations who are diagnosed with breast cancer. The theory is specific to, or grounded in, a particular study. It is not meant to be used to generate falsifiable statements about other women in other places.

Some useful primers are available for performing qualitative research. *The Sage Handbook of Qualitative Research,* edited by Denzin and Lincoln (2005a), is perhaps the most complete. A book by Silverman (2004) is the most thoughtful and thought provoking and is a good companion to the handbook. Thomas and Pollio (2002) provide a good view of qualitative research from a nursing perspective. Creswell (2007) has a useful review of the many traditions in qualitative research, from grounded theory to ethnography to phenomenology. Once a reader has chosen a tradition, he or she might want to read a book by Charmaz (2006), if grounded theory is the choice, or one specifically by oncology nurse scientists (Cohen, Kahn, & Steeves, 2000), if the choice is phenomenology.

Conducting a Qualitative Study

Generating Ideas

Ideas for qualitative oncology nursing research come from the same places as ideas for quantitative oncology nursing research: clinical experience, responses to the research of others, and noticing a gap in the literature. In coming up with the idea for the BC&IPA study, one of the three authors, Steeves, used his background in qualitative oncology nursing research (Cohen, Haberman, & Steeves, 1994; Cohen et al., 1998, 2000; Cohen, Kahn, & Steeves, 2002; Jones et al., 2007; Steeves, 2002), and Parker and Laughon used their experience in studying intimate partner violence. None of us remembers exactly how the question originated of how domestic abuse and cancer are experienced together. It seemed to be a natural question for the three of us to consider. We wondered how having cancer would affect the abusive relationship and how being in an abusive relationship would affect cancer care. Would women look at their lives anew with the threat of cancer and decide to escape the abusive relationship? Would they want to leave but be unable to because their abusive partner was the source of health insurance? Would an abusive partner refuse to take the patient to chemotherapy appointments or steal or hide her analgesics? We had heard from nursing colleagues about women who had experienced these things. We also had heard of women who were struck by their partners in their mastectomy incisions and of others who had said to their abusive husbands that they might have little time to live and were not going to spend it with someone who was abusive and left.

The Cutting-Edge Idea of Oncology Nursing Science and the Literature

Regardless of where they originate, the first place to take ideas for research projects is to the library, or more accurately, to a computer with access to scientific search software. Although opinions may exist to the contrary, all qualitative oncology nursing research, like quantitative oncology nursing research, begins with a thorough review of the literature.

Breast cancer was not an area of emphasis for any of us but was agreed on because almost all of those who have it are women, and the great majority of the victims of intimate partner abuse also are women. The chance of a woman developing invasive breast cancer during her lifetime is approximately 1 in 8 (12.28%) (American Cancer Society [ACS], 2007). According to ACS (2008), the incidence of breast cancer in the United States was 125.3 per 100,000 from 2000 to 2004. Unfortunately, statistics concerning abused women are more difficult to locate. They are not maintained and updated by a national group. We had to depend on the few studies in which abuse has been recorded. Rates of physical abuse of women by intimate partners during their lifetimes ranges from 25%–33% according to two large nationally representative studies (Plichta, 1997; Tjaden & Thoennes, 2000). Approximately 3%–12% of women have been assaulted physically in the past year. More than 7% of women have been sexually assaulted by an intimate partner in their lifetime (Tjaden & Thoennes). The fact that breast cancer and abuse must occur at the same time in a considerable number of women seemed clear to us.

We thought that perhaps someone had considered this possibility and had already done some research, but we were wrong. We looked at the domestic violence literature over the past 10 years and found references to abuse of older adults and individuals with mental and physical disabilities but no references to cancer. Curry, Hassouneh-Phillips, and Johnston-Silverberg (2001) provided an overview of abuse and disabilities. We looked at the cancer literature for studies of relationships between women with breast cancer and their partners. More than 75 research articles in this area have been published from 1997 to 2007, covering how to support the partners of the patients with cancer (Lewis et al., 2001; Lugton, 1997; Petrie, Logan, & DeGrasse, 2001), how partners could support the patients (Baider & DeNour, 1984; Ben-Zur, 2001; Ben-Zur, Gilbar, & Lev, 2001), and how their sexual lives will change (Ganz, Rowland, Desmond, Meyerowitz, & Wyatt, 1998; Meyerowitz, Desmond, Rowland, Wyatt, & Ganz, 1999; Wilmoth, 2001; Wimberly, Carver, Laurenceau, Harris, & Antoni, 2005).

However, only one paper was published that was based on clinical case studies grappling with the idea that some women with breast cancer might be in an abusive relationship (Schmidt, Woods, & Stewart, 2006). Our search of the literature made us well informed about patients with breast cancer and their partners and abused women with illnesses. It also told us that our question had not been answered. A gap in knowledge definitely existed, and when this occurs, research is needed.

The Specific Aim, or the Research Question

A research question or specific aim should be thought of as a contract that states the nature of the project and sets the basic parameters. Our specific aim for the BC&IPA study was best stated as a research question: What are the experiences of women who are in an abusive relationship when they are diagnosed with breast cancer? The two phenomena are presented, intimate partner abuse and breast cancer, as is the time frame: the abuse is to precede and overlap with the breast cancer treatment (the oncology topic). The fact that we use the word *experiences* tells the reader that we will be conducting a qualitative study. These are the terms of a contract on which we have agreed our study should be judged. We state that we will answer this question and only this question. The experience of these women is a broad topic and leaves us much room to talk about many aspects of their lives, but only their lives. Furthermore, by stating that we are interested in experience, we have said that we will not come back with a list of variables or cause-and-effect statements. Experience is much bigger and more complex than that (Cohen et al., 2000).

The Sample

In our BC&IPA study, we stated in our qualitative oncology nursing research question that we would research a sample of women who were in an abusive relationship when they were diagnosed with breast cancer. The specific aim does not call for comparison groups of women who had another disease or no disease, and it does not call for women who had breast cancer but were not in a relationship or were in a supportive relationship. One might think this goes without saying, but only people who are experiencing the phenomena being studied should be in the sample. Unfortunately, scientists often forget this basic principle.

The sample for a qualitative study is not meant to be representative; it is chosen on other criteria. Because qualitative oncology nursing research is meant to produce a thick description and a description of what is going on related to cancer at a specific time in a specific place, scientists do not attempt to say that the participants with cancer in a study are like other people at other times. The determination of how dissimilar or similar the participants in a qualitative study are to other groups of people is left for the reader to determine (Lincoln & Guba, 1985).

When we finish our oncology nursing study of BC&IPA, we will present our findings, and those findings either will be accepted as offering new insight and confirming or disconfirming existing beliefs or will not be accepted. The readers, those people who study or work clinically with or are interested in women, abuse, and breast cancer, will decide if we are correct. If the sample is a good sample, our readers will be able to decide if the findings apply to the women they encounter (Cohen et al., 2002).

The question then becomes What is a good sample? A good sample is one that allows for a thick description. If the women in our sample are able to provide nuanced, complex, and concrete data about their experiences, it is a good sample. If the women are able to provide a variety of points of view about a variety of different circumstances, it is a good sample. It is a good sample because our readers will be assured that we have covered the phenomena with enough depth that they can use our findings in understanding the women with whom they work. The time and place of the reader may be very different from what we experienced, and our findings may be judged as interesting but not applicable. That is how it should be, but if the reader is not able to compare our findings to the lives of the women with whom he or she works, we probably did not have a good sample because the description was not thick enough. Of course, other things can go wrong as well. The idea is to understand one situation in depth enough to allow the possibility of understanding similar situations (Geertz, 1973).

One could ask, "If we are looking for a variety of points of view and a variety of circumstances, why not recruit women who represent different points of view and circumstances?" For instance, why do we not recruit women with in situ breast cancer and women with stage-four cancer, older women and younger women, women in long-term marriages and women who are in new relationships? The answer is that we do not know if these are the right variables. If we decide in advance that the severity of the disease or the longevity of a relationship is the most important variable, we will not have allowed the women to speak for themselves and to tell us what is important. Women who look very much alike from the outside—stage of cancer, treatment regimen, marital relationship—may have very different experiences because of their understanding of who they are and what they want out of life (Denzin & Lincoln, 2005b).

In most cases, qualitative oncology nurse scientists begin by recruiting all those who volunteer for the study. As the study goes on, data analysis may reveal that participants differ in their experiences based on some identifiable characteristic. For example, if the women in our study had very unique experiences because they were evangelical Christians, then we might decide that religious beliefs were a large part of the sensibilities that were important in dealing with abuse and cancer. We would then try to recruit women with a variety of religious beliefs. Grounded theory has this technique built into its tradition. It is called *theoretical sampling* (Charmaz, 2006).

The Procedures

Perhaps the most useful way to think about the procedures of data collection in qualitative oncology nursing studies is to think about the production of a text. A verbal text (in the future, perhaps texts will be visual as well as verbal, as in video recordings) is the goal in qualitative oncology nursing studies as much as the collection of numbers is the goal in quantitative studies. This difference again points to a basic divergence of the goals of quantitative and qualitative research. Einstein wanted to be able to express the nature of the universe in an equation that was less than an inch long, thus $E = MC^2$. This is the ultimate goal in terms of creating a quantifiable theory about the nature of reality, specifically energy, matter, and time. On the other end is the multiple-volume novel by Proust, *In Search of Things Past* (1919/1992), which also describes the nature of time. Proust's verbal text is thick description at its thickest. Einstein's theory in which the letters are replaceable with numbers is description at its broadest.

The procedures of qualitative research are descriptions of how the text is created. In most qualitative research about oncology, the text is made up of interviews (Cohen et al., 2000). The semistructured interview is the most common technique. In most cases, the interview is recorded and then transcribed; a written text is the result.

In interviews, the questions being asked of the participant are vitally important. Because the goal is a thick description and that kind of description can only come from the person experiencing the phenomenon, the questions have to be general and not leading. For instance, we would not ask the participants in the BC&IPA study about how their religious beliefs affected their decision about whether to leave their abusive partner. First, a researcher wants to know if religious beliefs are important to the participants instead of planting the idea that they might be. A qualitative oncology nurse scientist has to trust that participants will bring up the important aspects of their lives if given the opportunity. Second, the question assumes that the decision to leave the partner was one the participant considered. On the other hand, questions cannot be so general that the participants do not know where to begin. We would not say to the women in our study, "Tell us about your life." Taking a middle-ground approach, we decided to ask questions in a chronologic order, starting with the history of the relationship. The questions we asked included

- How did you meet your partner?
- When did you begin to realize that you were in a difficult or troubled relationship? (Many women do not say they are in an "abusive" relationship even when the abuse is apparent.)
- What was the day you were diagnosed like?
- How did you feel when you learned the diagnosis?
- How did your partner learn about the diagnosis?
- Who has been supportive to you?

In the case of the BC&IPA study, the construction of the text is retrospective. We interviewed women who were looking back on their relationships and their breast cancer treatment. We could have conducted a prospective study instead of or in addition to the retrospective study. In quantitative studies, prospective studies are favored. When a retrospective study is completed, the fact that it was retrospective usually is given as a limitation on the findings. Quantitative scientists are interested in cause and effect, and that can only be established prospectively. Clinical trials are always prospective. In the case of qualitative oncology nursing research, whether prospective is better than retrospective is not clear. If we were to enroll women with abusive partners as they were diagnosed with breast cancer, we could follow them through the course of treatment and construct a text about what happens to them. Whether that would be a more accurate or in some other way a better description of the phenomena is undetermined. Perhaps participants better understand their experiences after they are complete. Looking back may afford important insights. Or perhaps, important parts of the experience are lost to memory over time. The two approaches certainly would produce different texts, but whether one would be superior to the other is unclear.

The texts produced in prospective studies are different from those produced in retrospective studies because in the former, the scientist usually is more involved in creating the text. In retrospective studies, the scientist is told about what happened; in prospective studies, the scientist may be able to watch what happens (Cohen et al., 2002). Watching what happens in a participant's life generally is referred to as *participant observation*. Many times the scientist is only minimally a participant, such as when a scientist might accompany a woman with breast cancer to her radiation appointment. In such cases, the participant may still, in an interview, explain what her treatment was like, but the scientist also would be able to record what he or she witnessed in field notes. Thus, the text for analysis is created by the observations of the scientist as well as by means of an interview with the participant. For anthropologists and many other social scientists who conduct qualitative research, participant observation is the most valued source of data. Nothing can compare to seeing things for oneself.

Both in planning qualitative oncology nursing research and in publishing the results, explicit detail as to exactly how the data were collected is vitally important. How much did the oncology nurse scientist witness and observe, and how much was told to the scientist by the participants? It is not that one data source is better than the other; scientists can misunderstand what they see just as easily as they can misunderstand what they are told. However, the two sources of data are different and need to be presented as such (Angrosino, 2005; Fontana & Fry, 2005).

Data Analysis

In qualitative research, analysis is a matter of taking texts from a number of different participants and perhaps from a number of different observations and making the thick description they present maximally understandable. One could argue that maximal understanding would be reached by simply publishing all the interviews and field notes. The reader would be immersed in the phenomenon. However, besides the obvious fact that people do not want to read that much about most phenomena, immersion is not the same as understanding. Scientists have an obligation to think hard about the texts and to try to tell their readers what they think it all means (Cohen et al., 2000).

The end results of data analysis in the varied types of qualitative research (e.g., grounded theory, phenomenology, critical theory) are all different (Guba & Lincoln, 2005). Sometimes, the end result is a theory, sometimes an interpretation, or sometimes a description of the experience or the themes that characterize the phenomenon. Regardless of the end result, the beginnings and middles of the analyses are very similar. In a stepwise fashion, the text has to be divided into small units that can stand alone and then is reassembled into groups of units with similar meanings. At first this seems rather silly and not a very useful thing to do, but it does allow the texts to be better understood. For example, in the BC&IPA study, we might identify every mention of people who came to the aid of participants. References to these helpers appear frequently in the text and are probably important. Using a computer program to help, we will mark all the references to people who helped as units and put them in the same file. (In the past, all of this was accomplished with scissors, glue, and index cards.) After we have all the references to support from other people in a file, we go back through that file and determine how the references can be grouped into smaller files. For instance, we found that in one case, a woman depended on the support of nurses when her husband told her he thought of her as deformed after the mastectomy. In another case, a woman's husband left her, and she depended on her daughter to do the things she had hoped he would do. As we find other examples of people who help, we may find that we have categories of family helpers and health-care helpers, and we may continue to keep separate files on women who help and men who help, or we may see that the difference is minor, and we will combine them.

Once the texts are broken apart into categories of statements about the same topics, the categories are arranged into bigger units. A good deal of creative thinking and trial and error are useful in arranging and rearranging the categories (Cohen et al., 2002). Perhaps the help that oncology nurses provide will become part of a larger category about what healthcare providers can and cannot do. Perhaps both nurse helpers and family helpers will become part of a category about gains and losses—husbands and breasts are lost, but daughters and kind nurses are gained.

In qualitative oncology nursing research, specific details about the steps of analysis are necessary. Although it might be possible to say in a report of quantitative research that an analysis of variance was conducted, nothing that simple will do in qualitative research. (Actually, in quantitative research, simply naming a mathematical operation without justifying its use is not acceptable either.) In qualitative research, the steps used in the analysis should be explicit and detailed with examples. If one reads only that a "phenomenologic analysis was performed," the whole enterprise should probably be called into question. Agar (1986) offers a comprehensive guide for this process in his monograph *Speaking of Ethnography*.

Rigor

Qualitative scientists may or may not talk about *reliability* and *validity* (Brink, 1989). The more common terms are *trustworthiness* or *rigor* (Cohen et al., 2000; Lincoln & Guba, 1985; Sandelowski, 1993). The approaches to establishing scientific rigor in qualitative research are numerous. The discussions of rigor usually are divided into concerns with data collection and concerns with data analysis. We already have discussed most of the issues that are a threat to rigor in data collection. In order to argue that a study is rigorous, the study must have a good sample, and the questions asked and the things observed have to be sufficiently broad to allow for a thick description, yet narrow enough to allow some direction.

Issues of rigor in data analysis can be addressed with a single principle: every decision must be open to inspection and revision. The decisions in qualitative analysis include what is going to be identified as a stand-alone unit of meaning, how those units are going to be categorized, and how the categories are going to be organized as a final product. Because we have a team of three investigators in the BC&IPA study, discussing every decision and calling into question each other's thinking has been easy for us to do. Sometimes, going outside the group of scientists and having others critique decisions is beneficial. In some cases, scientists form a panel of people with expertise to critique; in others, participants are asked to look at the categories or the final product and offer a critique. Decisions about the data should not be private or hidden (Lincoln & Guba, 1985).

The Future of Qualitative Science in Oncology Nursing

In 1983, Jeanne Quint Benoliel reviewed nursing research in oncology. She traced nurses' approach to advances in nursing education and the professionalization of nursing and, most importantly, to the traditional nursing concern for the well-being and comfort of patients. Her review was wide reaching and appears to be inclusive. Apropos to the present topic, what is most interesting in this review is that she never mentioned the role of qualitative work in her paper. She wrote about instrument development, testing, and sophisticated statistical techniques but not about grounded theory, ethnography, or phenomenology. This would not be so remarkable except for the fact that Benoliel herself was a qualitative oncology nurse scientist and taught the doctoral course on qualitative research at the University of Washington. Clearly, in 1983, qualitative research was not making a big impression in oncology nursing research. But, Benoliel and other oncology nurse scientists have been designated as Distinguished Researchers by the Oncology Nursing Society (see Chapter 2).

Today, by contrast, qualitative research has become a staple in cancer studies conducted by nurses. A brief perusal of the journals *Cancer Nursing* and *Oncology Nursing Forum* will show that qualitative studies by oncology nurses are plentiful. One qualitative research piece appeared in a recent issue of *Cancer Nursing* at the time of this writing (Koldjeski, Kirkpatrick, Everett, Brown, & Swanson, 2007), and three appear in recent issues of *Oncology Nursing Forum* (Houldin, 2007; Wilkins & Woodgate, 2007; Williams, 2007). The topics include colorectal cancer, bone marrow transplantation, and ovarian cancer. Some are longitudinal; one is concerned with family caregivers, whereas another looks at the professional staff. Just this small cross-sectional sample demonstrates how oncology nurse scientists continue to significantly contribute to qualitative nursing research.

As for the future of qualitative research in oncology, some trends are clear. The first trend is the move toward community participatory research, sometimes called *community action research* (Kemmis & McTaggart, 2005). This is qualitative research that includes the community where the study is to take place in every aspect of the research. In this approach, members of the community are asked what problem they would like to have studied and who they think would be good informants. Community members also are involved in analysis of the data inasmuch as they are asked to weigh in on whether the end result of the study reflects their understanding of the community. This approach has its positives in that the findings are more likely to be of practical use to those being studied, and access to key informants is easier when they are involved in the study from the beginning. The disadvantage of this approach is that communities may identify problems to be researched that are outside the scientists' area of expertise. If an oncology nurse scientist with expertise in early detection and prevention approaches a community, and the community identifies lack of adequate transportation to healthcare facilities as their major problem, then the scientist may have little to offer. Whether this approach becomes common in oncology research will be interesting to see.

The second issue currently facing qualitative oncology nurse scientists is that of narrative analysis (Chase, 2005; Riessman, 2007). This approach has become more popular over the past few years. Scientists ask participants to tell them the story of their treatment for cancer, for example. Techniques have been developed for analyzing narrative data that consider not only the content of the stories but the form of the stories as well. Narrative oncology nurse scientists argue that narratives offer a close and detailed look at the events in a person's life. Narrative data come close to revealing the way people understand their lives. However, some protest that narratives are a distortion of data. Clough (1992) argued that narratives are linear and rarely do a good job of revealing the lives of women. This methodologic argument probably will be the object of much investigation in the coming years. How and to what extent narratives may shape the gathering of qualitative data and whether a better approach to data collection exists are the questions that need to be addressed.

The third trend is that of technology, specifically, the collection of data other than through interviews and written field notes. This may include photographs and videos produced by the scientists or by the participants (Stanczak, 2007), and it also can include data derived from blogs or other kinds of sites on the Internet (Dicks, Mason, Coffey, & Atkinson, 2005). This trend is less controversial than the first two. Qualitative oncology nursing research must keep up with the way people communicate and live their lives.

Conclusion

Qualitative oncology nursing research is a science that can and should be conducted with care and rigor. When it is performed well, it offers an understanding of the world in the form of a thick description that cannot be achieved with quantitative research. Potentially, our review of the intersection of BC&IPA and other key qualitative studies conducted by Steeves and other qualitative oncology nurse scientists has had an important place in understanding those who suffer from cancer and the nurses who care for them. Additionally, qualitative research by oncology pioneers such as Dr. Benoliel and others cited in this chapter have advanced oncology nursing science.

References

Agar, M. (1986). *Speaking of ethnography.* Thousand Oaks, CA: Sage.

American Cancer Society. (2007). *Breast cancer facts and figures, 2007–2008.* Atlanta, GA: Author.

American Cancer Society. (2008). *Cancer facts and figures, 2008.* Atlanta, GA: Author.

Angrosino, M.V. (2005). Recontextualizing observation: Ethnography, pedagogy, and the prospects for a progressive political agenda. In N.K. Denzin & Y.S. Lincoln (Eds.), *The Sage handbook of qualitative research* (3rd ed., pp. 729–746). Thousand Oaks, CA: Sage.

Baider, L., & DeNour, A.K. (1984). Couples' reactions and adjustment to mastectomy: A preliminary report. *International Journal of Psychiatry in Medicine, 14*(3), 265–276.

Benoliel, J.Q. (1983). The historical development of cancer nursing research in the United States. *Cancer Nursing, 6*(4), 261–268.

Ben-Zur, H. (2001). Your coping strategy and my distress: Inter-spouse perceptions of coping and adjustment among breast cancer patients and their spouses. *Families, Systems and Health, 19*(1), 83–94.

Ben-Zur, H., Gilbar, O., & Lev, S. (2001). Coping with breast cancer: Patient, spouse, and dyad models. *Psychosomatic Medicine, 63*(1), 32–39.

Brink, P.J. (1989). Issues of reliability and validity. In J.M. Morse (Ed.), *Qualitative nursing research: A contemporary nursing dialogue.* Thousand Oaks, CA: Sage.

Charmaz, K. (2006). *Constructing grounded theory: A practical guide through qualitative analysis.* Thousand Oaks, CA: Sage.

Chase, S.E. (2005). Narrative inquiry: Multiple lenses, approaches, voices. In N.K. Denzin & Y.S. Lincoln (Eds.), *The Sage handbook of qualitative research* (3rd ed., pp. 651–680). Thousand Oaks, CA: Sage.

Clough, P. (1992). *The end(s) of ethnography: From realism to social criticism.* Newberry Park, CA: Sage.

Cohen, M.Z., Haberman, M.R., & Steeves, R. (1994). The meaning of oncology nursing: A phenomenological investigation. *Oncology Nursing Forum, 21*(Suppl. 8), 5–8.

Cohen, M.Z., Kahn, D.L., & Steeves, R.H. (1998). Beyond body image: The experience of breast cancer. *Oncology Nursing Forum, 25*(5), 835–841.

Cohen, M.Z., Kahn, D.L., & Steeves, R.H. (2000). *Hermeneutic phenomenological research.* Thousand Oaks, CA: Sage.

Cohen, M.Z., Kahn, D.L., & Steeves, R.H. (2002). Making use of qualitative research. *Western Journal of Nursing Research, 24*(4), 454–470.

Creswell, J.W. (2007). *Qualitative inquiry and research design: Choosing among five approaches* (2nd ed.). Thousand Oaks, CA: Sage.

Curry, M.A., Hassouneh-Phillips, D., & Johnston-Silverberg, A. (2001). Abuse of women with disabilities: An ecological model and review. *Violence Against Women, 7*(1), 60–79.

Denzin, N.K., & Lincoln, Y.S. (Eds.). (2005a). *The Sage handbook of qualitative research* (3rd ed.). Thousand Oaks, CA: Sage.

Denzin, N.K., & Lincoln, Y.S. (2005b). Introduction. In N.K. Denzin & Y.S. Lincoln (Eds.), *The Sage handbook of qualitative research* (3rd ed., pp. 1–32). Thousand Oaks, CA: Sage.

Dicks, B., Mason, B., Coffey, A.J., & Atkinson, P.A. (2005). *Qualitative research and hypermedia ethnography for the digital age.* Thousand Oaks, CA: Sage.

Fontana, A., & Fry, J.H. (2005). The interview: From neutral stance to political involvement. In N.K. Denzin & Y.S. Lincoln (Eds.), *The Sage handbook of qualitative research* (3rd ed., pp. 695–728). Thousand Oaks, CA: Sage.

Ganz, P.A., Rowland, J.H., Desmond, K., Meyerowitz, B.E., & Wyatt, G.E. (1998). Life after breast cancer: Understanding women's health-related quality of life and sexual functioning. *Journal of Clinical Oncology, 16*(2), 501–514.

Geertz, C. (1973). *The interpretation of cultures: Selected essays.* New York: Basic Books.

Guba, E., & Lincoln, Y.S. (2005). Paradigmatic controversies, contradictions, and emerging confluences. In N.K. Denzin & Y.S. Lincoln (Eds.), *The Sage handbook of qualitative research* (3rd ed., pp. 191–215). Thousand Oaks, CA: Sage.

Houldin, A.D. (2007). A qualitative study of caregivers' experiences with newly diagnosed advanced colorectal cancer. *Oncology Nursing Forum, 34*(2), 323–330.

Jones, R.A., Taylor, A.G., Bourguignon, C., Steeves, R., Fraser, G., Lippert, M., et al. (2007). Complementary and alternative medicine modality use and beliefs among African American prostate cancer survivors. *Oncology Nursing Forum, 34*(2), 359–364.

Kemmis, S., & McTaggart, R. (2005). Participatory action research: Communicative action and the public sphere. In N.K. Denzin & Y.S. Lincoln (Eds.), *The Sage handbook of qualitative research* (3rd ed., pp. 605–640). Thousand Oaks, CA: Sage.

Kockelmans, J.J. (1970). *Phenomenology and the natural sciences: Essays and translations.* Chicago: Northwestern University Press.

Koldjeski, D., Kirkpatrick, M.K., Everett, L., Brown, L., & Swanson, M. (2007). The ovarian cancer journey of families the first postdiagnostic year. *Cancer Nursing, 30*(3), 232–242.

Lewis, J.A., Manne, S.L., DuHamel, K.N., Vickburg, S.M., Bovbjerg, D.H., Currie, V., et al. (2001). Social support, intrusive thoughts, and quality of life in breast cancer survivors. *Journal of Behavioral Medicine, 24*(3), 231–245.

Lincoln, Y.S., & Guba, E. (1985). *Naturalistic inquiry.* Thousand Oaks, CA: Sage.

Lugton, J. (1997). The nature of social support as experienced by women treated for breast cancer. *Journal of Advanced Nursing, 25*(6), 1184–1191.

Merleau-Ponty, M. (1962). *Phenomenology of perception* (C. Smith, Trans.). New York: Routledge. (Original work published in 1945)

Meyerowitz, B.E., Desmond, K.A., Rowland, J., Wyatt, G.E., & Ganz, P.A. (1999). Sexuality following breast cancer. *Journal of Sex and Marital Therapy, 25*(3), 237–250.

Petrie, W., Logan, J., & DeGrasse, C. (2001). Research review of the supportive care needs of spouses of women with breast cancer. *Oncology Nursing Forum, 28*(10), 1601–1607.

Plichta, S. (1997). Violence, health and the use of health services. In M. Falik & K. Collins (Eds.), *Women's health: The Commonwealth Fund survey* (pp. 237–272). Baltimore: Johns Hopkins University Press.

Riessman, C.K. (2007). *Narrative methods for the human sciences.* Thousand Oaks, CA: Sage.

Sandelowski, M. (1993). Rigor or rigor mortis: The problem of rigor in qualitative research revisited. *Advances in Nursing Science, 16*(2), 1–8.

Schmidt, N.K., Woods, T.E., & Stewart, J.A. (2006). Domestic violence against women with cancer: Examples and review of the literature. *Journal of Supportive Oncology, 4*(1), 24–33.

Silverman, D. (2004). *Doing qualitative research: A practical handbook.* Thousand Oaks, CA: Sage.

Smith, P.H., Smith, J.B., & Earp, J.A. (1999). Beyond the measurement trap: A reconstructed conceptualization and measurement of woman battering. *Psychology of Women Quarterly, 23*(1), 177–193.

Stanczak, G.C. (2007). *Visual research methods: Image, society, and representation.* Thousand Oaks, CA: Sage.

Steeves, R.H. (2002). The rhythms of bereavement. *Family and Community Health, 25*(1), 1–10.

Thomas, S.P., & Pollio, H.R. (2002). *Listening to patients: A phenomenological approach to nursing research and practice.* New York: Springer.

Tjaden, P., & Thoennes, N. (2000). *Full report of the prevalence, incidence, and consequences of violence against women* [Rep. No. NCJ 183781]. Washington, DC: U.S. Department of Justice, Office of Justice Programs.

Wilkins, K.L., & Woodgate, R.L. (2007). An interruption in family life: Siblings' lived experience as they transition through the pediatric bone marrow transplant trajectory. *Oncology Nursing Forum, 34*(2), 311–312.

Williams, L.A. (2007). Whatever it takes: Informal caregiving dynamics in blood and marrow transplantation. *Oncology Nurisng Forum, 34*(2), 379–392.

Wilmoth, M.C. (2001). The aftermath of breast cancer: An altered sexual self. *Cancer Nursing, 24*(4), 278–286.

Wimberly, S.R., Carver, C.S., Laurenceau, J.P., Harris, S.D., & Antoni, M.H. (2005). Perceived partner reactions to diagnosis and treatment of breast cancer: Impact on psychosocial and psychosexual adjustment. *Journal of Consulting and Clinical Psychology, 73*(2), 300–311.

CHAPTER 19

Advancing Family-Focused Oncology Nursing Research

Frances Marcus Lewis, RN, MN, PhD, FAAN

Introduction

Cancer is not just a disease of the patient; it also is an illness of the family. It "invades" the family, similar to how it invades the patient. At first, things look well, but over time, cancer causes changes (Parkes, 1971, 1975). How can a disease "invade" a family? How can a disease of the patient be an illness of the family? In what ways can cancer be conceptualized as a family's experience, not just a patient's medical diagnosis?

This chapter has three main purposes: (a) to summarize the historical development of family-focused oncology nursing research, (b) to conceptualize cancer as a family's experience, and (c) to propose future directions that are needed for family-focused research in oncology nursing.

Historical Development of Family-Focused Oncology Nursing Research

Awareness has been growing that cancer is a family experience and not just the medical diagnosis of a lone patient. This awareness grew from early position or theoretical papers, including those written by nurses (Barckley, 1980; Hilkemeyer & Barckley, 1975), social scientists (Litman, 1974; Litman & Venters, 1979), and physicians (Ervin, 1973; Parkes, 1971, 1975). Family-focused research in oncology nursing only recently has been generated in research programs by a small group of nurse scientists, including Badger (Badger, Segrin, Meek, Lopez, & Bonham, 2005; Badger, Segrin, Meek, Lopez,

Bonham, & Sieger, 2005), Given (Given et al., 1993, 2006), Heiney (Heiney & Lesesne, 1996; Heiney, McWayne, Hurley, et al., 2003; Heiney, McWayne, Walker, et al., 2003), Hilton (Hilton, 1993a, 1993b, 1994, 1996; Hilton, Crawford, & Tarko, 2000), Hoskins (Hoskins, 1995a, 1995b, 1997; Hoskins, Baker, Budin, et al., 1996; Hoskins, Baker, Sherman, et al., 1996; Hoskins & Budin, 2000; Hoskins et al., 2001), Houldin (Houldin, 2007; Houldin & Lewis, 2006), Lewis (Lewis & Hammond, 1992, 1996; Lewis, Hammond, & Woods, 1993; Lewis, Woods, Hough, & Bensley, 1989; Lewis, Zahlis, Shands, Sinsheimer, & Hammond, 1996; Woods & Lewis, 1995), Mishel (Mishel et al., 2002), and Northouse (Northouse, 1989a, 1989b, 1992; Northouse, Dorris, & Charron-Moore, 1995; Northouse, Kershaw, Mood, & Schafenacker, 2004; Northouse, Laten, & Reddy, 1995; Northouse, Mood, Templin, Mellon, & George, 2000; Northouse & Swain, 1987; Northouse, Templin, Mood, & Oberst, 1998).

Family-focused research in oncology nursing has evolved from embryonic to adolescence. The earliest papers in nursing identified the importance of cancer's impact on the family (Barckley, 1980) but relied heavily on personal beliefs, values, and untested theory. The earliest clinical papers by physicians (Ervin, 1973) often emphasized psychopathology, were affected by extreme cases, or relied on psychoanalytic theory instead of data. The gift of these papers was to raise consciousness that cancer affects whole families, not merely patients.

The second generation of family-focused oncology nursing studies evolved in the 1970s, 1980s, and 1990s and primarily consisted of descriptive or hypothesis-testing studies. These types of studies continue to be important today. For example, recent research by scientists in other disciplines, especially psychology, continues to contribute to the second generation of studies. Although the research by Baider, Manne, Pistrang, and Ptacek is exemplary, this chapter is focused on oncology nursing science (Baider et al., 2004; Baider & Kaplan De-Nour, 1986, 1999; Baider & Sarell, 1984; Manne, 1994, 1999; Manne, Alfieri, Taylor, & Dougherty, 1999a, 1999b; Manne & Glassman, 2000; Manne et al., 2004; Pistrang & Barker, 1995, 1998; Pistrang, Barker, & Rutter, 1997; Ptacek, Pierce, Dodge, & Ptacek, 1997; Wellisch, Jamison, & Pasnau, 1978). Many early studies focused on the seriousness or magnitude of stress that cancer caused in family members, especially the spouse or caregiver. This second generation comprised two types of studies: those that derived from an empiric-analytic paradigm (quantitative) and measured specific concepts with standardized measures of psychosocial adjustment in family members and those that used an interpretive paradigm (qualitative) to discover and uncover the experience of family members.

In studies within the quantitative paradigm, most measures were borrowed from the psychiatric or social sciences to assess and describe the magnitude of disruption and distress in family members. These second-generation studies went substantially beyond the first-generation papers because they were based on data, were more theoretically informed, and used valid and reliable standardized measures. With few exceptions, the second-generation studies involved single-group designs and single-occasion data collection. Over time and with increasingly refined methodology, this second generation of studies systematically documented the experiences and concerns experienced by spouses and caregivers (Chekryn, 1984; Gotay, 1984; Samms, 1999; Zahlis & Shands, 1991), as well as school-age and adolescent children (Armsden & Lewis, 1994; Birenbaum, Yancy, Phillips, Chand, & Huster, 1999; Hymovich, 1993, 1995; Issel, Ersek, & Lewis, 1990; Lewis, Ellison, & Woods, 1985).

Qualitative studies during the second generation complemented results obtained from quantitative studies and were essential in helping oncology nurses to better understand, in the words of study participants, what family members' experiences with cancer were like (Shands, Lewis, Sinsheimer, & Cochrane, 2007). In addition, an increasing number of scientists began to systematically study the children of patients with cancer (Shands, Lewis, & Zahlis, 2000).

During the second generation, a small number of scientists incorporated longitudinal designs (studies that obtained data from multiple occasions over time) into their studies of families' behavior. The longitudinal designs better captured the complexity of the family's experience and the changing cancer trajectory for different family members. For example, Oberst and James (1985) studied the types of reported problems that 40 spouses experienced at 10, 30, and 60 days after hospital discharge. The pattern of responses across types of problems was clear: emotional concerns, uncertainty, impact on lifestyle, and spousal symptoms increased over time. In contrast, patients had a systematic decrease in these same areas.

Northouse was among the first to use longitudinal designs to study functioning over time with both patients and spouses facing recently diagnosed breast cancer (Northouse & Swain, 1987). Results revealed a pattern of responses that further heightened awareness of the complexity of family life. Often, the spouse's distress increased over time even as the patient's concerns decreased. Results from these longitudinal studies caused a radical shift in nurse scientists' understanding of families' experience with cancer. The notion that family members all experienced the patient's illness in the same way was no longer valid. Nurse scientists could no longer assume that the patients' responses and levels of adjustment reflected other members' functioning or type of responses. As simple as this seems, these results were major breakthroughs. They also meant, by implication, that nurses and nurse scientists could no longer rely on only one member of the family, including the patient, to be the valid reporter of the experiences and functioning of other members affected by cancer.

In the 1980s and 1990s, a third generation of family-focused studies substantially advanced oncology nursing science in several ways. Studies moved from primarily stress-adaptation-coping models to family systems models within which the family moved from mere "context" to foreground (Weihs, Fisher, & Baird, 2002). Family members' responses were no longer viewed as a backdrop to the patients' response. Family members' responses (e.g., perceptions, management behavior, household activities) began to be viewed as primary instead of secondary.

The third generation of studies also formally modeled the complexity of family life with a diagnosed family member. Formal modeling included measuring multiple variables that currently affected the family, such as tension in the marriage or pressures from the illness; allowed for divergent processes through which family members managed their lives as a family, as well as their lives with the cancer; and enabled the scientists to examine multiple outcomes (dependent variables) that reflected different and separate aspects of a family's adjustment. Data in the third-generation studies were not obtained from only one member of the family but were obtained concurrently from multiple family members, typically patients, as well as the children and spouses of the patients (Issel et al., 1990; Lewis et al., 1985).

Figure 19-1 provides an illustration of multivariate analysis that is relevant to the third generation of family studies. The model in the figure contains hypotheses within each occasion, across each occasion but on the same concept, and between occasions but across different concepts. Of the three hypotheses, one involves lagged, another cross-lagged, and the third unlagged variables, at three different time periods of measurement. The main concepts in the Relational Model of Family Adjustment to Cancer are shown as the unlagged variables within each of the three time periods.

Children in the households of diagnosed parents were incorporated into the formal models, enabling the scientists to understand their responses to parental cancer as well as their behaviors and adjustments as a systematic source of influence on the patients', caregivers', and total households' adjustments. Finally, the third-generation studies enabled nurse scientists to explicitly test the mediating or explanatory processes that described family members' differential responses and outcomes to cancer (Lewis & Hammond, 1996; Lewis et al., 1989, 1993).

In the third-generation studies that used a family systems model, simpler hypotheses about cancer-related stressors and their relationship to coping or adjustment were replaced by more complex sets of interrelated hypotheses that involved multiple family members (e.g., child, ill parent, non-ill parent), dyadic relationships between family members (e.g., marital dyad, parent-child relationship), and multiple measures of family member and household functioning. Two meta-assumptions within family systems theory were particularly important in these studies: equifinality and interdependence. Attention to these meta-assumptions forced scientists to hypothesize multiple mechanisms and processes by which household family members adjusted to cancer instead of just one (equifinality). Furthermore, scientists explicitly attended to the dyadic, triadic, or total household processes of its members and tested them as both mediators and predictors of household functioning (interdependence). The assumption of equifinality forced scientists to test divergent processes through which families adjusted to cancer, thereby ruling out as well as ruling in what helped or enhanced household functioning (Lewis, Casey, Brandt, Shands, & Zahlis, 2006; Lewis & Hammond, 1996; Lewis et al., 1989, 1993, 2008; Mishel et al., 2002; Northouse et

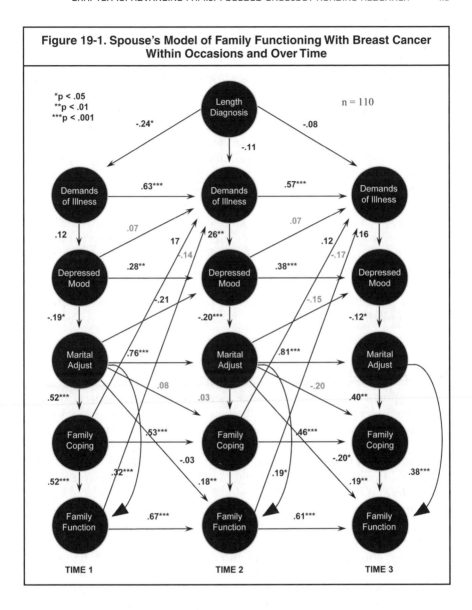

Figure 19-1. Spouse's Model of Family Functioning With Breast Cancer Within Occasions and Over Time

al., 2004; Woods & Lewis, 1995). The third generation of studies continues to the present.

The fourth generation of family-focused oncology nursing studies evolved from the 1990s and continues to current times. These studies are data-based, theory-informed intervention studies with the goal of improving family members' adjustment to cancer (Sidani & Braden, 1998). Intervention studies by nurse scientists include pilot studies, as well as experimental and quasi-experimental intervention studies.

Family-focused intervention studies in oncology nursing in this chapter are defined as including a dyad as the minimum unit. This definition includes interventions with family members that include the patient, other family members exclusive of the patient, and other dyads, including the healthy parent with young or adolescent children.

Interventions within the fourth-generation studies vary substantially on the extent to which the components explicitly address the mutable causes of the family's cancer experience. *Mutable causes* are the changeable factors that nurses potentially can alter. Interventions also vary greatly regarding the amount that a theory drives the operational components of the intervention. Although intervention studies in fourth-generation studies draw heavily from the prior three generations of research, they also utilize new channels (e.g., music videos), use new theories of family member behavior (Lewis, 1999), and make new assumptions about family member behavior. The interventions also range widely in the way they are structured, from broad, discretionary proto- cols to detailed, scripted text. The continuum of specificity to consider when designing an intervention moves from a manualized and scripted interven- tion, to a partially manualized, discretionary intervention, to a discretionary clinical model.

Cancer as a Family Experience

Conceptualizing cancer as a family experience requires a theoretical frame- work that integrates cancer within the family while being responsive to data- based studies about families' behavior with cancer. The Relational Model of Family Adjustment to Cancer, described in the following paragraph, offers a midrange theory that explains families' responses and adjustment to an adult member with cancer (Lewis, 1999, 2004). See Figure 19-2 for an intervention model derived from the Relational Model of Family Adjustment to Cancer, including the hypothesized relationships between the model's concepts.

The Relational Model derives from family systems theory and is based on the assumptions of interdependency (i.e., changes in one member affect other members), equifinality (i.e., optimum family functioning can be attained through multiple routes and means), morphogenesis (i.e., families learn to restructure their internal operations in order to be responsive to changes from the cancer and the family's environment), and nonsummativity (i.e., family members' individual responses are more complex than a simple additive sum of the behavior of the individual members—in other words, the whole is greater than the sum of its parts).

The Relational Model, similar to family systems theory, emphasizes the importance of families creating "requisite variety" (e.g., information, clarifica- tion) that facilitates their successful transformation of environmental input and "mapping" of their environment onto their operations as a family. The processes by which the family integrates new information are transformative

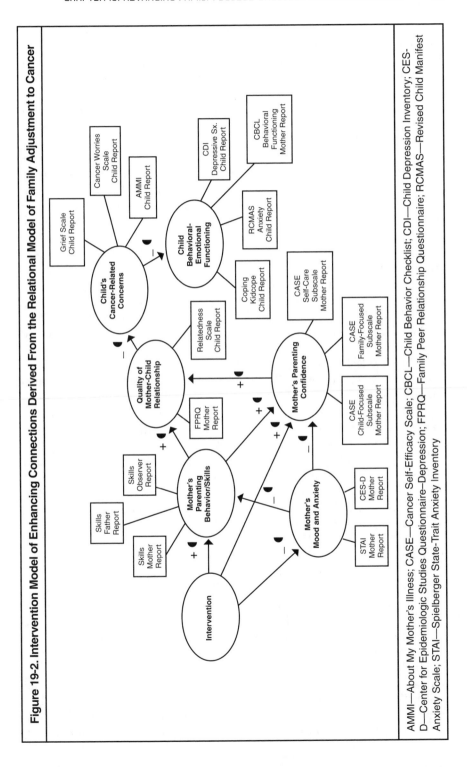

Figure 19-2. Intervention Model of Enhancing Connections Derived From the Relational Model of Family Adjustment to Cancer

AMMI—About My Mother's Illness; CASE—Cancer Self-Efficacy Scale; CBCL—Child Behavior Checklist; CDI—Child Depression Inventory; CES-D—Center for Epidemiologic Studies Questionnaire–Depression; FPRQ—Family Peer Relationship Questionnaire; RCMAS—Revised Child Manifest Anxiety Scale; STAI—Spielberger State-Trait Anxiety Inventory processes that enable the family to interpret, rearrange, reconfigure, and respond to the cancer and its effects on their internal operations and life as a family. In the Relational Model, the family is an active agent, not merely reacting or responding to the cancer. Therefore, the family is not a passive recipient of cancer's invasion but is instead an active agent acting on, interpreting, and modifying itself (morphogenesis) in response to how family members perceive and respond to the cancer and its contingencies.

Within the Relational Model, cancer is not viewed as an external "stressor" or set of "stressors," but as a multidimensional experience that produces multiple non-normative transitions that affect the families' internal operations, relationships, and core functions. In the Relational Model, the family concurrently has two lives: life as a family and life as a family with the cancer (Lewis, 2004). Problems can occur within the family system when families do not balance these two lives.

"Mapping" the cancer and its contingencies onto the family's operations involves multiple and often intense psychosocial transitions in family members. Psychosocial transitions are the cognitive-emotional processes by which members become involved and come to personal terms with the meaning of cancer, including its impact on oneself, as well as on the family (Lewis, 1993). Psychosocial transitions involve a confrontation of one's assumptive world during which values, orientation, and self-formulation are reevaluated (Lewis, 1993, Lewis & Daltroy, 1990; Parkes, 1971, 1975). These transitions are characterized by deep personal reflection and searching and involve existential questions such as "Why me?", "Why our family?", "Why us?", and "Why now?" (Houldin & Lewis, 2006; Lewis, 1993; Lewis & Deal, 1995). These psychosocial transitions often are not explicit and are conceptually mis-specified and overly reduced if they are viewed as merely "coping with the cancer."

In the process of "inputting" the cancer and reconfiguring around what is needed to "map" (i.e., integrating and reconfiguring around) the cancer in the family system, the family is dealing with both cancer-related distress and actual or potential destabilization. Like a biologic system, a high-functioning family is constantly modifying how it works and how it adjusts to the cancer and related contingencies. This process of self-regulation ideally enables the family to balance its family life and routines, even as it responds to the cancer's demands. However, self-regulation is not always successful. Escalating positive-amplifying or negative-amplifying feedback is known to occur, resulting in worsening conditions that threaten or destabilize an otherwise high-functioning family (see Lewis et al., 1989, for the earliest known evidence of this phenomenon). Substantial evidence exists that destabilization likely occurs in both the patient-spouse/partner dyad and the ill parent-child dyad. See Table 19-1 for examples of selected studies of adolescent children who were affected by parental cancers of different types. See Grabiak, Bender, and Puskar (2007) for the most recent analysis as of this writing of the published literature on adolescent children and parental cancer. As oncology nurse scientists who want to frame the cancer in positive ways, including its benefit-finding

Table 19-1. Selected Examples of Studies of Adolescents Affected by Parental Cancer

Source	Patient Diagnoses	Sample	Measures	Study Design/ Selected Goals
Compas et al., 1994	• Mixed cancers • 32% breast cancer • Mean = 2 months post-diagnosis • Stage I: 33%, stage II: 28%, stage III: 22%, stage IV: 17%	• 117 patients • 76 spouses • 34 young adults • 50 adolescents • 26 preadolescents	• YSR • BSI • IES • Control, seriousness, and stressfulness: four-point interval scale	Cross-sectional To examine anxiety/ depression and stress response in patients with cancer and their school-age, adolescent, and young adult children
Compas et al., 1996	• Mixed cancers • 28% breast cancer • Mean = 9.8 weeks post-diagnosis • Stage I: 36%, stage II: 24%, stage III: 21%, stage IV: 19%	• 134 patients (72% mothers, 28% fathers) • 45 young adults • 59 adolescents	• Control, seriousness, and stressfulness: four-point Likert scale • Coping: open-ended • YSR	Cross-sectional To examine coping styles in children, adolescents, and young adult children of parents with cancer
Grant & Compas, 1995	• Mixed cancers • 2 months post-diagnosis • Stage I: 36%, stage II: 24%, stage III: 21%, stage IV: 19%	• 55 adolescents • 21 girls with diagnosed mothers • 12 girls with diagnosed fathers • 12 boys with diagnosed mothers • 10 boys with diagnosed fathers	• APES • Coping: open-ended • YSR	Cross-sectional To examine the mechanisms that explain the risk to adolescent children of parents with cancer

(Continued on next page)

Table 19-1. Selected Examples of Studies of Adolescents Affected by Parental Cancer *(Continued)*

Source	Patient Diagnoses	Sample	Measures	Study Design/ Selected Goals
Lewis & Hammond, 1996	• Early-stage breast cancer • Mean time since diagnosis = 23.6 months (SD = 21.9)	• 70 women with breast cancer • 70 partners • 70 adolescents (mean age = 16.3 years)	• Rosenberg Self-Esteem • CES-D • Spanier Dyadic Adjustment • F-COPES • Child-Parent Attachment Subscale of the Relationships Scale	Cross-sectional To use path analysis to examine the impact of maternal breast cancer on adolescents and the family
Lewis et al., 1996	• Early-stage breast cancer • Median time since diagnosis = 18 months	• 22 single women with breast cancer and their 25 school-aged children • 101 married/ partnered women with breast cancer and their 106 school-aged children	• Rosenberg Self-Esteem • Child-Parent Attachment Subscale of the Relationships Scale • CES-D	Longitudinal To examine the functioning of adolescent and school-aged children of single women with breast cancer compared to married women
Lewis et al., 1989	• 13 women with type II diabetes • 19 women with nonmetastatic breast cancer • 16 women with fibrocystic breast disease • Mean illness length = 39.63 months	• 48 mothers • 48 fathers/ spouses • Children (ages 6–12)	• Spanier Dyadic Adjustment • Peer Relations subscale of Family Peer Relationships Questionnaire • CES-D	Cross-sectional To test a theoretical model using path analysis to examine the effects of maternal serious illness on the spouse and children

(Continued on next page)

Table 19-1. Selected Examples of Studies of Adolescents Affected by Parental Cancer *(Continued)*

Source	Patient Diagnoses	Sample	Measures	Study Design/ Selected Goals

Lichtman et al., 1985	• Breast cancer
	• Mean = 25.5 months post-diagnosis
	• Stage I: 31%, stage II: 55%, distant metastases: 14%
		• 68 mothers
		• 156 children (69 daughters, 87 sons), 30 living at home at diagnosis.
			• POMS
			• Rosenberg Self-Esteem
			• Index of Well-Being
			• Marital Adjustment Scale
			• Interview
			  – How has the relationship changed?
			  – Is change better, worse, or mixed?
				Retrospective cross-sectional
				To examine how the diagnosis of breast cancer affects the relationship between the mother and her children

Welch et al., 1996	• Mixed cancers • 37% breast cancer • Mean time since diagnosis = 9.7 weeks • Stage I: 29%, stage II: 36%, stage III: 22%, stage IV: 13%	• 54 patients (80% female) • 36 spouses • 55 adolescents • 34 preadolescents	• CBCL • YSR	Longitudinal To examine the effect of parental cancer on preadolescent and adolescent children 10 weeks post-diagnosis and at 4-week follow-up

Wellisch et al., 1991, 1992	Breast cancer	• 60 daughters (ages 18–65) with a history of mom's breast cancer
		• Daughter's age at diagnosis:
		  – 1–10 = 9
		  – 11–20 = 15
		  – 21+ = 36
		• 60 matched controls
			• Structured Questionnaire
			• BSI
			• Derogatis Sexual Function Inventory
			• Sexual Arousability Inventory
			• Ways of Coping Checklist
				Retrospective cross-sectional
				To examine the effects of a mother's breast cancer on her daughters and to compare the daughters with women with no history of maternal breast cancer

APES—Adolescent Perceived Events Scale; BSI—Brief Symptom Inventory; CBCL—Child Behavior Checklist; CES-D—Center for Epidemiologic Studies–Depression Scale; F-COPES—Family Crisis-Oriented Personal Evaluation Scales; IES—Impact of Events Scale; POMS—Profile of Mood States; SD—standard deviation; YSR—Youth Self Report aspects, it is important to remember that evidence suggests that families, even well-adjusted families, are always in the process of mapping the cancer and its changing contingencies onto their functioning as a family.

Destabilization of the family also is known to occur under multiple conditions: depressed mood in the diagnosed mother (Lewis & Darby, 2004; Lewis & Hammond, 1992); limited social support (Lewis et al.,1993); marital tension (not dissolution) (Lewis & Hammond, 1996; Lewis et al., 1989, 1993; Manne, 1999; Manne et al., 1999a, 1999b, 2004; Manne & Glassman, 2000); when the family decreases its ways of handling and reconfiguring its work around the cancer's changing conditions (Lewis & Hammond, 1992; Stetz, Lewis, & Primomo, 1986); poor parenting quality (Armsden & Lewis, 1993; Lewis & Darby, 2004); or when the parenting functions do not include interpreting, nurturing, or otherwise assisting vulnerable members with the cancer (Issel et al., 1990; Lewis & Darby, 2004; Zahlis & Lewis, 1998). These types of destabilization are known to occur at the time of initial diagnosis, as well as at recurring times during the illness trajectory (Lewis, 1997). This means that the work of families as family systems involves continual self-monitoring and self-regulating of their internal processes as well as their response to their external environment (i.e., information about disease recurrence, treatment failure, and disease remission, among other information they receive from the environment). Viewing the cancer as a stressor with which the family problem solves does not accurately depict their continuous, ongoing work (see Stetz et al. for additional details). Families' work with cancer is unending. A "cancer problem" is not ever completely solved and a total resolution never occurs (Stetz et al.).

Distress in family members is costly to individual family members and to the quality of the relationships they have with each other, and it negatively affects family members' ability to support patients (Holmes & Deb, 2003). Distress in family members is not the same as psychopathology, and destabilization is not the same as divorce or dissolution of a family. Both distress and destabilization in families are part of the natural history of families' cyclical experience with cancer (Lewis & Hammond, 1992). Distress and destabilization occur in well-adjusted marriages, in long-term relationships, in families with many resources, and in well-educated families (Lewis & Hammond, 1992, 1996; Lewis et al., 1989, 1993). In short, destabilization and distress are processes that occur in every family experiencing cancer, not just challenged or low-resource families. In oncology nursing, the goals in interventions need to focus on diminishing the intensity, duration, or consequences of families' distress and destabilization along the cancer trajectory. Most likely, oncology nurses will not be able to prevent distress but rather can diminish it, its intensity, its duration, and its deleterious consequences for families.

Distress can reach or exceed clinical levels. Even when distress (e.g., anxiety, depressed mood, marital adjustment, child behavioral-emotional functioning) is within normal range, it can have deleterious effects on family members' functioning. For example, the majority of school-age children worry that their diagnosed parent will die from cancer (Zahlis, 2001). One study of spouses of women with breast cancer showed the spouses were seriously concerned about their wives' well-being during active treatment. The spouses reported losing sleep, performing poorer at their jobs, feeling as though they were losing their wives to the cancer, and feeling marginalized by the medical team (Lewis, Fletcher, Cochrane, & Fann, 2008).

Core Processes of Families' Adjustment to Cancer in a Parent

We know the core processes that occur when a parent is diagnosed with cancer. Greater numbers and types of cancer-related pressures that family members attribute to the cancer result in greater symptoms of depressive mood. These elevated levels of depressed mood or greater numbers of illness pressures, in turn, negatively affect the quality of the marriage or the spouse-patient dyad. This means that the cancer is not a bounded event in the life of an individual patient but instead diffuses to the quality of the marriage or intimate partnership. When the marriage is not well adjusted, members of the household cope less frequently with their problems or challenges. When either marital quality is diminished or family members cope less with their problems, total household functioning diminishes (Lewis & Hammond, 1992).

In a system, most of the real activity to be studied or on which interventions are to be applied occurs at the junctures between units of the system, not at the level of the individual. By implication, relationships between family members, not the intra-individual methods of managing a cancer-related stressor, are one of the central focuses of family systems studies. Furthermore, studying and trying to affect these relational junctures includes minimizing or preventing both distress and destabilization. Key junctures in the cancer trajectory that are of particular importance to the family system are times of initial diagnosis, disease recurrence or progression, treatment failure, occurrence of escalating or unexplained symptoms, and termination of all forms of medical treatment for disease control (Lewis, 1997). Recent completed research on caregivers and symptom management have added to nurses' understanding of the complex relationships between symptoms, patient functional state, and caregiver and patient mood (Given, B., et al., 2006; Given, C.W., et al., 1993; Kurtz, Kurtz, Given, & Given, 1995).

Future Directions Needed for Research

Future research in family-focused oncology nursing must consider models, methods, machines, and sustainability. Each will now be discussed briefly.

Models

What a scientist sees depends on how and where the scientist looks: This is no simple claim; it is a statement about the power of a conceptual model or research paradigm to frame or constrain what is examined and the tested hypotheses. Future research needs to expand theories that are used to examine and frame families' experiences with cancer. Scientists should no longer overly rely on stress-adaptation-coping or self-regulation theories (Fawzy et al., 1990; Fawzy & Fawzy, 1994; Lazarus & Folkman, 1984; Wenzel, Glanz, & Lerman, 2002). Although these theories are essential in understanding what happens to the adjustment of individuals, they do not address sufficiently the complexity of issues that occur in the family as a total system, including the different and concurrent processes families use to manage both the cancer and their families' lives (Broderick & Smith, 1979; Hill, 1971; McCubbin & McCubbin, 1993; Wenzel et al.). They also do not help nurses or nurse scientists to understand what families as a unit do to regain or sustain their core functions (Lewis, 2004). Furthermore, coping-adaptation models are cognitive models. Cognitions are important, but family behavior is more complex than cognitions, and scientists have only begun to understand how different cultures, beliefs, traditions, and rituals, in addition to cognitions, affect how individuals and families respond and adjust to cancer. Future studies need to consider the addition of new conceptual models in both hypothesis testing and intervention studies.

What the scientist sees depends on the source of the data: Conceptual models implicitly or explicitly involve decisions about who in the family will be studied, how many times they will be observed, from whom data will be collected, and what concepts will be measured. If the scientist chooses to focus on the individual diagnosed with cancer, it will constrain what the researcher learns about families. If the scientist chooses to focus on a dyad in the family, that will enable examination of the dyad's behavior and adjustment processes and the individual members' behaviors and adjustment processes. The scientist can then triangulate among the types of data. However, studying diagnosed patients, even if they report on the family, is not family-focused research. An individual's view of the family is best understood as individual-level family data. Accumulated evidence from the first three generations of research revealed that one family member's view of the cancer will fail to account for the other family members' experiences with cancer and that one member reporting for other family members is not a reliable or valid source of information about the others. In short, do not do it.

Future studies need to consider the implications of integrating family systems theory or the Relational Model into their study. Adjustment processes involve multiple mechanisms through which cancer-related issues affect family members' adjustment and their interrelationships (e.g., marital and parenting relationships), as well as divergent strategies family members use to manage (e.g., map, transfigure around, modify internal operations) the effects of the cancer's impact. These multiple processes are consistent with concepts of morphogenesis and equifinality. If scientists limit themselves to studying caregivers' behavior, for example, they need not limit that research to outcomes in the patient that are hypothesized consequences of caregivers' behavior. They also can measure caregivers' impact on the patient-caregiver relationship and measure patients' views of the cancer, among other areas.

Why is this family-focused research important? From a family systems perspective, interventions with caregivers can produce changes in the quality of the patient-caregiver relationship, not just patient symptom outcomes. Changes in the quality of that relationship, as much as caregivers' competence in managing symptoms, may result in changes in patients' adjustment. Learning that changes in the patient's interpersonal environment have as much of an effect in enhancing the patient's adjustment as changes in the caregivers' symptom management would be remarkable.

Future research needs to attend to the two lives of a family affected by cancer: its life with the cancer and its life as a family. A family is about the business of being a family, not just about the business of dealing with the cancer. If oncology nurses and nurse scientists are to design programs and services to help families to heal, including protecting their core functions (i.e., their life as a family), they need to engage in research that is grounded in a healing paradigm, not merely a coping with cancer paradigm (Lewis, 2004).

Future research in family-focused oncology nursing needs to include other disciplines. This recommendation is consistent with the National Institutes of Health roadmap and recommendations by professional organizations. However, caution also is in order. Oncology nurse scientists must choose their intellectual bedfellows, they must not be co-opted. Disciplines that label families' adjustment and functioning as psychopathologic or as requiring "psychotherapy" may overly pathologize families' processes of adjustment (Greer et al., 1992; Lantz & Gregoire, 2000). Cancer in a family member involves a non-normative transition, not psychopathology (Lewis, 2007). Assisting families to integrate (i.e., map) the cancer into their everyday lives and relationships as a family will help its members to protect their core functions as well as to support the ill member.

Methods

Existing methods of studying individual family members need to include expanded measurement and data analysis systems. Self-report measures need to be complemented by other sources and types of measurement. The seminal paper by Fisher, Kokes, Ransom, Phillips, and Rudd (1985) distinguished among three types of family-level measurement: individual, interpersonal, and transactional. Scientists are only beginning to understand the meaning of measuring transactional family level data, including the exacting nature of coding that data and its importance in predicting dyadic quality. See Chen's (2007) dissertation as the seminal study enabling nursing science to move forward. Too many oncology nursing studies have relied on "individual family-level data" in which one member of the family reports on some characteristic of the family (e.g., conflict, cohesion).

Oncology nurse scientists may laud their success in the discipline, but intervention studies that are designed to help families are few. Furthermore, intervention studies of all kinds, even those directed at individual patients with cancer, still lag far behind descriptive studies (Cochrane & Lewis, 2005a, 2005b; Lewis, 1997). For example, in a recent analysis of intervention studies involving spouses or couples affected by cancer from 1983 to 2006, only four intervention studies met minimum criteria for scientific rigor and measured outcomes in spouse caregivers of women with breast cancer (Cochrane & Lewis, 2005b).

The lag needs to be shortened between study findings and implementing those findings. This does not mean that oncology nurse scientists need to be overzealous about interventions, but they do need to better balance timidity with action (Lewis, 2007). Describing the rocks is much easier than modifying the flow of the river. Descriptive research on families is about describing rocks; intervention research is about changing the flow of a river, that is, the families' behavior.

Families, by definition, are dynamic and deserve to be measured in ways that capture their dynamic. Understanding dynamic systems requires a minimum of three observation periods. Longitudinal designs need to be increasingly used (Woods & Lewis, 1992). Data analyses need to fit these dynamic models in order to statistically examine family members' behavior over time, as well as the mediation of family-level variables on both individual members' and families' functioning within and across occasions. See Lewis and Hammond (1992) for an example of analysis over time involving more than a hundred households using lagged, unlagged, and cross-lagged analyses to test within and across occasion hypotheses about families' adjustment processes.

Dynamic analyses require large study samples, which also beg for multisite studies. Study samples must be large enough to support structural equation modeling, latent growth curve analyses, and hierarchical linear modeling, among other multivariate dynamic analytic strategies.

Even as nurses develop increasingly informed interventions, descriptive, hypothesis-testing research still will be needed. Enormous holes exist in the understanding of what happens to families over time when an adult is diagnosed and survives cancer; what happens in families when the cancer trajectory is short-lived and characterized by intense symptoms; and what factors predict families who will have the greatest difficulty in managing as well as adjusting to cancer in a member. No known data-based studies exist of what happens to families when the disease trajectory is downward and fast. Scientists know little, if anything, about what happens to families when survivors go in and out of remission, have recurrences, and are repeatedly treated for cancer (Lewis, 2006). No one knows what an extended cancer trajectory costs or benefits the family (Lewis, 2006); however, scientists know that ongoing issues exist for the patient (Ganz et al., 1996, 2002). Nothing is known about school-age and adolescent children's experiences as they watch a parent deal with recurring bouts of cancer, retreatment, remissions, and disease recurrence (Lewis, 2007).

Most of the knowledge about cancer in families comes from studies of patients with breast cancer and a growing body of literature on prostate and colorectal cancers. However, few data-based studies have been performed with some cancer types, and large holes exist in the knowledge on the effects of advanced cancer on families, including colorectal cancer (Houldin, 2007; Houldin & Lewis, 2006).

Although studies in long-term survivors are an identified priority of the National Institutes of Health, the Oncology Nursing Society (ONS), and the Institute of Medicine, among others, very few studies involve family members and the ways in which they attend to, integrate, manage, or decide to not manage the issues that are part of long-term survivorship. The seminal work by Haberman's team raised awareness of the patient-centered issues of long-term survivorship for a population of cancer survivors, but comparable research with families is sorely needed (Bush, Haberman, Donaldson, & Sullivan, 1995; Haberman, Bush, Young, & Sullivan, 1993). In fact, no known study exists of families qua families and their experiences with long-term survivorship.

Future intervention studies should not be about merely doing things with, for, or to families. Family-focused interventions need to be built around theories of behavior and the mutable causes of what families experience. These may be relationship issues, parenting concerns, or symptom interpretation struggles, among others. The intervention should target the mutable causes of the issues. Efficacious interventions never directly address a problem; they address the *mutable causes* of the problem.

Future intervention studies need to be framed and informed by theories of health-related behavior (Sidani & Braden, 1998). Merely declaring that an intervention uses social cognitive theory is not enough. Claiming that the intervention dealt with "communication problems" or the "need to support" families is not enough, either. Declarative statements must be accompanied by theory-derived operational components of the intervention that tightly articulate the mutable causes of families' struggles.

Cancer involves the biology of the patient as well as the family. Literature that links patients' perceived social support with their T-cell proliferation in response to phytohemagglutinin and concanavalin A is slowly growing (Andersen et al., 2004). Future interventions that affect the quality of families' relationships or household environment (e.g., marital tension, support to the patient, quality of the patient-caregiver relationship) may affect patients' positive responses to treatment. Future research should consider the addition of biologic markers to evaluate the efficacy of interventions for families.

Cancer has a genetic component that can affect other members of the family. Beginning research exists on the families' response to a genetic alteration in one of its members. Existing studies about families and genetic risk have been framed as *communication* studies (studies that focus on family members communicating to other members about their risk for cancer). However, a genetic alteration or genetic risk in a family is much larger and more multidimensional than a "communication" problem. Future research needs to include studies of a genetic alteration's impact on family members and how family members' responses to the proband affect the proband as well as other family members.

Given's research programs, among others, are prototypes of programs that add to a diagnosed individual's or spouse-caregivers' abilities to self-manage cancer, including symptom management (Giesler et al., 2005; Given, B., et al., 2006; Given, C.W., et al., 1993). The science needs comparable research programs that help families to better self-manage, self-regulate, and thrive.

Most of what is known about survivorship emerged from studies of family members dealing with the first three years of a cancer diagnosis. Clearly, more studies are needed that describe long-term survivorship and the experiences of family members. These studies should not be limited to caregiver studies but should also include households.

Longitudinal research using mixed methods is needed (Woods & Lewis, 1992). Capturing a family at a single point in time is naïve; families are dynamic systems whose processes require multiple observation points. Mixed methods are needed that use the best of both interpretive and empiric-analytic paradigms.

Like the Beatles song "With A Little Help From My Friends," a little intervention can go a long way in helping families to adapt, manage, heal, and thrive. However, more is not always better (Stanton et al., 2005). Complex interventions that are offered at multiple occasions do not necessarily produce better results. Targeted, efficient interventions with essential core elements are needed that still are able to affect significant changes in the outcome variables of family members' adjustment.

Machines

Future research on families' experience with cancer should include the use of new channels, including the Internet (Kirsch & Lewis, 2004). Oncology nurse scientists have demonstrated that telephone-delivered interventions are effective for patients with serious medical illnesses, including cancer. Telephone-based interventions also hold promise under certain conditions, but their efficacy has only begun to be tested with certain patient populations and not with other family members. For example, see research programs by Badger (Badger, Segrin, Meek, Lopez, & Bonham, 2005; Badger, Segrin, Meek, Lopez, Bonham, et al., 2005), Dougherty (Dougherty, Johnson-Crowley, Lewis, & Thompson, 2001; Dougherty, Lewis, Thompson, Baer, & Kim, 2004; Dougherty, Thompson, & Lewis, 2005), and Mishel (Mishel et al., 2002). However, scientists do not know how best to engage multiple family members concurrently on the Internet.

Interventions with family members should expand beyond service-based settings to include community-based and public-service channels (Lewis, 1997). It would be remarkable if oncology nurse scientists could better harness the public library system, senior citizen centers, community centers, and other places where people gather and learn.

Sustainability

Whatever the content or form of family-focused interventions, they need to be sustainable. Family-focused oncology nurse scientists cannot afford to develop interventions that have no future within cost-sensitive environments. Scientists need to develop and test interventions that are sustainable over the long run. Scientists do no good, and perhaps cause potential harm, if they develop interventions that are efficacious but costly and not sustainable (Cochrane & Lewis, 2005b). With the goal of achieving sustainability, nurse scientists need to increasingly collaborate and partner with provider systems and agencies as scientific collaborators and as stakeholders. Efficacious interventions would then have a welcome "home" in which the intervention can be transferred and disseminated.

Family member behavior, interpersonal exchanges, affect, and mood are major direct and indirect sources of influence in patients' adjustment to cancer and long-term survivorship. To treat families as either context or background is technically naïve. Families establish the environment within which patients respond and adjust to cancer. Conversely, family members are themselves directly and indirectly affected by cancer in patients. The behavior, interpersonal activities, and exchanges between family members literally establish the environment within which each member struggles or flourishes.

Conclusion

Family is a ubiquitous part of people's lives, and the reality is that families are never simply context; they need to be foreground in oncology nursing research (Lewis, 1998; Weihs et al., 2002). Nurses, physicians, and other healthcare professionals want to "help" and value "family-focused" care, but they typically are not trained to conduct family-focused oncology research. Healthcare providers, likewise, do not know what to do or say to move from patient-centered to family-centered care and have little or no experience in engaging family members in dealing with cancer. At best, medical workers train a family member to be a caregiver or caretaker for the patient. At worse, they treat the family with benign neglect or view them as background or context, not foreground. Both extremes are bad: The family is known to struggle with how to deal with cancer, how to be supportive to the patient, and how to maintain and sustain the health and well-being of its core functions and family members (Lewis, 2004). Professional codes of practice do not help healthcare providers to know what to do, with what to assist families, or how to best assist families. All this argues for the importance and centrality of conducting family-focused oncology nursing research, from which evidence-based programs and services can evolve.

The reality is that cancer has the potential to cause "blood clots" in families. Even as I personally would hope otherwise, almost daily I receive a request to help a family to interpret, better manage, or address disrupted or tense family member relationships, all of which are attributed to the family member's cancer. Healing from cancer is much more than wound healing or biologic remission. To heal includes healing the family members, all of whom have been affected to some degree by the patient's cancer. "Blood clots" in a family represent damage, all or most of which can be prevented with short-term, brief interventions given directly to the family, not through or to only the patient. Toward that end, oncology nurse scientists can provide the essential studies to guide future programs and services, thereby being the stewards of the health of families affected by cancer.

Acknowledgments
....

Research reported in this chapter was made possible through grants from the National Institutes of Health (R01-NR-01000, R01-CA-78424, R01-CA-55347, R01-NR-04135), the Department of Defense Concept Award, and foundation research support, including the ONS Foundation, the Lance Armstrong Foundation, the Tennis Fund, the University of Washington School of Medicine, the Nesholm Family Foundation, the Dorothy S. O'Brien Special Projects Fund, Cancer Lifeline, the Puget Sound Affiliate of Susan G. Komen for the Cure, and the American Cancer Society. The author acknowledges the contributions of coprincipal investigators and subcontracting principal investigators on the Enhancing Connections: Helping the Mother With Breast Cancer Support Her Child multistate clinical trial: Patricia Brandt, Barbara Bean Cochrane, Marcia Grant, Joan Haase, Arlene Houldin, and Janice Post-White. Other members of the Family Functioning Research Team are Gay C. Armsden, PhD, Maggie W. Baker, RN, PhD, Connie Bellin, RN, PhD, Maryanne Bletscher, MS, Sue Bodurtha, RN, MN, Maryanne Bozette, RN, PhD, Patricia Buchsel, RN, MN, Patricia Carney, RN, PhD, Susan M. Casey, RN, PhD, Huei-Fang Chen, RN, PhD, Rochelle Crosby, RN, PhD, Lisa W. Deal, RN, MN, MPH, Cynthia Dougherty, RN, PhD, Mary T. Ersek, RN, PhD, Aileen Fink, RN, MN, Sharon C. Firsich, RN, MN, Rebecca Fiser, RN, MN, Melissa Gallison, RN, PhD, Jane Georges, RN, PhD, Mel R. Haberman, RN, PhD, Lisa E. Hales, BS, Mary A. Hammond, PhD, Blanche Hobs, RN, MN, Gail Houck, RN, PhD, Edith E. Hough, RN, EdD, L. Michele Issel, RN, PhD, Gail Kieckhefer, RN, PhD, Sallie Davis Kirsch, RN, PhD, Katherine Klaich, RN, PhD, Courtney A. Knox, Judy Kornell, RN, MN, Colleen Lucas, RN, MN, Katryna McCoy, RN, MN, Jean Moseley, RN, MN, Sandra Underhil Motzer, RN, PhD, Ingrid R. Nielsen, RN,

MN, Sandy O'Keefe, RN, MN, Nancy Packard, RN, PhD, Janet Primomo, RN, PhD, Connie V. Rousch, RN, MN, Marguerite Samms, RN, MN, Mary Ellen Shands, RN, MN, Terri Forshee Simpson, RN, PhD, Jan Sinsheimer, MS, Lillian B. Southwick, PhD, Rebecca Spirig, PhD, Kathy Stetz, RN, PhD, Viva J. Tapper, RN, PhD, Maye Thompson, RN, MN, Susan Turner, RN, MN, Lynn Wheeler, MSN, WHCNP, Nancy F. Woods, RN, PhD, Salene M. Wu, BA, Bernice Yates, RN, PhD, Ellen H. Zahlis, MN, and Gretchen Zunkel, RN, PhD.

References

Andersen, B.L., Farrar, W.B., Golden-Kreutz, D.M., Glaser, R., Emery, C.F., Crespin, T.R., et al. (2004). Psychological, behavioral, and immune changes after a psychological intervention: A clinical trial. *Journal of Clinical Oncology, 22*(17), 3570–3580.

Armsden, G.C., & Lewis, F.M. (1993). The child's adaptation to the mother's illness: Theory and clinical implications. *Patient Education and Counseling, 22*(3), 153–165.

Armsden, G.C., & Lewis, F.M. (1994). Behavioral adjustment and self-esteem among school-age children of mothers with breast cancer. *Oncology Nursing Forum, 21*(1), 39–45.

Badger, T., Segrin, C., Meek, P., Lopez, A.M., & Bonham, E. (2005). Profiles of women with breast cancer: Who responds to a telephone interpersonal counseling intervention? *Journal of Psychosocial Oncology, 23*(2–3), 79–100.

Badger, T., Segrin, C., Meek, P., Lopez, A.M., Bonham, E., & Sieger, A. (2005). Telephone interpersonal counseling for women with breast cancer: Symptom management and quality of life. *Oncology Nursing Forum, 32*(2), 273–279.

Baider, L., Andritsch, E., Goldzweig, G., Uziely, B., Ever-Hadani, P., Hofman, G., et al. (2004). Changes in psychological distress of women with breast cancer in long-term remission and their husbands. *Psychosomatics, 45*(1), 58–68.

Baider, L., & Kaplan De-Nour, A. (1986). Family perception and adjustment in postmastectomy women. *International Journal of Family Psychiatry, 7*(4), 439–447.

Baider, L., & Kaplan De-Nour, A. (1999). Psychological distress of cancer couples: A levelling effect. *New Trends in Experimental and Clinical Psychiatry, 15*(4), 197–204.

Baider, L., & Sarell, M. (1984). Couples in crisis: Patient-spouse differences in perception of interaction patterns and the illness situation. *Family Therapy, 11*(2), 115–122.

Barckley, V. (1980). *The family of the dying patient.* Geneva, Switzerland: International Union Against Cancer.

Birenbaum, L.K., Yancy, D.Z., Phillips, D.S., Chand, N., & Huster, G. (1999). School-age children's and adolescents' adjustment when a parent has cancer. *Oncology Nursing Forum, 26*(10), 1639–1645.

Broderick, C., & Smith, J. (1979). The general systems approach to the family. In W.R. Burr, R. Hill, F.I. Nye, & I.L. Reiss (Eds.), *Contemporary theories about the family* (Vol. 2, pp. 112–129). New York: The Free Press.

Bush, N., Haberman, M., Donaldson, G., & Sullivan, K. (1995). Quality of life of 125 adults surviving 6–18 years after bone marrow transplantation. *Social Science and Medicine, 40*(4), 479–490.

Chekryn, J. (1984). Cancer recurrence: Personal meaning, communication, and marital adjustment. *Cancer Nursing, 7*(6), 491–498.

Chen, H.-T. (2007). *Relational and transactional processes in couples' experience with breast cancer.* Unpublished doctoral dissertation, University of Washington, Seattle.

Cochrane, B., & Lewis, F.M. (2005a). Interventions for partners of breast cancer patients [Abstract]. *Oncology Nursing Forum, 32*(1), 153.

Cochrane, B.B., & Lewis, F.M. (2005b). The partner's adjustment to breast cancer: A critical analysis of intervention studies. *Health Psychology, 24*(3), 327–332.

Compas, B.E., Worsham, N.L., Epping-Jordan, J.E., Grant, K.E., Mireault, G., Howell, D.C., et al. (1994). When mom or dad has cancer: Markers of psychological distress in cancer patients, spouses, and children. *Health Psychology, 13*(6), 507–515.

Compas, B.E., Worsham, N.L., Ey, S., & Howell, D.C. (1996). When mom or dad has cancer II: Coping, cognitive appraisals, and psychological distress in children of cancer patients. *Health Psychology, 15*(3), 167–175.

Dougherty, C., Johnson-Crowley, N., Lewis, F.M., & Thompson, E.A. (2001). Theoretical development of nursing interventions for sudden cardiac survivors using social cognitive theory. *Advances in Nursing Science, 24*(1), 78–86.

Dougherty, C.M., Lewis, F.M., Thompson, E.T., Baer, J.D., & Kim, W. (2004). Short-term efficacy of a telephone intervention by expert nurses after an implantable cardioverter defibrillator. *Pacing and Cardiac Electrophysiology, 27*(12), 1594–1602.

Dougherty, C.M., Thompson, E.A., & Lewis, F.M. (2005). Long-term outcomes of a nursing intervention after an ICD. *Pacing and Cardiac Electrophysiology, 28*(11), 1157–1167.

Ervin, C., Jr. (1973). Psychologic adjustment to mastectomy. *Medical Aspects of Human Sexuality, 7*(2), 42–65.

Fawzy, F.I., Cousins, N., Fawzy, N.W., Kemeny, M.E., Elashoff, R., & Morton, D. (1990). A structured psychiatric intervention for cancer patients, I: Changes over time in methods of coping and affective disturbance. *Archives of General Psychiatry, 47*(8), 720–725.

Fawzy, F.I., & Fawzy, N.W. (1994). A structured psychoeducational intervention for cancer patients. *General Hospital Psychiatry, 16*(3), 149–192.

Fisher, L., Kokes, R.F., Ransom, D.C., Phillips, S.L., & Rudd, P. (1985). Alternative strategies for creating "relational" family data. *Family Process, 24*(2), 213–224.

Ganz, P.A., Coscarelli, A., Fred, C., Kahn, B., Polinsky, M.L., & Petersen, L. (1996). Breast cancer survivors: Psychosocial concerns and quality of life. *Breast Cancer Research and Treatment, 38*(2), 183–199.

Ganz, P.A., Desmond, K.A., Leedham, B., Rowland, J.H., Meyerowitz, B.E., & Belin, T.R. (2002). Quality of life in long-term, disease-free survivors of breast cancer: A follow-up study. *Journal of the National Cancer Institute, 94*(1), 39–49.

Giesler, R.B., Given, B., Given, C.W., Rawl, S., Monahan, P., Burns, D., et al. (2005). Improving the quality of life of patients with prostate carcinoma: A randomized trial testing the efficacy of a nurse-driven intervention. *Cancer, 104*(4), 752–762.

Given, B., Given, C.W., Sikorskii, A., Jeon, S., Sherwood, P., & Rahbar, M. (2006). The impact of providing symptom management assistance on caregiver reaction: Results of a randomized trial. *Journal of Pain and Symptom Management, 32*(5), 433–443.

Given, C.W., Strommel, M., Given, B., Osuch, J., Kurtz, M.E., & Kurtz, J.C. (1993). The influence of cancer patients' symptoms and functional states on patients' depression and family caregivers' reaction and depression. *Health Psychology, 12*(4), 277–285.

Gotay, C.C. (1984). The experience of cancer during early and advanced stages: The views of patients and their mates. *Social Science and Medicine, 18*(7), 605–613.

Grabiak, B.R., Bender, C.M., & Puskar, K.R. (2007). The impact of parental cancer on the adolescent: An analysis of the literature. *Psycho-Oncology, 16*(2), 127–137.

Grant, K.E., & Compas, B.E. (1995). Stress and anxious-depressed symptoms among adolescents: Searching for mechanisms of risk. *Journal of Consulting and Clinical Psychology, 63*(6), 1015–1021.

Greer, S., Moorey, S., Baruch, J.D.R., Watson, M., Robertson, B.M., Mason, A., et al. (1992). Adjuvant psychological therapy for patients with cancer: A prospective randomized trial. *BMJ, 304*(6828), 675–680.

Haberman, M., Bush, N., Young, K., & Sullivan, K.M. (1993). Quality of life of adult long-term survivors of bone marrow transplantation: A qualitative analysis of narrative data. *Oncology Nursing Forum, 20*(10), 1545–1553.

Heiney, S.P., & Lesesne, C.A. (1996). Quest: An intervention program for children whose parent or grandparent has cancer. *Cancer Practice, 4*(6), 324–329.

Heiney, S.P., McWayne, J., Hurley, T., Lamb, L., Bryant, L.H., & Butler, W. (2003). Efficacy of therapeutic group by telephone for women with breast cancer. *Cancer Nursing, 26*(6), 439–447.

Heiney, S.P., McWayne, J., Walker, S., Bryant, L., Howell, C., & Bridges, L. (2003). Evaluation of a therapeutic group by telephone for women with breast cancer. *Journal of Psychosocial Oncology, 21*(3), 63–80.

Hilkemeyer, R., & Barckley, V. (1975). *A cancer teaching unit for professional nurse instructors.* New York: American Cancer Society.

Hill, R. (1971). Modern systems theory and the family: A confrontation. *Social Science Information, 10*(5), 7–26.

Hilton, B.A. (1993a). Issues, problems, and challenges for families coping with breast cancer. *Seminars in Oncology Nursing, 9*(2), 88–100.

Hilton, B.A. (1993b). A study of couple communication patterns when coping with early stage breast cancer. *Canadian Oncology Nursing Journal, 3*(4), 159–166.

Hilton, B.A. (1994). Family communication patterns in coping with early breast cancer. *Western Journal of Nursing Research, 16*(4), 366–391.

Hilton, B.A. (1996). Getting back to normal: The family experience during early stage breast cancer. *Oncology Nursing Forum, 23*(4), 605–614.

Hilton, B.A., Crawford, J.A., & Tarko, M.A. (2000). Men's perspectives on individual and family coping with their wives' breast cancer and chemotherapy. *Western Journal of Nursing Research, 22*(4), 438–459.

Holmes, A.M., & Deb, P. (2003). The effect of chronic illness on the psychological health of family members. *Journal of Mental Health Policy and Economics, 6*(1), 13–22.

Hoskins, C.N. (1995a). Adjustment to breast cancer in couples. *Psychological Reports, 77*(2), 435–454.

Hoskins, C.N. (1995b). Patterns of adjustment among women with breast cancer and their partners. *Psychological Reports, 77*(3, Pt. 1), 1017–1018.

Hoskins, C.N. (1997). Differences in adjustment between women with breast cancer and their spouses: Implications for nursing interventions. *Clinical Effectiveness in Nursing, 1*(2), 105–111.

Hoskins, C.N., Baker, S., Budin, W., Ekstrom, D., Maislin, G., Sherman, D., et al. (1996). Adjustment among husbands of women with breast cancer. *Journal of Psychosocial Oncology, 4*(1), 41–69.

Hoskins, C.N., Baker, S., Sherman, D., Bohlander, J., Bookbinder, M., Budin, W., et al. (1996). Social support and patterns of adjustment to breast cancer. *Scholarly Inquiry for Nursing Practice, 10*(2), 99–123, 125–133.

Hoskins, C.N., & Budin, W.C. (2000). Measurement of psychological adjustment to breast cancer: A unidimensional or multidimensional construct? *Psychological Reports, 87*(2), 649–663.

Hoskins, C.N., Haber, J., Budin, W.C., Cartwright-Alcarese, F., Kowalski, M.O., Panke, J., et al. (2001). Breast cancer: Education, counseling, and adjustment—a pilot study. *Psychological Reports, 89*(3), 677–704.

Houldin, A.D. (2007). A qualitative study of caregivers' experiences with newly diagnosed advanced colorectal cancer. *Oncology Nursing Forum, 34*(2), 323–330.

Houldin, A.D., & Lewis, F.M. (2006). Salvaging their normal lives: A qualitative study of patients with recently diagnosed advanced colorectal cancer. *Oncology Nursing Forum, 33*(4), 719–725.

Hymovich, D.P. (1993). Child-rearing concerns of parents with cancer. *Oncology Nursing Forum, 20*(9), 1355–1360.

Hymovich, D.P. (1995). The meaning of cancer to children. *Seminars in Oncology Nursing, 11*(1), 51–58.

Issel, L.J., Ersek, M., & Lewis, F.M. (1990). How children cope with mother's breast cancer. *Oncology Nursing Forum, 17*(3), 5–13.

Kirsch, S.E., & Lewis, F.M. (2004). Using the World Wide Web in health-related intervention research: A review of controlled trials. *Computers, Informatics, Nursing, 22*(1), 8–18.

Kurtz, M.E., Kurtz, J.C., Given, C.W., & Given, B. (1995). Relationship of caregiver reactions and depression to cancer patients' symptoms, functional states and depression—a longitudinal view. *Social Science and Medicine, 40*(6), 837–846.

Lantz, J., & Gregoire, T. (2000). Existential psychotherapy with couples facing breast cancer: A twenty year report. *Contemporary Family Therapy, 22*(3), 315–327.

Lazarus, R.S., & Folkman, S. (1984). *Stress, appraisal, and coping.* New York: Springer.

Lewis, F.M. (1993). Psychosocial transitions and the family's work in adjusting to cancer. *Seminars in Oncology Nursing, 9*(2), 127–129.

Lewis, F.M. (1997). Behavioral research to enhance psychosocial adjustment and quality of life after cancer diagnosis. *Preventive Medicine, 26*(5), S19–S29.

Lewis, F.M. (1998). Family-level services in oncology nursing: Facts, fallacies, and realities revisited. *Oncology Nursing Forum, 25*(8), 1377–1388.

Lewis, F.M. (1999). Family issues in cancer care. In C. Miaskowski & P. Buchsel (Eds.), *Oncology nursing: Assessment and critical care* (pp. 319–331). St. Louis, MO: Mosby.

Lewis, F.M. (2004). Family-focused oncology nursing research: A healing paradigm for future studies. *Oncology Nursing Forum, 31*(2), 288–292.

Lewis, F.M. (2006). The effects of cancer survivorship on families and caregivers. More research is needed on long-term survivors. *American Journal of Nursing, 106*(Suppl. 3), 20–25.

Lewis, F.M. (2007). Parental cancer and dependent children: Selected issues for future research. *Psycho-Oncology, 16*(2), 97–98.

Lewis, F.M., Casey, S.M., Brandt, P.A., Shands, M.E., & Zahlis, E.H. (2006). The Enhancing Connections Program: A pilot evaluation of a cognitive-behavioral intervention for mothers and children affected by breast cancer. *Psycho-Oncology, 15*(6), 486–497.

Lewis, F.M., Cochrane, B.B., Fletcher, K.A., Zahlis, E.H., Shands, M.E., Gralow, J.R., et al. (2008). Helping her heal: A pilot study of an educational counseling intervention for spouses of women with breast cancer. *Psycho-Oncology, 17*(2), 131–137.

Lewis, F.M., & Daltroy, L. (1990). How causal explanations influence health behavior: Attribution theory. In K. Glanz, F.M. Lewis, & B. Rimer (Eds.), *Health behavior and health education: Theory, research, and practice* (pp. 92–114). San Francisco: Jossey-Bass.

Lewis, F.M., & Darby, E.L. (2004). Adolescent adjustment and maternal breast cancer: A test of the "Faucet Hypothesis." *Journal of Psychosocial Oncology, 21*(4), 83–106.

Lewis, F.M., & Deal, L.W. (1995). Balancing our lives: A study of the couples' experience with breast cancer recurrence. *Oncology Nursing Forum, 22*(6), 943–953.

Lewis, F.M., Ellison, E.S., & Woods, N.F. (1985). The impact of breast cancer on the family. *Seminars in Oncology Nursing, 1*(3), 206–213.

Lewis, F.M., Fletcher, K.A., Cochrane, B.B., & Fann, J.R. (2008). Predictors of depressed mood in spouses of women with breast cancer. *Journal of Clinical Oncology, 26*(8), 1289–1295.

Lewis, F.M., & Hammond, M.A. (1992). Psychosocial adjustment of the family to breast cancer: A longitudinal analysis. *Journal of the American Medical Women's Association, 47*(5), 194–200.

Lewis, F.M., & Hammond, M.A. (1996). The father's, mother's and adolescent's functioning with breast cancer. *Family Relations, 45*(4), 456–465.

Lewis, F.M., Hammond, M.A., & Woods, N.F. (1993). The family's functioning with newly diagnosed breast cancer in the mother: The development of an explanatory model. *Journal of Behavioral Medicine, 16*(4), 351–370.

Lewis, F.M., Woods, N.F., Hough, E.H., & Bensley, L.S. (1989). The family's functioning with chronic illness in the mother: The spouse's perspective. *Social Science and Medicine, 29*(11), 1261–1269.

Lewis, F.M., Zahlis, E.Z., Shands, M.E., Sinsheimer, J.A., & Hammond, M.A. (1996). The functioning of single women with breast cancer and their school-aged children. *Cancer Practice, 4*(1), 15–24.

Lichtman, R.R., Taylor, S.E., Wood, J.V., & Dosik, G.M. (1985). Relations with children after breast cancer: The mother-daughter relationship at risk. *Journal of Psychosocial Oncology, 2*(3–4), 1–19.

Litman, T.J. (1974). The family as a basic unit in health and medical care: A social-behavioral overview. *Social Science and Medicine, 8*(9–10), 495–519.

Litman, T.J., & Venters, M. (1979). Research on health care and the family: A methodological overview. *Social Science and Medicine, 13A*(4), 379–385.

Manne, S. (1994). Couples coping with cancer: Research issues and recent findings. *Journal of Clinical Psychology in Medical Settings, 1*(4), 317–330.

Manne, S., Alfieri, T., Taylor, K., & Dougherty, J. (1999a). Preferences for spousal support among individuals with cancer. *Journal of Applied Social Psychology, 29*(4), 722–749.

Manne, S., & Glassman, M. (2000). Perceived control, coping efficacy, and avoidance coping as mediators between spouses' unsupportive behaviors and cancer patients' psychological distress. *Health Psychology, 19*(2), 155–164.

Manne, S., Sherman, M.E., Ross, S., Ostroff, J., Heyman, R.E., & Fox, K. (2004). Couples' support-related communication, psychological distress, and relationship satisfaction among women with early stage breast cancer. *Journal of Consulting and Clinical Psychology, 72*(4), 660–670.

Manne, S.L. (1999). Intrusive thoughts and psychological distress among cancer patients: The role of spouse avoidance and criticism. *Journal of Consulting and Clinical Psychology, 67*(4), 539–546.

Manne, S.L., Alfieri, T., Taylor, K.L., & Dougherty, J. (1999). Spousal negative responses to cancer patients: The role of social restriction, spouse mood, and relationship satisfaction. *Journal of Consulting and Clinical Psychology, 67*(3), 352–361.

Mishel, M.H., Belyea, M., Germino, B.B., Stewart, J.L., Bailey, D.E., Jr., Robertson, C., et al. (2002). Helping patients with localized prostate carcinoma manage uncertainty and treatment side effects: Nurse-delivered psychoeducational intervention over the telephone. *Cancer, 94*(6), 1854–1866.

McCubbin, M.A., & McCubbin, H.I. (1993). Families coping with illness: The Resiliency Model of Family Stress, Adjustment, and Adaptation. In C.B. Danielson, B. Hamel-Bissell, & P. Winstead-Fry (Eds.), *Families, health and illness: Perspectives on coping and intervention* (pp. 21–65). St. Louis, MO: Mosby.

Northouse, L.L. (1989a). The impact of breast cancer on patients and husbands. *Cancer Nursing, 12*(5), 276–284.

Northouse, L.L. (1989b). A longitudinal study of the adjustment of patients and husbands to breast cancer. *Oncology Nursing Forum, 16*(4), 511–516.

Northouse, L.L. (1992). Psychological impact of the diagnosis of breast cancer on the patient and her family. *Journal of the American Medical Women's Association, 47*(5), 161–164.

Northouse, L.L., Dorris, G., & Charron-Moore, C. (1995). Factors affecting couples' adjustment to recurrent breast cancer. *Social Science and Medicine, 41*(1), 69–76.

Northouse, L.L., Kershaw, T., Mood, D., & Schafenacker, A. (2004). Effects of a family intervention on the quality of life of women with recurrent breast cancer and their family caregivers. *Psycho-Oncology, 14*(6), 478–491.

Northouse, L.L., Laten, D., & Reddy, P. (1995). Adjustment of women and their husbands to recurrent breast cancer. *Research in Nursing and Health, 18*(6), 515–524.

Northouse, L.L., Mood, D., Templin, T., Mellon, S., & George, T. (2000). Couples' patterns of adjustment to colon cancer. *Social Science and Medicine, 50*(2), 271–284.

Northouse, L.L., & Swain, M.A. (1987). Adjustment of patients and husbands to the initial impact of breast cancer. *Nursing Research, 36*(4), 221–225.

Northouse, L.L., Templin, T., Mood, D., & Oberst, M. (1998). Couples' adjustment to breast cancer and benign breast disease: A longitudinal analysis. *Psycho-Oncology, 7*(1), 37–48.

Oberst, M.T., & James, R.H. (1985). Going home: Patient and spouse adjustment following cancer surgery. *Topics in Clinical Nursing, 7*(1), 46–57.

Parkes, C.M. (1971). Psycho-social transitions: A field for study. *Social Science and Medicine, 5*(2), 101–115.

Parkes, C.M. (1975). The emotional impact of cancer on patients and their families. *Journal of Laryngology and Otolaryngology, 89*(12), 1271–1279.

Pistrang, N., & Barker, C. (1995). The partner relationship in psychological response to breast cancer. *Social Science and Medicine, 40*(6), 789–797.

Pistrang, N., & Barker, C. (1998). Partners and fellow patients: Two sources of emotional support for women with breast cancer. *American Journal of Community Psychology, 26*(3), 439–456.

Pistrang, N., Barker, C., & Rutter, C. (1997). Social support as conversation: Analyzing breast cancer patients' interactions with their partners. *Social Science and Medicine, 45*(5), 773–782.

Ptacek, J.T., Pierce, G.R., Dodge, K.L., & Ptacek, J.J. (1997). Social support in spouses of cancer patients: What do they get and to what end? *Personal Relationships, 4*(4), 431–449.

Samms, M. (1999). The husband's untold account of his wife's breast cancer: A chronological analysis. *Oncology Nursing Forum, 26*(8), 1351–1358.

Shands, M.E., Lewis, F.M., Sinsheimer, J., & Cochrane, B.B. (2007). Core concerns of couples living with early stage breast cancer. *Psycho-Oncology, 15*(12), 1055–1064.

Shands, M.E., Lewis, F.M., & Zahlis, E.H. (2000). Mother and child interactions about the mother's breast cancer: An interview study. *Oncology Nursing Forum, 27*(1), 77–85.

Sidani, S., & Braden, C.J. (1998). *Evaluating nursing interventions: A theory-driven approach.* Thousand Oaks, CA: Sage.

Stanton, A.L., Ganz, P.A., Kwan, L., Meyerowitz, B.E., Bower, J.E., Krupnick, J.L., et al. (2005). Outcomes from the Moving Beyond Cancer psychoeducational, randomized, controlled trial with breast cancer patients. *Journal of Clinical Oncology, 23*(25), 6009–6018.

Stetz, K.M., Lewis, F.M., & Primomo, J. (1986). Family coping strategies and chronic illness in the mother. *Family Relations, 35*(4), 515–522.

Weihs, K., Fisher, L., & Baird, M. (2002). Families, health and behavior: A section of the commissioned report by the Committee on Health and Behavior: Research, Practice, and Policy Division of Neuroscience and Behavioral Health and Division of Health Promotion and Disease Prevention, Institute of Medicine, National Academy of Sciences. *Families, Systems and Health, 20*(1), 7–46.

Welch, A.S., Wadsworth, M.E., & Compas, B.E. (1996). Adjustment of children and adolescents to parental cancer. Parents' and children's perspectives. *Cancer, 77*(7), 1409–1418.

Wellisch, D.K., Gritz, E.R., Schain, W., Wang, H.J., & Siau, J. (1991). Psychological functioning of daughters of breast cancer patients. Part I: Daughters and comparison subjects. *Psychosomatics, 32*(3), 324–336.

Wellisch, D.K., Gritz, E.R., Schain, W., Wang, H.J., & Siau, J. (1992). Psychological functioning of daughters of breast cancer patients. Part II: Characterizing the distressed daughter of the breast cancer patient. *Psychosomatics, 33*(2), 171–179.

Wellisch, D.K., Jamison, K.R., & Pasnau, R.O. (1978). Psychosocial aspects of mastectomy, II: The man's perspective. *American Journal of Psychiatry, 135*(5), 543–546.

Wenzel, L., Glanz, K., & Lerman, C. (2002). Stress, coping and health behavior. In K. Glanz, F.M. Lewis, & B.R. Rimer (Eds.), *Health behavior and health education: Theory, research and practice* (3rd ed., pp. 210–239). San Francisco: Jossey-Bass.

Woods, N.F., & Lewis, F.M. (1992). Design and measurement challenges in family research. *Western Journal of Nursing Research, 14*(3), 397–403.

Woods, N.F., & Lewis, F.M. (1995). Women with chronic illness: Their views of their families' adaptation. *Health Care for Women International, 16*(2), 135–148.

Zahlis, E.H. (2001). The child's worries about the mother's breast cancer: Sources of distress in school-age children. *Oncology Nursing Forum, 28*(6), 1019–1025.

Zahlis, E.H., & Lewis, F.M. (1998). The mother's story of the school-age child's experience with the mother's breast cancer. *Journal of Psychosocial Oncology, 16*(2), 25–43.

Zahlis, E.H., & Shands, M.E. (1991). Breast cancer: Demands of illness on the patient's partner. *Journal of Psychosocial Oncology, 9*(1), 75–93.

SELECTED RESOURCES FOR ADVANCING ONCOLOGY NURSING SCIENCE

CHAPTER 20

Introduction to Scholarly Writing

Elizabeth Tornquist, MA, FAAN

Introduction

Most scholarly writers enjoy writing: They find it exciting, even exhilarating—but they do not find it easy. People who are not accustomed to writing often expect it to be easy. They believe that writing a scholarly paper is a straightforward process in which the writer looks at the data, decides what it means, and then writes the paper from start to finish and sends the final product to a journal. Nothing could be further from reality. Writing is complex and difficult, and the only way to learn to do it well is to begin.

People who have had little experience in writing formal papers, however, often have no idea how to begin. This is a particular problem for those in scientific disciplines such as nursing. When they begin their undergraduate work, most students do not expect to become writers. They suffer through freshman English with the sense that writing is only for literary people and then take science courses requiring skills in memorization and an ability to handle multiple-choice examinations. Years later, when they are asked to write a paper, they feel lost, as if they suddenly had been told to make a speech in an unknown language. Yet, writing is a skill and a craft, and with practice, nearly everyone can learn to do it—and even come to like it.

Nurses have the first prerequisite for good writing—an endlessly fascinating subject: human beings. More than most other people, they see men, women, and children at their profoundest moments of fear, anger, and suffering; they watch over people; they help them to live and to die; they see everything that can go wrong; and they spend much of their working lives trying to prevent it from happening or, if that is not possible, to make it better or bearable. Nurses know the secrets of being ill, facing terrible choices, living with chronic illness, and looking at death. The problem is how to choose an approach that makes this world come alive for others.

No single correct way to write exists; however, a process is available that works for most people with some modifications, whether they are writing reviews of the literature, clinical articles, or research articles. This chapter describes that process, from the first idea for an article to the final draft.

Keeping a Notebook

No one becomes a writer without some tools for writing. The first, most basic tool is a notebook (or notebook file on the computer). The notebook allows the writer to capture ideas and insights that come up unexpectedly, as they likely are to do. These insights and ideas come clothed in words: They are concrete and precise. However, if not written down, the words soon disappear, leaving nothing but vague generalizations. The notebook provides a place to record the precise words that give an idea immediacy and vitality. In addition, the practice of writing things down sharpens the capacity to observe—when you write, you see more and learn to weed out the unimportant, leaving the essential core. That is because the very act of writing makes people more conscious of what they are doing and what matters.

Writing down reactions to what you have read, observations in the world of your work, and your thoughts and ideas about problems and solutions will soon lead to ideas for articles or even a research project. Not everything in the notebook will be usable, of course. Writers cull from their notebooks the best of what they have collected; they do not expect every thought to be important.

Selecting a Topic

The next step is selecting a subject for an article. The two cardinal rules for choosing a topic are to *write about something you care about* and *write about something you know.* An author's excitement about a topic enlivens the writing and keeps it from being tedious. Following these rules also makes the long process of perfecting an article for publication more bearable. The notebook will tell you what you find exciting—you will see it in the entries you have made. However, you also must know something about this topic, beyond empty generalizations and abstractions. Much of the work of writing comes before the actual construction of sentences and paragraphs; it involves digging for information in the literature, collecting physiologic or psychosocial data to evaluate a new intervention, or developing a survey instrument to find out what patients and their families think.

As you collect ideas and information, narrowing your topic to something manageable—and something that others have not written about extensively— is crucial. Often, the first thing that comes to mind is a topic so broad that it could not be covered in an article or even a book. The general subject of oncology nursing, for example, could take up a hundred volumes; and a short paper on that topic is unlikely to provide anything new or useful, but a description of a particular problem that oncology nurses face or a solution to that problem may be both new and interesting. Checking the current journals before beginning an article is always helpful to ensure that the topic has not been published already. You may find articles on similar topics, but if your work has something new to contribute, that will not be a problem.

Next, you have to decide what kind of article you are going to write. If you have completed a project or a formal study, that decision will not be difficult—you will write a research or project report. In addition, you can write a review paper on the subject, based on your reading for the research or project, and often you can write a clinical article on some new problem you are dealing with in practice or a new technique or type of equipment you are using. If you look at current journals, you will see the variety of types of articles you can write.

Making an Outline

Once you have a topic and a tentative decision about the type of article you are going to write, outlining the article before beginning is useful. An outline helps to build the logic of the paper and helps the author to see the paper in an organized way. An outline also shows where the gaps in your logic are and what you need to think about further, and where information is missing and additional data are needed.

Outlining can be difficult if you try to write down every point you will make in the article because writers often do not know in advance exactly what an article will contain—they learn that in the process of writing. Indeed, much of writing is a process of discovery; it makes people's thoughts visible and enables them to develop their thoughts; one idea leads to another. An outline is most useful when you already have a reasonably clear idea of what you want to say—when you are reporting on a project or a study you have conducted, for example. In such cases, you have already done much of the thinking about the project. You know what you did and the outcome, and writing involves putting that information on paper in the right order and interpreting it for readers. An outline should be considered just a broad approximation of that order, not a complete description of the article to be written. It may even be little more than a set of notes and jottings, topics or points you want to be sure to include, and some indication of the order in which you might present them.

Sometimes people skip the outline. They find it easier to plunge into the first draft of the article, which often is the case when the writer is unsure about the direction the paper will take, for the act of writing will help to develop the idea better than struggling with an outline. To find the method that works best for you and for the types of articles you are writing, try different approaches. If the organization of an article comes easily to mind, outlining will be useful in helping you to stay with that organization. If it does not, skip that step. Struggling to organize an outline when you do not know what you want to say is a waste of time.

Writing the First Draft

Writing is easier or more difficult depending on the conditions in which you write. The worst thing any author can do is procrastinate; avoiding a paper makes it far harder to write. Creating a writing schedule is very helpful. Set aside time for thinking, planning, and writing, and work at these routinely. Some people need a large block of time in which to write, and others work in short bursts. For those who need a long block of time, a half hour here and there is not enough to accomplish anything; a morning or afternoon or a whole day is necessary for progress because, in part, this kind of writer needs some warm-up time (otherwise known as *productive procrastination*)—time to sharpen pencils, to water the houseplants, to wash the car, or to do other mindless tasks that empty the mind of everything so that it is ready for the intense concentration required for writing. If you need that kind of preparation, allow time for it, but be sure to allocate enough time both to prepare and to write. Then, you will be able to work for hours. The other kind of writer generally needs no warm-up and can plunge straight into writing without any preparation; however, this kind of writer often can write for only 30 or 45 minutes before tiring. If you work best in short bursts, setting aside a long spell at the computer will be wasted. Instead, set aside a half hour a day and always use it for writing.

Observe yourself to see what works best for you, and then decide how to schedule your writing. Writing requires intense concentration; therefore, you want to do it when your mind is at its sharpest, and not when you are exhausted from a long day at work. Some people write best in the morning and others at night, although hardly anyone is at peak productivity between three and five in the afternoon.

Often, when people first sit down to write, nothing comes. Their thoughts vanish, and they stare at the blank sheet of paper or the blank computer screen in terror. That fear of the empty page is why people do not like beginning an article. However, if you already have some ideas written down in a notebook or you have an outline giving an approximate organization for the article, the project will not be so frightening, because you have a beginning. You can use the outline as topic sentences and then fill in the paragraphs that elaborate on those ideas. If you still have trouble finding the first words, writing down whatever comes into your mind often is helpful. Simply looking at the thoughts you have expressed will help you to focus them. Start with a thought or idea, write it down, and see where it leads. Perhaps the idea will be part of the beginning section of the article, or perhaps it will be the end, or it may fit somewhere in the middle. You may not know right away in which context it fits best, but you will discover that later.

The Beginning

If the thoughts that come to mind are not those that should begin the article, begin somewhere else. Inexperienced writers often think that writers must write from beginning to end. Few writers do. Writing is circular, serpentine, and exploratory; the process is not orderly. If you do begin at the beginning, and the opening seems awkward or unfocused, do not be dismayed. The first paragraph of an article is one of the two hardest paragraphs to write. The other is the closing paragraph. If you think about it, you will understand why: The opening paragraph invites the reader into the article and the closing paragraph sends the reader away with the message—the implications for practice. If readers do not like the beginning, they will stop reading; therefore, the opening paragraphs are crucial. They must interest readers, lead them into the article, and show them that it will be worth reading. Most writers have to struggle to make the opening accomplish all of that. Sometimes several revisions are required to perfect the opening, and often, it is the last paragraph to be completed. Some writers wait until the chapter or article is complete to draft the introduction and/or conclusion.

The Middle

Usually, starting in the middle is easier than starting at the beginning. The middle is easier to write because in most articles, it is the part that requires the least thinking. For example, if you are writing an article that reports research, the methods section is the easiest to begin because you have already done all the thinking there; the only tasks are deciding how much to say and how to organize it. Similarly, in a clinical article that describes an approach to caring for patients undergoing an experimental treatment for cancer, the introduction is much harder to write than the description of the care because you already know about caring for patients; you do it all the time.

Involvement in Writing

Once you have some paragraphs on paper, you can begin to see the structure they are creating, or you can fit them into the structure you have laid out in the outline. However, remembering that the outline may change as you write is important because writing is about discovery—often, people are not sure what they really want to say until they have put it on paper and can see it. Sometimes, after writing a few paragraphs, the author decides that this is not where the article should be going, and the original outline should be followed. Occasionally, however, the direction of the article will change so much that the original outline has to be abandoned. Eventually, the real subject of the article becomes clear. Writing becomes exciting when you suddenly realize what you have to say and how this insight can benefit readers.

Thinking and writing are tied together. When you write, you think more clearly, discover that you know things you were not aware you knew, have new ideas about a subject, and can put things together in new ways. That is why writing is exciting and also why it is difficult. The writing is not hard—the thinking is. When you write, you are not simply recording what you already know, you are discovering and creating, which is just as true of scholarly writing as it is of fiction and poetry.

Moreover, when you are deeply involved in writing something, your mind works on the subject around the clock, not only when you are sitting in front of the computer. Ideas for the article will come into your consciousness when you are doing other things or idly dreaming, driving home, or taking a shower. New points and examples to illustrate them seem to appear from nowhere because the unconscious is working for you. However, if you leave the article for too long and cease to think about it, you lose the advantages of that concentration; your mind works on something else and will bring up nothing for you. This is true of any project, not just writing. When you work on something steadily, it is exciting to take it up again each time you return to it because you have so many ideas about what to do or say. When you have been away from it for too long, you have to get beyond the blankness and reengage your mind with the subject before any ideas come.

For that reason, working on an article consistently is important—if not every day, at least every few days, until you have completed a draft. Schedule your writing time and go to the computer and wait for the words to come. One way to begin the flow of words each time you return to an article is to read over what you have written thus far, making changes or notes where you see problems. This bit of editing helps authors to ease into new material. However, if you use this method, you must quickly move to new material and not become obsessed with old problems. Finishing your draft, all of it, before you stop to seriously edit is important. If you worry constantly about particular words and sentences, you will never be able to see the general shape of the article or work on its coherence. So, keep your critical sense at bay, trust the process of composition, and write until you have a draft, no matter how rough. Experienced authors know that the first draft is merely the raw materials for an article, not the final product. Indeed, one of the obstacles to good writing is the notion that an article can be done well in one draft. An article almost never springs to life neatly organized and well written. Writers begin haltingly, and much of what they write at first goes into the wastebasket or is deleted. Few can write well in less than about three drafts, and many people will need more. The first draft simply provides something with which to work.

Rewriting, Revising, and Editing

The best way to become a good writer is to become a good editor. Happily, editing is a skill that you can learn, and doing it is the best way to learn it.

Another good way to learn to edit is to volunteer to be a reviewer for a journal, such as the *Oncology Nursing Forum*. Once you have a draft of an article, allow it to rest for a time. The act of writing is so intense that it produces a kind of euphoria, and when writers finish a draft, they experience a great feeling of satisfaction. Unfortunately, that good feeling gets in the way of their critical sense. When people finish something, they are certain that what is on the paper is exactly what they intended—and if they look at the article right away, they see only what they want to see. That is not the time to revise. A day or so away from the article will give you some perspective and will enable you to see what you actually wrote and recognize how far it is from what you had hoped to write. That is when revision begins.

Experienced writers often edit as they go, which becomes easier the more you get into the habit of editing your work. However, experienced writers also allow the first draft to rest a bit before beginning the serious work of revision. Editing requires some objectivity, and time away provides at least a modicum of that. Printing out the first draft also is important. The typed page is anonymous—my *y* looks just like your *y*, so nothing personal about the paper exists to attach it to the writer. Having the whole draft in front of you is essential when you begin editing so that you do not have to scroll back and forth to read it. The reason is this: When you read a draft, you may see something on page 10 that sounds suspiciously like the point you were making on page 2. The information may belong on page 2 or page 10 but is unlikely to belong in both places. If you have sheets of paper before you, you can look at pages 2 and 10 together and see where the point fits best, whereas if you have to scroll back and forth on the computer, you are less likely to fix this problem.

Your draft should be double spaced so that you have room to edit, write in new ideas, add information, and move paragraphs and sentences around in a way that you can follow. To edit well, you must be ruthless.

Revision for Clarity and Coherence

Every piece of scholarly writing is designed to inform, explain, and convince readers of the author's conclusions. Every article you write will use reasoning to convey more than facts alone. If authors were communicating only isolated facts, they simply could list them, but the relationships between facts, the synthesis they create, the writers' interpretation of those facts, and the conclusions they pinpoint make the argument in a paper. The aim of the first revision is to make this argument clear and coherent.

However, before you can make a coherent argument, you must be clear about your conclusions. Then, you can check the argument to see whether it is logical and makes a convincing case for readers. This requires close reading of your own article. The first step is to look at your conclusions: Where is the article going? Where are you trying to take readers? What do you want them to conclude? If you do not know where you are going, it is very hard to take others with you. If you are clear about the destination, it is much easier to show others the way.

Most first drafts are incoherent at best because, in part, writing thoughts in a clear, logical line is difficult. The mind tends to work in bursts and circles rather than a straightforward progression. Furthermore, people change course frequently as they write and say things they did not expect to say and had not thought about before writing; thus, the draft grows organically and not always linearly.

As a consequence, the first draft often contains some ideas that go nowhere, false starts that were never completed. Some sentences are half thoughts that might be important to an article but would require much more elaboration. These should be removed, and perhaps saved for another article. The first draft also may contain a mass of vague generalities with the germ or an idea of an article buried among them. People often begin with a topic that is too big, and they may not discover which aspect of the topic really interests them until they have poured out the generalities that tend to occupy the surface of their mind. To move from the first draft, you need to sift through all the material to see which of it is solid and what you want to do with it. You will need to throw out all the meaningless generalizations and then work the germ into a new draft on your real subject. Discarding much of what you have written may be difficult. If it is, try saving the ideas in a notebook so that you can review them later for usable elements.

Sentences and paragraphs will be present that simply are variations on a theme—the same idea or information in slightly different words on page 2 and page 10. Often, when writers have a great idea in their mind, it somehow seems weaker when they see it in words on the page. They may struggle with it a bit, trying to bring the words closer to what they want to say, but after a time give up. Then they may try again a few pages later—hence the repetition of page 2 on page 10. Combining the two and making the point only once, as best you can, is important.

Another problem with first drafts is that they often contain information that readers do not need. Writers know everything about the project or clinical problem or method they are describing, and sometimes deciding what is relevant for others—or easily generalized—and what is simply a detail the author knows but no one else cares about is difficult. For example, an article describing the development of a research group on an oncology floor might contain the information that the group always met on Tuesdays. But, no one cares about that. What matters is that the group met during work hours and regularly; Tuesday is irrelevant.

Another type of incoherence in first drafts is an illogical ordering of ideas and information. Articles need to be built block by block or idea by idea. They are like houses: You cannot put on the roof until you have the rafters. Unfortunately, thinking and writing logically is difficult, so sometimes people put information in an article in the order in which it occurred to them rather than the order in which readers should see it. If, for example, you are reporting a study of the effects of an innovative approach in caring for patients with cancer near the end of life, you will need to first tell readers what that innovative approach amounted to, and then describe how you tested it. Thus, you first describe the intervention and then the instruments or measures you used to test it. If you reverse that order and describe the measures before the intervention, it will make no sense to readers. Similarly, if you are writing a paper about a new concept, the reader needs a definition of the term the first time it is mentioned, not five pages later.

Finally, a major problem with first drafts is that writers do not always make their logic clear. They make a series of points and then grow silent: They do not stop thinking, but their logic does not appear in their writing. The consequence is a *logical leap*, when a reader must infer what the writer means. But, it is only the unfortunate reader who is leaping; the writer knows exactly what the logic is but did not say it. To deal with this kind of problem, you need to read your first draft very carefully and ensure that you have articulated your reasoning.

One way to deal with the question of logic and direction is to outline the draft as if someone else had written it, and then compare that outline to the original outline. You can see where you went off the track, or where the article changed direction because you had new ideas about how to present the information or new ideas about what it meant. When you see the shifts, you can decide what to do with them.

Even if you did not start with an outline, outlining the first draft often is helpful. Looking at the bare bones of the organization as it is presented in an outline, you quickly can see where it is logical and illogical, and it is much easier to deal with problems.

Organization

Several types of sequence or organization are available for articles, depending on their purpose. When you describe something that happened or explain a process or development of a process or procedure, you probably will use chronologic order. If you are describing a piece of equipment, you may use spatial arrangement as the organizing principle or may organize the article based on the functions of the parts. If you are describing a solution to a problem, as project or research articles often do, you should first indicate the problem. Then, describe the solution and how you measured the outcomes, and, finally, give the evidence of its effectiveness.

The organization will be clearer if you consider the reader. When writers compose a first draft, they frequently struggle to find the words to clearly express themselves, and that struggle is so intense that they often give no thought to what the reader might need. When you begin revising the first draft, take the reader's perspective. The reader does not have the information you have about the topic; he or she must obtain that information from the words you put on paper. If the information is not there, the reader cannot follow your argument. For example, if you are writing a review article, the reader must have some information about the studies being reviewed in order to understand your conclusions about the studies. If you are describing research that tested a new intervention, the reader must know how you measured outcomes in order to decide whether the intervention was useful.

As some writers revise their work, they find it helpful to think of a particular reader to whom they are trying to explain their main points. They think about what this reader will need in order to understand the information presented, and then they structure the paper accordingly. You might try imagining that you are explaining your article to a friend, or actually tell someone what you are writing. If the person cannot understand, ask what additional information you need to provide. Then, once you have made your argument clear, organize the paper as you organized your conversation, including all the information the reader needs and eliminating everything that was unnecessary.

Ask for Help in Revising

After you have done all the reorganizing that you think is needed and have reworked the paper to make it coherent and clear, asking a colleague to read your second draft is helpful. Ask the colleague to simply point out problems in the paper, and then you can correct them. The problems that slip by writers are not the problems that they know about but rather the problems that they do not see.

Editing: The Fine Points of Writing

The aim of good writing is to make understanding what you have to say as easy as possible for readers. To achieve that, every sentence must be clear, without ambiguity or confusion and without incomplete ideas or misplaced parts. Once you have a coherently organized draft, you need to go back through it to make sure that every sentence says exactly what you mean it to say.

Words have a life of their own and will do strange things to your thoughts if you are not careful with them. Indeed, when misused, they will make you appear foolish. Look at this sentence, for example: "The patient took some milk of amnesia before being admitted." Or try this one: "I can't hear you because of the noise of the celery I'm chewing in my ears." You do not want your sentences to look like that.

To write well, use words precisely and put them together following the conventions of the language. Precise usage requires an understanding of the meanings of words. When you are unsure about a word, the dictionary will tell you how to spell it, how to use it correctly, when to use it, and when not to use it. This resource also will help you to avoid using the word if it is altogether wrong—something the spell-checker cannot do. A dictionary thus will save you from countless misunderstandings. However, it will not always tell you about a word's connotations, that is, the shades of meaning or associations derived from the context in which the word is used. You learn those by reading and examining the use of words by others. Because words that have similar denotations, or dictionary definitions, may have quite different connotations, you must be careful about using a thesaurus. A thesaurus lists alternatives to a particular word, but these are rarely strict synonyms, and they often have different connotations. For example, you might find the word *aggressive* listed as an alternative for *assertive*, but the meanings of these words differ sharply; they cannot be used interchangeably.

In addition to using words precisely, you must put them together in a way that will produce coherent sentences. Therefore, you must have a basic understanding of English grammar and constantly work to enlarge your understanding of the language and the way it functions. The easiest way to improve your sentences is to listen to them. Languages are spoken: The written language simply is a set of signs and symbols to represent what the writer would say if the readers were listeners instead. The rules of grammar and the principles of rhetoric are designed to make communication clear and effective, and many of them represent what people do unconsciously when they speak. Unfortunately, when people sit down to write, they often forget how they would speak, and they use words as if writing and speaking were totally unrelated.

Read Aloud and Continue to Revise

The best way to become a good writer is to hear what you have written by reading aloud to yourself. Therefore, once you have developed an article to the point where it is clear and coherent, try reading it aloud to yourself or to a friend. "Does it sound right?" is the key question to ask about each sentence. When something does not sound right, your understanding of grammar will enable you to figure out what is wrong and fix it. However, if you do not give yourself the opportunity to hear the problems, you will not be able to solve them.

When you have made all your sentences clear, you need to edit one more time to eliminate unnecessary words. The aim of intellectual prose is to enable the reader to understand what you have to say as quickly as possible. Therefore, you want to write clearly but also concisely, with no extra words, no unnecessary repetitions, and no needless overlaps and redundancies. Every time you read what you have written, look for sentences, phrases, and words to cut. Often, you will find a few more unnecessary words even after you have gone over the article several times. The more unnecessary words that are eliminated, the crisper and cleaner your prose will be. As you learn the habit of editing, you will discover that making sentences clearer often means making them shorter. Confused thinking and wordiness go hand in hand. The best scientific writing is clean, clear, direct, and concise.

Conclusion

The more you write and revise your work, the easier it will become to see problems and find solutions. If you consistently work on what you have written, reshaping sentences, striving for greater precision, and eliminating unnecessary words, you will find that you steadily will improve as an editor and writer. Do not expect it to happen overnight, however. Find another oncology nurse to be your mentor in writing and editing. The Oncology Nursing Society offers the *Clinical Journal of Oncology Nursing* Mentor/Fellow Writing Program, in which novice writers can receive help from experienced writers. Becoming a better writer is a lifelong occupation and a continuing source of delight.

Bibliography

Strunk, W., White, E.B., & Angell, R. (1999). *The elements of style* (4th ed.). New York: Longman.

Tornquist, E.M. (1986). *From proposal to publication: An informal guide to writing about nursing research.* Menlo Park, CA: Addison-Wesley.

Truss, L. (2006). *Eats, shoots and leaves: The zero tolerance approach to punctuation.* New York: Gotham Books.

Williams, J. (2005). *Style: Ten lessons in clarity and grace* (8th ed.). New York: Pearson Longman.

CHAPTER 21

Launching an Oncology Nursing Research Career

Deborah B. McGuire, PhD, RN, FAAN

Introduction

The decision to pursue a career in oncology nursing science may be one of the most important and challenging that an individual will ever make in the course of a career. Why? First, this career choice takes nurses down a path that requires intense study, serious commitment, persistence, and at times, a separation from the world of nursing practice that may seem at odds with the reasons why most individuals became nurses. Second, the development of a program of research is an increasingly challenging career path given the current era of diminished federal funding, competitive forces from within and outside of the nursing profession, and the pressures of other job responsibilities. Third, pursuing a research program is a long-term proposition, necessitating focus, strategic planning, and comfort with delayed gratification. Finally, developing and maintaining a career as a successful oncology nurse scientist can require personal sacrifices that must be considered carefully and managed in order to have a balanced professional and personal life.

Despite these challenges, many rewards are inherent in pursuing a research career, as other authors in this book have attested. Thus, individuals who want to spend their careers contributing to oncology nursing science should embrace these challenges because with thoughtful planning and action, the challenges can be surmounted. The purpose of this chapter is to discuss the educational and professional elements that aspiring oncology nurse scientists should consider in launching a research career. Although the fact that many nurses have fulfilling careers in research as research coordinators or project managers is acknowledged, this chapter focuses on nurses who desire to pursue a research career as an independent investigator.

Although the concept of career can be construed as involving "advancement, professional status, and occupational stability," it also has been described as "more analogous to a journey than to a person's state of employment" (Miller, 2003, pp. 3–4). Because a research career is indeed a journey, this chapter is organized by four early phases of the journey:

- Considering a research career
- Selecting and obtaining admission to a doctoral program
- Progressing through the program
- Deciding what to do after completing the program.

Discussion of later phases of the journey unfortunately is beyond the scope of this chapter. Embedded in the discussion are practical guidance and direction, words of wisdom, and lessons learned from the author's individual experience, the experience of professional colleagues, and the literature.

Considering a Research Career

The point at which individual nurses begin to realize that research may become a major focus of their professional lives varies for each person. However, common characteristics of nurses who follow a research path appear to be curiosity about why things are the way they are and an intense desire to seek answers. Many nurse scientists cite a fascination with research concepts and processes that often dates back to their initial nursing education or to early clinical experiences in which they were exposed to research. Although these individuals cannot always articulate precisely what attracts them to research, they are clear about their predilection for the scientific process in the context of nursing. They also have a passion for improving nursing practice, and a conviction that they can make a difference to patients and others through research.

Nurses who have these characteristics naturally are drawn to research and intuitively seek research experiences as students and as practicing professionals. Nursing faculty can be good at recognizing such individuals and encouraging them to consider doctoral study, sometimes well before the nurses have fully recognized their own research interest, potential, or career possibilities. In some instances, recognition and encouragement by a faculty member or other professional colleague opens the door to a research career by revealing the possibility to the individual nurse and stimulating serious consideration. Once nurses begin to think about research as a career option, they should ask themselves a series of important questions.

Do I Like Research?

If a nurse is to spend a career doing research, liking research and having a realistic concept of what it involves are essential. Although being intrigued with the concepts and methods of research is easy, there is no substitute for actual experience. Seeking research opportunities can give the nurse experience that will be helpful in determining whether this is the right path. Involvement in research also can make a nurse more competitive when applying for admission to a doctoral program.

Am I Attracted to Clinical Problems for Which No Ready Answers or Little Information to Guide Practice Is Available, and Do I Have a Passion for Finding Answers?

The ability to ask why and to find answers through scholarly inquiry is one of the hallmarks of a scientist. As a practice profession, a solid foundation of research-based knowledge underlies evidence-based nursing practice (Melnyk & Fineout-Overholt, 2005). An interest in topics for which nursing has little knowledge, along with a commitment to generate such knowledge, bodes well for a productive scientific career, particularly if the clinical problem is important in scope and impact and is recognized as such by professional organizations and funding agencies. For instance, the Oncology Nursing Society (ONS, n.d.-c) research agenda for 2005–2009 identified the following six high-priority research content areas, each with numerous subtopics.

• Cancer symptoms and side effects
• Individual- and family-focused psychosocial and behavioral research
• Health promotion (primary and second prevention)
• Late effects of cancer treatment and long-term survivorship issues for patients and their families
• Nursing-sensitive patient outcomes
• Translational research to determine factors affecting clinical application of evidence-based guidelines

Similarly, the National Institute of Nursing Research (NINR, 2006) at the National Institutes of Health (NIH) lists its four areas of research emphasis in its strategic plan as

• Promoting health and preventing disease
• Improving quality of life
• Eliminating health disparities
• Setting directions for end-of-life research.

Nurses who can place their research interests in the context of such priorities will be better able to imagine and describe a potential research direction when applying to a doctoral program and more likely to be successful in developing a fundable and clinically relevant program of research over the long term.

Do I Feel That I Can Contribute to Patient Care in Ways Other Than at the Bedside, and Am I Comfortable With That?

A fulfilling career in nursing does not necessarily have to take place at the bedside. Indeed, one of the attractions of nursing as a career is the immense variability, intellectual stimulation, and challenges it presents (Wallace, 2003). As a practice profession, the focus of nursing is rightfully on promoting and restoring health in individuals or on supporting them through trajectories of illness, regardless of ultimate outcome. Not all nurses, however, spend their careers directly involved in practice. Some conduct clinical research in collaboration with clinicians, with the aim of improving care practices and nursing-sensitive patient outcomes (ONS, n.d.-b). Other nurses pursue teaching, management and administration, quality improvement, informatics, or other areas. For most of these activities, the primary focus and beneficiary of the nurse's effort is ultimately the patient and family. In research, the contribution to patient care occurs at a different level than direct care at the bedside, and the budding scientist needs to understand this and be comfortable with it. Although engaging in both research and practice are not mutually exclusive, mounting a successful program of research while at the same time engaging in full-time clinical practice is extremely challenging. To be successful, the scientist may need to restrict the time spent in practice or find other ways to remain engaged, such as collaborating with clinicians, serving on clinical advisory boards, or consulting.

Am I Detail-Oriented, Meticulous, and Persistent?

As a process, research is a precise, detail-laden activity. Often, what seems like an endless iteration and repetition can occur, as one formulates and reformulates ideas, designs studies, and writes grants or papers. The importance of clearly and adequately articulating the conceptual foundation of one's research, and the methods through which it will be accomplished, cannot be overstated. In this regard, the personality trait of compulsiveness is valuable, as it enables the scientist to construct adequately detailed research proposals, manuscripts, and other related documents that are conceptually and methodologically sound, as well as relevant to nursing. Thus, successful oncology nurse scientists generally are detail-oriented, meticulous, and able to persist through multiple iterations of proposals, to constructively deal with review and critique by others (e.g., colleagues, a grant review panel), and to handle unanticipated events that occur during one's research (e.g., the closure of a clinical program from which the scientist was planning to draw a study sample). These scientists are usually driven by clinical passions that led them to research in the first place, and because of their commitment and dedication, they are able to keep moving forward despite adversity along the way.

Can I Work Alone as Well as in Groups?

The research process is both highly solitary (e.g., writing a grant proposal or manuscript) and highly interactive (e.g., meeting with research team members or others in the planning and implementation of a study). To be successful, scientists must be comfortable with spending long periods of time alone to produce the necessary documents for research scholarship. In contrast, they also must be able to work effectively with groups and function in the leadership role of principal investigator or project director. In today's research funding arena, especially NIH, the ability to engage in interdisciplinary or transdisciplinary team science is essential (National Cancer Institute [NCI], 2006). Indeed, the research priorities of organizations such as ONS and NINR mandate collaborative interdisciplinary research; thus, scientists must be capable of developing and maintaining an interdisciplinary research team that focuses on problems of interest to nursing and nurses (McGuire, 1999).

Selecting and Obtaining Admission to a Doctoral Program

After answering the questions in the previous section and giving thoughtful consideration to the various ramifications of pursuing a research career, the budding scientist moves to the next phase of the journey—selecting and obtaining admission to a doctoral program. An extremely important consideration is the timing of this step. A nurse may decide on a research career but for personal or professional reasons may delay pursuing it until a later date. Because preparation to become a scientist is time consuming and at times arduous, aspiring scientists should enter a doctoral program when, and only when, the timing is right for them. In the past, the prevailing philosophy was that nurses needed clinical experience before going on to graduate school. As a result, many nurses waited to enter doctoral programs until they had practiced a while, had families, or achieved other personal goals. Given the amount of time required for research training, their subsequent careers in research were shorter than for other disciplines, whose members generally acquire doctorates relatively quickly after college. Happily, the current trend in nursing is for aspiring nurse scientists to enter doctoral programs earlier in their careers and at younger ages, so that their research careers can be longer and more productive. Thus, nurses considering a research career are strongly encouraged to embark on it as early as possible.

From a historical perspective, upward career mobility for nurses in some sectors (e.g., academia) has required doctoral degrees. Some nurses obtained doctoral degrees in fields related to nursing, for example, a doctorate in education (EdD) or a doctorate in philosophy (PhD) in a behavioral science, such as psychology. Many other nurses obtained PhD degrees in nursing not because they wanted a research career but because they needed the academic credential to achieve their career goals. In general, most of these individuals did not develop a long-term program of research because it was not among their career goals.

A doctorate in nursing practice (DNP), a practice-focused doctoral degree, is a recent development that offers a new alternative to nurses. Although a discussion of the rationale for and evolution of this degree is beyond the scope of this chapter, the DNP is designed "to prepare experts in specialized advanced nursing practice" (American Association of Colleges of Nursing [AACN], 2006, p. 3). Although AACN (2006) stated that both practice-focused and research-focused programs "share rigorous and demanding expectations: a scholarly approach to the discipline, and a commitment to the advancement of the profession" (p. 3), clear differences exist between the practice-focused DNP and research-focused doctorates. Specifically, research-focused programs emphasize theory, research methods, and statistics, whereas practice-focused programs emphasize advanced practice and the application of research to practice.

The most common research-focused degree offered by schools of nursing is the PhD degree, although some schools of nursing offer other research-oriented degrees (AACN, 2001). Because the PhD has long been the highest degree awarded in academia and is characterized by rigorous scholarship, theory development and testing, and the building of knowledge (or science), it is the preferred degree for a research career. In the remainder of this chapter, all discussion related to doctoral programs or a doctoral degree refers to a PhD unless otherwise noted. In general, the discussion also refers to PhD programs in nursing, although the research career goals of individual nurses may require seeking a PhD in another field, for example, neuroscience, health policy, or epidemiology.

Aspiring scientists need to consider several areas in selecting a doctoral program and gaining admission. As with any major life-altering decision, fact finding, consultation, and critical examination are important before moving forward. The following questions represent important factors in evaluating and selecting a doctoral program, and positioning oneself to be accepted into the program.

How Established Is the Program, and What Are Its Outcomes?

Most of the oldest doctoral programs in nursing were established in the 1970s or early 1980s (AACN, 2001). These programs naturally have a longer history and more graduates than newer programs. Most of them undergo periodic external peer review and often can provide potential applicants with data compiled for such review, including the typical profile of a successful applicant (e.g., grade point average, Graduate Record Examination® [GRE] scores), the admission and graduation rates, average length of time in the program, postdoctoral placements of its graduates, and so on. Newer doctoral programs obviously will have a much shorter track record because the initial class typically takes four or five years to graduate. Newer programs also may still be in the process of working out kinks in the program, both in the curriculum as well as in progression processes, and students can find this to be more challenging. Older programs usually have a well-oiled process in place, providing students with a smoother progression, although this is not always the case. Regardless of the age of the program under consideration, talking to current students is wise to ascertain their experiences and recommendations.

Meeting with the doctoral program director and the faculty in one's research interest area and examining the program's Web pages is prudent in order to gather information about the program, its requirements, and its outcomes. Be aware that outcomes include more than progression and graduation rates; they also include scholarly accomplishments of students and graduates and subsequent career paths.

Does the Program Encompass the Indicators of Quality in Research-Focused Doctoral Programs in Nursing Specified by the American Association of Colleges of Nursing?

AACN (2001) described five indicators of quality in research-focused doctoral programs in nursing. Because research-focused programs prepare students for rigorous scholarly inquiry aimed at expanding knowledge for practice, aspiring scientists must read the full AACN document and then carefully examine all programs under consideration for the presence and strength of the following five indicators.

Faculty: The faculty should present diverse backgrounds and experiences, have earned doctorates, be engaged actively in the conduct of research and scholarship, promote a culture of scholarship for students, be available for student guidance and mentorship, and assist in the development of students' programs of research both within the discipline of nursing and in the interdisciplinary arena.

Programs of study: The program of study should reflect the nursing discipline, the research focus of the program, and the university's mission. Faculty research areas usually drive the specific emphasis or focal areas offered in a program. Some schools have formalized centers of research excellence in specific areas, which may include federally funded institutional training grants for doctoral students, and sometimes postdoctoral fellows. Such centers provide an excellent culture of scholarship that fosters student and faculty interaction, research training, and career development. One of the most important criteria in selecting a program is the presence of research faculty available to mentor the applicant in his or her area of research interest (see Mentorship within this section for more detail). If this is not the case, the nurse may need to modify or change the interest area to fit with the research interest of faculty, or find a different program with a better fit, as the importance of fit between faculty and student research interests in facilitating successful scholarly development and career progression is becoming increasingly clear.

Resources: The resources offered by a program must encompass adequate faculty, staff, financial, and institutional support to enable the program to run. Examples include, but are not limited to, adequate research faculty with workloads that can accommodate student advisement and mentorship, an office of research administration, mechanisms that support students' development and progress, technical support, designated space, a culture of scholarship and inquiry, and an interdisciplinary environment at the university. AACN

(2001) also noted that schools of "exceptional quality" have centers of research excellence, endowed professorships, financial aid to support full-time study, and faculty who can assist students in preparing for faculty roles if they plan to seek these after graduation.

Students: The students in a doctoral program usually are selected from a competitive pool, as mentioned previously. Congruence of students' research goals and objectives with faculty members' research and with institutional resources is essential. Other important areas to investigate include availability of various forms of internal financial aid (e.g., scholarships, traineeships, loans), timely progression through the program, ratio of full-time to part-time students, and achievements such as internal and external grants, publications, presentations, collaborative opportunities with faculty, and so on. Establishment of a pattern of scholarly productivity when in the program lays a strong foundation for continued achievement throughout one's career.

Evaluation: Finally, evaluation of the program must be systematic and rigorous and should include both process and outcome data. Evaluation plans should involve students, faculty, and relevant others. External peer review, as described previously, should occur on a regular basis, with modifications made to programs based on input from both external review and internal process and outcome evaluations. Evidence that a program incorporates current trends in doctoral nursing education and in research is important, for example, in science policy (NIH, 2007) and in research priorities (NINR, 2006; ONS, n.d.-c) at the national level. No single program will be stellar in all five of these indicators, but the applicant should strive to find the program that best exemplifies them and that is feasible to attend.

Where Is the Program, and Is It Feasible for Me to Attend?

Historically, nurses attended programs that were located geographically close to them for a variety of personal, professional, and logistical reasons, even if the fit between their research interests and those of the faculty was poor. In more recent years, the development of weekend/summer, online, and distance doctoral programs has opened up more options for aspiring scientists. The trend toward earlier entry into doctoral programs by younger nurses enables them, if they have not yet established strong roots in a particular geographic area, to have more flexibility in selecting a program and therefore more options in finding the best fit. For most nurses, another important consideration is whether a program offers full-time or part-time study. Although full-time study is optimal for scholarly development, timely progression, and an easier and smoother launch to a research career, it is not always realistic for an individual's life circumstances. If part-time study is necessary, examining whether a structured plan of study can be developed is important to facilitate the most rapid completion possible. Data suggest that slow progression and interruptions to the plan of study can predict excessive time spent in the doctoral program or even failure to complete the program (K. Soeken, personal communication, May 15, 2007).

Will I Be a Competitive Applicant, and How Can I Best Present Myself to the Admissions Committee?

All doctoral programs publish their required admission criteria, and as noted previously, profiles of successful applicants are available, along with data on the number of applicants and number of acceptances. By virtue of reputation, ranking, research activity, and other factors, some programs are considerably more competitive than others. Such programs may place a high priority on specific criteria (e.g., a minimum GRE score, the fit of applicants' research interests with ongoing faculty research) and will not consider applicants who do not meet these criteria. Understanding the criteria essential for gaining admission to programs of interest and engaging in self-assessment in relation to these criteria are important. Another very important aspect of gaining admission is how the candidates position themselves to be competitive applicants. This positioning should begin with initial contacts with the program director or faculty (e.g., e-mail, phone, in person) and continue through the written application and interview process. This presentation goes beyond required admission criteria such as GRE score or prior academic record, or norms of courteous and appropriate social interaction. Rather, applicants need to demonstrate their awareness of the rigors of research-focused doctoral study, describe a clear area of research interest that fits with faculty/school research, and demonstrate evidence of experience with and commitment to research as a career path (e.g., participation in research, scholarly presentations or publications, membership in research-oriented organizations). Furthermore, applicants should be able to articulate a clear relationship between the specific doctoral program and their career goals. It will not bode well for the applicants if they appear to be naïve, uninformed, and unprepared for doctoral study. As noted earlier, all aspiring scientists can benefit from personally contacting the faculty at a program of interest to engage in conversation with them. Even better, the applicant should mention contact with these individuals in the written application. Asking questions of the program director and faculty about the program, and discussing how one could complete it, is strongly recommended. Faculty members with whom applicants interact in this manner are more likely to advocate for the applicant during the admissions process and eventually may mentor the accepted student.

Progressing Through the Program

Once accepted to a program of choice, nurses assume the role of doctoral student. For nurses who have been out of school for a while, this new role may cause them to feel like novice nurses again, uncertain of their ability to perform to their expectations or to those of the faculty. However, understanding the program's requirements, building a strong adviser-student relationship, and developing collegial relationships with fellow students will be helpful in adapting to this new role. Paul and Elder (2001) wrote a short monograph that explicated how to study and learn a discipline, and their advice is particularly germane for nursing doctoral students. They emphasized the importance of critical thinking as a key to learning, noting that it is "the kind of thinking—about any subject, content, or domain—that improves itself through disciplined analysis and assessment" (p. 6). The authors also suggested that in learning, one should look for interrelationships because learning is "figuring out the parts of an organized and intelligible *system*" (p. 8). For example, one can only understand a scientific experiment after one understands scientific theory. Students who approach doctoral study using their previously well-honed critical thinking skills, and understanding that almost all the material they learn is interrelated, will find it easier to make the transition from clinician to student and from student to scientist. Four major aspects of any doctoral program underlie preparation for a research career and are discussed briefly as follows.

Mentorship: How Do I Find a Mentor and Develop a Good Relationship?

Mentorship is fundamental to preparing for and launching a research career and may be the single most important factor contributing to an individual's success. Although the literature presents various definitions of this concept, a useful and succinct definition is "an intense, personal, and concentrated relationship with one or more experts with the aim of professional development" (Byrne & Keefe, 2002, p. 394). The mentor connection is a "collegial connection that potentiates and empowers each person" and through which "professionals share information, teach each other, and strengthen the profession by ensuring an adequate supply of competent practitioners and leaders" (Vance & Olson, 1998, p. 3). The mentor's multiple roles include those of adviser, supporter, tutor, master, sponsor, and model (Gaffney, 1995).

In selecting a doctoral program, the student presumably identified one or more faculty members who could serve as mentors because of the fit between their research and the interests of the student. Upon entering the program, the student usually is assigned to one of these individuals. Provided that the student's research area does not change and the relationship develops well, this person generally will become the student's primary research mentor and dissertation committee chair. It is extremely important that the mentoring relationship is characterized by mutual respect, trust, understanding, and empathy (National Academy of Sciences [NAS], National Academy of Engineering, & Institute of Medicine, 1997). Various authors have written about the responsibilities of both the mentor and the student, emphasizing that the common goal of each is to advance the student's professional growth and educational progress (NAS et al.). Mentors must become familiar with a student's learning needs and style, be objective, and be available. Students must understand their mentors' time constraints and professional pressures and not "view them as merely a means—or impediment—to their goal" (p. 4).

Even the most experienced nurses who are entering a doctoral program need a mentor, because good mentorship and socialization into the complex world of research can smooth their career path. For instance, interdisciplinary research is essential to the development of good science, and team science is a prerequisite for addressing complex research topics (NCI, 2006). The primary mentor must be able to facilitate the student's engagement with members of other disciplines relevant to the research problem at hand. The mentor ideally will introduce such individuals to the student, include them on exam and dissertation committees, and potentially share the mentorship role with one or more of them. The wise student will read about mentorship, including examples of good mentorship (Miller, 2003; Vance & Olson, 1998), and will strive to develop strong mentoring relationships during the program and beyond. Figure 21-1 presents a comprehensive overview of mentor and mentee characteristics and responsibilities and factors that are important to the development of a good mentoring relationship.

Coursework

What can I expect to find in the doctoral coursework? Research-focused doctoral programs generally consist of required theory, research, and statistics courses designed to provide a strong generic foundation; specialty or concentration courses designed to further prepare the student to study the problem of interest; research experiences (called rotation, residency, or practicum depending on the program); and dissertation research designed to help the student to learn to be part of a research team and to design and conduct the dissertation research project (AACN, 2006). Reading the doctoral program's handbook is essential to a smooth path through the program because it specifies precisely what courses must be taken and in what sequence, describes the goals and processes for program progression markers, and articulates all policies and other requirements.

Required theory, research, and statistics courses usually are offered in a recommended sequence that is designed to build knowledge and skills. Proceeding through these courses rapidly and taking the qualifying or preliminary examination based on these courses as soon as possible afterward are important to timely progression. A delay in taking the examination following completion of courses reduces mastery of the content and increases the risk of failure. Most content is interrelated, and it enhances success when students are able to understand how the theory, research, and statistical content in their various courses are related.

How do I gain the additional expertise necessary to study my topic? Specialty or concentration courses are those that support the student's research inter-

Figure 21-1. Mentors, Mentees, and Development of the Mentoring Relationship

Qualifications and Characteristics of a Good Mentor	Responsibilities of a Mentor	Characteristics and Responsibilities of a Good Mentee	Factors Important to a Good Mentoring Relationship
• Desire to mentor • Positive attitude and outlook • Caring personality • Available and has time to mentor • Experienced at mentoring • Seasoned veteran • Exemplifies excellence and integrity • Savvy insider • Good communicator • Good listener • Trustworthy • Able to provide constructive feedback • Able to provide leadership • Understands different learning styles	• Serves as a role model • Provides encouragement • Provides personal and career counseling • Protects mentee • Sponsors mentee • Provides exposure to others in the field • Teaches the job and formal and informal systems • Facilitates independence	• Motivated • Committed to excellence • Responsible • Stays in touch • Open to feedback • Persistent • Understands own strengths and limitations • Respects mentor's workload, time constraints, and schedule • Works independently • Asks for help if needed • Clearly communicates goals and desired timelines • Responds to mentor's requests promptly and completely	• Compatibility and personal chemistry • Shared research interests • Theoretical and methodologic compatibility • Congruent expectations • Mutual respect and trust • Good communication • Regular meetings • Focused on career development • Three phases: introduction, goal setting, and working

Note. Based on information from Bower, 2003; Byrne & Keefe, 2002; National Academy of Sciences et al., 1997; Vance & Olson, 1998.

ests. They are designed to build on the generic theory, research, and statistics courses and to provide the student with an enhanced level of expertise that will facilitate conduct of the dissertation research. This expertise encompasses content, theory, and methods, including statistics. For example, if a student is considering conducting a study that involves secondary analysis of a large data set, coursework in secondary analysis, advanced quantitative statistical analysis, and health services research might be helpful. Developing a plan of study for these courses with the mentor as early in the program as possible will allow for ample time to find and take relevant courses and to make alternate plans if certain courses are discontinued or not offered at a feasible time. Searching for courses both within and outside of nursing is advisable to enhance one's exposure to and comfort with the interdisciplinary research milieu. Taking such courses also is an ideal way to gain exposure to scientists outside of nursing, who may serve as additional mentors and members of a dissertation committee.

Will I gain exposure to any research experiences other than my dissertation? Courses that support learning how to do research, including the dissertation project, are fundamental to a research-focused doctoral program. In addition to the prescribed research rotations that are part of the curriculum, students should seek opportunities that enable them to work with active research teams (e.g., as a research assistant) in order to better understand how research teams function and gain additional research experience. Students also should attempt to work toward the dissertation proposal at every possible opportunity by using required curriculum courses or credits to identify and procure relevant literature, perform systematic analysis and reviews, and ultimately begin developing a dissertation proposal (with the mentor's input, of course).

How can I get teaching and related experience if my postdoctoral goals include taking a faculty position? Some doctoral programs have optional coursework or certificate programs in education or offer practical experience through graduate student teaching assistantships. If the student does not have previous academic teaching experience, coursework and guided experiences in teaching can be invaluable. Trying to learn the entire faculty role, including teaching, after graduation from a doctoral program can be challenging; thus, getting an early start makes sense. In addition, such experience may make the graduate more attractive to potential employers.

Progression Markers

What are the required components of a doctoral program besides the coursework? All doctoral programs have very specific progression markers that students must complete. Although some students view them as obstacles or "hoops" to jump through, these markers ought to be embraced as mechanisms for learning research content and skills and achieving objectives of the program. Understanding from the outset of the program what these markers are and when they occur is wise. As noted previously, the doctoral handbook will spell out the purpose and timing of each marker, along with policies and procedures. Most programs have an examination (often called preliminary or qualifying) that covers the initial required coursework and determines whether a student can continue in the program. Many also have a subsequent examination (sometimes called comprehensive) at the completion of all coursework, which assesses the student's ability to apply generic and specialty content to the research problem of interest. This examination often is a foundation for the student's dissertation because successful preparation and passing require mastery of theoretical and statistical research and specialty knowledge that bear directly on the doctoral research. After students pass this examination, they advance to *candidacy* and develop and defend the doctoral dissertation proposal, which is the next progression marker. At this stage, some students adopt the initials

PhD(c), but this is not a formally accepted academic designation or practice and should be discouraged because some people could interpret it as indicating that the student already has a PhD. The accepted practice simply is to use the highest *earned* degree until one actually completes, or *earns*, the PhD.

What happens after I complete these examinations? Immediately following successful completion of required examinations and advancement to candidacy, students must meet regularly with their mentor/research adviser to receive input on the dissertation proposal and the selection and formation of an interdisciplinary dissertation committee with complementary areas of expertise relevant to the topic. Regularly communicating with all committee members to determine the level of involvement each one wants, their individual style of interacting and providing feedback, time constraints, and preferences for reviewing and responding to written drafts is important. All committee members have other responsibilities and pressures, and students must be cognizant and respectful of these. Preparation of a timeline that is approved by the committee will be helpful in progressing smoothly. Following approval of the dissertation proposal, the students commence the dissertation study, including all relevant protection of human subjects and other review processes. Staying in touch with the mentor/adviser during this time is essential, both for providing regular progress reports as well as for seeking consultation if problems arise during the course of the research. Similarly, providing regular updates to all committee members is important as well, for they can assist with problem solving and other issues. This can be a lonely time for students, and continued contact and networking with other doctoral students is highly recommended. Once the dissertation is completed, including the analysis, interpretation, and writing phases (again conducted in close concert with the mentor/research adviser and committee), the students prepare for the final dissertation defense. This is an exciting time, and it marks the successful conclusion of the doctoral student phase of one's research career and progression to the next phase.

Professional Development

Socialization into the world of research and the development of a personal culture of scholarship are integral to one's development as a scientist. If the student does not have a track record of research and publications, the doctoral program is the ideal place in which to start this trajectory. A good mentor will guide the student, but the student must exhibit personal motivation and self-initiation. Students who enter a doctoral program with a track record of publications and other activities can expand these and focus them more specifically on their interest area, thus beginning to garner a reputation in the field. Important socialization activities include four major areas.

- Writing proposals for predoctoral scholarships (American Cancer Society, 2007; NINR, 2007; ONS, n.d.-a)

- Writing small grant proposals to support one's doctoral research (e.g., through the previous examples, Sigma Theta Tau International or a local chapter, American Nurses Foundation, ONS/ONS Foundation)
- Participating in professional dissemination activities such as formal presentations at conferences and publications in peer-reviewed journals
- Acquiring experience in scholarly pursuits such as working on a research team and learning the faculty role

How can I go about finding these experiences? Doctoral programs have various mechanisms for research socialization, and each program is different in this regard. Some programs place more emphasis on it than others. Common examples that address each of these four areas include but are not limited to the following.

- Faculty mentorship in development and submission of predoctoral training awards such as NIH career development awards (NINR, 2007) or American Cancer Society (2007) doctoral scholarships (Some schools require students to submit such applications.)
- Regularly scheduled research seminar series in which students, faculty, and visiting scientists present their work or conduct seminars on grant writing and similar activities
- Annual research programs with poster and podium presentations
- Financial and other support to attend and present at regional or national research conferences
- Required or optional manuscripts in lieu of the traditional written dissertation
- Individual mentorship from faculty
- Graduate assistantships in teaching or research

As noted previously, motivation and self-initiation are key variables; therefore, aspiring scientists will benefit by identifying opportunities that will address the four areas listed previously and become involved in them. Important caveats in considering graduate assistantships are to carefully explore the time and effort required and to try to determine whether the position might pull one away from a focus on the doctoral program. Each opportunity should be evaluated in terms of how it will support career development, as well as how it will pay the bills.

During the doctoral program, students may find it easy to become involved in interesting scholarly or clinical pursuits that are less relevant to the program and have the potential for sidetracking their progress. Although experienced nurses who have been active in professional organizations prior to entering the doctoral program may find this to be difficult, resisting these opportunities is an important skill to learn (especially for later when one enters the "real" world with its multiple competing demands on scientists). Students should evaluate each potential opportunity that comes along by asking Will this help me to finish my program? Will it give me an experience that can enhance my professional socialization *in research* or my reputation in my *area of research*? If the answer to *either* question is no, students should decline politely and suggest others who might be willing. If the answer to *both* questions is yes, then students should consult with their mentor/adviser before making a final decision and be prepared to articulate how the activity will advance their career as a scientist and will not interfere with their progress. Numerous opportunities exist that foster one's development as a scientist (e.g., being a guest editor of a journal issue, writing a systematic review on a research topic, serving on an ONS project team), but the wise student will be very judicious in making commitments of this sort.

Deciding What to Do After Completing the Program

Nurses who enter a research-focused doctoral program presumably were able to articulate long-term research career goals during the application process. Although these may change during the program, the process of planning for postgraduate directions should occur throughout the program. Assuming that the students remain committed to a research career, the mentors/advisers have a key role in helping students to learn about, consider, and decide on postgraduate options to advance their careers, ideally in plenty of time to act on the decisions prior to graduation. Other individuals, such as faculty and colleagues both in the school of nursing and outside of it (including outside the university), are excellent resources for career counseling, as well. In essence, aspiring oncology nurse scientists can take three paths upon graduation. Each is discussed in the following sections, along with factors to consider in selecting any of these paths. A decision to pursue a particular path should be based on individual circumstances, professional goals, family considerations, and other factors.

Postdoctoral Fellowship

A postdoctoral research fellowship is designed to expedite the development of the graduate's program of research by providing protected time devoted to publishing one's findings, designing and potentially procuring a grant to fund the next study, and acquiring additional research knowledge and skills. Fellowships usually are designed to last from one to three years and generally are done at a university under the tutelage of faculty with expertise in the new scientist's interest area. They are important in retaining talented graduates and increasing the quality of the budding scientist's program of research (Sigmon & Grady, 2001). Although considered standard in disciplines outside of nursing for years, postdoctoral research fellowships have not been common in nursing until relatively recently. Reasons for this include that (a) nurses are older than doctoral graduates in other fields, (b) nurses are unable or unwilling to relocate for fellowships because of personal or family reasons, (c) fellowships in nursing are variable and sometimes do not meet individual needs, (d) research is not emphasized in some schools of nursing, thus graduates are not encouraged to follow this path, and (e) qualified mentors and other postdoctoral fellows are scarce (Sigmon & Grady).

Because postdoctoral fellowships commonly are viewed as the single best way to advance a research career, nursing has embraced them as the next logical step in launching a research career. An NINR work group met in 2001 to address strategies and collaborative approaches for increasing postdoctoral research training opportunities (Sigmon & Grady, 2001). The group viewed such training as a "pipeline" for producing well-trained scientists capable of conducting complex interdisciplinary research in basic, translational, clinical, and outcomes research. It emphasized the importance of early identification and recruitment of potential scientists at younger ages, encouragement to take personal responsibility for professional development, facilitation of the transition from student to scientist through postdoctoral study, identification of qualified mentors, improvement of the fit between research areas of fellows and mentors, development of specific outcome criteria for postdoctoral fellowship experiences, improvement in the commitment of institutions and schools to research training, and promotion of collaboration across institutions (Sigmon & Grady).

What are the advantages and disadvantages of a postdoctoral fellowship? The major advantage of a fellowship is that it provides a defined period of support in which the nurse can focus on strengthening the research program with guidance from mentors without the distractions of an academic or other position. As a result, the nurse can be highly productive in terms of publishing papers from the dissertation research, writing research grants, developing long-term interdisciplinary collaborative relationships, and engaging in additional formal or informal research training. It is an invaluable opportunity to lay a strong foundation for a research career. If the fellowship is done in an environment where a group of faculty members and fellows are focused on a specific area of oncology research, the learning experience is enriched considerably and career-long relationships may develop. Disadvantages of postdoctoral fellowships include a relatively low salary, lack of oncology-focused research training programs in one's geographic region, and lack of accessible mentors. Although postdoctoral fellowships are wonderful mechanisms for moving a research career forward more rapidly, unfortunately, they are not for everyone because of geographic location, personal or professional commitments, financial situation, and other factors.

How do I find a fellowship, and what should I be looking for in a postdoctoral fellowship? Fellowships are advertised in the professional literature, at professional conferences, on Web sites of academic and other institutions, through personal contact and networking, and in one's own doctoral program. Sources of funding for fellowships include the federal government, nonprofit organizations, institutional funds, industry, and more. NIH has individual postdoctoral fellowships, for which students must compete under the sponsorship of a primary mentor, or institutional training grants, in which students apply for a position in a research training program based at a university (NINR, 2007). If the nurse is able to do a fellowship, several areas are important to consider in selecting an institution, mentor, and/or institutional training program. First, nurses should explore availability, competitiveness, and fit between the training opportunities and research interests by talking with faculty. Second, it is important to ask about retention and outcomes of current fellows, particularly in terms of research productivity such as publications and grants. Third, it is advisable to visit the institution and attend research seminars and other training opportunities to get a feel for faculty, students, and available research training experiences. Fourth, potential fellows should talk with current fellows to determine their perceptions of the quality of research training, mentorship, and support. Bear in mind that the single most important aspect of a postdoctoral fellowship is working with mentors whose research is similar to the aspiring fellows' research. Finally, nurses should talk with their doctoral program mentors to receive input on the options being explored. This deliberative process should enable aspiring scientists to identify one or more viable options for a postdoctoral fellowship.

Academic Faculty Position

For many new doctoral graduates, taking a full-time faculty position immediately after completing the program is another common option, and perhaps the only one available. In this case, however, applicants must negotiate regarding things that will help or hinder their short- and long-term success as a scientist (Burroughs Wellcome Fund [BWF] & Howard Hughes Medical Institute [HHMI], 2006).

What things are important in my negotiations? Assuming that the new scientist has identified desirable and appropriate positions (through mechanisms such as institutional Web sites, professional publications, and networking), has applied for them, has been invited to visit, and has been offered a position, the negotiation phase begins. One's strongest bargaining position during this phase is common knowledge; thus, careful consideration of factors important to career success is advised. Evaluating any offer in terms of the details (e.g., rank, term of appointment, tenure status, source of funding in terms of grants or guaranteed "hard" money), the match of one's own priorities with the proffered position, acceptability of the salary and benefits package, and availability of necessary resources to succeed in research is important (BWF & HHMI, 2006). BWF and HHMI published a handbook in 2006 (BWF & HHMI) (viewable online at www.hhmi.org/resources/labmanagement/moves.html) that thoroughly covers the details of what to ask, where to find information such as competitive salaries, and how to negotiate. Negotiation involves reaching agreement on (a) salary and other forms of compensation such as benefits or bonuses, (b) a start-up package to support research and scholarship (e.g., space, computers and software, research assistants, funds for professional travel), (c) service within the university (e.g., committees),

(d) teaching responsibilities and teaching load, (e) rank and tenure policies and procedures, and (f) release time for research. Schools of nursing that value research are more likely to provide new faculty with protected research time for one or more years, thus enabling them to acquire research grants. If the nurse is seriously committed to a research career, another highly critical negotiation item is the teaching workload. If it is too heavy, it can be time consuming and can hinder development of a research program. One often overlooked item to consider is whether the school has a mechanism in place for senior faculty mentorship in learning the faculty role. The transition from new doctoral student to full-fledged faculty member can be challenging, but guidance from someone who knows the ropes can ease this transition.

Alternative Paths

Not everyone who seeks a research career is able to take a postdoctoral fellowship or wants to be a faculty member. Some nurses, by virtue of personal situation, financial necessity, geographic location, professional issues, or other factors, must find alternate paths to launching a career as a scientist. Generally speaking, such individuals may not be able to put forth substantial effort toward developing their own research trajectory because of job responsibilities, but they find ways in which to build on their dissertation and continue active involvement in research. Mechanisms can include small studies, interdisciplinary collaborative research, intramural research sponsored by their employers, or clinical effectives (outcomes) research using available databases. Several examples of these alternative career options in oncology nursing are shown in Table 21-1. Although alternative paths may not lead immediately to a full-blown research career, they can help to maintain research momentum and position individuals for more focused efforts when timing and circumstances are favorable.

Conclusion

A career in oncology nursing research can be very fulfilling. One only has to review the research programs of ONS Distinguished Researchers (see Chapter 2) to understand the tremendous contributions that research can make to practice in areas such as coping with cancer treatment, caring for loved ones with cancer, managing symptoms, and engaging in self-care (McGuire & Ropka, 2000). Each of these individuals, as well as all the other oncology nurse scientists who are active today, became researchers through a wide variety of career trajectories—some described in this chapter and some not. The current state of nursing science argues for a more direct and focused path to becoming a researcher in order to maximize the likelihood of a long, strong, and productive career. The career phases that are discussed in this chapter will guide the journey of developing oncology nurse scientists toward their goal of improving care for patients with cancer and their families.

Table 21-1. Examples of Alternative Paths to a Research Career

Individual/ Doctoral Preparation	Initial Postdoctoral Position	First Research Activities	Subsequent Research Activities
Person #1/ PhD in nursing	Remained in a position in the quality improvement department	Served as coinvestigator on a federally funded grant; wrote a small grant application to Oncology Nursing Society for a study building on position-related clinical responsibilities	Submitted an R-series grant application to National Institutes of Health working with experienced collaborators
Person #2/ DNSc in nursing	Took a joint position as coordinator of nursing research in a hospital and faculty member in a school of nursing	Developed small research studies in conjunction with nursing staff	Submitted own research proposals for small and large external grants; took a full-time faculty position
Person #3/ PhD in nursing	Took a position coordinating a cancer center–based patient-oriented program	Developed a research agenda for the program; initiated small studies	Continued development of a research program; obtained an adjunct faculty appointment

References

American Association of Colleges of Nursing. (2001, November). *Indicators of quality in research-focused doctoral programs in nursing.* Retrieved August 15, 2007, from http://www.aacn.nche.edu/Publications/positions/qualityindicators.htm

American Association of Colleges of Nursing. (2006, October 30). *The essentials of doctoral education for advanced nursing practice.* Washington, DC: Author. Retrieved August 6, 2008, from http://www.aacn.nche.edu/dnp/pdf/Essentials.pdf

American Cancer Society. (2007). *Doctoral degree scholarships in cancer nursing.* Retrieved August 23, 2007, from http://www.cancer.org/docroot/RES/content/RES_5_2x_Doctoral_Degree_Scholarships_in_Cancer_Nursing.asp?sitearea=RES

Bower, F.L. (2003). Mentoring. In T.W. Miller (Ed.), *Building and managing a career in nursing* (pp. 379–396). Indianapolis, IN: Sigma Theta Tau International.

Burroughs Wellcome Fund & Howard Hughes Medical Institute. (2006). *Making the right moves: A practical guide to scientific management for postdocs and new faculty* (2nd ed.). Research Triangle Park, NC, & Chevy Chase, MD: Authors.

Byrne, M.M., & Keefe, M.R. (2002). Building research competence in nursing through mentoring. *Journal of Nursing Scholarship, 34*(4), 391–396.

Gaffney, N. (Ed.). (1995). *A conversation about mentoring: Trends and models.* Washington, DC: Council of Graduate Schools.

McGuire, D.B. (1999). Building and maintaining an interdisciplinary research team. *Alzheimer Disease and Associated Disorders, 13*(Suppl. 1), S17–S21.

McGuire, D.B., & Ropka, M.E. (2000). Research and oncology nursing practice. *Seminars in Oncology Nursing, 16*(1), 35–46.

Melnyk, B.M., & Fineout-Overholt, E. (2005). *Evidence-based practice in nursing and healthcare: A guide to best practice.* Philadelphia: Lippincott Williams & Wilkins.

Miller, T.W. (2003). Work versus career. In T.W. Miller (Ed.), *Building and managing a career in nursing* (pp. 3–18). Indianapolis, IN: Sigma Theta Tau International.

National Academy of Sciences, National Academy of Engineering, & Institute of Medicine. (1997). *Adviser, teacher, role model, friend: On being a mentor to students in science and engineering.* Washington, DC: National Academies Press.

National Cancer Institute. (2006, October). *The science of team science: Assessing the value of transdisciplinary research.* Retrieved August 23, 2007, from http://cancercontrol.cancer .gov/brp/scienceteam/intro_stokols_etal.pdf

National Institute of Nursing Research. (2006, October). *Changing practice, changing lives: The NINR strategic plan.* Retrieved April 20, 2007, http://www.ninr.nih.gov/NR/ rdonlyres/9021E5EB-B2BA-47EA-B5DB-1E4DB11B1289/4894/NINR_Strategic PlanWebsite.pdf

National Institute of Nursing Research. (2007, September). *Training.* Retrieved August 23, 2007, from http://www.ninr.nih.gov/training

National Institutes of Health. (2007). *NIH roadmap for medical research.* Retrieved August 23, 2007, from http://www.nihroadmap.nih.gov

Oncology Nursing Society. (n.d.-a). *Awards, grants, and scholarships.* Retrieved August 23, 2007, from http://www.ons.org/awards

Oncology Nursing Society. (n.d.-b). *Nursing-sensitive patient outcomes resources.* Retrieved August 23, 2007, from http://www.ons.org/research/outcomes/measuring.shtml

Oncology Nursing Society. (n.d.-c). *ONS research agenda and priorities.* Retrieved August 20, 2007, from http://www.ons.org/research/information/agenda.shtml

Paul, R., & Elder, L. (2001). *How to study and learn a discipline using critical thinking concepts and tools.* Dillon Beach, CA: Foundation for Critical Thinking.

Sigmon, H.D., & Grady, P.A. (2001). Increasing nursing postdoctoral opportunities: National Institute of Nursing Research Spring Science Work Group. *Nursing Outlook, 49*(4), 179–181.

Vance, C., & Olson, R.K. (1998). Mentorship and nursing. In C. Vance & R.K. Olson (Eds.), *The mentor connection in nursing* (pp. 3–10). New York: Springer.

Wallace, A. (2003). Career opportunities. In T.W. Miller (Ed.), *Building and managing a career in nursing* (pp. 99–110). Indianapolis, IN: Sigma Theta Tau International.

CHAPTER 22

Obtaining Support for a Career in Oncology Nursing Research

Martha L. Hare, PhD, RN

Introduction

The purpose of this chapter is to assist the reader in building a career in oncology nursing research. It will explore issues related to securing funding at different points along the research career trajectory. The chapter is written mainly for the scientist seeking support from the National Institutes of Health (NIH, www.nih.gov). However, information on other resources also is included. This chapter cannot be fully comprehensive, and the information is likely to change very quickly. Therefore, the references and tables contain a number of useful Web sites for readers to explore for further information.

The most important step for any scientist is to begin the process of developing a program of research. All decisions about seeking funding should be closely related to the program of research. One mistake that scientists make—both novice and experienced—is to allow the available funding determine the research idea pursued, which is the reverse of what should occur. Of course, a scientist should be savvy and should understand what kinds of studies different agencies, such as NIH, are seeking. At the same time, agencies respond to input from scientific communities, and one scientist's unusual idea may be cutting-edge research in the not-too-distant future. Also, if one agency is

The chapter was written while the author was employed by the National Institutes of Health/National Institute of Nursing Research. The information shared is part of the public domain. The information does not imply endorsement of any funding source and was accurate at the time of submission for publication.

not able to support an idea, another one may. Scientists live with a project for anywhere from two to five years. They publish findings that may be cited for many years after that; therefore, the topic for any individual research project must be one that the scientist finds exciting, interesting, and important.

Furthermore, each project should contribute to a body of work that is associated with the scientist (i.e., a program of research). This does not mean that novice scientists need to narrowly develop their careers and never deviate from early plans. Most people know of scientists and other scholars who made fairly dramatic shifts in their careers to meet changes in knowledge or in their own interests. Instead, a program of research is meant to ensure that the scientists stick with an area of science that they can remain passionate about over a long period of time. Of course, they will work with mentors to make needed corrections, while also keeping up with the literature and remaining flexible enough to move away from dead ends or to develop new skills and knowledge when indicated. However, scientists should not develop a project simply to obtain funds. The remainder of the chapter will discuss different types of funding and how to match support to the research idea and to the research career level.

Research Career Trajectory

A research career is divided into a number of phases beginning with predoctoral training, followed by postdoctoral training, further career development, and independence as a scientist. In fact, career development is a lifelong process, and funding agencies such as NIH recognize this by having awards available for those who wish to obtain new knowledge and skills throughout their research careers. For example, a predoctoral scientist may obtain a predoctoral fellowship, a novice scientist may obtain a postdoctoral fellowship, and an established investigator seeking training in a new area of science may apply for a senior fellowship.

Often seen as a next step after receiving a predoctoral or postdoctoral fellowship, the career development award actually can be used at any point during the research career depending on the type of career development award. Most frequently, the career development award is used when serving as a junior faculty or junior research scientist and involves mentoring both in the process of conducting research and in a substantive scientific area. Many types of career development awards are available as shown on the NIH K Kiosk (NIH Office of Extramural Research, n.d.-a).

Table 22-1 presents information on the kind of funding that is available at different points in the scientist's career. This table focuses on NIH funding. However, readers can explore the other sources of funding discussed toward the end of the chapter and incorporate these resources into their strategies for securing funds.

Aside from competing directly for fellowships and grants from NIH, other routes are available to build a research career. Many readers of this chapter

Table 22-1. Common Types of Funding Available From the National Institutes of Health

Career Phase	Funding Mechanism	Description
Predoctoral student Postdoctoral student	Ruth Kirschstein Institutional National Research Service Award (NRSA) (T32)	Provides research mentoring and experience to predoctoral and postdoctoral students through a focused award (e.g., symptom management, health disparities) granted to an institution. Students may develop small projects or work with the mentors on their research studies.
Predoctoral fellow	Ruth Kirschstein Individual NRSA (F31)	Supports predoctoral research through a coherent training plan, research project, and mentoring team.
Postdoctoral fellow Advanced fellow	Ruth Kirschstein Individual NRSA (F32, F33)	Provides limited funding to assist a beginning or midcareer scientist in obtaining mentored research experience in a new area of science. This may be a method or content area that the fellow deems necessary for fulfilling career goals.
Junior scientist	National Institutes of Health Career Development Awards (K01, K07, K22, K23, etc.)	Supports scientists, usually beginning within five years of obtaining doctorate, for three to five years as they obtain advanced training and mentoring and pursue a research program that is preliminary to submitting an R01. Requirements and type of award vary by institute but generally require a 75% time commitment.
Midcareer scientist	National Institutes of Health Career Development Awards (K02, K05, K24, etc.)	Supports highly productive or promising scientists, enabling them to further advance their careers and provide mentoring to others. Requirements and type of award vary by institute but generally require a 75% time commitment.
Independent scientist	Research Program Grants (R01, R03, R21, etc.)	Research grants are used to answer discrete research questions and test hypotheses, thereby forming the building blocks of the independent research career. Size of funding varies from $50,000 in direct costs for two years to $250,000–$500,000 for four to five years.

Note. Based on information from National Institutes of Health Office of Extramural Research, 2008.

already will have experience as a research assistant or other staff in a senior investigator's project, a critical first step in developing a research career. Later in their careers, scientists will have many opportunities to participate in the research of colleagues as key personnel or as consultants. Balancing the workload is crucial. Participating in colleagues' research is an excellent way to learn from each other and to build important relationships. On the other hand, an overreliance on research opportunities through others can slow down scientists in building their own program of research. Investigators' arrangements for receiving credit as authors on research-related publications on all projects in which they have meaningful participation also is imperative.

In 2007, NIH began to allow more than one principal investigator (PI) for research applications (NIH, 2006a). This should not be done as a matter of course. All multiple-PI applications need to contain a plan stating the scientific leadership role for each named PI. If a member of the team is not leading a discrete scientific area, best practice is to not include that person as a PI.

As the investigator grows as a scientist, opportunities other than training, career development, or research awards may present themselves. These may include leading or helping to establish a research center (e.g., through the P20 Exploratory Center, P30 Program Center awards). Centers build infrastructure for concentrated research on an area of science, such as symptom management, end of life, or health disparities, and afford more junior scientists the opportunity to engage in pilot research. For junior investigators, participating in a center as the PI for a small center-funded pilot study is an excellent way to transition from mentored to independent research.

Many scientists become involved with *cooperative agreements* (U mechanisms), in which the scientist works collaboratively with NIH staff. These mechanisms often are used for high-profile projects and/or for when a large amount of funding is required. Clinical trials and large-scale surveys often are supported through cooperative agreements. They can be an outstanding source of support for a career, yielding data for many important scientific advances and publications.

Another form of support is the mechanism for Small Business Innovation Research (SBIR) or Small Business Technology Transfer Research (STTR). The federal government sets aside funding for independent entrepreneurs for advances in biomedical technology. Oncology nurse scientists in academic settings can team with an entrepreneur to develop a product that is compatible with their program of research. Requirements for the SBIR and STTR program are somewhat different from the standard research grants, so readers should familiarize themselves with the SBIR/STTR Web site (NIH Office of Extramural Research, 2008).

Encouraging Diversity Among Scientific Investigators

Several categories of scientists may qualify for targeted funding at NIH and also should seek similar types of funding through other funding agencies. The purpose of such funding is to maintain a diverse scientific workforce and to ensure that scientists who need to take time away from research for compelling reasons are able to reignite their careers. This latter category often is unaware that specific support for their needs is available.

Many scientists' careers do not move in a linear fashion. To begin with, many nurses spend a number of years in practice before considering a research career. Some take time away from their program of research because of other critical obligations. A scientist should not interrupt a research career, if at all possible. For example, if accepting an academic position with a large teaching or service load, be sure to carve out protected time for research. Mining data also is possible so that the publication record continues to grow. Even so, special awards, such as midcareer fellowships, or the award known as "Supplements to Promote Reentry Into Biomedical or Behavioral Research Awards" may be useful. These awards are targeted to scientists who took time off for childrearing, other family responsibilities, health concerns, or similar personal issues. The PI, of a funded grant (known as the "parent grant") prepares an application for submission to the NIH institute that is funding it. Therefore, if considering such funding, a candidate needs to contact the PI, who should, in turn, discuss the supplement with the program director for the parent grant.

Similarly, NIH supports supplements to existing grant awards in order to enhance diversity in the scientific workforce. This program, known as "Research to Promote Diversity in Health-Related Research," is available to individuals from ethnic and racial minorities, people with disabilities, or those who can demonstrate that their education was affected by being from a low socioeconomic group. Again, the candidate does not apply directly but rather through a PI with a funded research project of interest to the candidate. One of the unique features of this opportunity is that it is available to high school students, undergraduate students, graduate students, junior scientists who have interrupted their graduate education, postdoctoral scientists, and junior faculty. The expectations vary according to the academic or professional level of the diversity candidate, so PIs and candidates must read the funding announcement carefully, and PIs must discuss their plans with the program director for the parent grant before submitting an application.

Mentoring and Publication: Ingredients for Success

The key factor in the special supplements is the quality of mentoring. Mentoring also is a crucial component of training and career development awards. In fact, successful careers include mentoring throughout their entire life span. Mentors are needed at every transition, and functioning both as a mentor and a mentee at any point in a career is common.

The other critical component of a successful research career is publication. As students, novice scientists should be mentored to submit abstracts for presentations and manuscripts for publication, initially as a member of a team. Later, graduate students may publish as a lead author in areas of developing competence. By the time that a candidate is applying for a career development award, some publications are expected, although the number of data-based publications with the candidate as lead author may be understandably limited. With time, the applicant for funding will be judged increasingly by the number and quality of publications. Negotiating for time to publish and to work with fellow scientists on a plan that will allow for several publications from each grant with varied lead authors is always important.

Obtaining Support From the National Institutes of Health

In this section, the National Institute of Nursing Research (NINR) will serve as an exemplar with regard to obtaining support for a program of research. Following the discussion of NINR, information on other components of NIH will be presented. Because NIH and other organizations use many acronyms, Table 22-2 summarizes those used in this chapter, and the acronyms are provided in the text to familiarize readers with them.

Many readers of this chapter may be familiar with NINR, and this institute would be a natural choice when seeking support for research. Staying familiar with news and events at NINR through its Web site (www.ninr.nih.gov) is a good idea, as it is updated regularly. For example, the Web site features pages with current funding opportunity announcements (FOAs), contact people (program directors) for scientific discussion and guidance, and information on various opportunities specific to nurse scientists. In 2006, NINR unveiled its strategic plan for 2006–2010, which can be accessed through the Web site (NINR, n.d.-a). The plan includes the NINR mission and research priorities for the remainder of the current decade. Figure 22-1 summarizes key points from NINR Strategic Plan.

NINR has supported a number of successful investigators, and some of their work is discussed in other chapters. Up-to-date information on funded research can be found in an NIH database, known as CRISP, or the Computer Retrieval Information on Scientific Projects database (NINR CRISP, n.d.). In addition, NINR highlights recent findings and publications on its Web site (NINR, n.d.-b) and provides a link to current funding opportunities.

Familiarity with the NINR Web site and with other Web pages at NIH is important because many investigators are not aware of the breadth of opportunities available to them, as well as some constraints. For example, NINR has an interest in supporting investigators from many disciplines who meet its mission. Conversely, an investigator from a school of nursing who has an interest in an area that is not within the NINR mission may be successful in another institute or center at NIH or at another federal agency, such as the Agency for Healthcare Research and Quality (AHRQ). This is one reason why

Table 22-2. Acronyms Commonly Used by Federal Agencies That Support Cancer-Related Research

Acronym	Definition	Explanation
AHRQ	Agency for Healthcare Research and Quality www.ahrq.gov/fund/ragendix .htm	The agency concerned primarily with quality improvement and health services research
CDC	Centers for Disease Control and Prevention www.cdc.gov/cancer/dcpc /about/programs.htm	The agency responsible for protecting the public health
CSR	Center for Scientific Review http://cms.csr.nih.gov	The central location at NIH responsible for initial acceptance of grant applications and overseeing the review process
DHHS	U.S. Department of Health and Human Services www.hhs.gov/search	A department of the executive branch of the U.S. government responsible for overseeing a number of agencies (e.g., AHRQ, FDA, HRSA, CDC, NIH) that are concerned with the health and welfare of U.S. citizens
DoD	U.S. Department of Defense www.defenselink.mil/faq /pis/21.html	A military department that supports cancer-related research
DSMB	Data and Safety Monitoring Board	A board of experts in the science under study who oversee the DSMP and evaluate the safety of phase III clinical trials
DSMP	Data and Safety Monitoring Plan	A plan for ensuring that data are monitored for safety during the course of a phase I or II clinical trial
FDA	U.S. Food and Drug Administration www.fda.gov	The agency concerned with regulating food, drugs, and medical devices
FOA	Funding Opportunity Announcement	Generic term for all U.S. federal government announcements seeking responses to opportunities for funds. This includes but is not limited to requests for applications (RFAs), program announcements (PAs), and requests for proposals (RFPs)
HRSA	Health Resources and Services Administration www.hrsa.gov/grants	The agency charged with ensuring access to health care for vulnerable Americans

(Continued on next page)

Table 22-2. Acronyms Commonly Used by Federal Agencies That Support Cancer-Related Research *(Continued)*

Acronym	Definition	Explanation
IACUC	Institutional Animal Care Use Committee	The entity at the performance site and/or PI's home institution that is responsible for ensuring ethical conduct of research involving animals
I/C	Institutes and Centers	An abbreviation used to refer to the 27 institutes and centers that form the NIH
IRB	Institutional Review Board	The entity at the performance site and/or PI's home institution that is responsible for ensuring ethical conduct of research involving human subjects
IRG	Integrated Review Group	A group of study sections that reviews grants dealing with a particular area of science. IRGs are divided into study sections.
NCI	National Cancer Institute www.cancer.gov	The institute within NIH charged with overseeing research on all aspects of cancer
NGA	Notice of Grant Award	The legal document in which NIH specifies the terms of a grant, contract, or cooperative agreement
NIH	National Institutes of Health www.nih.gov	The federal agency charged with biomedical research
NINR	National Institute of Nursing Research www.ninr.nih.gov	The NIH institute that supports research on patient, family, and community health outcomes throughout the lifespan
OPASI	Office of Portfolio Analysis and Strategic Initiatives http://opasi.nih.gov	An office of the NIH director responsible for overseeing the NIH Roadmap for Medical Research, and other interdisciplinary trans-NIH initiatives
PA	Program Announcement	The most common type of FOA for grant applications, meant to stimulate an area of science. The PA does not include set-aside funds.
PI	Principal Investigator	The individual(s) identified as the scientific leader(s) of the research project
RFA	Request for Applications	Similar to a PA, the RFA has a limited time duration and allocated funds.

(Continued on next page)

Table 22-2. Acronyms Commonly Used by Federal Agencies That Support Cancer-Related Research (Continued)

Acronym	Definition	Explanation
SBIR	Small Business Innovation Research http://grants2.nih.gov/grants /funding/sbir.htm	A set-aside program for domestic small business concerns to engage in research/ research and development (R/R&D) that has the potential for commercialization
SEP	Special Emphasis Panel	A study section created for a special need, such as review of an RFA
SRO	Scientific Review Officer	The NIH scientific employee responsible for overseeing a study section
STTR	Small Business Technology Transfer Research http://grants2.nih.gov/grants /funding/sbir.htm	Similar to SBIR, but requires research partners at universities or other nonprofit research firms
VA	U.S. Department of Veterans Affairs www.va.gov	Primarily a healthcare organization for veterans and their families, the VA con- ducts surveillance and other research and evaluation studies.

Figure 22-1. Key Components of the National Institute of Nursing Research 2006–2010 Strategic Plan

National Institute of Nursing Research (NINR) Mission
The mission of NINR is to promote and improve the health of individuals, families, com- munities, and populations. NINR supports and conducts clinical and basic research and research training on illness across the life span.

Strategies to Advance Science
- Integrating biology and behavior
- Designing and using new technology
- Developing new tools
- Preparing the next generation of nurse scientists

Areas of Research Emphasis
- Promoting health and preventing disease
- Improving quality of life
  - Self-management
  - Symptom management
  - Caregiving
- Eliminating health disparities
- Setting directions for end-of-life research

Note. Based on information from National Institute of Nursing Research, n.d.-a.

building a relationship with the scientific program staff person, known as the program director at NINR, or the counterpart at any other funding agency of interest to a potential research funding applicant is important.

Each applicant should consider the program director to be a primary resource throughout the life cycle of a grant. Potential applicants are encouraged to contact the program director covering their area of scientific interest early, well before an application is submitted. The appropriate program director can be identified in one of two ways: either through the NINR Web site or through the list of contacts at the end of an FOA. Usually, the relationship with a program director is initiated through sending a concept paper via e-mail, although phone calls or discussions at professional conferences also are good means for establishing contact. At this stage of development, program directors can provide insight into the appropriateness of the concept for the institute and the best funding mechanism for the research proposed (e.g., R03, R01) and can raise general issues about content and design.

Because of concerns about fairness, program directors are limited as to the specific recommendations that they can give with regard to a grant application. However, they can offer a good deal of general advice and support. Once the application has been reviewed, the program director is available to discuss the summary statement with the applicant.

Table 22-3 summarizes the grant application process. The tool developed by Crain and Broome (2000) is another excellent resource that provides a handy guide to the grant application process.

Program directors do not select applications for funding. Once the review process is complete, however, the program director monitors the progress of the grants that are funded. The Notice of Grant Award may stipulate issues that are monitored, and, in general, contacting the program director is a good idea whenever a change in aims or scope or a major change in research personnel, methods, or sample is contemplated. The program director also is eager to hear about successes. Program staff members are responsible for informing others at NINR, NIH, and elsewhere about the continuing progress in nursing science. They track publications, and contacting the program director always is useful when an article based on findings developed from an NINR-supported (that includes cofunded) grant has been accepted for publication. Thus, the relationship between program directors and PIs can last for many years, as findings are published and new research applications are contemplated.

The *grants specialist* is another category of important staff at NINR and other NIH institutes. Grants specialists are responsible for fiscal oversight of grants. At times, a program director will refer an applicant or grantee to the grants specialist in order to clarify a fiscal or policy question. As with the program director, scientists should consider their grants specialists as sources of support for them because they can help with numerous issues that arise in administering a grant. Occasionally, issues need to be resolved between the PI's institutional business official and the grants specialist. The fact that awards

Table 22-3. The National Institutes of Health (NIH) Grant Application Process

Task	Time Frame	Resources
Develop concept for research project.	Several months to a year (or more) prior to applying for funding	Scientific literature NIH institute Web sites NIH program directors Mentors and colleagues
Register on the Electronic Research Administration (eRA) Commons.	Any time prior to submitting an application. *This is required.*	eRA Commons Web site
Identify Funding Opportunity Announcement (FOA). (See Table 22-2 for types of FOAs.)	Several months to a year prior to applying for funding	NIH Web sites Federal guide Grants.gov Dean, mentors, and colleagues NIH program directors
Write the application.	Varies, but enough time should be allotted to hold a mock review at the applicant's home institution and possibly to send the application to other outside reviewers for comment.	NIH Web sites Grants.gov Dean, mentors, and colleagues The applicant's business office (Office of Sponsored Programs)
Submit the application.	Posted submission dates. Allow time to correct for errors.	Office of Extramural Research Submission Dates Web site (http://grants2.nih.gov/grants/dates.htm) Grants.gov
Track the progress of the application.	The time from submission through review can range from several weeks to several months depending on the type of application.	eRA Commons If problems arise: • Grants.gov • Scientific Review Officer • Applicant's business office
Initial review of application	Several weeks to several months after submission. Summary statements are then posted about a month after completion of review.	eRA Commons Program director after the summary statement is posted
Secondary review of application	About two months after initial review, meritorious applications are reviewed at the council for the institute.	Program director contacts grantee for additional information, if needed.
Funding decisions	Several weeks after conclusion of the council	Program director Grants specialist
Monitoring of grant	Life of the grant	Program director Grants specialist

Note. Based on information from National Institutes of Health Office of Extramural Research, n.d.-a.

are made to institutions, not individuals, is important to remember, although institutions recognize the scientific leadership of the PI.

One source of common confusion with regard to NIH grants is the review process. Most grants are not reviewed in the institute to which they are assigned; therefore, the review process will be discussed in a separate section of this chapter. Another source of common confusion is how the decision is made with regard to the percent of applications that can be funded in any year. The federal budget year begins on October 1 and ends on September 30. Different institutes and agencies may have their own ways of communicating these decisions to the public. Each year, the proportion of applications that receive financial support varies, depending in large part on the federal budget but also on scientific priorities and other issues that cannot always be foreseen. The reality is that a certain amount of patience is needed in building a research career, and this includes patience in awaiting a funding decision.

NINR offers many resources for potential grant applicants and for funded grantees or PIs. Although the grant application process is complex and can be lengthy, scientists with good scientific ideas are encouraged to pursue them. All scientists, from the neophyte to the seasoned investigator, should become familiar with the NINR Web site and check it frequently and should build a relationship with the program director responsible for their science area and, once funded, with their grants specialist.

Other Resources at the National Institutes of Health

The National Cancer Institute (NCI) is a logical resource for readers of this chapter. Many similarities exist between NCI and NINR with regard to policies and procedures, but many differences exist, too. Therefore, potential applicants must familiarize themselves with NCI's Web site (www.cancer.gov) and with one or more NCI program directors. NINR and NCI program directors have a strong history of working together to the benefit of grant applicants. Also, NCI has a Web site devoted to step-by-step grant help (NCI Division of Cancer Control and Population Sciences, n.d.), which contains information on grant writing.

Potential applicants also should consider other NIH institutes and centers (I/Cs), all of which can be located through the NIH Web page, Institutes, Centers and Offices (www.nih.gov/icd). For example, the National Institute on Aging (NIA) or the National Institute on Child Health and Human Development may be appropriate for research that focuses on a person's developmental stage in relation to cancer. The National Institute of Mental Health, National Institute on Drug Abuse, and National Institute on Alcohol Abuse and Alcoholism may be funding resources for studies that combine mental health or substance use issues with cancer prevention, treatment experience, or survivorship. The National Center for Complementary and Alternative Medicine may be a resource for complementary and alternative medicine research in oncology, as would

NCI's Office of Cancer Complementary and Alternative Medicine. Basic genetics-related studies may find a home at either the National Human Genome Research Institute or the National Institute of General Medical Sciences. Although both NINR and NCI are strongly supportive of symptom-related research, an often-overlooked resource for research on pain or mucositis is the National Institute of Dental and Craniofacial Research (NIDCR).

Applications are sent to NIH and disseminated to the I/Cs through the Center for Scientific Review (CSR). CSR (2006) makes this determination based on a set of guidelines. However, the applicant may submit a cover letter requesting assignment to one or more I/Cs. For example, an applicant may be studying an intervention for pain in older adults with head and neck cancer. That applicant may write a cover letter indicating NINR as the institute for primary assignment and NCI as the institute for secondary assignment and also may request consideration by NIA and NIDCR. The number and order of requested institutes could be different for this same application depending upon conversations with the program directors and their suggestions. This flexibility allows more than one institute to cofund a grant. When two or more I/Cs cofund a grant, the PI's acknowledgment of each funding institute on publications and other products resulting from the grant is very important.

Since the early 2000s, NIH has encouraged the development of interdisciplinary research, in particular through the development of the NIH Roadmap for Medical Research (NIH, 2006b). Many nurse scientists recognize that their research is inherently interdisciplinary and can position themselves for the kinds of initiatives that the roadmap has supported. Since late 2006, roadmap activities have been administered through the NIH Office of Portfolio Analysis and Strategic Initiatives (OPASI). The roadmap has led to numerous opportunities to build teams of scientists across disciplines, some of which have strengthened the nurse scientists' careers. Because the roadmap is meant to be fast-moving, readers of this chapter should consult the NIH Roadmap Web page (http://nihroadmap.nih.gov) and the OPASI Web page (http://opasi.nih.gov) directly.

Two of the most essential Web sites for anyone seeking funding from the federal government are Grants.gov and the eRA Commons. Grants.gov (2007) is the single federal Web site for obtaining FOAs. The eRA Commons (NIH Electronic Research Administration, n.d.) is the central location for tracking all matters related to grant applications and funded grants. Individual investigators register with the Commons and then have confidential access to information concerning their own grant. Anyone contemplating a grant application should register well ahead of the due date.

Grant Review at the National Institutes of Health

NIH, like many funding agencies, uses a peer-review system. The review process was in a period of rapid development during the mid- to late-2000s largely because of the technology available to increase efficiency in a system that reviews tens of thousands of applications each year. Therefore, readers should add the CSR Web site (http://cms.csr.nih.gov) to their list of favorites or bookmarks in order to stay up to date on issues related to scientific review of applications.

A common cause of confusion is which entity is responsible for review of applications. The vast majority of applications are assigned to a study section through CSR. Study sections are grouped into Integrated Review Groups (IRGs). For example, the study sections Nursing Science of Adults and Older Adults and Nursing Science of Children and Families are part of the larger IRG, Health of Populations (CSR, 2006). Neither the IRGs nor the study sections are a part of NINR or any other institute. In fact, NIH is very careful to keep the review process distinct from program staff in order to avoid bias because program directors and scientific applicants often develop long-term relationships. And although constraints on bias are built into the program director role, this is balanced with the aspects of the role that involve scientific mentoring and advocacy.

Applications from nurse scientists may be assigned to a variety of study sections based on the predominance of the science as described in the application's specific aims. In other words, nurse scientists should not assume that their applications will be assigned to a study section with the designation *nursing science.* Conversely, applications from investigators concerned with questions that are particularly germane to the science of nursing may be assigned to a nursing science study section, even if the scientists hail from a variety of other disciplines.

Each study section is led by two people. One is an employee of NIH, the scientific review officer (SRO), and the other is an extramural scientist who is an expert in the specific field under review and in the interpersonal skills needed to lead a large group of peer reviewers. The extramural scientist is the chair of the IRG. The SRO is the main NIH resource from when the grant application is assigned to an IRG to when the review is completed. The SRO does not give advice on scientific content but can be helpful with specific questions on assignments or on the review process.

Another category of study section is known as the Special Emphasis Panel (SEP). SEPs are established for special types of reviews, and some are located within an I/C. For example, many I/Cs develop a SEP to review each request for applications (RFA) developed by staff at the I/C. Some institutes have SEPs for the review of training and career development grants. The NIH staff member in charge of the SEP is always an SRO and not the program director.

At other times, CSR establishes a SEP. These SEPs can be established for a variety of reasons, from the need for a very specific type of expertise to the need to hold a meeting of reviewers who are not in conflict with applications to one of the standing study sections. Generally speaking, if the FOA is of the type known as a Program Announcement with special Review (PAR), then all applications to the PAR will be assigned to a SEP established for that PAR.

Review Criteria

Because the NIH review process is modified from time to time, readers should stay apprised of changes posted on the NIH Grants and CSR Web sites. They also should glean carefully any criteria specifically written into the FOA to which they decide to apply. In general, the review criteria for research applications include significance of the research, innovation, scientific approach, expertise of the PI and research team, and the quality of the research environment. The majority of the application is devoted to the scientific approach, but a targeted literature review is very important for establishing the significance of the research. Overall, the sections of the application and the criteria are not distinct, and the applicant should be careful to weave information addressing the review criteria into several sections of the application. The discussion here focuses on the R01 research application. Similarities and variations exist for many of the other kinds of FOAs.

Research applications usually begin with a project overview, and then a section describing budget, personnel, and the research environment. Often, applicants use the budget justification section as a space to talk about the qualifications of personnel; however, plenty of room is available for this in the biosketches that are included in the personnel section of the application. Rather, the applicant should use the budget justification section to clarify the level of effort requested for personnel and the rationale for all other budget items. The scientific discussion begins with the presentation of the study aims. This should include the overall purpose and goal of the study, along with any hypotheses attached to the aims. Sometimes, applicants choose to use research questions instead of hypotheses. This choice should be justified scientifically. For example, a hypothesis may not be appropriate for a qualitative study, but a research question might.

The section on background and significance should include a focused literature review. The next section is concerned with preliminary data, which are critical for R01 applications. Subsequently, the applicant describes the research and data collection methods and data analysis plan. Finally, human subject issues are addressed. Most FOAs allow the applicant to include appendices, but applicants should be very careful to stay within the guidelines for both the number of pages and the type of material (e.g., photographs, article reprints) allowed in the appendix. These guidelines change occasionally, and the applicant is responsible for searching for this information in the FOA and on the relevant NIH Web sites. Under no circumstances should an applicant use an appendix to include information that does not fit into the page limit for the main portion of the application. Most reviewers and some staff do not have ready access to the appendices, and the primary reviewers, who do have such access, may be annoyed by having to search for critical information outside the prescribed sections. Scores are based upon an evaluation of the information in the prescribed sections of the application.

Human subject information is a critical part of the application, but neither human subject information nor budget information is germane to the score. (At times, human subject issues are tied critically to the research design and therefore may have an impact upon the score.) However, if a portion of the human subject information is not addressed or is inadequately addressed, then the applicant is barred from funding until this is corrected. Study section members flag human subject concerns, and then program directors are responsible for ensuring that the concerns are fully addressed. Program directors, grants specialists, and other NIH staff members also can flag concerns, even when reviewers have decided against doing so. In general, human subject issues include confidentiality, other protections of human subjects, and a discussion of informed consent. The informed consent forms are not part of the human subject section of the application but may be included as an appendix. Studies that are clinical trials must include a Data and Safety Monitoring Plan (DSMP), and phase III clinical trials must have a Data and Safety Monitoring Board (DSMB). The NIH Data/Safety Monitoring Guidelines were established in 2000 (NIH, 2000), but individual I/Cs may have updates and modifications that can be obtained by doing a search on the term *data/safety monitoring* or by asking I/C program staff.

When human subjects are part of the research, then the applicant also must provide information on the recruitment of women, children, and minorities (NIH Office of Extramural Research, n.d.-b). The children category includes individuals between the ages of 18 and 21. At times, the appropriate category for a study will be obvious. For example, a study of prostate cancer will only include adult men. However, including a statement as to why certain populations are not included in a study is always best. Having a reasonable recruitment plan that includes members of all populations affected by the research problem also is critical. Sometimes, in pilot studies or in intensive grounded theory studies, the sample is restricted even when the problem under study affects a broad cross-section of people. If this is the case, the applicant must discuss the reason for restricting the study population. Most types of applications involving human subjects require a form that specifies the number of women and ethnic/racial minorities to be included. This form is part of the application packet that is obtained online from Grants.gov.

Applicants do not need institutional review board (IRB) approval at the time that they submit their applications, but they must obtain this approval prior to engaging in data collection from human subjects. Similarly, investigators engaging in animal studies need to have institutional animal care and use committee approval prior to receiving a funding award, but they do not need to have this in place when submitting their application. Again, applicants should use the NIH Web site for updates to policies concerning human subjects or animal care.

Study sections comment on budgets and may recommend an adjustment based on the budget justification in light of the scientific aims and methods. A realistic budget for the proposed research is imperative, meaning that it should not be "padded," and proposing less than what is needed provides no advantage.

Applicants also need to be aware of the funding limits for each mechanism (e.g., the amount allowable under the small grant program, the limit at which special permission is required for a larger application) and follow those guidelines faithfully. Aside from NIH program and grants staff, the applicant's own business officials are invaluable resources. Creating a draft budget early in the development of the grant application and then revising it as the application is finalized generally is the best practice. Overall, the scientific research should dictate the budget required, but certainly times arise when difficult scientific choices need to be made to stay within budget guidelines. Applicants do not want to discover such choices are required shortly before the application deadline.

The discussion in this section has focused on the research (R-series applications). Many readers of this chapter likely would be interested in training and career development awards. Budgets allowed for such awards tend to be slim, and the guidelines on the kinds of other funding that can be pursued while a recipient of the "F" or "K" award tend to be strict, but awardees find that such mentored awards are worthwhile. In terms of scientific review, the candidate is evaluated on the training or career development plan and the faculty sponsors, as well as the criteria described previously. Further guidance should be obtained from the academic sponsor and other mentors when applying for these awards.

Once the review of an application is completed, the SRO for the study section generates a summary statement that consists of the critiques of the two to four assigned reviewers from the study section. All applications, regardless of whether they were scored, receive a summary statement. Once the summary statement is generated, contacting the program director for an appointment to discuss the major points of the critique is a good idea. Any decision about whether to revise and resubmit always is the applicant's decision, so long as the application has not reached the specified limit for resubmission, which usually includes one initial application and two revisions.

Other Federal Resources

NIH is only one of several federal agencies that funds oncology research. Each agency has its own focus, and potential applicants should obtain guidance from the staff at the agency. The discussion that follows is not comprehensive, and readers should refer to material posted by the U.S. Department of Health and Human Services (n.d.).

Agency for Healthcare Research and Quality

AHRQ supports research that improves "quality, safety, efficiency, and effectiveness of health care for all Americans" (AHRQ, n.d.). Research programs are divided into cross-cutting portfolios, such as patient safety, long-term care, health information technology, and others of interest to oncology nurse scientists. Annual priorities and program contacts also are posted on the AHRQ

Web site (www.ahrq.gov), an excellent resource for scientists whose primary concerns involve health systems and organizational issues.

Centers for Disease Control and Prevention

The Centers for Disease Control and Prevention (CDC) is mandated by Congress to protect the public health (CDC, 2008). Often associated with infectious disease prevention and case finding, the CDC has many programs in place to prevent and control chronic diseases, including cancer. For example, long-standing programs are available to promote breast and cervical cancer early detection (Lantz et al., 2000), as well as programs in cancer surveillance, colorectal cancer screening, and tobacco control, among others. Since 2000, the CDC has worked closely with states and tribal organizations to establish comprehensive cancer control strategic plans (Hare et al., 2001). Funding opportunities at the CDC may be administered directly through the CDC or through contracts with other entities, such as states, tribal organizations, universities, or nonprofit research or service organizations.

U.S. Food and Drug Administration

The U.S. Food and Drug Administration (FDA) is primarily a regulatory agency. In order to carry out its regulatory mission, research is required on drugs and devices. Recently, the FDA has become interested in patient-related outcomes, an area of great concern to many nurse scientists (Bren, 2006).

Health Resources and Services Administration

The Health Resources and Services Administration (HRSA) is the primary governmental agency for improving access to healthcare services for uninsured, isolated, or medically vulnerable individuals (HRSA, 2007). Most programs deal with issues related to health disparities and underserved populations and can provide opportunities for interesting service-related projects or leads on collaborations for scientists involved with the populations that HRSA grantees serve.

Other Federal Agencies

Aside from agencies within DHHS, other federal agencies also support cancer-related research. Again, any federal agency is required to post its FOAs on Grants.gov. The U.S. Department of Defense is one supporter of oncology research. Calls for research tend to be cancer site–specific. The U.S. Department of Veterans Affairs also supports research and evaluation studies. Interested investigators may want to contact their local Veterans Affairs facility to discuss collaboration on projects of mutual interest.

Nurse scientists should be creative in thinking about funding resources. They should explore as many federal agencies as seem relevant to their program of research. This could include those involved with education, energy, occupational health, and the environment. Because priorities change, readers are encouraged to use this chapter as a starting point in their funding search but not as a complete or final guide to funds for oncology nursing research.

Nongovernmental Resources

Funds from foundations, nonprofit and other organizations, and industry are exceedingly important to developing a program of research. These resources, with the exception of many industry-related resources, often are associated with small studies and are very useful to novice scientists. However, nongovernmental resources are important at any phase of a career.

Home Institutions

One of the first places that investigators should consider in the early stages of a study is their own home institutions. Often, universities can provide direct seed money through a limited competition. This is especially true of fellowships but also can be true for scientists at any stage of their career. For example, an investigator may apply for a small amount of funding from his or her university to determine the feasibility of one aspect of the study before applying for funding from an outside agency.

Oncology Nursing Society and ONS Foundation

Most readers of this chapter are familiar with the Oncology Nursing Society (ONS). ONS is a major supporter of oncology nursing research. ONS conducts a membership research priorities survey every four years and updates the ONS Research Agenda every two years at the ONS National Cancer Nursing Research Conference. ONS offers research mentorship to beginning scientists. The ONS Foundation (www.onsfoundation.org) administers major research grants, fellowships, and small research grants. Some of the small research grants are specific to a type of cancer or cancer-related problem, so the reader should check this Web site regularly. Many successful oncology nurse scientists intersperse ONS funding with NIH and other funding throughout their careers. Grant applications are peer reviewed. The ONS Foundation (www.onsfoundation.org/funding.shtml) also offers individual or conference scholarships and other types of awards (ONS Foundation, n.d.).

American Cancer Society

The American Cancer Society (ACS) has a varied portfolio of research activities. Research applications are investigator-initiated and peer-reviewed, may be in areas such as cancer prevention or behavioral research and can be domestic or international. In addition, ACS posts priority areas for research on its Web site (www.cancer.org) (ACS, n.d.); research priorities may be cancer site–specific or topical (e.g., childhood cancer).

Other Cancer-Related Organizations

Although ACS is the largest cancer-related voluntary organization in the United States, other organizations exist that deal with cancer-related issues and provide funds for research. One well-known example is Susan G. Komen for the Cure (2008). Its Web site provides information on a broad range of support in basic, clinical, and translational research; breast cancer health disparities research; and support for postdoctoral fellows. One of the best known organizations concerned with the cancer survivor population is the Lance Armstrong Foundation (LAF). LAF supports cancer survivorship centers and research grants. The centers have a strong service component, and research grants are available for both new and experienced investigators (LAF, n.d.). These are only two of many possible sources.

Foundations

Nurse scientists additionally may utilize the resources of foundations specific to nursing science that are not specific to oncology. Among the best known are the American Nurses Foundation (2008) and Sigma Theta Tau International (n.d.). Numerous foundations outside of nursing exist that may be useful for nurse scientists. The John A. Hartford Foundation (n.d.) offers grants specific to nurses as well as for interdisciplinary training. Support is available at the undergraduate through postdoctoral levels. The Robert Wood Johnson Foundation (RWJF) is known for stimulating cutting-edge programs of research. Potential applicants should check the RWJF Web site (www.rwjf.org) (RWJF, n.d.) for its annual interest areas. In order to identify other foundations, readers are encouraged to follow leads that are related to subjects such as women's health, ethics, gerontology, childhood disabilities, or any others that are related to their research program.

Industry

Industry is a critical source of funding for oncology research. Industry usually is associated with pharmaceuticals and devices. Nurses have a long history as data collectors or other team members on studies that test these products. As nurses increase their involvement with technology, industry sponsors may prove invaluable for nursing investigators who are either developing technologies needed to conduct research or testing and evaluating the technology itself. Nurse scientists also should consider PI roles in some types of pharmaceutical studies. These can include studies related to adherence and quality of life, as well as interventions specific to symptom management and supportive care. Familiarity with the relevant FDA regulations is critical for any nurse who is leading a study that involves testing a pharmaceutical or clinical device. Herbal or other interventions that are not considered medications by the lay public may still be regulated when part of a research study.

Resources for Grant Writing

The purpose of this chapter has been to provide information on securing funding for research. NIH also provides technical resources to assist applicants. Occasionally, when stimulating a very new area of research, a program announcement or RFA will include an opportunity for technical assistance. Some NIH institutes publish their own materials to assist applicants with grant writing. The National Institute of Allergy and Infectious Diseases (2008) offers very popular and useful tutorials.

Coursework and mentoring are primary resources for technical assistance with grant writing. *Proposals That Work* (Locke, Spirduso, & Silverman, 2007) is a textbook for junior investigators that offers detailed instruction on all phases of proposal writing. Scientists also must stay current with literature targeted to nurse scientists outside of oncology.

Grey (2000) highlighted key points that stand the test of time. These research tips can be summarized as

- The importance of maintaining the scientist's dreams and enjoying the grant-writing process
- The need to be realistic about steps needed to reach one's dreams
- The importance of being thorough and clear in writing the grant application.

Conclusion

The process of securing funding for research can be lengthy and arduous but is well worth the effort. Nursing science has evolved over the past few decades as signified by the 2006 recognition of NINR's 20th anniversary (NINR, n.d.-a). Scientific advances have improved the lives of patients, families, and communities. However, much more needs to be done. With new technologic approaches and increased recognition of the need for interdisciplinary collaboration to answer the challenging questions facing a diverse and aging population, nurses are well positioned to lead important studies that will have an impact on the lives of patients with cancer, their caregivers, and the communities in which they live.

References

Agency for Healthcare Research and Quality. (n.d.). *AHRQ research agenda.* Retrieved October 26, 2007, from http://www.ahrq.gov/fund/ragendix.htm

American Cancer Society. (n.d.). *Research programs and funding.* Retrieved July 7, 2008, from http://www.cancer.org/docroot/RES/RES_0.asp

American Nurses Foundation. (2008). *Nursing research grants.* Retrieved July 7, 2008, from http://www.anfonline.org/anf/nrggrant.htm

Bren, L. (2006). The importance of patient-reported outcomes . . . It's all about the patients. *FDA Consumer Magazine, 40*(6), 26–32. Retrieved October 26, 2007, from http://www.fda.gov/fdac/features/2006/606_patients.html

Center for Scientific Review. (2006, January 6). *Scientific areas of integrated review groups (IRGs).* Retrieved October 26, 2007, from http://cms.csr.nih.gov/PeerReviewMeetings/CSRIRGDescription/HOPIRG/HOPIRGAll.htm

Centers for Disease Control and Prevention. (2008). *About CDC.* Retrieved July 7, 2008, from http://www.cdc.gov/about

Crain, H.C., & Broome, M.E. (2000). Tool for planning the grant application process. *Nursing Outlook, 48*(6), 288–293.

Grants.gov. (n.d.). *Find. Apply. Succeed.* Retrieved October 26, 2007, from http://www.grants.gov

Grey, M. (2000). Top 10 tips for successful grantsmanship. *Research in Nursing and Health, 23*(2), 91–92.

Hare, M.L., Wijesinha, S., Rose, J., Orians, C., Candreia, M., & Odell Butler, M. (2001). *Organizational design options for state cancer planning: Development model comprehensive state cancer plans.* Report to Centers for Disease Control and Prevention.

Health Resources and Services Administration. (2007). *About HRSA.* Retrieved October 26, 2007, from http://www.hrsa.gov/about/default.htm

John A. Hartford Foundation. (n.d.). *Grant programs.* Retrieved October 26, 2007, from http://www.jhartfound.org/program/index.asp

Lance Armstrong Foundation. (n.d.). *Grants and programs: Research.* Retrieved October 26, 2007, from http://www.livestrong.org/site/c.jvKZLbMRIsG/b.739079/k.DC18/Research.htm

Lantz, P.M., Richardson, L.C., Sever, L.E., Macklem, D.J., Hare, M.L., Orians, C.E., et al. (2000). Mass screening in low-income populations: The challenges of securing diagnostic and treatment services in a national cancer screening program. *Journal of Health Politics, Policy and Law, 25*(3), 451–471.

Locke, L.F., Spirduso, W.W., & Silverman, S.J. (2007). *Proposals that work: A guide for planning dissertations and grant proposals* (5th ed.). Thousand Oaks, CA: Sage.

National Cancer Institute Division of Cancer Control and Population Sciences. (n.d.). *Step-by-step grant help.* Retrieved April 18, 2007, from http://cancercontrol.cancer.gov/grant_help/learn_resources.html

National Institute of Allergy and Infectious Diseases. (2008, April 1). *All about grants tutorials.* Retrieved July 7, 2008, from http://www.niaid.nih.gov/ncn/grants/default.htm

National Institute of Nursing Research. (n.d.-a). *Changing practice, changing lives: The NINR Strategic Plan.* Retrieved October 26, 2007, from http://www.ninr.nih.gov/NR/rdonlyres/9021E5EB-B2BA-47EA-B5DB-1E4DB11B1289/4894/NINR_StrategicPlanWebsite.pdf

National Institute of Nursing Research. (n.d.-b). *Nursing research: Changing practice, changing lives.* Retrieved July 29, 2008, from http://www.ninr.nih.gov

National Institutes of Health. (2000). *Further guidance on data and safety monitoring for phase I and phase II trials.* Retrieved October 26, 2007, from http://grants2.nih.gov/grants/guide/notice-files/NOT-OD-00-038.html

National Institutes of Health. (2006a, May 11). *Multiple PI implementation update.* Retrieved October 26, 2007, from http://grants2.nih.gov/grants/guide/notice-files/NOT-OD-06-069.html

National Institutes of Health. (2006b, August). *NIH roadmap for medical research.* Retrieved October 26, 2007, from http://nihroadmap.nih.gov/pdf/NIHRoadmap-FactSheet-Aug06.pdf

National Institutes of Health. (n.d.). *National Institutes of Health: The nation's medical research agency.* Retrieved October 26, 2007, from http://www.nih.gov

National Institutes of Health CRISP (Computer Retrieval of Information on Scientific Projects). (n.d.). *eRA Commons computer retrieval of information on scientific projects.* Retrieved October 26, 2007, from http://crisp.cit.nih.gov

National Institutes of Health Electronic Research Administration. (n.d.). *eRA Commons.* Retrieved October 26, 2007, from https://commons.era.nih.gov/commons

National Institutes of Health Office of Extramural Research. (2008). *Small business funding opportunities.* Retrieved July 7, 2008, from http://grants2.nih.gov/grants/funding/sbir.htm

National Institutes of Health Office of Extramural Research. (n.d.-a). *Grant application basics.* Retrieved July 7, 2007, from http://grants.nih.gov/grants/grant_basics.htm

National Institutes of Health Office of Extramural Research. (n.d.-b). *Research involving human subjects.* Retrieved October 26, 2007, from http://grants.nih.gov/grants/policy/hs

ONS Foundation. (n.d.). *Home.* Retrieved July 14, 2008, from http://www.onsfoundation.org

Robert Wood Johnson Foundation. (n.d.). *Grants.* Retrieved July 7, 2008, from http://www.rwjf.org/grants

Sigma Theta Tau International. (n.d.). *Research/library.* Retrieved October 26, 2007, from http://www.nursingsociety.org/research/main.html

Susan G. Komen for the Cure. (2008). *Grants program.* Retrieved July 7, 2008, from http://cms.komen.org/komen/GrantsProgram/index.htm

U.S. Department of Health and Human Services. (n.d.). *HHS.gov: Improving the health, safety, and well-being of America.* Retrieved October 26, 2007, from http://www.hhs.gov

Looking Into the Future

Janice Phillips, PhD, MS, RN, FAAN

The previous chapters provide testimonies to oncology nurse scientists' contributions to advancing the science and thereby advancing the specialty of oncology nursing. As we continue to move forward, the projected trends and advancements in cancer care will provide numerous opportunities for oncology nurse scientists to conduct nursing research across the cancer continuum. Although numerous oncology nurse scientists have already developed a considerable body of knowledge in a variety of areas, we must continue to build on these areas and identify additional areas for future research. In doing so, generating knowledge that is applicable and translatable into practice must remain a high priority.

Along with discussing future considerations for advancing oncology nursing science, acknowledging a number of areas that are not discussed in this first edition of *Advancing Oncology Nursing Science* is important. Although these areas are not fully represented in this edition, they continue to be fruitful areas for nursing research. A number of oncology nurse scientists have already laid the foundation, thus setting the tone for ongoing work. A few are highlighted here.

Pediatric Oncology Research

Oncology nurse scientists are making substantive contributions to enhance our knowledge in areas such as pediatric end-of-life and palliative care, quality of life for children with cancer, neurocognitive problems associated with childhood cancer treatments, and individual and family responses to a diagnosis of childhood cancer. A major accomplishment in pediatric oncology nursing research is the integration of nursing research into pediatric oncology cooperative groups, such as the Children's Oncology Group. This integrative approach to pediatric oncology nursing research continues to show great promise for enhancing nursing research visibility and value, as well as facilitating the dissemination of nursing research findings.

Behavioral Oncology Research

Behavioral research across the cancer continuum will require ongoing attention. From prevention to end of life and cancer survivorship, oncology nurse scientists are well positioned to add to the growing body of knowledge in behavioral oncology research. Oncology nurse scientists are already making progress in this area by conducting descriptive and interventional behavioral oncology studies. They have set the stage for success by creating interdisciplinary networks to help to advance knowledge and enhance the dissemination and application of research findings.

Genetic Research

The introduction of the Human Genome Project provides evidence of the increasing role of genetics and genomics in today's healthcare arena. Genetic scientific advancements from cancer risk identification to cancer recurrence estimation, among others, are revolutionizing the way that we treat and counsel high-risk individuals and those living with cancer. In collaboration with multiple disciplines, oncology nurse scientists continue to enhance our understanding of genetic uncertainty, genetic susceptibility, genetic testing, and the psychosocial responses to genetic findings.

Cancer Survivorship

Recent reports revealed that more than 10 million people are now living with a cancer diagnosis or history of cancer (American Cancer Society, 2008). Increasingly, as cancer becomes a chronic condition, each phase of the survivorship experience will provide oncology nurse scientists with ongoing opportunities to advance knowledge and improve the quality of life for cancer survivors and their families. Oncology nurse scientists are already assuming leadership in this area of research and advancing knowledge on topics such as the effects of cancer survivorship on individuals, families, and caregivers, transitional issues from treatment to survivorship, racial and ethnic perspectives related to cancer survivorship, and myriad quality-of-life concerns among cancer survivors across various cancer sites and stages.

The Next Generation of Oncology Nurse Scientists

Moving forward, the next generation of oncology nurse scientists will be standing on the shoulders of many pioneers who have established a foundation for continued advancements in oncology nursing science. As the next generation emerges, it will be challenged to keep the ball rolling by creating and seizing opportunities to engage in team science, conduct global health research, foster the translation of research findings into oncology nursing practice, improve scientific rigor, and conduct and integrate biologic and behavioral oncology research. Oncology nurse scientists, along with other members of the oncology community, have already articulated an agenda for advancing oncology nursing science. This agenda will take us well into the future. In order to successfully address these and others areas, we must continue to devote our energies and resources to ensure an ample supply of well-prepared oncology nurse scientists.

This brief look at our future only begins to scratch the surface. No doubt, scientific advances in oncology along with societal needs will help to guide our future efforts. As we look to the future, we must remain vigilant in building and disseminating oncology nursing science. Advancing our science is a professional imperative for our specialty, our profession, and the many patients and families we serve.

> *The future is not a result of choices among alternative paths offered by the present, but a place that is created—created first in the mind and will, created next in activity. The future is not some place we are going to, but one we are creating. The paths are not to be found, but made, and the activity of making them, changes both the maker and the destination.*
>
> —John Schaar, PhD, Scholar and Political Theorist

Reference

American Cancer Society. (2008). *Cancer facts and figures, 2008*. Atlanta, GA: Author.

APPENDIX

Oncology Nursing Science Resources

A number of resources are available to assist individuals who are interested in oncology nursing science. Professional and specialty organizations, nonprofit organizations, and governmental agencies provide many resources for both scientists and research consumers. Many of these organizations and agencies have been instrumental in shaping oncology nursing science through research development, dissemination, funding, health policy development, and supportive cancer care.

Organization	Web Site
Cancer Organizations, Foundations, and Agencies	
American Association for Cancer Research	www.aacr.org
American Cancer Society	www.cancer.org
American Society of Clinical Oncology	www.asco.org
International Union Against Cancer	www.uicc.org
Lance Armstrong Foundation	www.livestrong.org
National Coalition for Cancer Survivorship	www.canceradvocacy.org
Prevent Cancer Foundation	www.preventcancer.org
Robert Wood Johnson Foundation	www.rwjf.org/services
Susan G. Komen for the Cure®	www.komen.org
Clinical Trials	
CancerGuide: Clinical Trials and Experimental Treatments	http://cancerguide.org/internet _trials.html
Genentech BioOncology Clinical Trials	www.biooncology.com/bioonc/trials/ index.m

(Continued on next page)

Organization	Web Site
National Cancer Institute (NCI) Cancer Clinical Trials	http://cancertrials.nci.nih.gov
NCI Clinical Trials Cooperative Groups Program	www.cancer.gov/cancertopics /factsheet/NCI/clinical-trials -cooperative-group
PDQ®—NCI's Comprehensive Cancer Database	www.cancer.gov/cancerinfo/pdq /cancerdatabase
Evidence-Based Resources	
Cochrane Database of Systematic Reviews	www.cochrane.org/reviews
Evidence-Based Nursing	http://ebn.bmj.com
Joanna Briggs Institute	www.joannabriggs.edu.au/about /home.php
National Guideline Clearinghouse	www.guideline.gov
Oncology Nursing Society (ONS) Evidence-Based Practice Resource Area	http://onsopcontent.ons.org/toolkits /evidence
University of Texas Health Science Center at San Antonio Academic Center for Evidence-Based Nursing	www.acestar.uthscsa.edu
Government Agencies	
Agency for Healthcare Research and Quality	www.ahrq.gov
Centers for Disease Control and Prevention	www.cdc.gov
Center to Reduce Cancer Health Disparities	http://crchd.cancer.gov
National Center on Minority Health and Health Disparities	www.ncmhd.nih.gov
NCI	www.nci.nih.gov
Health Databases	
NCI CancerLit	www.cancer.gov/search/cancer _literature
CINAHL®	www.cinahl.com
Combined Health Information Database	http://www.chid.nih.gov (The database has been discontinued, but this Web site provides links to other sites that were formerly included in the database.)

(Continued on next page)

Organization	Web Site
PubMed/MEDLINE®	www.ncbi.nlm.nih.gov/entrez
Nursing-Related Organizations	
Association of Pediatric Hematology/Oncology Nurses	www.apon.org
Eastern Nursing Research Society	www.enrs-go.org
International Society of Nurses in Cancer Care	www.isncc.org
International Society of Nurses in Genetics	www.isong.org
Midwest Nursing Research Society	www.mnrs.org
National Institute of Nursing Research	www.ninr.nih.gov
Oncology Nursing Society	www.ons.org
Sigma Theta Tau International	www.nursingsociety.org
Southern Nursing Research Society	www.snrs.org
Western Institute of Nursing	www.ohsu.edu/son/win/index.shtml
Additional Web Sites of Interest	
Cancer Control P.L.A.N.E.T. (Plan, Link, Act, Network with Evidence-based Tools)	http://cancercontrolplanet.cancer.gov
National Institutes of Health (NIH) Computer Retrieval of Information on Scientific Projects (CRISP)	http://crisp.cit.nih.gov
NIH Office of Human Subjects Research	http://ohsr.od.nih.gov
NCI Statistical Resources	http://cancer.gov/statistics
ONS Oncology Nursing Research Agenda 2005–2009	www.ons.org/research/information/agenda.shtml

Additional Resources

Fitzpatrick, J.J., & Montgomery, K.S. (Eds.). (2004). *Internet for nursing research: A guide to strategies, skills and resources.* New York: Springer.

Frank-Stromborg, M., & Olsen, S.J. (Eds.). (2004). *Instruments for clinical health-care research* (3rd ed.). Sudbury, MA: Jones and Bartlett.

Given, C.W., Given, B., Champion, V.L., Kozachik, S., & DeVoss, D.N. (Eds.). (2003). *Evidence-based cancer care and prevention: Behavioral interventions.* New York: Springer.

Klimaszewski, A.D., Bacon, M., Deininger, H.E., Ford, B., & Westendorp, J.G. (Eds.). (2008). *Manual for clinical trials nursing* (2nd ed.). Pittsburgh, PA: Oncology Nursing Society.

Index

The letter f after a page number indicates that relevant content appears in a figure; the letter t, in a table.